Scott-Brown's
Essential
Otorhinolaryngology
Head & Neck Surgery

Scott-Brown's
Essential
Otorhinolaryngology
Head & Neck Surgery

Editors

R James A England MD FRCS (ORL-HNS)

Consultant Otolaryngologist Head and Neck and Thyroid Surgeon,
Honorary Senior Lecturer, Hull University Teaching Hospitals NHS Trust, Hull, UK

Eamon Shamil MBBS, MRes, FRCS (ORL-HNS)

ST8 - Specialist Trainee in Otorhinolaryngology,
Guy's and St Thomas' NHS Foundation Trust, London, UK

Section Editors

Rajeev Mathew PhD FRCS (ORL-HNS)

Post CCST Fellow in Neurotology and Skull Base Surgery,
Addenbrooke's Hospital, Cambridge, UK

Manohar Bance FRCSC, FRCS

Professor of Otology and Skull Base Surgery, University of Cambridge
Honorary Consultant, Cambridge Universities Hospitals Foundation Trust,
Cambridge, UK

Pavol Surda MD

Consultant ENT Surgeon, Guy's and St Thomas' NHS Foundation Trust, London, UK

Jemy Jose MBBS, MS, FRCS (ORL-HNS)

Consultant ENT Head & Neck Surgeon, Hull University Teaching Hospitals
NHS Trust, Hull, UK

Omar Hilmi MB ChB, FRCS, FRCS (ORL HNS)

Consultant ENT Surgeon, Glasgow Royal Infirmary, Glasgow, Scotland, UK

Adam J Donne PhD FRCS (ORL-HNS)

Consultant Paediatric ENT Surgeon, Alder Hey Children's NHS Foundation
Trust, Liverpool, UK

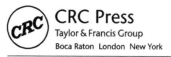

CRC Press
Taylor & Francis Group
Boca Raton London New York

CRC Press is an imprint of the
Taylor & Francis Group, an **informa** business

First edition published 2022
by CRC Press
6000 Broken Sound Parkway NW, Suite 300, Boca Raton, FL 33487-2742

and by CRC Press
2 Park Square, Milton Park, Abingdon, Oxon, OX14 4RN

© 2022 Taylor & Francis Group, LLC

CRC Press is an imprint of Taylor & Francis Group, LLC

Library of Congress Cataloging-in-Publication Data

Names: England, R. James A., editor. | Shamil, Eamon, editor.
Title: Scott-Brown's essential otorhinolaryngology, head & neck surgery / editors, R. James A. England, Eamon Shamil.
Other titles: Essential otorhinolarnygology, head & neck surgery | Scott-Brown's otorhinolaryngology head and neck surgery. Description: First edition. | Boca Raton : CRC Press, 2021. | Abridgement of Scott-Brown's otorhinolaryngology head and neck surgery. Eighth edition. [2019] | Includes bibliographical references and index. |
Summary: 'A portable handbook that provides a concise summary of ENT surgery based on Scott-Brown's Otorhinolaryngology, Head & Neck Surgery 8e. Of practical use in clinics, the ward and the operating room, and of interest to a wide range of clinicians'-- Provided by publisher.
Identifiers: LCCN 2021011043 (print) | LCCN 2021011044 (ebook) | ISBN 9781138608481 (paperback) | ISBN 9781032008301 (hardback) | ISBN 9781003175995 (ebook)
Subjects: MESH: Otolaryngology--methods | Otorhinolaryngologic Diseases--surgery | Head--surgery | Neck--surgery | Otorhinolaryngologic Surgical Procedures--methods | Handbook
Classification: LCC RF46 (print) | LCC RF46 (ebook) | NLM WV 39 | DDC 617.5/1--dc23
LC record available at https://lccn.loc.gov/2021011043
LC ebook record available at https://lccn.loc.gov/2021011044

ISBN: 978-1-032-00830-1 (hbk)
ISBN: 978-1-138-60848-1 (pbk)
ISBN: 978-1-003-17599-5 (ebk)

Typeset in Minion Pro
by KnowledgeWorks Global Ltd.

DEDICATION

"For my parents, whose living example and love give me the strength to stay true and kind"

—Eamon Shamil

"For Katie, Charlotte, Laura, Samuel and Isabelle, keep smiling!"

—James England

CONTENTS

SECTION 1
The Ear

SECTION 2
Rhinology and Facial Plastic Surgery

SECTION 3
Head and Neck

SECTION 4
Head and Neck Endocrine Surgery

SECTION 5
Paediatric Otolaryngology

PREFACE

It is our pleasure to introduce the first edition of *Scott-Brown's Essential Otorhinolaryngology, Head and Neck Surgery*.

The award-winning three-volume text *Scott-Brown's Otorhinolaryngology Head and Neck Surgery, Eighth Edition* (CRC Press 2018) has been recognised as the primary ENT reference manual for nearly 70 years. Its exhaustive text has provided a definitive resource for generations of ENT Surgeons.

The inception of this new textbook emanated from the demand for an up-to-date, evidenced-based textbook that is easily accessible and portable. Trainees sitting exams will find *Essential Scott-Brown's Otorhinolaryngology, Head & Neck Surgery* a useful primary textbook, and consultants will have it on their bookshelves to serve as a ready reference resource. We also anticipate other specialists, GPs and allied healthcare professionals will use it to demystify common but complex topics.

This book provides an abbreviated version of the 8th edition of the parent textbook, with additional new content and diagrams, and we have included updated guidelines where appropriate. We would like to thank our contributing authors, who include a combination of trainees and leaders in their field. We chose our subeditors based on their love of teaching, as well as their clinical rigour; their work speaks for itself. We also thank the Editors and authors of *Scott-Brown's Otorhinolaryngology Head and Neck Surgery, Eighth Edition*, for providing content that helped produce this textbook.

Putting together this textbook has been truly enjoyable. Amidst the grey cloud of the COVID-19 pandemic, our silver lining has been a reminder of how wonderfully diverse, evolving and stimulating our specialty is. We look forward to the positive impact of our readership on the future of otorhinolaryngology.

James and Eamon
2022

COMPANION WEBSITE

The Companion Website to this book, www.scottbrownent.com, contains numerous supplemental resources that will enhance the reader's understanding of this text.

Jonathan Abbas
Specialist Registrar in Otolaryngology,
Northwest Deanery, Royal Manchester
Children's Hospital, Manchester, UK

Shahzada K. Ahmed
Consultant Rhinologist and Skull Base
Surgeon, Queen Elizabeth Hospital,
Birmingham, UK

Mikkel Alanin
Rhinology Fellow, Guy's and St Thomas'
NHS Foundation Trust, London, UK

Christopher P. Aldren
Consultant Otolaryngologist, Wexham
Park Hospital and Windsor ENT

Victoria Alexander
Consultant Otologist, St. George's
Hospitals NHS Foundation Trust and
Epsom and St Helier University Hospitals,
Epsom, UK

Shahram Anari
Consultant ENT Surgeon, University
Hospitals Birmingham NHS Foundation
Trust, Birmingham, UK

Patrick Axon
Department of ENT Surgery,
Addenbrooke's Hospital, Cambridge, UK

David M. Baguley
NIHR Nottingham Biomedical Research
Centre, Nottingham University NHS Trust,
Nottingham, UK

Stephen Ball
ENT Surgeon, Auckland DHB & The
University of Auckland, Auckland,
New Zealand

Doris-Eva Bamiou
Professor in Neuroaudiology and Honorary
Consultant in Audiovestibular Medicine,
UCL Ear Institute, London, UK

Martyn L. Barnes
Consultant Rhinologist, Mid and South
Essex NHS Foundation Trust, Essex, UK

Florian Bast
Consultant ENT Surgeon, Guy's and
St Thomas's NHS Foundation Trust,
London, UK

Warren O. Bennett
Locum Consultant ENT, University
Hospitals Bristol and Weston NHS
Foundation Trust, Bristol, UK

Rajiv K. Bhalla
Consultant Rhinologist and Skull Base
Surgeon, Manchester Royal Infirmary and
Salford Royal Hospital, Manchester, UK

Mahmood F. Bhutta
Chair in ENT Surgery, Brighton & Sussex
Medical School, Brighton, UK

Kamal Bisarya
Consultant Plastic & Reconstructive
Surgeon, University Hospitals of North
Midlands NHS Trust, Stoke-on-Trent, UK

Daniele Borsetto
ENT/Skull Base Department, Guy's and
St Thomas' NHS Foundation Trust, London,
UK

Alex Bowen
Interface Fellow in Head & Neck Surgical
Oncology, Manchester Royal Infirmary &
The Christie NHS Foundation Trusts,
Manchester, UK

Steven M. Bromley
Smell & Taste Center, University
of Pennsylvania Medical Center,
Pennsylvania, USA

Adolfo Bronstein
Professor of Clinical Neuro-otology &
Consultant Neurologist, Imperial College
London and UCLH, London, UK

George Browning
Emeritus Professor of Otolaryngology Head
and Neck Surgery, University of Glasgow,
Glasgow, Scotland

A. Simon Carney
Professor of Otorhinolaryngology and
Consultant Surgeon, Flinders University,
Adelaide, Australia

Sean Carrie
Consultant ENT Surgeon, Freeman
Hospital and University of Newcastle,
Newcastle upon Tyne, UK

Samuel Chan
Clinical Research Fellow & ENT Specialty
Registrar, St George's University Hospital &
Royal Marsden Hospital, London, UK

Linnea Cheung
Specialty Registrar in ENT Surgery,
University Hospitals Bristol NHS Trust,
Bristol, UK

Stephen Connor
Consultant Neuroradiologist and Head and
Neck Radiologist, Guy's and St Thomas'
NHS Foundation Trust, London, UK

Alwyn D'Souza
Consultant ENT and Facial Plastic Surgeon
President European Academy Facial Plastic
Surgery, London, UK

Dustin M. Dalgorf
Lecturer, Department of Otolaryngology-
Head & Neck Surgery, University of
Toronto, Toronto, Canada

Katharine Davies
Head and Neck Consultant, Liverpool
University Hospital NHS Foundation Trust,
Liverpool, UK

Sarah Dawes
Liverpool University Hospitals NHS
Foundation Trust, Liverpool, UK

Harvey Dillon
University of Manchester, Manchester, UK

Neil Donnelly
Consultant Otologist and Skull Base
Surgeon, Cambridge University Hospitals,
Cambridge, UK

Richard L. Doty
Smell & Taste Center, University
of Pennsylvania Medical Center,
Pennsylvania, USA

Catriona Douglas
Consultant ENT/Head and Neck Surgeon,
Queen Elizabeth University Hospital,
Glasgow, UK

Ronald Eccles
School of Biosciences, Cardiff University,
Cardiff, UK

Juan C. Fernandez-Miranda
Professor of Neurosurgery, Stanford
University Medical Center, California, USA

Andrew Forge
Emeritus Professor of Auditory Cell
Biology, UCL Ear Institute, London, UK

Jonathan Gale
Professor of Auditory Cell Biology,
Director, UCL Ear Institute, London, UK

Tira Galm
Consultant ENT Surgeon, Gloucestershire
Royal Hospital, Gloucestershire, UK

Quentin Gardiner
Consultant ENT Surgeon, University of
Dundee, Dundee, UK

Paul A. Gardner
Professor, Department of Neurological
Surgery, Stanford University School of
Medicine, California, USA

Emily Gauzzo
Department of Otology and Skull Base
Surgery, Cambridge University Hospitals,
Cambridge, UK

Manish George
ENT Registrar, Imperial College Healthcare
NHS Trust, London, UK

Jennifer Gilchrist
ENT, Royal Blackburn Hospital,
Blackburn, UK

Emma Gosnell
Otolaryngology Specialty Trainee,
Manchester University NHS Foundation
Trust, Manchester, UK

Ayeshah Abdul Hamid
Oxford University Hospitals NHS
Foundation Trust, Oxford, UK

Lucy Handscomb
UCL Ear Institute, London, UK

Andrew Harris
TIG Fellow in Head and Neck Surgical
Oncology, The Churchill Hospital, Oxford,
UK

Anna Harrison
Paediatric ENT, Royal Manchester Children's
Hospital, Manchester, UK

Richard J. Harvey
Clinical Professor Rhinology / Skull Base
Surgery, Macquarie University, NSW,
Australia

Anastasha Herman
Department of Otorhinolaryngology,
Pennine Acute Hospitals, Crumpsall, UK

Claire Hopkins
Professor of Rhinology at King's College
and Consultant ENT Surgeon, Guy's
and St Thomas' NHS Foundation Trust,
London, UK

Charlie Huins
Consultant ENT Surgeon, Queen Elizabeth
Hospital Birmingham, Birmingham, UK

Hiro Ishii
ENT Specialist Registrar, Gloucestershire
Hospitals NHS Foundation Trust,
Gloucestershire, UK

Thomas Jacques
Consultant ENT Surgeon, St. George's
University Hospitals NHS Foundation
Trust, London, UK

Todd Kanzara
ENT Specialty Trainee Mersey LETB,
Liverpool, UK

Andrew Kelly
Consultant ENT Surgeon, Antrim Area
Hospital, Antrim, Ireland

Maha Khan
ENT Specialty Trainee, Blackpool Teaching
Hospitals NHS Foundation Trust,
Blackpool, UK

Jeremy Lavy
Consultant Ear Surgeon, Royal National
ENT Hospital, London, UK

Samuel Leong
Rhinologist and Skull Base Consultant,
Aintree University Hospital NHS
Foundation Trust, Liverpool, UK

Simon K. W. Lloyd
Manchester University Hospitals NHS
Foundation Trust, Manchester, UK

Valerie Lund
Professor of Rhinology, Ear Institute,
University College London, London, UK

Samuel MacKeith
Consultant ENT Surgeon, Oxford
University Hospitals, Oxford, UK

Josephine Marriage
Director of Chear Ltd, Cambridge, UK

Andrew McCombe
Consultant ENT Surgeon, City Hospital
Mohammed bin Rashid University Medical
School, Dubai, UAE

Don McFerran
British Tinnitus Association, Sheffield, UK

Gerald McGarry
Consultant Surgeon Head and Neck and
Anterior Skull Base Surgery, Glasgow Royal
infirmary, Glasgow, UK

Nishchay Mehta
Consultant ENT Surgeon, University
College Hospitals London NHS Foundation
Trust, London, UK

Louise Melia
Rhinology & Anterior Skull Base
Consultant, Queen Elizabeth University
Hospital, Glasgow, Scotland, UK

Omar Mirza
Advanced Head & Neck Surgical Oncology
Fellow, Memorial Sloan Kettering Cancer
Center, New York, USA

David K. Morrissey
Consultant ENT Surgeon Hospital,
Toowoomba Hospital, Queensland,
Australia

Louisa Murdin
Consultant Audiovestibular Physician and
Associate Professor, Guy's and St Thomas'
NHS Foundation Trust and UCL Ear
Institute, London, UK

Cristina F. B. Murphy
Specialist Audiologist, Bupa Cromwell
Hospital, London, UK

Jameel Muzaffar
TWJ Foundation Fellow in Otology and
Auditory Implantation, University of
Cambridge and Cambridge University
Hospitals NHS Foundation Trust,
Cambridge, UK

Paresh Naik
Rhinology/Anterior Skull Base Fellow
University Hospitals Birmingham NHS
Trust, Birmingham, UK

Robert Nash
Consultant Otologist and Cochlear
Implant Surgeon, Great Ormond Street
Hospital, London, UK

Ravinder Singh Natt
Consultant ENT surgeon, Royal Free
London NHS Foundation Trust, London,
UK

Hannah Nieto
Academic Clinical Lecturer, University of
Birmingham, Birmingham, UK

Rupert Obholzer
Consultant ENT/Skull Base Surgeon, Guy's
and St Thomas' NHS Foundation Trust,
London, UK

Saleh Okhovat
Specialist Registrar in ENT Surgery, Royal
Hospital for Children, Glasgow, UK

Babatunde Oremule
ENT Registrar, Royal Manchester
Children's Hospital, Manchester, UK

Irumee Pai
Consultant Otologist and Auditory
Implant Surgeon, Guy's and St Thomas'
NHS Foundation Trust, London, UK

Arun Pajaniappane
Consultant Audiovestibular Physician,
St George's University Hospitals NHS
Foundation Trust, London, UK

Parag Patel
Consultant Otologist and Skull Base
Surgeon, St. George's Hospitals NHS
Foundation Trust, Kingston, UK

Neil Patel
Registrar Endocrine and General Surgery,
University Hospital of Wales, Cardiff, UK

Santdeep H. Paun
Consultant Otorhinolaryngologist /
Facial Plastic Surgeon, Barts Health NHS
Trust, London, UK

John Phillips
Consultant ENT Surgeon, Norfolk and
Norwich University Hospital NHS
Foundation Trust, Norwich, UK

Carl Philpott
Professor of Rhinology & Olfactology,
James Paget and Norfolk & Norwich
University Hospitals, Norwich, UK

Rohan Pinto
Specialist Registrar in Otolaryngology,
Alder Hey Children's Hospital, Liverpool,
UK

Harry Powell
Consultant Otologist and Auditory Implant
Surgeon, Guy's and St Thomas' NHS
Foundation Trust, London, UK

Alkis J. Psaltis
Head of Department of Otolaryngology
Head & Neck Surgery Queen Elizabeth
Hospital, Adelaide, Australia

Jason Ramsingh
Consultant General and Endocrine
Surgeon Royal Victoria Infirmary,
Newcastle Upon Tyne Hospital NHS
Foundation Trust, Newcastle Upon Tyne,
UK

Catherine Rennie
Consultant ENT Surgeon, Imperial College
Healthcare NHS Trust, London, UK

Joanne Rimmer
Consultant Otolaryngologist/Rhinologist,
Monash Health, Melbourne, Australia

Elizabeth Ross
Head and Neck Surgical Oncology Fellow,
Castle Hill hospital, Hull, UK

Anthony Rotman
Consultant ENT Surgeon, Monash Medical
Centre, Melbourne, Australia

Raymond Sacks
Professor and Head of Otolaryngology—
Head & Neck Surgery, Macquarie
University, Sydney, Australia

Raguwinder Bindy Sahota
Consultant Head and Neck/ ENT surgeon,
Royal Derby Hospital, Derby, UK

Hesham Saleh
Consultant Rhinologist and Professor
of Practice in Rhinology, Charing Cross
Hospital, London, UK

Marina Salorio-Corbetto
Research Associate at Cambridge
Hearing Group, University of Cambridge,
Cambridge, UK

Christopher Skilbeck
Consultant ENT and Skull Base Surgeon,
Guy's & St Thomas' NHS Foundation Trust,
London, UK

Anna D. Slovick
SpR Otolaryngology, Barts Health NHS
Trust, London, UK

Matthew Smith
Otology Fellow, Cambridge University
Hospitals, Cambridge, UK

Caroline P. Smith
Advanced Rhinology Fellow, Manchester
Royal Infirmary, Manchester, UK

Carl H. Snyderman
Professor, Department of Otolaryngology,
Stanford University School of Medicine,
California, USA

Kirsten Stewart
ENT Specialty Registrar, East of Scotland,
UK

Andrew C. Swift
Consultant ENT Surgeon and Rhinologist,
Aintree University Hospital NHS
Foundation Trust, Liverpool, UK

Hitesh Tailor
ENT Registrar, Greater Glasgow & Clyde
NHS, Glasgow, UK

Theofano Tikka
ENT Registrar, Queen Elizabeth University
Hospital, Glasgow, UK

Sara Timms
Specialist Registrar, ENT, Royal
Manchester Children's Hospital,
Manchester, UK

Neil S. Tolley
Consultant ENT & Thyroid Surgeon,
Imperial College Healthcare NHS Trust,
London, UK

Abbad Toma
Consultant ENT and Rhinoplasty Surgeon,
Kingston Hospital, London, UK

Chrysostomos Tornari
Fellow in Head and Neck Surgery, Guy's
and Thomas' NHS Foundation Trust,
London, UK

Phillip Touska
Consultant Head and Neck Radiologist,
Guy's and St Thomas' NHS Foun`dation
Trust, London, UK

Stephen C. Toynton
Consultant Otolaryngologist, Hawke's
Bay Fallen Soldiers' Memorial Hospital,
Hastings, New Zealand

Mathieu Trudel
Manchester Skull Base Unit, Salford Royal
NHS Foundation Trust, Manchester, UK

James R. Tysome
Consultant ENT and Skull Base Surgeon,
Cambridge University Hospitals,
Cambridge, UK

Peter Valentine
Consultant Otologist and ENT Surgeon,
Royal Surrey County Hospital, Guildford,
UK

Nimisha Vallabh
Specialist Trainee in Otolaryngology,
Salford Royal NHS Foundation Trust,
Salford, UK

Deborah Vickers
Department of Clinical Neurosciences,
University of Cambridge, Cambridge, UK

Ananth Vijendren
Consultant Otologist and ENT Surgeon,
Lister Hospital, East and North Herts NHS
Trust, Stevenage, UK

William Wakeford
ENT Specialist Registrar, Colchester
Hospital, Colchester, UK

Hussein Walijee
Specialist Registrar in Otolaryngology,
Leighton Hospital, Crewe, UK

Eric W. Wang
Associate Professor, University of
Pittsburgh Medical Center, Pennsylvania,
USA

Paul S. White
Consultant ENT Surgeon and Rhinologist,
Dundee, UK

Andrew Williamson
Specialist ENT Registrar, NHS Greater
Glasgow, UK

Tim Woolford
Consultant ENT SurgeonManchester Royal
Infirmary, Manchester, UK

Robert Wotherspoon
Specialist Registrar Oral and Maxillofacial
Surgery, Leeds General Infirmary, Leeds,
UK

Rosanna Wright
Specialist Trainee in Otolaryngology,
Health Education North West, Manchester,
UK

Kirsty Young
Consultant Pathologist, Queen Elizabeth
University Hospital, Glasgow, UK

ACKNOWLEDGEMENTS

We thank all the Section Editors and contributors for the time and effort that they have given to this project, and especially those who contributed to *Scott-Brown's Otorhinolaryngology Head and Neck Surgery 8th edition,* on which this *Essential* handbook is based.

Chapter 1, Anatomy and physiology of hearing, contains some material from Volume 2, Chapters 46: by Peter Valentine and Tony Wright, 47: by Jonathan Gale and Andrew Forge and 48: by Soumit Dasgupta and Michael Maslin

Chapter 2, Anatomy and physiology of balance, contains some material from Volume 2 Chapters 47: by Jonathan Gale and Andrew Forge and 49: by Floris L. Wuyts, Leen K. Maes and An Boudewyns

Chapter 3, Clinical examination of the ear and hearing, contains some material from Volume 2 Chapter 73: by George G. Browning and Peter-John Wormald

Chapter 4, Psychoacoustic and objective assessment of hearing, contains some material from Volume 2 Chapters 51: by Josephine E. Marriage and Marina Salorio-Corbetto and 52: by Jeffrey Weihing and Nicholas Leahy

Chapter 6, Vestibular disorders and rehabilitation, contains some material from Volume 2 Chapters 63: by Vincent W.F.M. van Romapaey, 64: by Yougan Saman and Doris-Eva Bamiou, 65: by Harry R.F. Powell and Shakeel R. Saeed, 67: by Louisa Murdin and Lina Luxon, 68: by Marousa Pavlou and 72: by Julius Bourke, Georgia Jackson and Gerald Libby

Chapter 7, Conditions of the external ear, contains some material from Volume 2 Chapters 74: by Malcolm P. Hilton, 75: by Samuel A.C. MacKeith, 76: by Tristram H.J. Lesser, 77: Jonathan P. Harcourt, 78: by Simon Carney, 79: by James W. Loock, 80: by Phillip J. Robinson and Sophie J. Hollis, 81: by James W. Loock, 92: by Philip D. Yates and 114: by Cheka R. Spencer and Peter Monksfield

Chapter 8, Eustachian tube dysfunction, contains some material from Volume 2 Chapter 86: by Holger H. Sudhoff

Chapter 9, Acute otitis media and otitis media with effusion in adults, contains some material from Volume 2 Chapter 82: by Anil Banerjee

Chapter 10, Chronic otitis media, contains some material from Volume 2 Chapter 83: by George G. Browning, Justin Weir, Gerard Kelly and Iain R.C. Swan

Chapter 11, Ossiculoplasty and myringoplasty, contains some material from Volume 2 Chapters 84: by Charlie Huins and Jeremy Lavy and 85: by Daniel Moualed, Alison Hunt and Christopher P. Aldren

Chapter 12, Otosclerosis, contains some material from Volume 2 Chapters 89: by Christopher P. Aldren, Thanos Bibas, Arnold J.N. Bittermann, George G. Browning, Wilko Grolman, Peter A. Rea, Rinze A. Tange and Inge Wegner

Chapter 13, Bone conduction and middle ear implants, contains some material from Volume 2 Chapters 93: by James Ramsden and Chris H. Raine and 95: by Maarten J.F. de Wolf and Richard M. Irving

Chapter 14, Sensorineural hearing loss, contains some material from Volume 2 Chapters 56: by Linnea Cheung, David M. Baguley and Andrew McCombe, 57: by Andrew McCombe and David M Baguley, 58: by Polona Le Quesne Stabej and Maria Bitner-Glindzicz and 59: by Andy Forge and 60: by Tony Narula and Catherine Rennie

Chapter 15, Tinnitus and hyperacusis, contains some material from Volume 2 Chapters 61: by Don McFerran and John Phillips and 70: by Laurence McKenna, Elizabeth Marks and David Scott

Chapter 16, Auditory neuropathy spectrum disorder and auditory processing disorder, contains some material from Volume 2 Chapters 69: by Rosalyn A. Davies and Raj Nandi and 71: by Doris-Eva Bamiou and Cristina Ferraz B. Murphy

Chapter 17, Hearing aids and auditory rehabilitation, contains some material from Volume 2 Chapters 54: by Harvey Dillon and 55: by Lucy Handscombe

Chapter 18, Cochlear implants and auditory brainstem implants, contains some material from Volume 2 Chapters 94: by Andrew Marshall and Stephen Broomfield and 96: by Shakeel R. Saeed and Harry R.F. Powell

Chapter 19, Ear trauma, contains some material from Volume 2 Chapter 91: by Stephen C. Toynton

Chapter 20, Metabolic bone disease and systemic disorders of the temporal bone, contains some material from Volume 2 Chapters 88: by Ameet Kishore and 90: by Ian D. Bottrill

Chapter 21, The facial nerve, contains some material from Volume 2 Chapters 112: by Michael Gleeson and 113: by Patrick R. Axon and Samuel A.C. MacKeith

Chapter 22, Vestibular schwannoma, contains some material from Volume 2 Chapters 101: by Mirko Tos, Sven-Eric Stangerup and Per Caye-Thomasen, 102: by Shakeel R. Saeed and Christopher J. Skilbeck, 103: by Paul Sanghera, Geoffrey Heyes, Helen Howard, Rosemary Simmons and Helen Benghiat and 104: by Gareth Evans

Chapter 23, Lesions of the cerebellopontine angle, petrous apex and jugular foramen, contains some material from Volume 2 Chapters 105: by Simon K.W. Lloyd and Scott A. Rutherford, 107: by Rupert Obholzer and 108: Petrous apex lesions by Michael Gleeson

Chapter 24, Temporal bone tumours, contains some material from Volume 2 Chapters 110: by Marcus Atlas, Noweed Ahmad and Peter O'Sullivan and 115: by Liam Masterton and Neil Donnelly

Chapter 26, Physiology of the nose and paranasal sinuses, contains some material from Volume 1 Chapter 89 by Tira Galm and Shahzada Ahmed

Chapter 29, Imaging in rhinology, contains some material from Volume 1 Chapter 117: by Gregory O'Neill

Chapter 31, Allergic rhinitis, contains some material from Volume 1 Chapters 14: by Sai H.K. Murng and 15: by Moira Thomas, Elizabeth Drewe and Richard J. Powell

Chapter 32, Non-allergic rhinitis, contains some material from Volume 1 Chapters 14: by Sai H.K. Murng and 15: by Moira Thomas, Elizabeth Drewe and Richard J. Powell

Chapter 35, Medical management of CRS, contains some material from Volume 1 Chapters 28: by Wendy Smith and 97: by Claire Hopkins

Chapter 36, Surgical management of CRS, contains some material from Volume 1 Chapters 98: by A. Simon Carney and Raymond Sacks, 99: by Salil Nair and 100: by Darlene E. Lubbe

Chapter 41, Nasal fractures, contains some material from Volume 1 Chapter 107: by Dae Kim and Simon Holmes

Chapter 45, Diagnosis and management of facial pain, contains some material from Volume 1 Chapter 112: by Rajiv K. Bhalla and Timothy J. Woolford

Chapter 46, Pre-assessment for rhinoplasty, contains some material from Volume 3 Chapters 80: by David Chadwick, 81: by Barney Harrison, 82: by Sean Carrie, John Hill and Andrew James, 83: by Thozhukat Sathyapalan and Stephen L. Atkin, 84: by Christopher M. Jones and John Ayuk and 85: by Mihir R. Patel, Leo F.S. Ditzel Filho, Daniel M. Prevedello, Bradley A. Otto and Ricardo L. Carrau

Chapter 47, Rhinoplasty following nasal trauma, contains some material from Volume 3 Chapters 80: by David Chadwick, 81: by Barney Harrison, 82: by Sean Carrie, John Hill and Andrew James, 83: by Thozhukat Sathyapalan and Stephen L. Atkin, 84: by Christopher M. Jones and John Ayuk and 85: by Mihir R. Patel, Leo F.S. Ditzel Filho, Daniel M. Prevedello, Bradley A. Otto and Ricardo L. Carrau

Chapter 48, External rhinoplasty, contains some material from Volume 3 Chapters 80: by David Chadwick, 81: by Barney Harrison, 82: by Sean Carrie, John Hill and Andrew James, 83: by Thozhukat Sathyapalan and Stephen L. Atkin, 84: by Christopher M. Jones and John Ayuk and 85: by Mihir R. Patel, Leo F.S. Ditzel Filho, Daniel M. Prevedello, Bradley A. Otto and Ricardo L. Carrau

Chapter 49, Cosmetic facial interventions, contains some material from Volume 3 Chapters 86: by Andy Levy, 87: by Dustin M. Dalgorf and Richard J. Harvey, 88: by Martyn L. Barnes and Paul S. White and 89: by Tira Galm and Shahzada K. Ahmed

Chapter 50, Surgical anatomy of the neck, contains some material from Volume 3 Chapters 35: by Laura Warner, Christopher Jennings and John C. Watkinson, 43: by Stuart Winter and Brian Fish, 47: by Joanna Matthan and Vinidh Paleri and 58: by Nimesh N. Patel and Shane Lester

Chapter 51, Aetiology of head and neck cancer, contains some material from Volume 3 Chapter 2: by Pablo H. Montero, Snehal G. Patel and Ian Ganly

Chapter 52, Molecular biology and gene therapy, contains some material from Volume 1 Chapters 1: by Michael Kuo, Richard M. Irving and Eric K. Parkinson and 3: by Seiji B. Shibata and Scott M. Graham

Chapter 53, Imaging of the neck, contains some material from Volume 3 Chapters 37: by Ivan Zammit-Maempel and 45: by Daren Gibson and Steve Colley

Chapter 54, Management of laryngotracheal trauma, contains some material from Volume 3 Chapter 71: by Carsten E. Palme, Malcolm A. Buchanan, Shruti Jyothi, Faruque Riffat, Ralph W. Gilbert and Patrick Gullane

Chapter 55, Pharyngitis, contains some material from Volume 3 Chapter 51: by Sharan Jayaram and Conor Marnane

Chapter 56, Upper airway obstruction and tracheostomy, contains some material from Volume 3 Chapters 72: by Paul Pracy and Peter Conboy and 76: by Guri S. Sandhu and S.A. Reza Nouraei

Chapter 57, Voice disorders and laryngitis, contains some material from Volume 3 Chapters 61: by Jean-Pierre Jeannon and Enyinnaya Ofo, 63: by Yakubu Gadzama Karagama and Julian A. McGlashan, 65: by Declan Costello and Meredydd Harries, 66: by Marianne E. Bos-Clark and Paul Carding, 67: by Abie Mendelsohn and Marc Remacle, 68: by Declan Costello and John S. Rubin, 69: by Sanjai Sood, Karan Kapoor and Richard Oakley and 70: by Kenneth MacKenzie

Chapter 58, Dysphagia and aspiration, contains some material from Volume 3 Chapters 49: by Helen Cocks and Jemy Jose, 50: by Joanne Patterson and Jason Powell, 51: by Sharan Jayaram and Conor Marnane, 52: by Nimesh N. Patel and T. Singh, 53: by Shajahan Wahed and S. Michael Griffin, 54: by Kim Ah-See and Miles Bannister, 55: by Maggie-Lee Huckabee and Sebastian Doeltgen and 56: by Guri S. Sandhu and Khalid Ghufoor

Chapter 59, Salivary gland tumours, contains some material from Volume 3 Chapter 9: by Jarrod Homer and Andy Robson and 10: by Vincent Vander Poorten and Patrick J. Bradley

Chapter 60, Parapharyngeal space, contains some material from Volume 3 Chapter 11: by Suren Krishnan

Chapter 61, Staging of head and neck cancer, contains some material from Volume 3 Chapter 4: by Nicholas J. Roland

Chapter 62, Laryngeal malignancy, contains some material from Volume 3 Chapters 14: by Vinidh Paleri, Stuart Winter, Hannah Fox and Nachi Palaniappan, 15: by Yvonne Edels and Peter Clarke, 22: by Mark Sayles, Stephanie L. Koonce, Michael L. Hinni and David G. Grant and 27: by Volkert Wreesman, Jatin Shah and Ian Ganly

Chapter 63, Hypopharynx, contains some material from Volume 3 Chapter 16: by Prathamesh Pai, Deepa Nair, Sarbani Ghosh Laskar and Kumar Prabhash

Chapter 64, Oropharynx, contains some material from Volume 3 Chapters 13: by Terry M. Jones with Mererid Evans and 29: by Chris Holsinger, Chafeek Tomeh and Eric M. Genden

Chapter 65, Nasopharyngeal carcinoma, contains some material from Volume 3 Chapter 8: by Raymond King-Yin Tsang and Dora Lai-Wan Kwong

Chapter 66, Nasal and sinus malignancy, contains some material from Volume 3 Chapter 7: by Cyrus Kerawala, Peter Clarke and Kate Newbold

Chapter 67, Benign and malignant disease of the oral cavity, contains some material from Volume 3 Chapters 12: by Tim Martin and Omar A. Ahmed and 42: by Konrad S. Staines and Alexander Crighton

Chapter 68, Management of the unknown primary in head and neck cancer, contains some material from Volume 3 Chapter 17: by Ricard Simo, Jean-Pierre Jeannon and Maria Teresa Guerrero Urbano

Chapter 69, Metastatic neck disease, contains some material from Volume 3 Chapter 18: by Vinidh Paleri and James O'Hara

Chapter 70, Prosthetic management of oral and facial defects, contains some material from Volume 3 Chapter 31: by Chris Butterworth

Chapter 71, Grafts and flaps in head and neck reconstruction, contains some material from Volume 3 Chapters 91: by Kenneth Kok and Nicholas White, 92: by Ralph W. Gilbert and John C. Watkinson and 93: by John C. Watkinson and Ralph W. Gilbert

Chapter 72, Radiotherapy and chemotherapy, contains some material from Volume 3 Chapters 19: by Sara Meade and Andrew Hartley and 24: Chemotherapy by Charles G. Kelly

Chapter 73, Immunotherapy in head and neck cancer, contains some material from Volume 3 Chapter 30: by Kevin J Herrington and Magnus T. Dillon

Chapter 74, Quality of life, survivorship, and outcomes in head and neck cancer, contains some material from Volume 3 Chapters 20: by Simon Rogers and Steve Thomas and 28: by Helen Cocks, Raghav C. Dwivedi and Aoife M. I. Waters

Chapter 76, Benign and malignant conditions of the skin, contains some material from Volume 3 Chapter 94: by Murtaza Khan and Agustin Martin-Clavijo

Chapter 77, Anatomy and physiology of head and neck endocrine glands, contains some material from Volume 1 Chapters 53: by Julian A. McGlashan and 55: by Martin O. Weickert

Chapter 78, Thyroid and parathyroid pathology, contains some material from Volume 1 Chapter 58: by Ram Moorthy, Sonia Kumar and Adrian T. Warfield

Chapter 79, Endocrine imaging, contains some material from Volume 1 Chapter 57: by Steve Colley and Sabena Fareedi

Chapter 80, Evaluation and investigation of thyroid disease, contains some material from Volume 1 Chapters 59: by Andrew Coatesworth and Sebastian Wallis, 60: by Anthony P. Weetman and 61: by Christopher M. Jones and Kristien Boelaert

Chapter 81, Benign thyroid disease, contains some material from Volume 1 Chapter 61: by Christopher M. Jones and Kristien Boelaert

Chapter 82, Management of differentiated Thyroid cancer, contains some material from Volume 1 Chapters 62: by Hisham M. Mehanna, Kristien Boelaert and Neil Sharma, 65: by Iain J. Nixon and Ashok R. Shaha and 66: by Laura Moss

Chapter 83, Management of medullary thyroid cancers, contains some material from Volume 1 Chapter 63: by Barney Harrison

Chapter 84, Management of anaplastic thyroid cancer and lymphoma, contains some material from Volume 1 Chapter 64: by James D. Brierley and Richard W. Tsang

Chapter 85, Thyroidectomy, contains some material from Volume 1 Chapters 67: by Ricard Simo, Iain J. Nixon and Ralph P. Tufano, 69: by Neil S. Tolley and 70: by Neeraj Sethi, Josh Lodhia and R. James A. England

Chapter 86, Surgery for metastatic and locally advanced thyroid cancer, contains some material from Volume 1 Chapter 68: by Joel Anthony Smith and John C. Watkinson

Chapter 87, Investigation of hypercalcemia, contains some material from Volume 1 Chapter 71: by Mo Aye and Thozhukat Sathyapalan

Chapter 88, Management of hyperparathyroidism, contains some material from Volume 1 Chapter 73: by Neil J. L. Gittoes and John Ayuk

Chapter 89, Parathyroid surgery, contains some material from Volume 1 Chapters 76: by R. James A. England and Nick McIvor and 77: by Parameswaran Rajeev and Gregory P. Sadler

Chapter 90, Medicolegal aspects of thyroid and parathyroid surgery, contains some material from Volume 1 Chapter 81 by Barney Harrison

Chapter 91, Evaluation and investigation of pituitary disease, contains some material from Volume 1 Chapters 82: by Sean Carrie, John Hill and Andrew James and 83: by Thozhukat Sathyapalan and Stephen L. Atkin

Chapter 92, Primary pituitary disease, contains some material from Volume 1 Chapter 84: by Christopher M. Jones and John Ayuk

Chapter 93, Management of pituitary disease, contains some material from Volume 1 Chapters 85: by Mihir R. Patel, Leo F.S. Ditzel Filho, Daniel M., 86: by Andy Levy and 115: by Philip G. Chen and Peter-John Wormald

Chapter 94, The paediatric consultation, contains some material from Volume 2 Chapters 1: by Raymond W. Clarke, 2: by Raymond W. Clarke and 3: by Julian Gaskin, Raymond W. Clarke and Claire Westrope

Chapter 95, Paediatric anaesthesia, contains some material from Volume 2 Chapter 4: by Crispin Best

Chapter 96, Hearing testing, contains some material from Volume 2 Chapters 8: by Sally A.Wood and 9: by Glynis Parker

Chapter 97, Management of the hearing-impaired child, contains some material from Volume 1 Chapters 2: by Mohammed-Iqbal Syed, Volume 2 Chapter 10: by Chris H. Raine, Sue Archbold, Tony Sirimanna and Soumit Dasgoupta and 12: by Jonathan P. Harcourt

Chapter 98, Otitis media, contains some material from Volume 2 Chapters 14: by Peter A. Rea and Natalie Ronan and 15: by William P.L. Hellier

Chapter 99, Embryological developmental disorders, contains some material from Volume 2 Chapters 16: by Iain Bruce and Jaya Nichani, 18: by David M. Wynne and Louisa Ferguson, 19: by Benjamin Robertson, Sujata De, Astrid Webber and Ajay Sinha, 30: by Chris Jephson and 42: by Daniel J. Tweedie and Benjamin E.J. Hartley

Chapter 100, Imbalance, contains some material from Volume 2 Chapter 20: by Louisa Murdin and Gavin A.J. Morrison

Chapter 101, Nasal obstruction, contains some material from Volume 2 Chapters 23: by Michelle Wyatt and 26: by Peter J. Robb. Tunde Oremule is also acknowledged for his assistance

Chapter 102, Rhinosinusitis and lacrimal disorders, contains some material from Volume 2 Chapters 24: by Daniel J. Tweedie and 25: by Caroline J. MacEwen and Paul S. White

Chapter 103, Adenotonsillar conditions and obstructive sleep apnoea, contains some material from Volume 2 Chapters 26: by Peter J. Robb, 27: by Steven Powell and 38: by Yogesh Bajaj and Ian Hore

Chapter 104, Acquired laryngotracheal stenosis, contains some material from Volume 2 Chapters 31: by Michael J. Rutter, Alessandro de Alarcón and Catherine K. Hart and 32: by Rania Mehanna and Michael Kuo

Chapter 105, Stridor, contains some material from Volume 2 Chapters 28: by Kate Stephenson and David Albert and 29: by Lesley Cochrane

Chapter 106, Foreign bodies in the ear, nose and throat, contains some material from Volume 2 Chapter 34: by Adam J. Donne and Katharine Davies

Chapter 107, Childhood malignancies, cysts, and sinuses of the head and neck, contains some material from Volume 2 Chapters 40: by Fiona McGregor and James Hayden and 41: by Keith G. Trimble and Luke McCadden

Chapter 108, Drooling, aspiration, and oesophageal problems, contains some material from Volume 2 Chapters 43: by Haytham Kubba and Katherine Ong, 44: by Ravi Thevasagayam and 45: by Graham Haddock

Chapter 109, Paediatric tracheostomy and paediatric airway management, contains some material from Volume 2 Chapters 35: by Mike Saunders and 36: by Pensée Wu, May M.C. Yaneza, Haytham Kubba, W. Andrew Clement and Alan D. Cameron

Chapter 110, Pinnaplasty, contains some material from Volume 1, Chapter 86 by Victoria Harries and Simon Watts

THE EAR

1. ANATOMY AND PHYSIOLOGY OF HEARING

Anatomy of Hearing

External Ear

The auricle (pinna) is the outermost projection of the ear with its lateral surface character-ised by prominences and depressions (Figure 1.1a). The body is composed of elastic fibro-cartilage and is a continuous plate except for a narrow band between the tragus and anterior crus of the helix where endaural incisions can be made. The auricle functions to collect acoustic energy and direct it into the external auditory canal (EAC), and to create incident angle–dependent modifications that help with sound localisation. The EAC is a 2.4-cm-long passage formed from cartilage in the lateral third and bone in the medial two-thirds. It is lined with keratinising squamous epithelium, which facilitates migration of desquamated cells toward the external opening of the canal at a rate of 0.1 mm/day.[1] The mixture of these desquamated cells, cerumen, and sebum forms wax.

Both the pinna and EAC derive their blood supply from branches of the external carotid artery (posterior auricular, superficial temporal artery, and internal maxillary arteries). Venous drainage is into the external jugular vein, maxillary veins, and pterygoid plexus while lymphatic drainage is to the nodes at the mastoid tip, pre-auricular nodes, and upper deep cervical nodes. The EAC receives sensory innervation from the trigeminal, facial and vagus nerves. Innervation of the pinna is shown in Figure 1.2.

Middle Ear

The middle ear consists of the tympanic cavity (TC), Eustachian tube (ET) (see Chapter 8) and the mastoid air cell (MAC) system. The mastoid antrum is an air-filled sinus within the petrous temporal bone that communicates with the middle ear by way of the aditus. The MAC system is largely developed by the age of 6.

Tympanic Cavity (TC)

The TC is bounded by the tympanic membrane (TM) laterally and the osseous labyrinth medially (Figure 1.2a). The TM is divided into the pars tensa and pars flaccida, which sit, respectively, below and above the malleolar folds at the level of the lateral process of the mal-leus. The TM consists of three layers: an outer epithelial layer, middle fibrous layer (deficient in the pars flaccida), and an inner mucosal layer. It receives sensory innervation from the auriculotemporal nerve, auricular branch of the vagus nerve (Arnold's nerve), and the tym-panic branch of the glossopharyngeal nerve (Jacobsen's nerve).

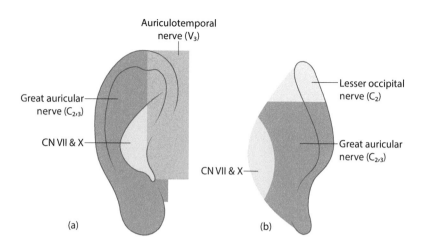

Figure 1.1 (a) Anatomy and (b) innervation of the anterior and posterior surfaces of the pinna.

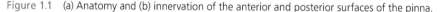

The TC is divided into the following sections by mucosal folds:

1 *Epitympanum*: It is also known as attic located above the malleolar folds. A bony crest known as the cog projects from the tegmen tympani caudally and divides the epitympanum into a larger posterior and smaller anterior space where residual cholesteatoma may be left in canal wall up surgery. The anterior and posterior isthmus tympani are gaps in mucosal folds that provide the only route of ventilation for the epitympanic space from the mesotympanum. Prussak's space is found between the pars flaccida and the neck of malleus and is an important site for cholesteatoma formation.

2 *Mesotympanum*: This is the part of the middle ear visible through the external canal with a microscope. The promontory is a rounded elevation, which occupies most of the medial wall, consisting of the basal turn of the cochlea.

3 *Hypotympanum*: This lies below the level of the inferior part of tympanic sulcus. The floor is made up of the bony covering of the jugular bulb, which can be dehiscent and should be kept in mind when raising the inferior portion of the tympanomeatal flap.

4 *Retrotympanum*: This is an area posterior to mesotympanum. The round window niche is separated from the promontory by two bony ridges arising from the promontory known as the ponticulus and subiculum (Figure 1.2b). The sinus tympani is a posterior extension of the mesotympanum and lies deep to the facial nerve and pyramid, making it difficult to access during surgery. The facial recess is a groove, which lies between the pyramid, facial nerve medially. and annulus of the TM laterally.

5 *Protympanum*: This is anterior to the promontory and contiguous with the tympanic portion of the ET. It's contents include the following:

  (i) *Ossicular chain*: The **malleus, incus, and stapes** connect the TM to the oval window.

  (ii) *Muscles*: The **tensor tympani** is supplied by the mandibular nerve. It arises from a bony canal lying above the ET, passes backward into processus cochleariformis, and turns at a right angle to insert into the malleus handle. The **stapedius** is supplied by the facial nerve, arises from the pyramidal eminence, and inserts onto the stapes superstructure.

  (iii) *Nerves*: The **chorda tympani** is a branch of the facial nerve. It runs across the medial surface of the TM between the mucosal and fibrous layers and passes

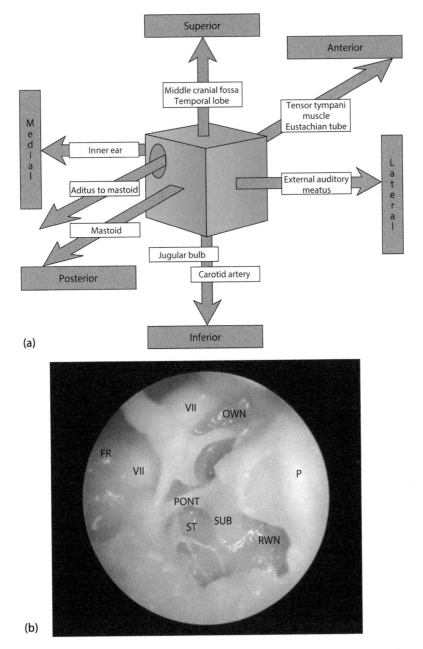

(a)

(b)

Figure 1.2   Relationships of the middle ear as shown in a schematic drawing (a) and endoscopic image (b).

medial to the malleus handle above the tensor tympani tendon. It leaves the TC through the petrotympanic fissure. The **tympanic plexus** is formed by Jacobsen's nerve and caroticotympanic nerves on the promontory, providing sensory and parasympathetic branches to the middle ear.

(iv)   *Mucosa*: The middle ear consists of ciliated mucus-secreting respiratory mucosa. The mucociliary pathways coalesce at the tympanic orifice of the ET.

Table 1.1   Pattern of structures within the otic capsule

Bony covering	Membranous duct suspended in perilymph and filled with endolymph	Sensory hair receptor cells with a dominant kinocilia
Cochlea	Cochlea duct	Inner hair cell on basilar membrane
Vestibule	Utricle and saccule	Hair cell in macula
Semicircular canal	Semicircular duct	Hair cells in crista ampulla

Inner Ear

The inner ear delivers sensory information relating to hearing via the cochlea and balance via the vestibular system. It is formed of

1 Dense bony covering (also called the otic capsule or bony labyrinth),
2 Membranous ducts, and
3 Sensory organs within these ducts (Table 1.1).

The space between the bony and membranous labyrinth is filled with perilymph. This contains high sodium and low potassium ion content (similar to extracellular fluid) and communicates variably with cerebrospinal fluid via the cochlear aqueduct. The fluid within the membranous labyrinth is known as endolymph and contains high potassium and low sodium ion content (similar to intracellular fluid).

Cochlea

The cochlea is formed of three parallel scalae (vestibula, media, and tympani) coiled in a spiral around a central modiolus in two and a half turns (Figure 1.3).

Both the scala vestibuli (SV) and scala tympani (ST) are filled with perilymph, whereas the central scala media (SM) is filled with endolymph. Within the SM is the sensory epithelium of the cochlea, called the organ of Corti. This is a strip of cells coiled in a spiral, resting on the basilar membrane (BM), and overlain by the gelatinous tectorial membrane. Ion transportation within the cochlea is mediated by the stria vascularis, which forms the lateral wall of the SM.

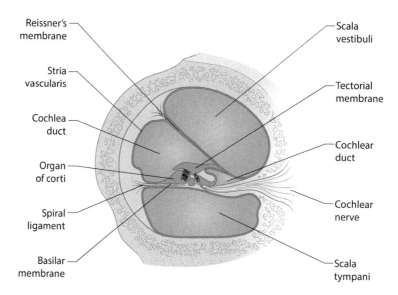

Figure 1.3   Cross section of the cochlea.

It contains the Na$^+$/K$^+$-ATPase, which maintains the high endolymphatic K$^+$ concentration and the +80-mV electrical potential of the cochlea endolymph, relative to the perilymph.

The cochlea's blood supply is the spiral modiolar artery, which is a branch from an end artery called the vestibulocochlear artery (VCA) from the anteroinferior cerebellar artery.

The organ of Corti contains the cylindrical-shaped outer hair cells (OHCs) and goblet-shaped inner hair cells (IHCs). There are four times more OHCs, which form three rows, compared with one row of IHCs. The IHCs form the primary receptor cell, innervated by the majority of cochlear afferent nerves. The OHCs play more of an efferent and modulating role. They respond to BM motion to amplify signal and improve frequency selectivity reaching the IHCs.

The hair cells have rows of motile microvilli-like structures called stereocilia, which increase in height in one particular direction (see Chapter 2 for further details of hair cell microanatomy).

The spiral ganglion is the collection of cell bodies from two types of afferent nerve fibres, namely:

- *Type 1 neurons (myelinated)*: They innervate IHCs, have large diameters, and constitute 95% of the nerve fibre population. One type 1 fibre innervates one IHC, but one IHC may synapse with several nerve fibres.
- *Type 2 neurons (unmyelinated)*: They innervate OHCs and are smaller than type 1 neurons. One type 2 fibre innervates many OHCs.

The afferent auditory pathway involves spiral ganglion central axons projecting via the cochlear nerve, into the cochlear nucleus of the brainstem. From here auditory information is conveyed *bilaterally* to the superior olivary nuclei (SON) in the pons, and then to the lateral lemniscus and inferior colliculus of the midbrain, medial geniculate nucleus of the thalamus, and the primary auditory cortex in the Sylvian fissure of the temporal lobe (Brodmann area 41, Heschl's gyrus, also known as the transverse temporal gyrus). Functional magnetic resonance imaging (MRI) studies indicate the presence of two broad cortical processing pathways: an anterior 'what sound' pathway and a posterior 'where is it coming from' pathway.

Connections from the SON to the facial nuclei mediate the stapedius reflex, which occurs in response to loud sounds (70–90 dB above threshold).

The efferent auditory pathway arises from projections from both the lateral olive and the medial olivary complex, which synapse mostly with type 1 and 2 spiral ganglion cells, respectively, and thus connect to both the IHCs and the OHCs. The efferent fibres are carried by the inferior vestibular nerve and meet at the anastomosis of Oort through the saccular branch of the nerve to join up with the cochlear nerve, forming the vestibulocochlear nerve. The cochlear nerve traverses the internal auditory canal (IAC), which is roughly 1 cm in length and its contents are shown in Figure 1.4.

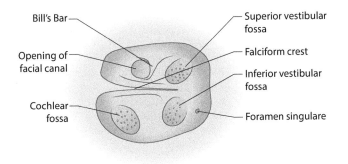

Figure 1.4   Contents of the internal auditory canal (IAC). A, anterior, P, posterior; S, superior; I inferior.

Table 1.2   Derivatives of first and second branchial arch

Cartilage	Nerve	Artery	Muscle
First branchial arch derivatives			
Meckel's cartilage Malleus Incus 'Mandible' Anterior malleolar ligament Sphenomandibular ligament	Mandibular branch of trigeminal nerve		Tensor tympani
Second arch derivatives			
Reichert's cartilage Stapes superstructure Styloid process Lesser cornu of hyoid Stylohyoid ligament	Facial nerve	Stapedial	Stapedius

Eighty percent of these efferent fibres synapse directly with OHCs, with the remainder terminating on afferent nerve fibres. The ratio of efferent to afferent fibres in the OHC is 1:2, whereas those in the IHCs is 1:7. This suggests efferent function is mainly to biologically amplify sound, modulate signals (protective damping of loud sounds), and frequency selectivity, via the OHCs. The medial system innervates both ears while the lateral system supplies only the ipsilateral cochlea. Both project to the different parts of the ventral cochlear nucleus.

Embryology of the Ear

The pinna develops from hillocks (swellings) on the first and second pharyngeal arches. Abnormalities of the pinna may therefore be associated with abnormalities of other first and second arch derivatives. The EAC develops from the ectoderm of the first branchial groove (cleft) while the ET and middle ear are derived from the second branchial pouch. The ossicular chain and middle ear muscles are derived from the first and second branchial arches (Table 1.2).

The inner ear develops independently of the middle and external ears. The otic capsule (containing the cochlea, vestibule, and three semicircular canals) develops from the mesoderm, whereas the membranous labyrinth develops from an ectodermal thickening (otic placode) on the side of the head between days 22 and 35 and is fully formed by 25 weeks of gestation to an adult state.

Physiology of the Hearing

The human ear has a huge dynamic range and is able to hear frequencies of 2–20 kHz and intensities up to 120 dB. The ears are most sensitive to frequencies between 2 and 5 kHz.

The pinna reflects sound from various directions into the EAC. The acoustic signal then travels down the EAC where it undergoes a resonance boost between 2.5 and 3.5 kHz in adults.

The middle ear acts as an efficient transformer to conduct acoustic energy from the low-impedance high-velocity TM, to the high-impedance, low-velocity fluid-filled cochlea. The impedance difference is mainly matched by the ratio of the surface area of the TM to the stapes footplate (approximately 18:1, or about 25 dB). A much smaller part is played by the lever action of the ossicles. The stapedius muscle plays a role in reflex contraction and stiffening of the ossicular chain to protect the cochlea's sensory epithelium from high-amplitude sounds (see below). In humans, the role of the tensor tympani is unknown, but it does not normally contract in response to sound. Aside from air conduction, the cochlea can also be directly stimulated by vibration of the bony skull (through the bone of the EAC, ossicles or cochlea). The middle ear has a resonant frequency around 1–3 kHz. If this resonance is reduced by a mechanical problem in the ossicular chain (e.g. fixation), the ossicular component of bone conduction is affected and results in a drop in the bone-conduction threshold. This classically appears at 2 kHz as Carhart's notch in the bone-conduction threshold in otosclerosis; however, Carhart's effect may be present between 1 and 4 kHz in any pathology affecting the ossicles.

Once sound is delivered into the cochlea through the stapes-oval window interface, a cochlear traveling wave is generated that traverses the BM. The arrangement of organ of Corti and basilar and tectorial membranes across the length of the cochlea gives rise to a 'tonotopic' relationship due to the variations in stiffness, thickness, and mass along these structures from base to apex. High-frequency sounds are best represented at the basal end and low frequencies at the apex. The movement of the BM creates relative motion between the tectorial membrane and the stereocilia of the IHCs. This allows ion channels to open and depolarise the cell, resulting in synaptic release of glutamate and firing of afferent nerve fibres.

Afferent nerve fibres on OHCs form a feedback loop with efferent fibres, which result in a change in the shape of OHCs and active modification of BM motion. This results in signal amplification at low intensity levels, improving hearing sensitivity and also improves spectral resolution. The OHCs are responsible for otoacoustic emissions and the cochlear microphonic potential.

Information on timing, frequency, and intensity of sound is encoded by the rate, number, location, and timing of auditory nerves firing. For sound localisation, encoding of interaural time differences (for low-frequency sounds) and interaural level differences (high-frequency sounds) in the auditory pathway are important.

KEY POINTS

- The external and middle ear develops from the first and second branchial arches, whereas the inner ear arises independently from an ectodermal thickening.
- The middle ear provides critical modifications and matches the change of impedance of sound as it moves between differing mediums, mainly by the ratio of the surface area of the TM to the stapes footplate (18:1).
- The BM within the cochlear is tonotopic, with high-frequency sounds producing displacement toward the base of the cochlea and low-frequency sounds toward the apex. These are influenced by active mechanisms of the OHC and the passive arrangement of the BM.
- Sound from the auditory nerve is propagated to the cochlear nucleus, SON, inferior colliculus, medial geniculate nucleus, and finally the auditory cortex.

Further Reading

1. Pickles JO. *An Introduction to the Physiology of Hearing.* 4th ed. Boston, MA: Brill; 2013.
2. Ahveninen J, Kopčo N, Jääskeläinen IP. Psychophysics and neuronal bases of sound localization in humans. *Hear Res.* 2014;307:86–97. doi:10.1016/j.heares.013.07.008.

2. ANATOMY AND PHYSIOLOGY OF BALANCE

Introduction

The role of the vestibular system is to maintain visual fixation and posture by (1) detecting changes in head motion, position, and spatial orientation and (2) stabilising eye, head, and body position.

The vestibular system is housed in the labyrinth of each ear. The main components of the vestibular system are three semicircular canals and two otolith organs (utricle and saccule). The three semicircular canals (superior, posterior, and lateral) detect angular acceleration in orthogonal planes. The utricle and saccule detect linear acceleration in primarily horizontal and vertical planes, respectively, as well as head position in relation to gravity.

Anatomy

Bony Labyrinthine Anatomy

The bony labyrinth lies within the petrous temporal bone, which is the densest bone in the body. The bony labyrinth (otic capsule) has three main components: the cochlea (anteriorly), vestibule (centrally), and semicircular canals (posteriorly) (Figure 2.1).

On the medial surface of the vestibule there is a further bony extension that projects posteriorly called the vestibular aqueduct. The vestibule has two openings on its lateral surface, the oval window superiorly and round window inferiorly.

The posterior limb of the superior canal and medial limb of the posterior canal join to become the common crus as they enter the vestibule. Each semicircular canal has a bony dilatation, called the ampulla, which houses its sensory organ. The semicircular canals are arranged in orthogonal planes (see Figures 2.1 and 2.2). The superior and posterior canals both lie 45° from the sagittal plane. Therefore, the superior canal of the right ear lies parallel to the posterior canal of the left ear, and vice versa.

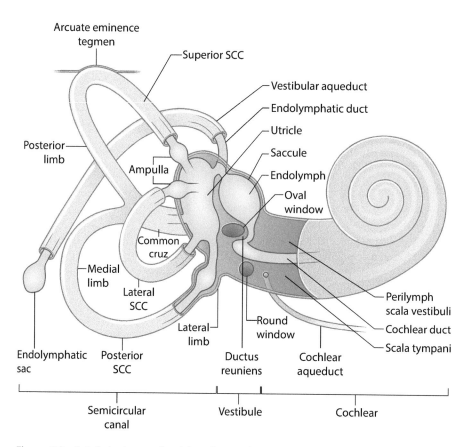

Figure 2.1 Detailed scheme of a right otic capsule's medial surface demonstrating the bony covering and internal ducts. Locations of oval and round windows are demonstrated. SCC, semicircular canal.

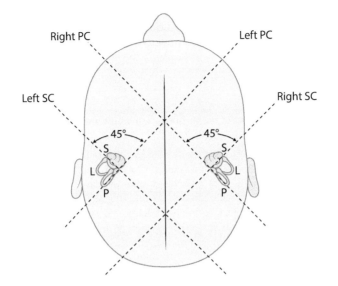

Figure 2.2   This figure demonstrates the orthogonal relationship of the semicircular canals. The superior and posterior canals (SC and PC) are 45° from the sagittal plane. Additionally the left superior semicircular canal is in a parallel plane to the right posterior semicircular canal. L, lateral; P, posterior; S, superior.

The superior semicircular canal abuts the mastoid tegmen, with a corresponding intracranial projection called the arcuate eminence. The thin bone of the tegmen that separates the canal from the dura at this point can be less than 1 mm in diameter.

Ductal Anatomy

The cochlear, utricle, and saccule semicircular and endolymphatic ducts are the membranous ducts of the four bony coverings. The ducts are filled with endolymphatic fluid that is potassium rich (similar to intracellular fluid, see Chapter 1). Anatomically, there appear to be two distinct membranous systems with implications on function and disease. The cochlear duct joins the saccule via the ductus reuniens, whilst the semicircular ducts branch directly off the utricle. Intense acoustic stimulation can inadvertently activate the saccule causing the sensation of movement (vertigo) in some people, called the Tullio's phenomenon, particularly if fluid pressure wave pathways are abnormal, for instance, in inner ear 'third window' syndromes, such as superior semicircular canal dehiscence.

The saccule lies in a spherical recess, anterior and inferior in the vestibule, ~0.6 mm deep to the anterior surface of the stapes footplate. This relationship is important for stapes surgery where an overlong piston inserted beyond the footplate can stimulate the saccule. The saccule is united with the cochlear duct from its anterior surface and endolymphatic duct on its posteromedial surface. The saccular macula contains the sensory hair cells, present in a cellular layer on its anterior surface.

The utricle is more oblong in shape, lies posterosuperior in the vestibule, and is ~0.8 mm deep to the posterior edge of the stapes footplate. The five semicircular ducts are projections of the utricle. The endolymphatic duct exits from its anteromedial surface. The utricular macula, containing the sensory cells, lies in its floor and is orientated primarily in a horizontal plane. The saccular macula lies on the medial surface of the saccule and is orientated primarily in a vertical plane.

The endolymphatic duct is formed from smaller ducts leading off the medial surfaces of the utricle and saccule and travels in the vestibular aqueduct. It courses behind the arcs of the posterior semicircular canal and narrows at its isthmus before it leads to the endolymphatic sac, which is a highly complex structure of interconnecting tubules, cisterns, and crypts. The distal, extraosseous portion of the sac rests on the posterior wall of the petrous bone, between layers of dura.

Microanatomy

Hair cells are the main receptors of the vestibular apparatus and occur in both the maculae (Figure 2.3) and crista ampullaris (Figure 2.4).

The apical surface of a hair cell is covered by large, actin-rich, rod-like microvillar projections called stereocilia, grouped in a bundle (the 'hair bundle'), wherein stereocilia progressively increase in length, like a staircase, with one large microtubule-based true cilium called the kinocilium positioned behind the longest row of stereocilia. The hair bundle staircase and position of the kinocilium define the axis of sensitivity or 'polarity' of the hair bundle (note the kinocilium, although present in early embryonic development, is absent in mature cochlear hair cell bundles). The tips of each shorter stereocilium is linked to the shaft of its neighbouring taller stereocilium by a thin proteinaceous filament, the tip link. Tip links are composed of two linear proteins joined end to end: cadherin 23 and protocadherin 15. Defects in one of these proteins are associated with different forms of Usher's syndrome. All of the hair cells in a crista are orientated in a single direction, along the plane of the semicircular duct, whereas hair cells in the maculae are arranged in a multiplanar orientation.

The hair bundles, which are bathed in endolymph, are covered by acellular membrane structures. In the maculae, the otolithic membrane is covered with *otoconia,* which are white crystalline particles composed predominantly of calcium carbonate. In semicircular canals, the hair cells of cristae protrude into a barrel-shaped gelatinous cap (termed the cupula) that lacks otoconia.

Sensory afferents of the saccule and the posterior semicircular canal are formed into the inferior vestibular nerve and those of the utricle; lateral and superior semicircular canals are formed into the superior vestibular nerve. The vestibular nerves travel medially in the internal auditory canal to the vestibular nuclei at the medullary-pontine junction. There is cross communication of nuclei on each side. In addition, each nucleus sends fibres to the nuclei of the ipsilateral and contralateral abducens, trochlear and oculomotor nerves, cerebellum, and descending fibres to the vestibulo-spinal tracts.

Physiology

The otolith organs sense gravity and linear translation of the head, and the semicircular canals sense angular acceleration of the head. Standing upright, in the absence of movement, the semicircular canals, utricles, and saccules of both the left and right ears cause firing of the right and left vestibular nerves at an equivalent baseline rate. Perception of movement and spatial position are a consequence of how these organs *change* the firing rate in the vestibular nerves from their basal rate and in relation to each other.

Movements of the head are synonymous with movements of the embedded bony labyrinth, The endolymphatic fluid lags behind owing to inertial forces and the viscous drag between the fluid and the duct wall. The 'lagging' endolymph deflects the cupula, which in turn deflects the stereocilia of the hair cell. If the stereocilia are pushed towards the kinocilia, then the tip links at the tips of stereocilia are stretched and thus 'gate open' mechanotransducer ion channels allow cations (mostly potassium) from the endolymph to enter the hair cell. The resulting depolarisation of the hair cell triggers pre-synaptic calcium influx and neurotransmitter release at the basal end of the cell and a post-synaptic depolarisation and thus increased firing rate of afferent nerve fibres. If the head movement is in the opposite direction

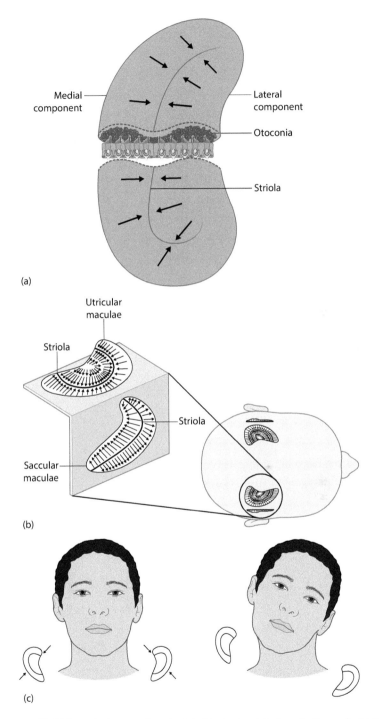

Figure 2.3 (A) Right utricular macula orientated in horizontal plane in floor of utricle. (B) A striola is a strip with no hair cells that separates the polarity of the hair cells on the medial and lateral components. The otoliths sit on an otolithic membrane which the hair cells project into. (C) Tilting head to the right will cause the otoconia to fall to the right, causing stereocilia to deflect to the right. The lateral component of the macula will thus become hyperpolarised and the medial component depolarised.

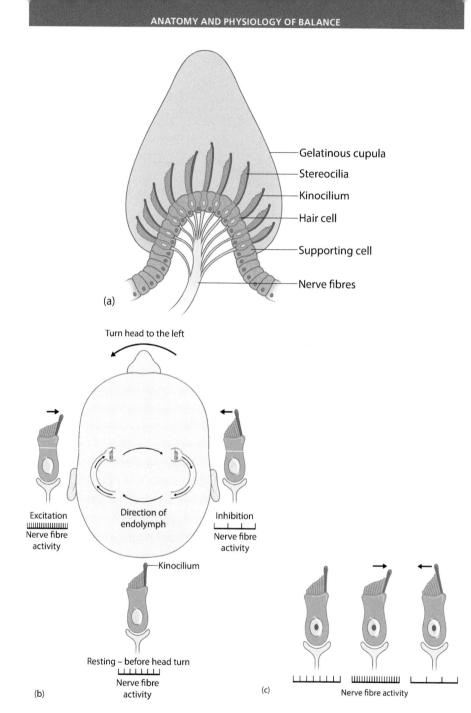

Figure 2.4 (A) Crista ampullaris of a left lateral semicircular duct. This shows the hair cells enveloped within the gelatinous cupula. Endolymphatic fluid surrounds the cupula. (B) Blow up demonstrates movement of head to the left. Inertia of the endolymph pushes cupula to the right; the stereocilia move towards the kinocilia and thus the cell becomes active on the left, increasing the firing rate of associated nerve fibres. (C) The stereocilia move away from the kinocilia on the right and thus firing rate decreases on the right. The differential firing between right and left semicircular canals provides an accurate awareness of head movement.

and the endolymph pushes stereocilia away from the kinocilia, this closes mechanotransducer channels, hyperpolarises the cell, and reduces firing in the afferent fibres.

Semicircular Canals

The semicircular canals are orientated so that they provide complementary information about angular movement. Anti-clockwise head rotation (turning your head to the left) increases the nerve-fibre firing rate of the left lateral semicircular canal and decreases the firing rate of fibres from the right lateral semicircular canal. The perception of head rotation is the net result of differential firing rates between these complementary lateral semicircular canals (see Figure 2.4). The superior and posterior canals of opposing ears lie in the same plane. Therefore, with the head rotated 45° to right, head flexion results in an increased fibre firing rate of the right superior semicircular canal and decreased firing rate of the left posterior semicircular canal. With the head rotated 45° to right, head extension causes reversal in this pattern of activation, between the right superior and left posterior semicircular canals.

The semicircular canals are integral in maintaining visual target fixation during movement, through the very short latency vestibulo-ocular reflex (VOR).

Differential firing of nerve fibres from each semicircular canal is communicated through the vestibular nerves from the vestibular nuclei to the abducens and oculomotor nuclei through a series of interneurons. When the head is rotated to the right, this fast reflex causes the left lateral rectus and right medial rectus to move both orbits to the left at the same rate and degree of the head turn, allowing visual fixation despite movement. Using differential information delivered from all six semicircular canals, the VOR allows visual stabilisation despite movements of the head in all planes. Unilateral vestibular lesions cause conjugate eye movement towards the affected ear (due to unopposed action from the healthy vestibular side) and a corrective (fast-phase nystagmus) movement back to the centre (away from the lesion).

Utricle and Saccule

The stereocilia within the maculae are embedded in a gelatinous matrix covered by otoconia. These crystals have a large specific gravity relative to endolymph, and thus pull the matrix to align with the gravitational vector, keeping it deflected post-movement. In addition, linear translation causes acceleration either horizontally or vertically, which also results in inertial deflection of the otoconia.

Since each hair cell is specialised to detect movement in one direction (movement that pushes the stereocilia towards the kinocilium), the hair cells within the maculae are arranged such that there are individual hair cells oriented to detect virtually any head position or direction of acceleration. This is accomplished by a complex three-dimensional arrangement of each macula and of the hair cells within the maculae (see Figure 2.3).

The arrangement of the saccule is such that anteroposterior translation is best detected (e.g. breaking at a red traffic light in a car). In addition, the saccule provides continuous information about vertical body position in relation to gravitational centre (e.g. awaking from sleep, lying flat on back). This allows one to detect that they are tilted backwards off the vertical, and perhaps about to fall. The saccule is therefore a key sensory input for the vestibulo-colic reflex (VCR) and the vestibulo-spinal reflex (VSR). These reflexes activate extensor muscles to maintain posture.

The orientation of hair cells in the utricle are such that horizontal translation (e.g. standing face forward on a skateboard and being pulled to the left or right) is best detected. In addition, the utricle provides continuous information about horizontal body position in relation to gravitational centre (e.g. awaking from sleep lying on side). This allows one to detect that they are tilted sideways off the vertical. The utricle provides sensory input for the utriculo-ocular reflex that causes eyes to move in the opposite direction to the side of lateral translation and maintain visual fixation. The ocular vestibular myogenic evoked potential (VEMP) is a test of the utriculo-ocular reflex, and the cervical VEMP is likely more dominated by the saccule.

KEY POINTS

- Movements that cause hair bundles to move 'towards' the kinocilia cause vestibular hair cells to depolarise and this increases the firing rate of afferent nerve fibres. Movements that cause hair bundles to move 'away' from kinocilia cause hair cells to hyperpolarise and reduce the firing rate of nerve fibres.
- Perception of movement is detected by the *change* in firing rate, and the relative difference between firing rates from complementary organs on either side.
- Lateral canals of each ear are complementary and detect head rotation (yaw). The superior canal of the right ear is complementary to posterior canal of the left ear (and vice versa) and together they detect non-horizontal head movements (pitch and roll).
- The otolithic organs, the utricle and saccule, are housed in the vestibule (main body) of the labyrinth. The saccule is closely related to the cochlear duct and as a result can be activated by intense acoustic stimuli. The saccule detects vertical translation and forward-backward tilt. It activates the VCR and VSR.
- The utricle is closely related to the semicircular canal. It detects horizontal translation and side-to-side tilt. It activates the utriculo-ocular reflex. Dislodged otoconia can pass from the utricle into the semicircular canals and cause an intense sense of vertigo on head movement (benign paroxysmal positional vertigo).

Further Reading

1. Alan Desmond. *Vestibular Function Clinical and Practice Management*, 2nd Ed. April 2011, Chapter 2, E-Book ISBN: 9781604063622.

2. Michael Gresty. *Clinical Neurophysiology of the Vestibular System*, 3rd Ed., April 2002, New York: Oxford University Press.

3. CLINICAL EXAMINATION OF THE EAR AND HEARING

Examination of the Ear

If ear surgery has been performed, external scars (endaural or postauricular) are looked for. The external ear skin is assessed for dermatological conditions.

Examination of the external auditory, pars tensa, and flaccida requires illumination and a speculum. Microsuction should be available to clear debris. Magnification with a handheld auriscope or microscope allows pathology to be assessed in greater detail. Pulling the pinna upward and back slightly will straighten the cartilaginous part of the external canal to enable the largest speculum to be inserted.

Rod endoscopes can be used to gain a wider view (Figure 3.1A), photographically record pathology, and allow electronic communication with others. Endoscopes with variable magnification can be fitted to a smartphone and have the potential of artificial intelligence (AI) to make a diagnosis. However performed, it is important to record the otoscopic findings, in detail, in case notes or letters of communication.

If a structured approach to otoscopy is taught, diagnostic skills improve and disease patterns are more easily recognised and appropriately dealt with.[1] In most ears, the most recognisable feature is the handle of malleus (Figure 3.2). The umbo and lateral process should be identified and the adjacent tympanic membrane visualised. The pars tensa and pars flaccida should

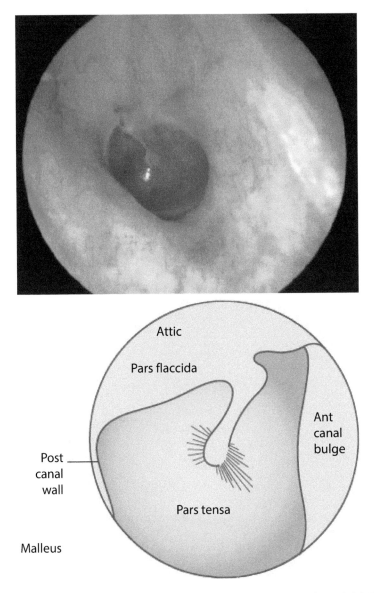

Figure 3.1 Endoscopic view of the tympanic membrane (A) with labeled schematic (B). The pars flaccida is located above the malleolar folds and is deficient of a middle fibrous layer.

be inspected (see Figure 3.1B). The examiner should decide if the pars tensa is intact and if so whether it is in its normal position. Clues as to its normal position should be sought in identifying the angle of the handle of the malleus. Foreshortening indicates retraction of the tympanic membrane medially as does lipping around the annulus creating a 'neo-annulus' (Figure 3.2.1). Mobility of the pars tensa can be assessed by getting the patient to perform a Valsalva manoeuvre or use of a pneumatic Siegel closed speculum. Immobility would suggest middle ear fluid.

The tympanic membrane is normally a grey, slightly translucent colour. Hyaline degeneration of the fibrous layer sometimes associated with calcium deposition occurs as a consequence of previous episodes of middle ear inflammation. This increases the whiteness of the tympanic membrane and can be either a diffuse thickening of the tympanic membrane or

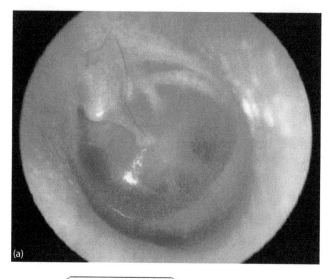

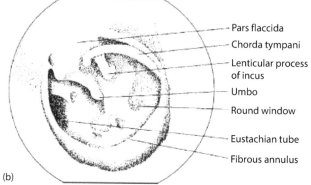

- Pars flaccida
- Chorda tympani
- Lenticular process of incus
- Umbo
- Round window
- Eustachian tube
- Fibrous annulus

(b)

Figure 3.2 Normal tympanic membrane with labeled middle ear structures.

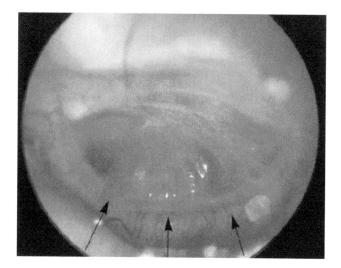

Figure 3.2.1 Severely retracted position of the malleus handle in otitis media with effusion (left ear). As retraction develops, a neoannular fold may form (arrows).

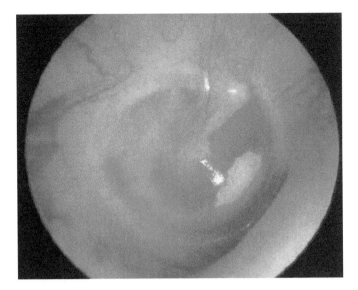

Figure 3.2.2   Chalk patch on the anterior pars tensa (right ear).

occur as isolated, tympanosclerotic plaques (Figure 3.2.2). Previous grommet insertion produces a rather characteristic crescent-shaped deposition of calcium in about 30% of patients (Figure 3.2.3). Tympanosclerosis may also fixate the ossicles with a resultant conductive impairment. If the tympanic membrane is perforated posteriorly, the ossicular chain may be visible (Figure 3.3).

It should be routine to angle the vision to have a full view of the pars flaccida particularly if the ear has had surgery (Figure 3.3.1). The extent of any attic defect requires assessment after any contents have been removed and deciding whether they are from active mucosal or squamous disease.

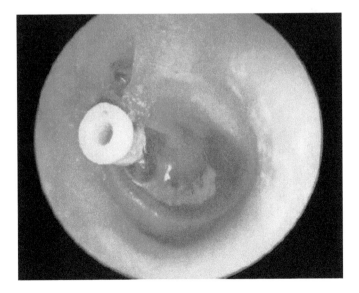

Figure 3.2.3   Extruded ventilating tube with otoscopic recurrence of middle ear fluid. Left ear retracted and yellow.

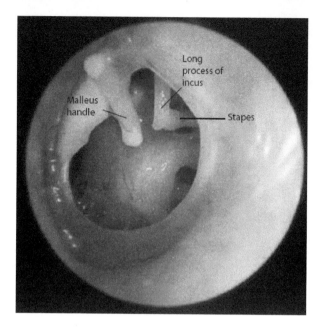

Figure 3.3 Subtotal perforation with visible middle ear contents.

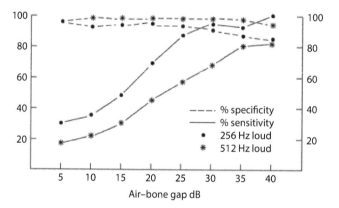

Figure 3.3.1 A comparison of the sensitivity and specificity of the 256 Hz fork using a loudness comparison method against the 512 Hz fork using a threshold method, in detecting air–bone gaps of various magnitudes. Redrawn with permission from Browning et al. Clinical role of informal tests of hearing. *J Laryngol Otol* 1989; 103: 7–11.

Clinical Assessment of Hearing

Clinical assessment of the hearing in each ear should be done in all patients presenting with ear problems irrespective of whether hearing impairment is a symptom. Free-field speech testing is reliable[2] (Table 3.1) and can act as a screening tool to determine whether pure-tone audiometry is required.

General Technique of Free-Field Speech Testing

The examiner explains to the patient that a combination of letters and numbers are going to be whispered or spoken and the patient's task is to try and repeat them. A number-letter combination is chosen as this has a reasonable mix of consonants that allows a relatively broad range of frequencies to be tested. For less experienced testers, a list of these to read from allows

Table 3.1 Comparison of free-field voice thresholds and pure-tone average (PTA) over 0.5, 1, 2 and 4kHz

Voice level	Distance (cm)	Loudness (dBA)	PTA mean percentiles	
			5th	95th
Whisper	60	12	–	27
	15	34	20	47
Conversation	60	48	38	60
	15	56	48	67
Loud	60	76	67	87

Source: From Swan IRC, Browning GG. The whispered voice as a screening test for hearing loss. *J R Coll Gen Pract* 1985; 35: 197.

a more consistent voice level to be produced. The examiner then positions themselves behind the patient so that the subject cannot lip-read and in a loud voice confirms that they understand the task by saying very recognisable numbers such as '99.' The non-test ear can be masked by tragal rubbing where the tragus is positioned over the canal and rubbed; this produces a masking level of around 40 dBA. When standing behind at arm's length, if the subject cannot repeat more than 50% of the words spoken in a whispered voice they will have a hearing impairment of at least 25 dB hearing loss (HL) in that ear. Varying the distance from 60 to 15 cm and the voice level can thereafter determine the likely degree of hearing impairment.

Tuning Fork Tests

These are of minimal value when accurate pure-tone audiometry, with both air and bone conduction, is available. The most commonly used forks are the 256 and 512 Hz with the former giving more reliable results. They are best activated by striking them gently on the elbow giving a sound of ~70 dBA when presented to the ear.

Rinne Test

With the tuning fork activated, the patient is asked to say which of the following sounds louder: the fork placed within 2 cm of the external auditory canal (air conduction [AC]) or placed firmly on the flat bone of the mastoid behind the pinna (bone conduction [BC]). To aid bone contact with the tuning fork, the patient's head is held with the other hand to prevent it from moving. In normal ears and those with a pure sensorineural impairment, AC will be reported as louder than BC. When this is not the case, then a conductive defect is suggested. BC can also be louder than AC due to a severe-profound HL in the test ear, with BC being detected in the contralateral better-hearing ear.

If the ear is otoscopically normal and there is a hearing impairment, the Rinne tuning fork test is insufficiently sensitive to diagnose otosclerosis with an air-bone gap of less than 30–40 dB[2] (Table 3.2). It will only suggest a conductive loss in ears with a 20-dB air-bone gap in ~50% of ears.

Weber Test

This is only applicable to those with unilateral or asymmetric hearing. An activated tuning fork base is firmly placed in the midline over the forehead, incisor teeth, or skull vertex. The patient is asked to report where in the head the sound is loudest. If heard in the 'better-hearing' ear there is a sensorineural impairment in the contralateral ear. If heard in the poorer ear then it has a conductive impairment. The Weber test has a low sensitivity and specificity and is marginally better than chance at determining whether a HL is sensorineural or conductive in nature.

Table 3.2 Size of air-bone gap (dB) which would be correctly identified by Rinne test on various percentages of occasions. (See *Scott-Brown's Otorhinolaryngology*, 8th edition, Chapter 73, for full references)

Fork	Study	Confidence limits		
		50%	75%	>90%
256 Hz	Crowley & Kaufmann (1966)[17]	25 dB		30 dB
	Gelfand (1977)[17]		40 dB	
	Browning et al. (1989)[13]	15 dB	20 dB	30 dB
512 Hz	Crowley & Kaufmann (1966)[17]	25 dB		30 dB
	Wilson & Woods (1975)[18]			40 dB
	Gelfand (1977)[20]		40 dB	
	Golabed & Stephens (1979)[19]	19 dB		
	Browning et al. (1989)[13]	20 dB	25 dB	40 dB

KEY POINTS

- Otoscopy is best performed backed up by microscopic-aided suction to improve visualisation of all areas including the attic and surgical defects.
- The largest speculum available should be used to visualise the tympanic membrane; an oval one is better than a round one.
- Free-field speech tests with a whispered voice at 60 cm from the ear can be used as a screening test for a hearing impairment if audiometry is not available.
- If the tympanic membrane is normal the Rinne tuning fork test will only detect an air-bone gap of 20 dB in 50% of cases.
- If otoscopy suggests the possibility of a conductive impairment, full audiometry is required to assess the magnitude of the air-bone gap if any.

Further Reading

1. Wormald PJ, Browning GG, *Otoscopy: A Structured Approach*. 1996, London: Hodder Arnold.
2. Browning GG, Swan IRC, Chew KK, Clinical role of informal tests of hearing *Journal of Laryngology and Otology*, 1989, 103, 7–11.

4. PSYCHOACOUSTIC AND OBJECTIVE ASSESSMENT OF HEARING

Psychoacoustic Audiometry

Audiometry is the measurement of hearing detection levels for pure tones in each ear across frequencies. Results indicate the type and degree of hearing loss and give a basic indication of the impact of ear pathology on hearing.

Audiometry results are recorded on a chart called the pure-tone audiogram (PTA).[1] Sound levels are represented on the y-axis of the PTA in decibels (dBs). The number of decibels is 20 times the logarithm of the ratio of two sound pressure levels (SPLs). A logarithmic

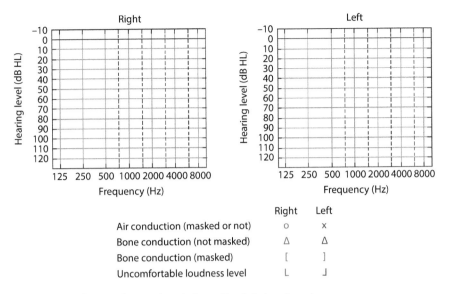

Figure 4.1   Audiogram chart and symbols used in clinical audiometry.

unit is used due to the wide dynamic range of human hearing (120 dB). The unit 'dB hearing level' or dB HL is used for ease of reading, as the normal hearing threshold varies across frequencies when measured in SPL. The 0 dB HL line on the PTA represents average thresholds for otologically normal young adults at each frequency. The higher up the chart the better are the HLs. Negative numbers indicate that thresholds are better than average. Pure tones are used to measure HLs as they are easily characterised in terms of frequency and level. The x-axis displays the frequencies of pure-tone signals typically at octave intervals and encompasses a range important for speech understanding (250, 500, 1000, 2000, 4000 and 8000 Hz). The name of the patient, date, tester, and audiometer are recorded. The convention for symbols used to record the outcomes of audiometry are shown in Figure 4.1.

The procedures and calibration of audiometry equipment are specified by international and national standards. The characteristics of the test environment are defined to reduce external and internal competing noise sources.

Testing of absolute thresholds is done using air conduction (AC), using headphones or insert earphones, and bone conduction (BC), using a transducer placed on the mastoid. The sensitivity for detecting mechanical vibrations produced in BC testing depends largely on the inner ear with reduced influence of the outer and middle ears.

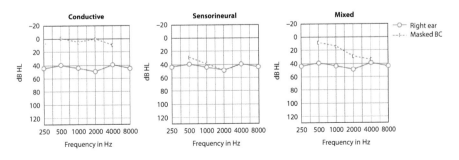

Figure 4.2   Types of hearing loss.

Following otoscopic examination, headphones or insert earphones are positioned on the ears. Patients are asked if they have had exposure to loud sounds in the last 24 hours, and whether they have tinnitus, in which case the sound signal can be changed to warble tones to make it easier to distinguish from tinnitus.

Patients respond by pressing a button or raising a finger for the duration of the presented tone. The order of testing is typically started at 1000 Hz in the better-hearing ear, followed by 2000, 4000, 8000, 500, and 250 Hz. The first frequency is repeated at the end of testing of the first ear to ensure test-retest consistency of 5 dB or less. The second ear is then tested.

Starting at an easily audible level, the signals are systematically reduced in volume in 10-dB steps until the signal is inaudible. When the patient no longer responds, the signal is increased in steps of 5 dB until the patient responds again. This is a bracketing technique, which is also called the '10 dB-down, 5 dB-up technique'. The 'absolute threshold' is defined as the lowest sound level that a person responds to on two out of three presentations and it is used to quantify the degree of hearing loss, which can be mild (21–40 dB HL), moderate (41–70 dB HL), severe (71–95 dB HL), or profound (above 95 dB HL). Differences of 10 dB or greater across tests are considered significant.

Next, BC thresholds are tested at frequencies from 500, 1000, 2000, and 4000 Hz. The bone transducer is placed to avoid it touching the pinna and hair. The test-retest reliability of BC thresholds is poorer than that for AC. In moderate-to-profound hearing loss, some low-frequency BC signals may be felt as vibration, giving the impression of a conductive component of hearing loss in low frequencies. The type of hearing loss is defined as either sensorineural (AC and BC loss differ by less than 20 dB, known as air-bone gap [ABG]), conductive (AC loss greater than BC loss by 20 dB or more), or mixed.

There are occasions when the test signal may be perceived in the non-test or contralateral ear through transcranial transmission (via BC). In AC, this tends to occur when there is an interaural difference of 40 dB or more, in thresholds derived with supra-aural headphones, or over 55 dB with insert earphones. Ear-specific thresholds are obtained by 'masking' the non-test ear by presenting a continuous narrow band of noise centred around the test signal frequency (Table 4.1). Masking noise is calibrated in the decibel-effective masking level (dB EML). The

Table 4.1   Rules for the use of clinical masking

'Rule'	Situation	What to do
1	The not-masked AC thresholds differ by 10dB or more when using supra-or circum-aural headphones, or by 55dB when using insert earphones.	Retest the AC threshold of the worse ear masking the contralateral ear.
2	The not-masked BC threshold of one ear is better than the AC threshold of either ear by 10dB or more.	Retest the BC threshold of the ear with the worse AC threshold masking the contralateral ear. Use clinical judgement. Is it critical to diagnosis to apply this rule (e.g. when there are only small BC thresholds)? If the masked BC threshold has changed little (i.e. up to 10dB), it may be necessary to retest the BC threshold of the ear with better AC threshold masking the contralateral ear.
3	Rule 1 was bit applicable, but the BC threshold of one ear (ear A) is 40 dB (for supra- or circum-aural headphones) or 55dB (for insertion earphones) better than the not masked AC threshold for the other ear (ear B).	Retest the AC threshold of ear B masking ear A.

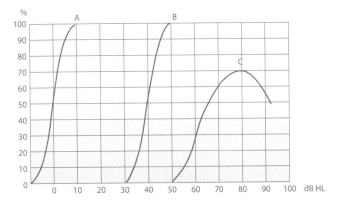

Figure 4.3 Example of speech discrimination score curves. Curve A represents normal hearing and Curve B is typical of a conductive hearing loss, whereas the pattern in Curve C may be seen with a retrocochlear hearing loss.

level of the masking noise is increased in 10-dB steps and the threshold for the pure-tone signal is re-evaluated. The hearing threshold is recorded as the level at which the threshold remains unchanged across three 10-dB step increments of masking. It is not always possible to derive masked thresholds in case of severe conductive hearing loss due to constraints in masking levels. For BC, unmasked thresholds indicate detection levels in the better-hearing cochlea, so masking is generally recommended whenever quantification of ABG is needed.

There are known distortions that occur in auditory perception for people with cochlear impairment and reduced HLs, for example, loudness recruitment (an abnormal increase in loudness perception between the detection level and maximum comfort level of sound), or loss of frequency selectivity, among others. These are not tested in PTA. Thus, people with similar PTAs may have a very different experience of hearing in everyday life.

Speech-Perception Testing

To understand the impact of hearing loss on communication, speech audiometry is required. Testing using real words at a range of intensities in each ear provides the performance intensity function. The optimum discrimination score (ODS) gives a measure of speech discrimination and the cochlear reserve in a mixed hearing loss. A lack of improvement with increasing intensity may indicate impaired cochlear function. A marked rollover (worsening speech recognition with increased intensity, Figure 4.3, Curve C) is usually indicative of vestibular schwannoma or other neural pathology.

Objective Assessment of the Ears and Hearing

Tympanometry

Tympanometry is used to assess middle ear function. The test is conducted by placing a probe in the ear canal, which is surrounded by a soft tip. The probe is composed of a loudspeaker, a microphone, and a pump. The soft tip should seal the ear canal so that the pump introduces controlled variations of the air pressure in the ear canal. The loudspeaker delivers a tone, usually 226 Hz, and the microphone monitors the sound level in the ear canal. With this probe, the compliance (or admittance) of the middle ear is measured as a function of the air pressure in the ear canal.

The result is shown on a chart called a tympanogram, which includes parameters of middle ear compliance/pressure, and the ear canal volume (ECV). The norms for compliance peak are values of 0.3 (or 0.2 for children) to 1.6 cm^3 for adults. Low compliance indicates abnormal stiffness of the middle ear (i.e. otosclerosis or malleus fixation). Abnormally high compliance may indicate ossicular discontinuity or atrophic scarring of the eardrum. Different

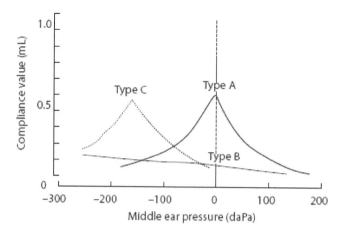

Figure 4.4 Different types of tympanogram traces. Normal middle ear pressure values are between ±50 daPa in adults (Type A tympanogram). Values around −200 daPa indicate significant Eustachian tube dysfunction (negative middle ear pressure: Type C tympanogram). If the trace is flat (Type B tympanogram), the test confirms the presence of middle ear effusion if the ear canal volume (ECV) is normal (between 0.6 and 2.5 cm³ for adults and between 0.4 and 1 cm³ for children). It is important to consider the ECV: a flat trace with a small ECV may indicate that the probe was blocked, and a value that is large may indicate a tympanic perforation.

types of tympanogram traces are shown in Figure 4.4. Additional testing through the use of tympanometry includes long time-based tympanometry (Chapter 8) and the acoustic stapedial reflex. The latter is elicited by brief pure tones or noise bursts. The lowest intensity of sound that triggers the reflex is the acoustic reflex threshold (ART). An absent or abnormal stapedial reflex with normal middle ear pressure occurs in otosclerosis.

OAEs
Otoacoustic emissions (OAEs) are low-level sounds that reflect the active mechanism of the outer hair cells (OHCs) in the cochlea. They can be recorded in the ear canal. OEAs can be spontaneous or evoked. Evoked OAEs with clinical relevance are classified into the following:

- *Transient evoked OAEs (TEOAEs)*: These are evoked by a transient stimulus (click or burst) and recorded in the ear canal after a short delay. The outcomes are assessed in terms of reproducibility, level, and signal-to-noise ratio. TEOAEs are typically absent or abnormal with cochlear hearing losses above 30 dB HL.
- *Distortion-product OAEs (DPOAEs)*: These are evoked by the simultaneous presentation of two pure tones (called 'primaries' with frequencies f1 and f2). If f1 and f2 are close in frequency, they lead to the production of distortion products in ears with a healthy basilar membrane. The highest amplitude distortion product is usually 2f1-f2; therefore, it is assessed clinically. DPOAEs are typically absent or abnormal with cochlear hearing losses above 40–50 dB HL.

It is advised that the measurement of OAEs is combined with tympanometry, especially in cases where OAEs are absent, because middle ear problems can interfere with the recording of OAEs. A key application of OAEs is the diagnosis of auditory neuropathy (Chapter 16). The newborn hearing screening programme (NHSP) uses automated OAE recordings in babies together with automated auditory brainstem responses (ABRs).

Auditory Evoked Potentials (AEPs)   Sound stimuli result in activation of the auditory pathway, and this electrical activity can be recorded from the scalp. An analysis of response characteristics, such as latency and amplitude of the resulting waveform, gives important diagnostic information about the integrity of the peripheral and central auditory system. Recordings are performed with a minimum of three electrodes: an active electrode, a reference electrode, and a ground electrode. Biological and electric noise are reduced by averaging responses to repeated stimulation. While noise occurs randomly, the auditory evoked potential (AEP) occurs at a constant latency to the stimulus onset. Signal processing techniques including filtering are typically also used to reduce noise. Common sound stimuli are clicks (square wave pulses) and tone bursts (sinusoidal).

Cochlear Microphonics (CM) CM is a pre-neural response from cochlear OHCs that mirrors the waveform of the stimulus. It is often measured in children, as part of the auditory neuropathy test battery. Similar to OAEs, the CM indicates OHC function. However, the CM is less vulnerable to the effect of a conductive hearing loss than OAEs.

Electrocochleography (ECOG) ECOG is a technique of assessing cochlear and auditory nerve function. The active electrode is placed on the tympanic membrane, through the tympanic membrane on the promontory or in the cochlea. The response has several components including (1) the CM; (2) the summating potential (SP), which is a direct current response from hair cells; and (3) the auditory nerve action potential (AP). A high SP:AP ratio is associated with Meniere's disease. AP measurements can also be used to indicate the presence of a functioning auditory nerve prior to cochlear implantation.

Auditory Brainstem Response (ABR) The ABR arises from the auditory nerve and low brainstem within 10 ms from the onset of the click stimulus and comprises five waves, labeled from I to V. The generators of each wave are thought to be for I the distal portion of the auditory nerve, for II the proximal portion of the auditory nerve, for III the cochlear nucleus, for IV the superior olivary complex and lateral lemniscus, and for V the lateral lemniscus and possibly the inferior colliculus.

By measuring the lowest sound signal at which the ABR response can be detected, the hearing threshold can be estimated for different frequencies for both air and bone conduction. It must be noted that the 95% confidence intervals for estimated HLs are fairly large (up to 30 dB at low frequencies). However, the great advantage of ABR is that a robust response can be measured even during sleep or general anaesthesia. This makes it particularly suitable for hearing-threshold estimation for patients in whom behavioural audiometry is not possible. ABRs are important in the diagnosis of auditory neuropathy, which is characterised by normal OAE/CM but absent or abnormal suprathreshold ABRs.

Auditory Late Response (ALR) The ALR is cortical in origin and the neural generator is thought to include Heschl's gyrus. The response is recorded at a latency of approximately 50–290 ms after stimulus onset. ALRs assess the auditory pathway at the level of the auditory cortex and are less susceptible to muscle activity compared with ABR. They are typically used for hearing threshold estimation in adults with suspected non-organic hearing loss and to indicate whether young children with hearing loss are obtaining benefit from their hearing aids.

KEY POINTS

- Performance on a PTA relies on sound detection; therefore, it does not characterise other deficits that have a significant impact on hearing for speech.
- Speech audiometry is essential in the assessment of the impact of hearing loss on communication.
- AEP can be used to assess the peripheral and central auditory pathways.
- Patients who are difficult to test by behavioural audiometry can have their hearing thresholds quantified using the threshold ABR.

Further Reading

1. British Society of Audiology. Pure-Tone Air-Conduction and Bone-Conduction Threshold Audiometry with and without Masking. British Society of Audiology Recommended Procedures and Publications. Reading, UK: British Society of Audiology; 2011.

2. British Society of Audiology. Recommended Procedure for Tympanometry. Reading, UK: British Society of Audiology; 2013.

3. Katz J, Medwetsky L, Burkhard R, et al. (eds). *Handbook of Clinical Audiology.* 6th ed. Baltimore: Lippincott, Williams & Wilkins; 2009.

4. Musiek F, Josey A, Glasscock M. Auditory brainstem response: interwave measurements in acoustic neuroma. *Ear Hear.* 1986;7:100–105.

5. EVALUATION OF BALANCE

Symptoms in Balance Disorders

Vertigo and Dizziness

Dizziness, vertigo, and unsteadiness accounts for one-fifth of referrals to ear, nose, and throat (ENT) and neurology clinics, and the rise in the ageing population will increase this further. Despite many developments in vestibular science, nothing replaces a good clinical history.

Vertigo is a reliable vestibular symptom, but lesions can be anywhere from the semicircular canals to vestibular cortex. Additional symptoms allow localisation (Table 5.1). Duration is indicative, lasting seconds in benign paroxysmal positional vertigo (BPPV); minutes to

Table 5.1 Additional symptoms helpful in the topographical diagnosis of balance disorders

Site of lesion	Symptom	Comment
Peripheral (labyrinth or VIII nerve)	Tinnitus	
	Hearing loss	
Special cases		
- Labyrinthine	Ear fullness	Meniere's disease
- Cerebellopontine angle	V, VI, and VII cranial nerves	Extra-canalicular growth
- VII + VIII neuritis	External auditory canal vesicles + VII	Ramsay Hunt syndrome (herpes zoster oticus)
Brainstem	Diplopia (III, IV, VI, or skew deviation*)	
	Facial numbness (V) weakness (VII)	
	Difficulty swallowing, choking (IX, X)	
	Slurred speech (XII, cerebellum)	
	Uni-bilateral numbness, weakness, ataxia (long tracts, cerebellum)	
	Unilateral deafness (+ ataxia)	AICA infarct

* Skew deviation (elevation of one eye and depression of the other) is caused by unilateral lesion in brainstem vestibular structures.

Note: AICA, anterior inferior cerebellar artery, from where the labyrinthine artery branches off.

Table 5.2   Some non-vestibular causes of dizziness

Type	Possible causes
Endocrine	Hypoglycaemia, adrenal failure, pheochromocytoma
Cardiovascular	Vasovagal syncope, orthostatic hypotension, embolic disease, cardiac dysrhythmias
Haematological	Hyperviscosity syndromes, anaemias
Psychological	Anxiety, phobias, panic attacks, PPPD

Note: PPPD, persistent perceptual postural dizziness, is a common functional balance disorder.

many hours in migraine-associated vertigo (vestibular migraine); a few hours in Meniere's disease; and days in acute vestibular neuritis and stroke.

Non-rotational 'dizziness', rocking sensations, light-headedness, and feeling detached can be vestibular or non-vestibular (Table 5.2). Some patients are 'unsteady' or 'off-balance' but 'not dizzy in the head' or feeling fine if seated or lying down; indeed, patients with a neurological gait disorder perceive their own disequilibrium and can report it as dizziness.

Vertigo Presentations

The three main presentations of vertigo are single episode (acute vertigo), recurrent (episodic), or chronic dizziness (Bronstein and Lempert 2017).

Acute vertigo is severe and disabling, with autonomic symptoms such as nausea, vomiting, pallor, and sweating. The key syndromes are

1 Acute vestibulopathy/neuritis (no hearing or neurological symptoms),
2 A vascular or inflammatory disorder of the VIII nerve or labyrinth (hearing loss), and
3 A cerebellar-brainstem stroke (central nervous system [CNS] symptoms) (Table 5.3).

Differentiate *positional increase* of vertigo (as in conditions above) from *truly positional* vertigo where vertigo stops, if motionless.

Inquire actively about additional hearing or cerebellar-brainstem symptoms as they may not be volunteered. Distinguishing peripheral and central acute vertigo is crucial because a stroke requires urgent treatment, hence the 'red flags' are described in Box 5.1.

Table 5.3   Vertigo presentations: episodic or recurrent vertigo, accompanying features

Accompanying feature	Possible cause
Positional	Benign paroxysmal positional vertigo (on lying or turning in bed)
Postural	Orthostatic hypotension (on standing)
Paroxysmal	Vestibular paroxysmia
Migraine features (headache, photophobia)	Vestibular and basilar migraine
Hearing disorder	Meniere's syndrome or hydrops
Ataxia	Episodic ataxias
Brainstem symptoms	Transient ischaemic attacks (TIA)
Autonomic-anxiety-avoidance	Panic attacks
Faintness	Heart disease, vasovagal syncope
No accompanying features	Benign recurrent vertigo*

* Benign recurrent vertigo, recurrent peripheral vestibular disorder, or vestibular Meniere's disease are names given to patients with recurrent peripheral vertigo that do not fall into well-defined categories such as Meniere's disease or migraine.

Source: Modified from Bronstein and Lempert (2017) (see further reading).

Triggers are critically important for diagnosis in patients with **recurrent symptoms**. Incorrectly, clinicians may believe neck movement–related dizziness indicates dubious entities like cervical vertigo, before excluding common vestibular disorders, particularly BPPV. Tables 5.3 and 5.4 list triggers and associated symptoms.

Most patients with a single acute vertigo attack recover fully and most patients with recurrent vertigo are free of symptoms between attacks, but not all. Given vertigo's prevalence, the small proportion of not fully recovered patients develop **chronic dizziness,** contributing significantly to specialist clinics. Chronic dizziness may result from many factors interfering with the process of central vestibular compensation (Box 5.2).

Examination of the Dizzy Patient

Clinical assessment includes auroscopy (Chapter 3), eye movements, and positional (Chapter 6) and gait examination.

Table 5.4 Vertigo presentations: symptom triggers in patients with episodic vertigo

Trigger	Possible cause
Lying down, turning over in bed	Benign paroxysmal positional vertigo
Standing up	Orthostatic hypotension
Neck movements	Any vestibular disorder
Pressure changes/Valsalva	Fistulas, superior canal dehiscence
Loud sounds	Tullio's phenomenon, superior canal dehiscence
Alcohol, exercise	Episodic ataxias
Sleep deprivation, alcohol, foods, bright lights	Vestibular migraine

BOX 5.2 FACTORS INTERFERING WITH CENTRAL VESTIBULAR COMPENSATION

- Fluctuating vestibular disorder (Meniere's disease, vestibular migraine)
- Additional disorder:
    - Central nervous system
    - Peripheral nerve
    - Cervical spine
    - Visual
- Lack of mobility
- Drugs
- Visual dependence ('visual vertigo')
- Psychosocial issues
- Old age (+ many of the factors above)

Eye Movements

The vestibular system provides a powerful input to the oculomotor system so eye movements must be examined in detail (see Bronstein and Lempert 2017 for videos). The examination has two broad aims:

1 To search for direct signs of a peripheral vestibular disorder, e.g. nystagmus, BPPV, or a positive head thrust test.
2 To ensure non-vestibular mediated eye movements (saccades, pursuit) are normal, excluding CNS lesions; patients must be clearly instructed to focus on a predetermined object with their eyes well illuminated.

The examination should assess six areas (see below). Diplopia or disconjugate appearance of the eyes mandates formal cranial nerve III-IV-VI examination.

1 **Spontaneous nystagmus** is observed in primary (straight-ahead) eye position. Document the waveform as sawtooth or jerky (and the fast-phase beat direction), which is usually vestibular (peripheral or central), or pendular, quasi-sinusoidal nystagmus, without fast phases, which is central and non-vestibular.

Peripheral unilateral lesions induce vestibular tone bias between labyrinths and the eyes *slowly* drift (just as the body) *ipsilesionally*. Quick-phase resetting the eyes straight ahead perpetuates the nystagmus cycle, hence peripheral lesions are characterised by *fast-phase* 'beating' *contralesionally*. Vestibular nuclei lesions can follow this pattern, although, instead of being binocularly conjugate and mostly horizontal, nystagmus often shows major torsional (rotatory) components.

2 **Gaze-evoked nystagmus** is identified through patients fixating on an object approximately 30° up-down and right-left; only very asymmetric nystagmus is pathological in extreme gaze positions. Following an *acute peripheral vestibular lesion*, nystagmus severity is classified as the following:
   - First-degree (on gaze deviation in direction of fast phase).
   - Second-degree (also present in primary gaze).
   - Third-degree (present even with gaze deviation to opposite direction to fast phase).
   - Nystagmus on gaze deviation can also indicate *central* lesions, frequently called 'gaze-paretic' because there is difficulty holding an eccentric gaze. This can be present in all gaze directions, as with cerebellar degenerations.

3 **Smooth pursuit** is examined with the patient tracking a slowly moving object that they can see well. Abnormal pursuit means too many saccades to catch up with the target, appearing jerky. Move the target slowly, otherwise everybody shows 'broken pursuit'. In principle normal pursuit rules out central vestibular disorders. Pursuit *performance decays significantly* with *cerebellar-brainstem disease*, age, alcohol and CNS-acting drugs. Small horizontal plane asymmetries, if consistent, are significant; vertical plane asymmetries are common in normal subjects.

4 **Saccades** (fast eye movements) shift gaze between objects. Examine them with patients keeping the head still and watching a pen or finger flick 20–30° up-down and right-left. The three independent properties to assess are velocity (normal/slow/absent, i.e. gaze palsy), accuracy (normo-/hypo-/hypermetric), and binocular conjugacy (conjugate/disconjugate, as internuclear ophthalmoplegia). A small degree of hypometricity can be normal; otherwise abnormalities are a strong sign of *central* disease.

The **optokinetic nystagmus** (OKN) system is not a truly separate oculomotor system. When repetitive visual patterns, such as traffic, move before our eyes, they follow an object with smooth pursuit but intermittently the eyes are reset by fast, saccadic components. This sequence of slow ipsidirectional following and fast contradirectional resetting movements can be elicited with a rotating drum in front of the patient. Abnormalities of OKN follow saccadic and pursuit movement rules, but slight oculomotor asymmetries are easier to see in OKN. Peripheral vestibular lesions usually leave OKN *unaffected*.

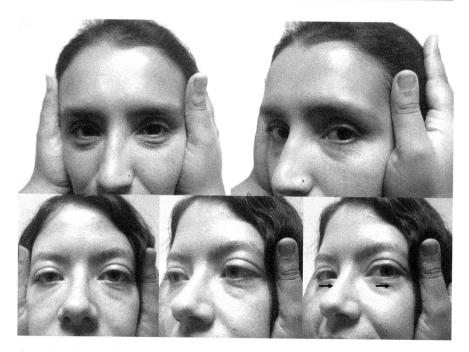

Figure 5.1 The head-impulse test. The examiner holds the patient's head with two hands and delivers brisk head turns to one side and then the other, after resting for a couple of seconds. Top: a normal response shows the eyes remain fixed on the examiners nose. Bottom: abnormal response, or positive HIT, is caused by lack of vestibular function. On the right labyrinth the eyes are carried with the head and, in order to refixate on the examiner's nose, a catch-up saccade has to be produced.

5 **Vestibulo-ocular reflex (VOR)** acts to stabilise gaze during head movements through slow-phase eye movements of equal velocity, but opposite direction, to head movement. VOR allows clear vision when walking, running, or head turning. Bouncing images (oscillopsia) during such activities indicate *bilateral* vestibular function loss. Manoeuvres assessing VOR in clinic use a fast version of the doll's eyes-head manoeuvre – the 'head thrust' or 'head-impulse' test (HIT) (Figure 5.1). Sit the patient in front of you and ask him or her to fixate a target on your face, e.g. nose. Hold the patient's head firmly and deliver fast, sudden head turns 10–15° on either side. Catch-up saccades towards the target immediately after head turns indicate failure of the horizontal canal in the head turn's direction.

The test identifies acute and/or large unilateral peripheral vestibular deficits, e.g. vestibular neuritis. Chronic, compensated, incomplete unilateral lesions often give negative or inconclusive results.

6 **Positional manoeuvres** are perhaps the single most important component of vestibular examination. BPPV is the most common and easily treated cause of vertigo, as discussed in Chapter 6.

Clinical Examination of Postural Balance

Unsteadiness is associated with many disorders but if never associated with vertigo, dizziness, oscillopsia, or hearing disorder it is unlikely due to vestibular disease (see Bronstein and Lempert 2017 for videos).

During **Romberg's test** patients stand with feet as close together as possible and then close their eyes. A Romberg-positive patient may actually fall, unlike normal subjects and patients with balance problems who only show some increase in body sway. It is positive in patients with dorsal column disease, severe afferent polyneuropathy, and during the hyper-acute phase of peripheral vestibulopathy, usually falling ipsilesionally. The most dramatic Romberg's tests are seen in functional (psychogenic) disease. Always show patients that you are ready to catch them should they fall.

Postural reflexes become important in examination of patient's dizziness, which cannot be explained by the vestibular system. They are elicited by pushing and pulling the upper trunk, whilst standing behind the patient (avoiding anticipation). Postural responses may be absent in parkinsonian patients who can fall log-like unless caught; a few shuffling steps prevent this in early stages. In cerebellar syndromes, trunk pulls may unmask trunk tituba-tion. Elderly patients with fear of falling exhibit a startle response. Vestibular patients may be unsteady, but the response pattern is preserved.

During **gait examination**, neurological balance disorders show problems with step initiation (frontal lesions, parkinsonism), steady-state stepping (parkinsonism, spasticity), broad-base gait (cerebellar, bilateral vestibular failure), or arm movements (parkinsonism). Patients with fear of falling reach out arms as if expecting to fall and step with apparent unnecessary care; this may be a psychogenic reaction often triggered by a vestibular, vascular, or fall episode. If gait is normal, examine tandem walking (heel to toe) or with eyes closed. In unilateral vestib-ular lesions, particularly the acute stage, patients may deviate ipsilesionally. In Unterberger's test, on-the-spot eyes-closed walking reveals an ipsilesional deviation.

Laboratory Assessment of Vestibular and Oculomotor Function

Most balance disorder patients do not require eye movement recordings (oculography or nystagmography). Recordings may be useful to

1 Establish if spontaneous nystagmus is acquired or congenital,
2 Ascertain a potentially significant abnormality, e.g. internuclear ophthalmoplegia if clinical examination of eye movements cannot, and
3 Measure vestibular function.

Vestibular conditions diagnosed clinically or with other investigations (audiograms, mag-netic resonance imaging [MRI] scans) do not necessitate oculography, e.g. BPPV, vestibular neuritis, vestibular migraine, Meniere's disease, and vestibular schwannomas.

Caloric tests activate the horizontal semicircular canal via temperature changes in the external auditory canal. Irrigation can be water or air, usually at 30°C and 44°C. Air irrigation allows testing with eardrum perforations, but responses are less consistent. The supine subject has the head raised 30° so the horizontal canal assumes an approximately vertical position. Cold irrigation induces horizontal nystagmus beating the opposite direction, and ipsilaterally during warm irrigation (cold-opposite-warm-same; COWS). Computerised measurements are taken of the slow-phase velocity of the nystagmus but naked-eye measurement of nystagmus duration is reliable. There are four main abnor-malities of caloric responses:

1 Bilateral absence: Ototoxicity, post-meningitis, idiopathic, artefact due to poor tech-nique or wax.
2 Unilateral canal paresis: One ear shows reduced/absent response (vestibular schwan-noma or vestibular neuritis).
3 Directional preponderance (DP) of nystagmus: This is essentially a right-left asym-metry in VOR. An acute left vestibular neuritis initially shows left canal paresis and spontaneous right-beating nystagmus but, after recovery, may only show right DP. DP is a non-specific finding with poor localisation value.
4 Abnormal VOR suppression: Vestibular nystagmus is suppressed by visual fixation, so lack of suppression is a good central sign. To do this the caloric response has to be measured comparatively in the dark and under visual fixation.

Computer-controlled chairs for **rotational testing** are available in few specialised depart-ments. However, patients can be rotated on any swivel chair for 30 seconds, timing the nys-tagmus on stopping rotation. Rotational tests are a good way of measuring the overall level of vestibular function, e.g. remaining vestibular function following ototoxicity.

Video head-impulse test (vHIT) systems are now commercially available. Detecting cor-rective 'catch-up' saccades after an operator-delivered head thrust becomes easier, thus indicating vestibular insufficiency. The gain of the VOR (peak eye velocity/peak head velocity) is also measured. Discrepancies between clinical HIT, vHIT, and caloric tests is not always due to technical problems; vHIT tests high-frequency VOR whereas the caloric test examines the low-frequency response. Thus, a patient with Meniere's disease may have abnormal caloric results but normal vHIT. Three-dimensional (3D) vHIT systems assess all six semicircular canals, but this adds little to the day-to-day management of most ves-tibular patients.

Posturography and Vemps

Posturography records postural sway usually with force platforms. Recordings with eyes open and closed quantify the Romberg's test. Dynamic posturography adds balance stimuli (moving platform, visual stimuli). Posturography advances understanding of postural sys-tems but offers limited day-to-day clinical value.

Cervical vestibular myogenic evoked potential (cVEMP) is the only routine test of ves-tibulo-spinal function. VEMPs are electromyographic potentials elicited in sternomastoid muscles by loud clicks delivered to each ear individually. Conductive deafness prevents clicks reaching the labyrinth, abolishing the response, so otoscopy and audiometry are necessary. VEMPs identify Tullio's phenomenon and third window disorders, such as superior canal dehiscence, where the symptomatic ear generates low-threshold, high-amplitude potentials. It is argued that the main structure activated by sound is the saccule, so cVEMPs are considered an otolith test. Ocular VEMPs may be mediated via the utricle more than the saccule. Ideally, absent VEMPs would imply a selective otolithic disorder but, unfortunately, the meaning of an isolated VEMP abnormality is unclear, particularly in older patients.

Acknowledgements

The author is grateful to Drs. Alex Charlton and Simon Cole for their useful feedback and suggestions.

KEY POINTS

- Dizziness may indicate vestibular disease but equally general medical, cardiovascular, or neurological disorders can be the cause.
- Rotational vertigo usually indicates vestibular system disease, but the lesion may be anywhere from the semicircular canals up to the cerebral hemispheres.
- History taking is the key to diagnosis, but examination of the eye movements, the positional manoeuvre, and hearing levels are a close second.
- Audio-vestibular tests are not essential for diagnosis in most cases.
- A summary of examination findings and tests is as follows:
  - Positional manoeuvres are perhaps the single most important component of vestibular examination.
  - During spontaneous nystagmus, in peripheral unilateral vestibular lesions, the eyes *slowly* drift (just as the body) *ipsilesionally*, with eye resetting by *fast-phase* 'beating' *contralesionally.*
  - Smooth pursuit, saccades, and OKN become impaired with central (cerebellar-brainstem) disease. Peripheral vestibular lesions usually leave these unaffected.
- VOR (measured by 'head thrust' or HIT) is impaired in acute and/or large unilateral peripheral vestibular deficits, e.g. vestibular neuritis.

- cVEMPS are the only routine test of vestibulo-spinal function to identify third window disorders such as superior canal dehiscence with low-threshold, high-amplitude potentials. They are absent in conductive hearing loss.
- Romberg's test is positive if a patient falls ipsilesionally in hyper-acute peripheral vestibulopathy, dorsal column spinal disease, and afferent polyneuropathy.
- Caloric tests activate the lateral semicircular canal via temperature changes (30°C and 44°C). Cold irrigation induces horizontal nystagmus beating the opposite direction, and ipsilaterally during warm irrigation.
- vHIT detects vestibular insufficiency through corrective catch-up saccades. It tests high-frequency VOR, whereas the caloric test examines the low-frequency response. Meniere's disease demonstrates abnormal caloric results but normal vHIT.

Further Reading

1. Bronstein A and Lempert T. *Dizziness, a Practical Approach to Diagnosis and Management*. 2nd ed., Cambridge, UK: Cambridge University Press, 2017.

2. Lee SH, Kim JS. Differential diagnosis of acute vascular vertigo. *Curr Opin Neurol*. 2020, 33(1):142–149. doi: 10.1097/WCO.0000000000000776.

3. Seemungal BM, Bronstein AM. A practical approach to acute vertigo. *Pract Neurol*. 2008, 8(4):211–21. doi: 10.1136/jnnp.2008.154799. Review. Erratum in: Pract Neurol. 2009, 9(1). doi: 10.1136/jnnp.2008.154799corr1.

6. VESTIBULAR DISORDERS AND REHABILITATION

Acute Unilateral Peripheral Vestibulopathy (AUPVP)

Acute unilateral peripheral vestibulopathy (AUPVP) is a clinical syndrome caused by acute vertigo (onset over hours or days) with nausea and vomiting, oscillopsia, ipsilateral latero-pulsion, and gait instability, occurring as a result of vestibular tone imbalance.

On examination the unilateral loss of vestibular function is associated with a positive head thrust test ipsilaterally, and horizontal-torsional nystagmus beating ipsilaterally. Hearing is preserved.

Pathophysiology

The pathophysiology of AUPVP is not fully understood. There is some circumstantial evidence for a viral aetiology, from autopsy studies, from animal models, and from genome-wide association studies. There is also evidence of vascular aetiology in some cases, including evidence of pro-inflammatory state and associations with specific HLA subtypes. The term AUPVP incorporates both neural and end-organ pathologies, rather than using terms which presuppose a specific site of lesion or pathophysiology (vestibular neuritis, vestibular neuronitis).

Clinical assessment of the nystagmus and head impulse abnormality, supplemented by vestibular diagnostic tests (video head-impulse test, caloric, ocular, and cervical video evoked myogenic potential) can allow the differentiation into isolated superior or inferior vestibular nerve pathology, or complete varieties (see Chapter 5). These subtypes have differing presentations, prognoses, and rates of complications such as benign paroxysmal positional vertigo (BPPV). Imaging is usually normal, although in exceptional cases neuritis can be seen on magnetic resonance imaging (MRI).

Management

Management is largely supportive, with medical management of nausea and vomiting. Expert consensus is to recommend early mobilisation and/or vestibular rehabilitation (VR) as tolerated, and to minimise use of vestibular sedatives, since this is believed to slow recovery. The use of corticosteroids is controversial and further evidence is awaited from ongoing trials.

Prognosis

The prognosis is variable with persistent symptoms in a significant proportion. Predictors of poor recovery include visual dependency, high levels of anxiety, and maladaptive illness beliefs. The relapse rates for AUPVP seem to be very low (around 2% in 5 years), meaning recurrent episodes should arouse suspicion of another disorder such as vestibular migraine (VM).

Meniere's Disease (MD)

Meniere's disease (MD) is an idiopathic inner ear disorder characterised by recurrent spontaneous vertigo episodes characteristically at least 30 minutes long. It is accompanied by fluctuating or progressive sensorineural hearing loss (SNHL), tinnitus, and aural fullness in the affected ear.

MD is highly linked to endolymphatic hydrops (ELH), although ELH is not pathognomonic of MD. Autoimmune, viral, allergic, and vascular hypotheses have all been proposed as underlying causes and all have some circumstantial support, but a single unifying aetiology remains elusive. The condition is most common during the working adult age range. A minority of cases (<15%) appear to be familial and there are a number of candidate genes, some of which link to ion transport.

Diagnosis

Diagnosis is based on a set of criteria derived from expert opinion. Diagnostic criteria for 'definite' and 'probable' cases are shown in Table 6.1.[1]

There is associated nystagmus when the patient is seen around the time of an attack. In the *irritative* phase, the fast phase of nystagmus will beat *towards* the affected ear in a horizontal or horizontal-torsional direction, a finding which usually lasts less than 1 hour. In the *paretic*

Table 6.1   Diagnostic criteria for Meniere's disease and vestibular migraine from The International Headache Society (IHS) 2018[2]

Diagnosis	Criteria
Definite Meniere's disease	1 ≥2 definitive spontaneous episodes of vertigo lasting 20 minutes to 12 hours + 2 Audiometrically documented low-to medium-frequency sensorineural hearing loss in the affected ear on at least one occasion before, during, or after one of the episodes of vertigo + 3 Fluctuating aural symptoms (hearing, tinnitus or fullness) in the affected ear
Probable Meniere's disease	1 ≥2 episodes of vertigo or dizziness, each lasting 20 minutes to 24 hours + 2 Fluctuating aural symptoms (hearing, tinnitus or fullness) in the affected ear
Vestibular migraine	1 At least five episodes with vestibular symptoms of moderate or severe intensity lasting 5 minutes to 72 hours 2 History of migraine according to IHS classification 3 Migraine feature with >50% of attacks: • Headache with two of: unilateral, throbbing, moderate–severe • Aggravation by movement • Photo- and phonophobia • Visual aura 4 Not better accounted for by another disorder

phase, the fast phase of nystagmus will beat *away* from the affected ear and last hours to days. In the recovery phase the nystagmus again beats towards the affected side because peripheral vestibular function recovers.

SNHL characteristically affects the low frequencies. Occasionally patients experience drop attacks (also called Turmarkin or otolithic crisis) where there is a sudden drop to the ground without loss of consciousness, or associated vertigo. Bilateral MD does occur, but in the majority of cases the condition is unilateral, at least initially. Estimates of rate of bilateral disease are highly variable; one estimate is 47% within 20 years of onset.

Other investigations can include an MRI of the brain and internal auditory meatus (mainly to rule out retrocochlear causes) and electrocochleography (an increased summation potential:action potential ratio (>0.45) is supportive of the diagnosis). Use of gadolinium-enhanced MRI to image ELH directly is a promising and evolving technique.

Management
Dietary restrictions on sodium and caffeine are traditionally advised, although not proven. There is mixed evidence for the use of betahistine in MD, although it does have a favourable safety profile and is well tolerated, so it is often used. A Cochrane review concluded that there is no evidence to demonstrate the effectiveness of positive transtympanic low-pressure therapy. Diuretics have also been recommended, although the evidence base is weak and there is potential for significant unwanted effects in relation to salt homeostasis and renal function.

There is some evidence to support the effectiveness of intratympanic steroids. Endolymphatic duct surgery and vestibular nerve section are surgical options for refractory cases that allow hearing preservation. Intratympanic gentamicin and labyrinthectomy tend to be reserved for patients with significant SNHL or refractory symptoms due to the risks of worsening hearing (3–21% rate of hearing loss for low-dose gentamicin injections, complete hearing loss for labyrinthectomy) or causing persistent vestibular dysfunction.

Supportive treatments for hearing loss, tinnitus, and persistent interictal vestibular symptoms (VR) should be offered where applicable.

Benign Paroxysmal Positional Vertigo (BPPV)
BPPV is a common cause of episodic vertigo with a lifetime prevalence of 2.5%. It is a disorder of the otoconia, which are calcium carbonate crystals normally embedded in the macula of the utricle and saccule.

There are two theories about how BPPV occurs: canalolithiasis and cupulolithiasis. Canalolithiasis is thought to be more common, and it occurs when the detached otoconia are free floating, but these cause cupula deformation by exerting a plunger effect on the endolymph when stimulated to move by gravity. In cupulolithiasis, degenerative otoconia adhere to the cupula making it more gravity sensitive.

All three horizontal canals can be affected in BPPV, but the majority of cases (over 93%) occur in the posterior canal (PC-BPPV), with the horizontal canal affected in around 5%. Anterior canal BPPV is very rare. This distribution is explained by the natural anatomical orientation of the canals.

The hallmark of PC-BPPV is vertigo lasting seconds on lying down, sitting up from the lying position, or rolling in bed and when extending or flexing the neck.

These symptoms can present in clusters with several attacks per day. In between attacks or shortly after successful treatment, patients are either symptom free or experience a sensation of imbalance. However, some patients may report atypical symptoms, and it is worthwhile conducting the positional tests in all patients presenting with episodic vertigo, older adults with falls or imbalance, or after a head injury.

BPPV can occur in isolation or in association with other conditions like AUPVP, MD, or head injury.

Diagnosis

Diagnosis is made on the basis of typical signs (nystagmus) and symptoms (vertigo) provoked by specific positional tests in each plane for each pair of canals: left anterior and right posterior (LARP), right anterior and left posterior (RALP), and the horizontal canals.

The posterior and anterior canal pairs are stimulated when performing the Dix-Hallpike test (Figure 6.1). The patient is seated along the couch, feet up, and the head is turned 45° towards the side being tested, aligning the vertical canals with the sagittal plane. The head is

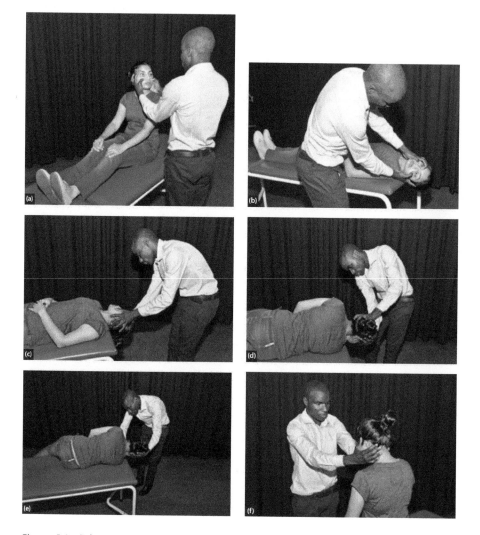

Figure 6.1   Epley's repositioning manoeuvre. Left posterior canal BPPV. The patient is sat on the table with the head turned 45° to the left side (affected side) **(a)**, and **(b)** brought down rapidly with the head still turned 45° to the affected side and extended over the edge of the table, 30° below the horizontal plane. Note that the neck is well supported (inquire about neck pathology before the test). **(c)** The head is then turned 90° to the opposite side (right). **(d)** This is followed by rotating the head and body 90° facing downwards (135° from the supine position). **(e)** The legs are then displaced over the side of the table in anticipation of a return to a seated position, and **(f)** the patient is brought to a sitting position with the head turned forward.

brought down briskly over the end of the couch to lie 30° below the horizontal while maintaining a position 45° to the side being tested. Patients should be counselled prior to the test to expect vertigo, but they still need to try and maintain their eyes open for examination. In PC-BPPV, the fast phase of the resultant nystagmus is upwards and outwards (upbeating geotropic-torsional nystagmus), whereas in anterior canal BPPV the nystagmus is downward and inwards. The LARP canals are stimulated during the right Dix-Hallpike test and the RALP canals in the left Dix-Hallpike test.

Lateral canal BPPV is assessed using the roll test. The head is flexed 30°, bringing the horizontal canal into the vertical plane, and it is then briskly rolled to one side. The same is repeated on the opposite side. In the majority of cases the nystagmus will be horizontal and geotropic and towards the ear being tested, and it will be present on rolling both sides, even with a unilateral lesion.

It is important to discriminate BPPV from positional vertigo arising from central pathology. Neurological disorders that can cause positional vertigo include VM, vertebrobasilar insufficiency, demyelinating lesions, and central nervous system (CNS) lesions. Drugs can also cause positional vertigo.

An MRI of the brain including the posterior fossa and internal auditory meatus is required when

- Nystagmus is atypical for any of the BPPV syndromes.
- Brainstem or cerebellar signs are present.
- Positional vertigo does not resolve with repeated therapeutic manoeuvres.

Management

The canalith repositioning procedure (CRP) is based on the theory of 'canalolithiasis' and seeks to move the particles from the PC into the utricle via the common crus. A recent Cochrane meta-analysis has found that the CRP on its own is effective in almost 80% of cases. The Epley manoeuvre is described in Figure 6.1. There are alternative effective manoeuvres for PC-BPPV (e.g. modified Semont) and for lateral canal BPPV (log roll or barbecue manoeuvre). Brandt Daroff exercises are well known but are less effective than repositioning manoeuvres, so they should not be considered as a first-line treatment. Recurrence of BPPV is common, so patients should be educated on what to do in this eventuality. Surgery (semicircular canal occlusion) is considered in a very small number of refractory cases. Although effective, this procedure has risks of SNHL and chronic imbalance.

Vestibular Migraine (VM)

Migraine is common and almost everyone will either have experienced the condition personally or have friends, family, or other acquaintances who are sufferers. Migraine is a neurovascular condition in which the headache is thought to originate via activation of the trigeminovascular reflex; the trigeminal nerve innervates the meninges mediating the pain that is migraine's most notorious clinical feature. VM is a subtype of migraine in which vestibular symptoms predominate.

Diagnosis

Diagnosis is made according to clinical criteria (Table 6.1) based around the presence of episodic vertigo with associated migrainous features including headache and sensory sensitivity (photophobia, phonophobia) and aura.[2]

The physical examination of patients with VM in the interictal period is usually normal. However, some patients report significant visual motion intolerance that can be detected during eye movement examination. One study of patients with VM in the acute setting found a range of eye movement abnormalities including positional nystagmus, spontaneous nystagmus, and mixed and central type patterns. The presence of interictal eye movement abnormalities should alert the examiner to consider the possibility of either a different disorder altogether (e.g. episodic ataxia type 2) or an underlying neurological disorder causing a migraine phenotype. Pure-tone audiometry is usually normal in VM and can be helpful in differentiating VM from MD. In cases where the history is typical and examination findings are normal, MRI scanning to exclude secondary causes may not be required.

Management

A clear explanation to the patient about the nature of the condition is essential since VM is frequently chronic and patients need to become expert in self-management. The evidence base for management of VM as a specific subtype is generally weak, and recommendations are generally made on the basis of management of migraine in general.

Migraine headache should be managed along standard lines with analgesics or migraine-specific relief medicines such as the 5-hydroxytryptamine receptor 1-B/D (5-HT1B/D) agonists ('triptans'), taking care to avoid analgesic-overuse headache. Acute symptoms of vertigo can be managed with vestibular sedatives such as prochlorperazine, cyclizine, or cinnarizine. When symptoms of headache and vertigo together are sufficiently intrusive/frequent to justify the risk of adverse effects, migraine prophylactic agents can be considered. Evidence-based guidelines should be followed; beta blockers and tricyclics remain frequently recommended, but there are many options. VR may be useful in patients with sensitivity to self- and visual motion.

Superior Semicircular Canal Dehiscence (SSCD)

Superior semicircular canal dehiscence syndrome (SSCD) is the dehiscence of otic capsule bone overlying the superior semicircular canal. It encompasses a wide variety of vestibular and auditory symptoms, and it creates a third cochlea window in addition to the oval and round window.

Typical third window symptoms are a result of movement at the dehiscence from raised intracranial pressure, or at the oval or round windows, from loud sounds or straining (e.g. Valsalva manoeuvre). Alterations in inner ear fluid dynamics due to the third window cause increased firing of vestibular afferents and transient momentary vertigo.

Diagnosis

A 0.5–0.6% prevalence of SSCD has been observed in histological studies of cadaveric temporal bones. In comparison, reported prevalence from studies reviewing high-resolution temporal bone computed tomography (CT) scans was 4–8%. Dehiscence alone is therefore not sufficient to cause the syndrome. SSCDS could be congenital, acquired, or a combination where a genetic predisposition followed by a secondary event triggers SSCDS.

Symptoms can include hearing loss (typically a low-frequency conductive hearing loss, with supranormal bone conduction), autophony, pulsatile tinnitus, and a description of hearing their eye movements or footfall. Transient vertigo, imbalance, and oscillopsia can all occur with loud sounds (Tullio's phenomenon) or intracranial/middle ear pressure changes. Generalised imbalance can also occur.

High-resolution CT is the gold standard for identification of SSCD. Patients with SSCDS also have ocular or cervical vestibular evoked myogenic responses present with lower thresholds or higher amplitudes than normal for the affected ear.

Management

Patients with mild symptoms that are not intrusive or bothersome should be treated conservatively and given advice on avoidance of triggers. Surgery via either a transmastoid or middle fossa approach can be offered where symptoms are persistent/disabling, and techniques include plugging, capping, and resurfacing of the SSC. Surgery typically does not improve hearing, and it can be complicated by SNHL and chronic imbalance. There is some evidence to support patching of the round window to reduce third window symptoms.

Neuropsychiatric Aspects of Vestibular Disorders

It has long been recognised that psychological factors can play a significant role in the genesis of dizziness.

The concepts of phobic positional vertigo, space motion discomfort, and chronic subjective dizziness were brought together to produce the entity known as persistent perceptual postural dizziness (PPPD), referring to dizziness, unsteadiness, or non-spinning vertigo that are present pervasively over 3 months or more and that are exacerbated by upright posture, active or passive movement, and exposure to moving or complex visual stimuli and thought to be a functional disorder. Models for explaining PPPD have been drawn from anatomical, neurochemical, and cognitive behavioural theories, and it is considered to be a functional neurological disorder.[3] Anxiety and major depressive disorders are common in patients with PPPD but do not occur in all cases.

Management

Uncontrolled trials indicate that selective serotonin reuptake inhibitors (SSRIs) and serotonin-noradrenaline (norepinephrine) reuptake inhibitors (SNRIs) may be of benefit for chronic dizziness with or without co-existing anxiety and depression. Psychotherapy (cognitive behavioural therapy [CBT]) also appears to be a helpful intervention. VR is effective in PPPD for hypersensitivity to motion, improving balance confidence, and reduction of avoidance behaviour. Outcomes appear to be variable. A multidisciplinary approach is recommended.

Vestibular Rehabilitation (VR)

VR is offered for patients with head or visual motion intolerance, or imbalance, related to vestibular disorders. VR is based on principles of vestibular compensation including habituation, adaptation, substitution, and/or sensory reweighting (table 6.2).

Table 6.2 Examples of commonly prescribed exercises in vestibular rehabilitation

Type of exercise	Examples
Head exercises (performed with eyes open and eyes closed)	Bend head backwards and forwards Turn head from side to side
Eye movement exercises	Head stationary follow movement of finger left and right/up and down Head movement to look back and forth between two vertical or horizontal targets
Visual fixation exercises	Perform head exercises while fixating stationary target Perform head exercises while fixating moving target
Positioning exercises (performed with eyes open and closed)	While seated, bend down to touch the floor While seated, turn to look over shoulder to left and then right Bend down with head turned first to one side and then the other Lying down, roll from one side to the other Sit up from lying supine and on each side
Postural exercises (performed with eyes open; eyes closed under supervision)	Practise static stance with feet as close together as possible Practise standing on one leg, and heel to toe Repeat head and fixation exercises while standing and then walking Practise walking in circles, pivot turns, up slopes, upstairs, and around obstacles Stand and walk in environments with altered surface and/or visual conditions with and without head and fixation exercises Aerobic exercises, e.g. alternate touching the fingers to the toes, trunk bends, and rotation

Although components of the pioneering exercise programme by Cawthorne and Cooksey may still be used today, good practice is now considered to be a customised programme based on individual deficits.

A VR assessment will include validated questionnaires around symptoms and disability, objective and subjective tests to identify functional deficit, and objective static and dynamic balance tests and gait measures.

Treatment goals are devised to address each person's individual subjective symptoms (i.e. dizziness, giddiness, nausea) and objective symptoms (postural and gait instability, falls).

Various authors have discussed the potential benefit of virtual reality as a therapeutic protocol to improve postural and gait stability, vestibulo-ocular reflex (VOR) gain, and subjective symptoms. Benefits over standard approaches so far are not very striking, but the experience may be more enjoyable with more sustained engagement as a result.

Outcome in VR can be influenced by a number of factors which should be sought and addressed especially if progress with therapy is limited (see Box 2, Chapter 5).

The Law and Vertigo

In the United Kingdom, the Driver and Vehicle Licensing Authority (DVLA) requires that drivers declare any ongoing liability to sudden and unprovoked attacks of disabling vertigo, because these could lead to loss of vehicle control while driving. It is the responsibility of the driver to inform the DVLA, although clinicians have a responsibility to make patients aware of this regulation.

The nature of the regulations means that some, but not all, individuals with vestibular paroxysmia, MD, PPPD, and VM may need to declare their condition. PC-BPPV would not normally cause problems when driving, because when driving head movement is mainly in the horizontal plane.

KEY POINTS

- MD causes episodes of incapacitating vertigo with unilateral auditory symptoms, and treatment can be medical in the first instance, or with intratympanic steroids or gentamicin.
- BPPV is a common cause of episodic vertigo, which is diagnosed with positional manoeuvres; management includes particle repositioning procedures that are highly effective.
- VM is a common cause of episodic vertigo, and treatment of frequent or disabling symptoms is usually with medical management.
- PPPD is a functional dizziness disorder.
- VR is offered for patients with head or visual motion intolerance, or imbalance, related to vestibular disorders.

Further Reading

1. Lopez-Escamez JA, Carey J, Chung WH, et al. Diagnostic criteria for Meniere's disease according to the Classification Committee of the Barany Society. *HNO* 2017;65(11): 887–93. doi: 10.1007/s00106-017-0387-z.

2. IHS. Headache Classification Committee of the International Headache Society (IHS) The International Classification of Headache Disorders, 3rd edition. *Cephalalgia* 2018; 38(1):1–211. doi: 10.1177/0333102417738202.

3. Popkirov S, Staab JP, Stone J. Persistent postural-perceptual dizziness (PPPD): a common, characteristic and treatable cause of chronic dizziness. *Practical Neurology* 2018; 18(1):5–13. doi: 10.1136/practneurol-2017-001809.

7. CONDITIONS OF THE EXTERNAL EAR

Wax

Wax is a combination of desquamated skin and cerumen, formed by glands in the base of the hair follicles of hair-bearing skin, in the lateral third of the external auditory canal (EAC). Most external canals are self-cleaning, but a common finding on otoscopy is partial occlusion of the canal that is usually asymptomatic. Wax is amenable to removal by non-specialists by water syringing most commonly using a pressure-controlled irrigator. Specialists prefer to remove wax under direct vision with the aid of a headlight, microscope, or endoscope, via a speculum with ear wax hooks or similar instruments, or suction. Various wax-softening agents including olive oil and sodium bicarbonate are frequently used to ease removal. However, there is no evidence to support the use of one agent over another.[1]

Otitis Externa

Otitis externa (OE) is characterised by erythema and oedema of the EAC, associated with itch, pain, discharge, and debris in the meatus. Predisposing factors include a narrow/obstructed EAC, dermatological conditions of the ear canal (e.g. eczema or psoriasis), maceration of the skin, excessive moisture (swimming or bathing), and active chronic otitis media. OE affects approximately 10% of the population during their lifetime. Water and moisture are thought to change the flora in the ear from predominantly gram-positive organisms to gram-negative organisms. Most patients will culture multiple organisms, with *Pseudomonas aeruginosa* being the most prevalent.

The main treatment of OE is a combination of regular topical medications, with or without an oto-wick/aural toileting, and prevention of aetiological factors. A topical combination of antibiotic/steroid drops or spray, for a minimum of 7 days, is regarded as the best first-line treatment; however, randomised trials comparing treatments are few and with small patient numbers.[2] Systemic antibiotics are indicated for patients with pinna cellulitis or evidence of necrotising OE (see later). Most otolaryngologists reserve microbiological investigations for refractory cases. Water precautions using cotton wool with petroleum jelly or custom moulds can be helpful in patients with recurrent infections. In patients with refractory OE, sensitivity to topical agents including steroid drops may contribute to ongoing symptoms. Patients with recurrent OE that is exacerbated by air-conduction hearing aids may benefit from bone conduction devices or middle ear implants, depending on the inner ear function.

Otomycosis

Otomycosis or fungal OE accounts for approximately 10% of OE cases. It is more common in hot, humid climates or following prolonged treatment with topical antibiotics. The diagnosis must be considered in patients with OE who fail to respond to appropriate treatment. *Aspergillus* accounts for 80–90% of cases, with *Candida* accounting for the remaining cases. The most common finding is discharge with debris and occasionally visible fungal hyphae or spores. Treatment is similar to OE but with topical antifungal drops, and longer courses of treatment are typically required.

Furunculosis

Furunculosis is an infection of a single hair follicle. The lateral aspect of the EAC, which has hair follicles, is the site of furunculosis. Bacterial infection of the hair follicle can progress from a deep skin infection to form a local abscess with associated cellulitis and oedema.

Symptoms can be similar to severe OE; however, characteristically oedema and inflammation are restricted to the lateral canal. *Staphylococcus aureus* is the most common organism. Recurrent furunculosis may result from colonisation of the external nares by *S. aureus* and decolonisation therapy should be considered in these cases.

Treatment choices include the following:

- Aspiration or incision and drainage for an abscess
- Oral or intravenous anti-staphylococcal antibiotics
- Topical antibiotics/antiseptics

Perichondritis

Perichondritis is an infection or inflammation involving the perichondrium of the external ear. It occurs usually secondary to trauma and is mostly caused by *P. aeruginosa* but can be polymicrobial. It should be differentiated from cellulitis of the ear, classically by being lobule sparing.

The presentation is usually with dull pain increasing in severity, and there is inflammation of the cartilaginous pinna. Relapsing polychondritis is an autoimmune condition, and it may present similarly but is differentiated on the basis of the systemic nature of the condition, which may also affect joints, the eye, and cartilage of the nose and airway. Perichondritis is treated with prompt broad-spectrum antibiotics with anti-pseudomonal cover, ideally intravenously. If there is a subperichondrial abscess it should be drained. If perichondritis is untreated, it could result in avascular necrosis of the cartilage and deformity of the pinna.

Myringitis

Myringitis is inflammation of the tympanic membrane (TM). Acute bullous myringitis (BM) and chronic granular myringitis (GM) are different clinical entities.

BM is characterised by bullae or vesicles on the TM, which are believed to develop between the middle fibrous and outer squamous layers. The aetiological pathogens are similar to acute otitis media (AOM) such as *Streptococcus pneumoniae, Haemophilus influenzae,* and respiratory viruses. It is more common in winter and in children between the ages of 2 and 8 years. This differs from AOM, which is more common in children under 2 years.

Patients typically present with unilateral sudden-onset severe otalgia lasting for 1–2 days. There is a high incidence of associated middle ear effusion resulting in a conductive loss. However inner ear involvement with sensorineural hearing loss (SNHL) and vertigo is not uncommon and usually resolves spontaneously. As BM is usually self-limiting the treatment is usually symptomatic.

GM is a chronic inflammation characterised by the de-epithelialisation of the outer (squamous) layer of the TM being replaced by granulation tissue, with the absence of middle ear disease. The aetiology is unknown, but there is a high incidence following myringoplasty. It usually presents with otorrhoea and granulation on the TM. Treatment of GM includes microsuction/debridement with topical antimicrobial, steroid, or astringent preparations for prolonged periods. Laser resurfacing and surgical excision + grafting are usually reserved for recalcitrant cases.

Acquired Canal Atresia

Acquired canal atresia is progressive stenosis leading to closure of the EAC resulting in a blind sac. This is usually following chronic inflammation and occurs in the medial aspect of the EAC.

Solid atresia consists of a continuous block of fibrosis from the TM. Membranous atresia is typified by a fibrous tissue that has a covering of canal skin on both sides, separating the ear canal into two segments. The medial segment inevitably collects keratin, which may become erosive. Stenosis may also cause this. Atresia may be caused by the following processes:

- Inflammation
  - Chronic OE
  - Chronic otitis media
- Trauma
- Burns
- Surgery especially involving a meatal approach

It is useful to use computed tomography (CT) imaging to help identify the extent of atresia and ascertaining the presence of middle ear pathology.

Patients with atresia will have a conductive hearing loss. This may be managed in some cases with a conventional behind-the-ear hearing aid (especially when the atresia is medial), a bone-conducting device, a middle ear implant, or surgical treatment. Surgery involves removing the fibrosed segment, down to the lamina propria of the TM. The exposed bone and TM is sometimes grafted with a split-thickness skin graft. These patients require intensive post-operative aural toilet and restenosis is not uncommon.

Exostosis

Exostoses are benign growths of the periosteal bone in the medial aspect of the external ear canal. Exostoses are usually multiple and bilateral. They are usually found incidentally and are associated with a history of prolonged cold-water exposure.

The diagnosis of exostosis is made clinically and can be differentiated from osteomas, which are generally unilateral, solitary, arise from the lateral EAC, and can often be pedunculated as opposed to the sessile base of exostoses. Most exostoses are incidentally found and are asymptomatic; however, more severe cases may result in keratin accumulation, recurrent OE, and rarely cholesteatoma. Treatment may include regular aural toilet or surgical excision. Avoidance of cold water may help prevent progression.

Keratosis Obturans and External Auditory Canal Cholesteatoma

Keratosis obturans (KO) results from failure of epithelial migration, which causes accumulation of keratin in the medial bony EAC with expansion and remodelling.

EAC cholesteatoma is characterised by invasion of squamous epithelium into bone (Table 7.1 and Figure 7.1).

Table 7.1   Differential diagnosis of non-neoplastic conditions eroding the bony EAC

	Keratosis obturans	External auditory canal cholesteatoma	Necrotising otitis externa
Aetiology	Abnormal epithelial migration	Abnormal bone leading to epithelial migration into bone	Immunocompromise Patient with necrotic bone in ear canal
Symptoms and findings	Severe otalgia Conductive hearing loss Lung or sinus disease Younger Occasionally bilateral	Otalgia mild No hearing loss Itchiness Older Usually unilateral	Severe penetrating pain Cranial nerve palsy Diabetic/renal failure or otherwise immunosuppressed Raised inflammatory markers
Pathology	Keratin plug Tympanic membrane thickened Widened deep canal Hyperaemia of skin canal with granulations	Keratin in random pattern Tympanic membrane normal Localised osteitis/erosion of ear canal usually posteroinferior Sequestration of bone	Chronic inflammation *Pseudomonas aeruginosa*
Treatment	Remove plug Treat granulations Occasionally biopsy Canaloplasty	Surgically remove cholesteatoma graft with cartilage and fascia Biopsy	Treat cause of immunosuppression High-dose long-term antibiotics Surgical debridement
Differential diagnosis	Wax impaction with infection Otitis externa Neoplasm	Necrotising otitis externa Neoplasm	Malignant neoplasm

Source: Modified from Shire JR, Donegan JO. Cholesteatoma of the external auditory canal and keratosis obturans. *Am J Otol* 1986; 7: 361–364.

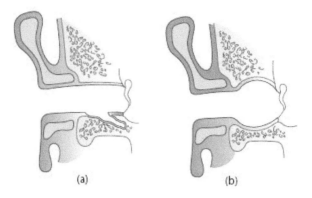

Figure 7.1   (a) Canal cholesteatoma – a sac of canal skin invades bone. (b) Keratosis obturans – the bony canal is widened.

Necrotising Otitis Externa

Necrotising otitis externa (NOE) is a skull base osteomyelitis of the temporal bone occurring as a complication of OE. It was previously termed malignant OE due to its associated mortality. Whilst often described as a rare condition there is evidence of increasing incidence, the cause of which is unclear. There is no universally agreed diagnostic criteria; however, most would agree that the condition presents with otalgia, often severe and nocturnal; otorrhoea; and evidence of ear canal inflammation, frequently with granulation tissue inferiorly. It is almost invariably seen in immunocompromised individuals either due to age, diabetes, or other causes.

Progression of disease can result in cranial neuropathies, including facial and bulbar nerves. Diagnosis is clinical combined with radiological assessment which may utilise CT (showing bone erosion) and contrast magnetic resonance imaging (MRI) and bone scans. Biopsy of granulation tissue should be considered to exclude malignancy. Treatment should be guided by microbial sampling. *P. aeruginosa* is the most common pathogen and therefore agents should target this. Anti-microbial treatment is usually prolonged, typically lasting 6–12 weeks, and may benefit from a multidisciplinary guidance by microbiology colleagues. Rarely NOE can be fungal. Treatment response is assessed clinically (most importantly resolution of pain), with inflammatory markers and in some units with imaging (nuclear medicine scans or MRI). The role of surgery is limited to obtaining microbiological samples, removing bony sequestra, and draining abscesses. There is evidence from cases series for the therapeutic benefit of hyperbaric oxygen in NOE.

Osteoradionecrosis of the Temporal Bone

Osteoradionecrosis of the temporal bone is defined as necrosis of a previously irradiated petrous temporal bone which fails to heal. The temporal bone is dense, which results in greater absorption of radiation than soft tissue. The tympanic ring is particularly susceptible, likely due to its poor vascular supply.[3] Often there is loss of skin and soft tissue exposing bone, bony sequestration, and secondary infections. In an established case, ruling out an underlying recurrence of malignancy is vital.

Localised disease can be managed with regular aural toileting of the sequestra and topical antibiotic treatments. For more extensive cases or those complicated by chronic infection, prolonged antibiotic treatment and surgical debridement with possible reconstruction using vascularised tissue may be required.

Otalgia

Otalgia can be primary, arising from the ear, or secondary/referred, as a result of pathology elsewhere. In children otalgia is usually otogenic; however, in adults referred otalgia is more common. The sensory supply to the ear is complex and therefore the potential origin of the referred otalgia is widely distributed, which can cause diagnostic difficulty (Figure 7.2).

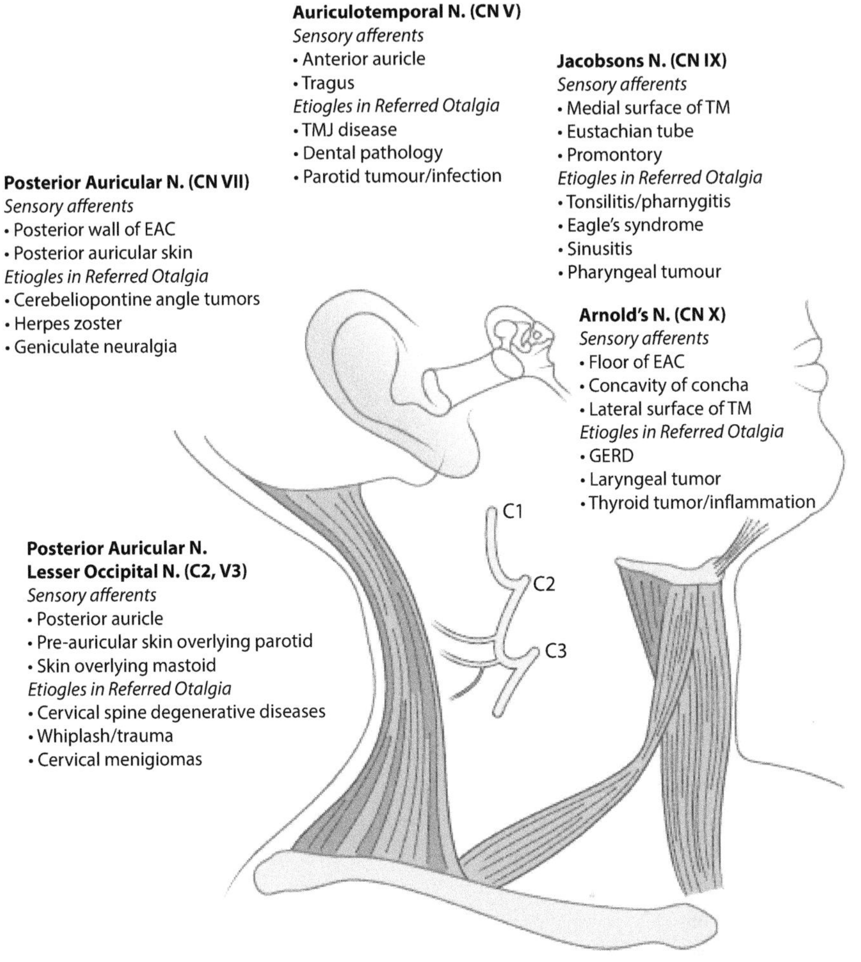

Auriculotemporal N. (CN V)
Sensory afferents
• Anterior auricle
• Tragus
Etiogles in Referred Otalgia
• TMJ disease
• Dental pathology
• Parotid tumour/infection

Jacobsons N. (CN IX)
Sensory afferents
• Medial surface of TM
• Eustachian tube
• Promontory
Etiogles in Referred Otalgia
• Tonsilitis/pharnygitis
• Eagle's syndrome
• Sinusitis
• Pharyngeal tumour

Posterior Auricular N. (CN VII)
Sensory afferents
• Posterior wall of EAC
• Posterior auricular skin
Etiogles in Referred Otalgia
• Cerebeliopontine angle tumors
• Herpes zoster
• Geniculate neuralgia

Arnold's N. (CN X)
Sensory afferents
• Floor of EAC
• Concavity of concha
• Lateral surface of TM
Etiogles in Referred Otalgia
• GERD
• Laryngeal tumor
• Thyroid tumor/inflammation

C1

C2

C3

Posterior Auricular N.
Lesser Occipital N. (C2, V3)
Sensory afferents
• Posterior auricle
• Pre-auricular skin overlying parotid
• Skin overlying mastoid
Etiogles in Referred Otalgia
• Cervical spine degenerative diseases
• Whiplash/trauma
• Cervical menigiomas

Figure 7.2   The origin of referred pain can be grouped into the following: **Malignancy:** Malignant tumours of the upper aerodigestive tract can present with otalgia as part of a symptom complex or can be the sole symptom. Therefore, a full examination of the oral cavity and flexible nasoendoscopy is essential for patients with unexplained otalgia. **Dental:** Dental causes are the most common cause of referred otalgia and can be referred from the teeth, periodontal tissues, or the temporo-mandibular joint (TMJ). The pain in acute apical abscess tends to be severe and can be localised; however, if the inflammation is mild and chronic, localisation may be poor. In TMJ dysfunction there is diffuse pain in or around the TMJ joint, including tenderness of the masticatory muscles. Intraoral palpation of the lateral and medial pterygoids frequently reveals tenderness in patients with referred otalgia. Treatment of TMJ pain includes a soft diet and analgesics including non-steroidal anti-inflammatories. Other treatment options include tricyclic antidepressants, occlusal splints, and TMJ surgery. **Cervical:** Cervical spine degenerative disease is an increasingly common cause of referred otalgia. The pain is usually retroauricular or infra-auricular and related to neck movement. **Neuralgia:** Numerous neuralgias have been implicated as causes of referred otalgia, but all are rare. Trigeminal and post-herpetic neuralgias are the most common. In glossopharyngeal neuralgia, there can be severe transient pain in the ear usually triggered by swallowing. Jacobsen's nerve has been implicated as well. If there is an elongated styloid process or mineralisation of the stylohyoid ligament it can result in neuralgia known as Eagle's syndrome. Depending on the cause of neuralgia, treatment options include neuropathic pain killers, styloidectomy, section of the tympanic branch of the glossopharyngeal nerve, or microvascular decompression. Neurology and pain team consultations may be helpful in management. For patients with a unilateral otalgia and unclear cause, further imaging with contrast enhanced magnetic resonance imaging scan should be considered.

Otalgia in the absence of discharge, hearing loss or otoscopic abnormality should raise suspicion of referred otalgia.

KEY POINTS

- The incidence of NOE appears to be increasing, and the complex management of these patients may benefit from an multidisciplinary team approach.
- Underlying malignancy should be excluded in patients presenting with granulation or bone erosion in the EAC.
- Patients with unilateral otalgia should have a full head and neck examination; if cause is not identified imaging with contrast-enhanced MRI should be considered.

Further Reading

1. Roland PS, Smith TL, Schwartz SR, et al. Clinical practice guideline: cerumen impaction. *Otolaryngol Head Neck Surg* 2008; 139(3 Suppl 2), S1–S21.

2. Rosenfeld RM, Schwartz SR, Cannon CR, et al. Clinical practice guideline: acute otitis externa. *Otolaryngol Head Neck Surg* 2014; 150(1 Suppl), S1–S24.

3. Ramsden RT, Bulman CH, Lorigan BP. Osteoradionecrosis of the temporal bone. *J Laryngol Otol* 1975; 89, 941–55.

---

8. EUSTACHIAN TUBE DYSFUNCTION

Introduction

The Eustachian tube (ET) is a narrow passage approximately 40 mm in length that connects the nasopharynx and the middle ear (ME). The medial two-thirds is formed from cartilage and other soft tissue, whilst the lateral third is within the temporal bone. The lumen of the ET is lined with respiratory-type cuboidal epithelium and has an hourglass shape, with the anatomical isthmus located within the cartilaginous portion, approximately 20 mm from the nasopharyngeal ostium. In the healthy state the cartilaginous ET lumen is collapsed for a 5- to 10-mm long segment, usually located a few millimetres from the isthmus.

The ET opening may be active or passive. Active opening typically lasts 300–600 ms and is due to contraction of paratubal muscles, predominantly the tensor veli palatini. Most active opening is involuntary and due to swallowing. Passive ET opening occurs if the nasopharyngeal or ME pressure exceeds the periluminal pressure that holds the lumen closed, for example, during a Valsalva (forcible exhalation with the nose and mouth occluded).

The ET is shorter and more horizontal and compliant in children, which may contribute to an increased incidence of ME disease in children.

ETD in Clinical Practice

The ET has three primary functions: (1) gas transfer and pressure equalisation between the ME and nasopharynx; (2) clearance of ME secretions via both muscular action and mucociliary transport; and (3) prevention of sound, fluid, and pathogen reflux into the ME from the nasopharynx.

ET dysfunction (ETD) is usually caused by failure of the tube to adequately open or close. It is important to recognise ET function as a continuous spectrum, with a permanently open

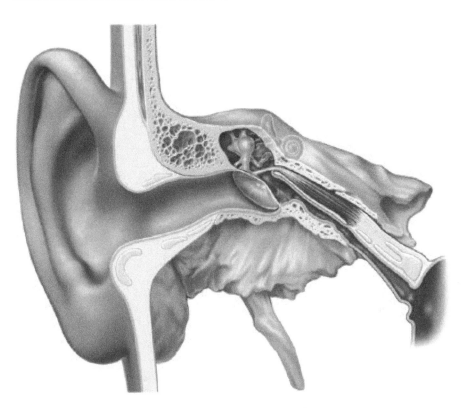

Figure 8.1   Cross section along the length of the Eustachian tube.

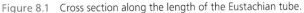

(patulous) tube at one end, and a permanently closed (obstructed) tube at the other. The healthy state falls in the middle of this spectrum.

Obstructive ETD, due to inadequate ET opening, is estimated to affect 0.9% of British adults. Reported symptoms are typically aural fullness or pressure, popping or crackling sounds, tinnitus, muffled hearing, and otalgia. Some patients with obstructive ETD only experience symptoms in situations of rapid ambient pressure change, such as when ascending or descending in a plane, or undertaking scuba diving. This may represent a milder form of the disorder, although objective testing does not fully support this. Most ME disorders have a multifactorial etiology; however, an association has been demonstrated between obstructive ETD and otitis media with effusion, chronic otitis media, tympanic membrane retraction, and cholesteatoma.

Patulous ETD, due to inadequate ET closure, is estimated to affect 0.3% of the population, although with screening, prevalence has been found to be as high as 6.6% in adults. Symptoms are similar to those for obstructive ETD, although often with a heightened awareness of the patient's own voice (autophony) and breath sounds (aerophony). Patulous ETD is usually intermittent, with symptoms often worse with exercise and better when supine. Sequelae of patulous ETD include atelectasis, retraction pockets, perforations, and cholesteatoma as ME pressure can vary from negative to positive with sniffing and Valsalva, respectively.

It is useful to classify ETD as acute or chronic if present for more than 3 months. There have been further attempts to develop a classification for ETD, notably making a distinction between baro-challenge induced and other forms of obstructive ETD.

The pathogenesis of ETD is poorly understood. Chronic obstructive ETD is often attributed to mucosal inflammation, and it has been associated with gastroesophageal reflux, allergy, rhinosinusitis, and smoking, though to date evidence of a causal relationship is lacking. Failure of active ET opening appears to account for the association between cleft palate and obstructive ETD. Patulous ETD is more likely to have a structural cause with loss of soft tissue, and it is associated with acute weight loss in one-third of cases. Other associations include pregnancy, allergy, haemodialysis, neurological disorders, and local radiotherapy, although in one-third or more of cases no cause is identified.

Assessment and Diagnosis

ETD provides a diagnostic challenge, as the presenting symptoms are non-specific and similar to many otological conditions, as well as temporomandibular joint disorders, and even chronic rhinosinusitis. It is important to note that autophony can be caused by other disorders, such as superior canal dehiscence. Furthermore, patient symptoms correlate poorly with the underlying ET function and should not be used in isolation when deciding on management.[1]

Symptom severity may be quantified through the use of one of the disease-specific questionnaires, the Cambridge ETD Assessment (CETDA) or the ETD questionnaire (ETDQ-7). While useful in tracking changes in symptoms and as outcome measures, these tools have very low specificity and therefore a limited role in diagnosis. A subgroup of patients with patulous ETD that provides a particular diagnostic challenge are those with a closed ET but low ET opening pressure. These individuals tend to sniff regularly to generate a negative ME pressure, stiffening an atelectatic tympanic membrane to improve hearing and symptoms of autophony and aural fullness. This habit can generate a negative ME pressure, leading to misdiagnosis if tympanometry alone is used to diagnose ETD.

Examination should focus on the assessment of ET function using tests that measure ET opening and ME pressure equalisation.

ET opening can be assessed with the patient sitting during Valsalva or Toynbee (swallowing with a pinched nose and closed mouth) manoeuvres by watching the tympanic membrane for deflection, which is seen in 80–85% of healthy individuals. If patulous ETD is suspected, the tympanic membrane is observed as the patient breathes to look for synchronous deflection. If no movement is seen, the patient is asked to occlude the contralateral nostril and breathe forcefully. If still negative, the patient should be asked to exercise (jog on the spot or climb a staircase) prior to examination as intermittent patulous ETD may be provoked.

Tympanometry provides a useful indicator of ET function. An ME pressure below −50 daPa suggests obstructive ETD with a specificity close to 100%, but sensitivity of only 50%.[1] This relies on excluding patulous ETD and sniff-induced negative ME pressure, which may be suggested by the history or a high compliance. It should also be noted that ME pressure should be measured before asking the patient to perform Valsalva or Toynbee. Continuous recording of tympanic impedance (long time base or reflex-decay tympanometer settings) detects synchronous movement of the tympanic membrane with breathing in patulous ETD.

Although not widely available, specialist tests such as tubomanometry and sonotubometry have been shown to have good sensitivity and specificity for ETD, providing a quantitative assessment of ET opening. Table 8.1 summarises the methods of ET function assessment.

Treatment of Obstructive ETD

The majority of patients with obstructive ETD do not require treatment following reassurance. Most treatments for obstructive ETD (summarised in Table 8.2) lack an evidence base, including nasal steroids.[2] Tympanostomy tubes provide short-term relief in patients with a predominance of symptoms on baro-challenge, but other symptoms may fail to improve. Surgery with laser ablation of the mucosa and submucosa around the nasopharyngeal ET ostium has been shown to improve symptoms and ET function at least in the short term, but most recent work has focussed on balloon dilation of the ET (BDET).

Table 8.1   Methods of assessing ET function to investigate obstructive or patulous ETD

Method of assessment	Indicator of ET function
• Tympanometry	ME pressure in relation to ambient pressure at rest
• Patient-reported ME pressure change • TM movement on otoscopy • Continuous tympanic impedance monitoring • Ear canal pressure monitoring (TTAG)	ME pressure changes on ET opening with Valsalva, Toynbee, or heavy breathing
• Nine-step equilibration test (intact TM) • Forced-response test (perforated TM)	ME pressure equalisation after applied external canal pressure
• Tubomanometry *(a sealed nosepiece for pressure delivery and ear canal pressure sensor)*	ME pressure changes on ET opening with an induced high nasopharyngeal pressure synchronised with swallowing
• Sonotubometry *(a speaker held at the nostril and microphone within an ear canal probe)*	Degree of sound transmission along the ET with opening during swallowing or heavy breathing
• Rigid or flexible endoscopy	Extent of ET movement on swallowing and atrophy or swelling of ET soft tissues

Note: ET, Eustachian tube; ME, middle ear; TM, tympanic membrane; TTAG, tubo-tympano-aerodynamic-graphy.

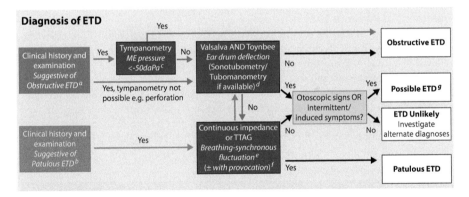

Figure 8.2   Diagnostic flowchart for Eustachian tube dysfunction (modified from Smith et al. 2018[1]).(a,b) Clinical assessment may not be diagnostic of ETD, but remains a means to identify patients for investigation. (c) Effort should be made during assessment of the clinical history to identify habitual sniffing, as a negative middle ear pressure in these individuals may not indicate obstructive ETD, and further testing should be undertaken. (d) Valsalva and Toynbee represent simple tests of ET opening available to any clinician, though more sophisticated tests of ET opening such as sonotubometry and tubomanometry may provide higher accuracy and repeatability. (e) Tubo-tympano-aerodynamic-graphy (TTAG) is an alternate method recommended if a tympanic membrane perforation is present. (f) A simple provocation test for use in clinic is asking the patient to exercise prior to testing. (g) This group could contain healthy patients, or those with patulous or obstructive ETD. ET function may vary over a relatively short time period. Tests may be repeated on a separate occasion to improve sensitivity in patients with variable ET function. Patients with baro-challenge-induced obstructive ETD may present here with normal test results in the absence of significant pressure change.

Table 8.2   Management of obstructive ETD

Management of obstructive ETD
Medical/Conservative
• Topical nasal steroids
• Antihistamines
• Management of acid reflux
Surgical
• Tympanostomy tubes
• Laser removal of mucosa and submucosa ± cartilage scoring
• Microdebrider removal of tissue at the ostium
• Balloon dilation (transnasal or transtympanic)

BDET uses a high-pressure balloon passed into the ET to dilate the tube and improve opening. The balloon is typically inserted with an introducer via a nasal approach, guided using a 30° endoscope, although transtympanic approaches have been described. Improvement in patient symptoms, tympanometry results, ability to Valsalva, and some objective measures of ET function have been reported up to 24 months, but long-term data are lacking. BDET has been used less in children, but some reports suggest it has a role in the management of otitis media with effusion.

There is no widespread consensus on patient selection criteria for BDET. Several groups have published criteria, which stress the importance of careful pre-operative diagnosis, and suggest on the basis of current evidence that BDET may provide benefit to patients with chronic symptoms, serous otitis media, and baro-challenge-induced discomfort. The benefit of BDET as an adjunct to ME surgery has not been determined.

Treatment of Patulous ETD

As with obstructive ETD, the evidence supporting treatments for patulous ETD is often limited to small case series. Techniques are summarised in Table 8.3. As many symptoms are believed to be due to tympanic membrane movement, mass loading of the membrane has been used as a treatment, and this may also explain the beneficial effect of tympanostomy tubes. Before embarking on surgery, many surgeons place Blu-Tack or cream on the tympanic membrane in clinic to assess its effect on symptoms. Increasing evidence suggests good and sustained results from use of a silicone (Kobayashi) plug or wax-filled catheter inserted into the ET via either a tympanic or nasal approach. While bulking agents injected around

Table 8.3   Management of patulous ETD

Management of patulous ETD
Medical/Conservative
• Cessation of nasal steroids or decongestants
• Increased weight
• Nasal saline spray
• Nasally applied salicylic or boric acid powder, or dilute hydrochloric acid
Surgical
• Tympanostomy tubes
• Mass loading of the tympanic membrane:
• Paper patches applied to the tympanic membrane
• KTP laser resurfacing of the tympanic membrane
• Cartilage tympanoplasty
• Occlusion of the Eustachian tube lumen:
• Intraluminal occlusion with a silicone plug or blocked catheter
• Injection of bulking agent (Teflon, silicone, calcium hydroxyapatite)
• Cartilage grafting (harvested from nasal septum)

the nasopharyngeal ET orifice appear to be successful in improving symptoms, the long-term results are poor and some patients need multiple injections.

> **KEY POINTS**
>
> - The ET opening is mediated by intermittent active or passive opening.
> - ET disorders are common, with patulous and obstructive dysfunction at either end of a spectrum of ET function.
> - Presenting symptoms and signs are non-specific.
> - Tests of ET function are required to distinguish patulous from obstructive dysfunction.
> - BDET is increasingly used to treat obstructive ETD, with a body of evidence to suggest improvements to patient symptoms and objective outcomes.
> - Uncertainty remains in relation to patient selection for BDET and long-term outcomes.
> - Patulous ETD may be treated by several methods to obstruct the ET lumen or reduce tympanic membrane movement.

Further Reading

1. Smith ME, Takwoingi Y, Deeks J, et al. Eustachian tube dysfunction: a diagnostic accuracy study and proposed diagnostic pathway. *PLoS One* 2018; 13:e0206946.

2. Norman G, Llewellyn A, Harden M, et al. Systematic review of the limited evidence base for treatments of Eustachian tube dysfunction: a health technology assessment. *Clin Otolaryngol* 2014; 39:6–21.

9. ACUTE OTITIS MEDIA AND OTITIS MEDIA WITH EFFUSION IN ADULTS

Acute Otitis Media

Definition

The term *otitis media* describes inflammation of the middle ear space. 'Acute' otitis media indicates a time frame of inflammation resolution within 12 weeks. Clearly, timely diagnosis is required to manage such conditions, and thus in practice the term *acute otitis media* (AOM) is used to describe an acute infection of the middle ear space. Clinical differentiation of AOM from an initial presentation of otitis media with effusion (OME) is important, as overtreatment of OME with antibiotics in primary or secondary care is common.

Incidence

AOM occurs most commonly in children; however, it is seen in adults – a large international multicentre primary care study recorded that 16% of patients with AOM were aged >15 years. In a study of U.S. veterans, the incidence of AOM in adults leading to a presentation at a veterans' medical centre was 2.6/1000/yr.

Aetiology

Much of our understanding of the aetiology of AOM is based on its clinical presentation in children. AOM is thought to be caused by a combination of Eustachian tube anatomy, disordered Eustachian tube function, immune status, and infective organisms.

Eustachian tube dysfunction (ETD) may be caused by a viral upper respiratory tract infection (URTI) which may also cause infection within the middle ear cleft. ETD can also be associated with smoking. Immune function is most relevant in patients with immunodeficiency.

People with human immunodeficiency virus (HIV) have an incidence of AOM four times higher than age-matched controls, and around 50% of patients with common variable immunodeficiency have had AOM episodes. The higher incidence of AOM in children is thought to be due to anatomical differences of the Eustachian tube (it is shorter and more horizontal) and their less mature immune system.

Bacteria are identified in the vast majority of middle ear aspirates, with the most common organisms identified as *Streptococcus pneumoniae*, *Haemophilus influenzae*, and *Moraxella catarrhalis*. There is an increasing recognition of polymicrobial disease – with both bacterial and viral pathogens found in approximately 66% of cases. The most common viruses identified are rhinovirus and respiratory syncytial virus.

Diagnosis

History

The characteristic symptoms of AOM are otalgia, hearing loss, and systemic upset. Secondary symptoms include balance disturbance, general malaise, pyrexia, and headache. Otorrhoea may occur with tympanic membrane perforation, which typically resolves the otalgia and systemic illness – such cases may need to be differentiated from bullous myringitis.

Examination

Otoscopy may be challenging as the bulging red tympanic membrane may prove difficult to focus on until the examiner realises the drum is more lateral than usual, and withdraws the otoscope slightly to allow the drum to appear in focus. The bulging of the tympanic membrane is the most reliable otoscopic indicator of AOM.

Other signs include perforation and pus in the ear canal. Swelling of the posterior ear canal is a sign of mastoiditis.

Differential Diagnosis

Bullous myringitis mimics AOM most closely. Otitis externa may have similar symptoms and abnormal examination. Temporomandibular joint dysfunction may also cause otalgia with normal examination findings.

Examination findings of AOM can be similar to those seen in OME, middle ear paraganglioma, or aberrant middle ear vasculature.

Management

Although most cases will resolve spontaneously and only analgesia/antipyretics are required, AOM is still the most common cause of antibiotic prescription in the United States. In the United Kingdom, the National Institute of Health and Care Excellence recommends withholding antibiotic treatment for 3 days in the majority of cases, and reserving antibiotics for cases that do not improve, for those who are systemically unwell, and for younger children with bilateral AOM. This is based on evidence showing that antibiotics have limited efficacy in AOM in all patients, and with particularly limited evidence in the adult population. The recommended first-line agent is a 5- to 7-day course of amoxicillin, or a macrolide such as clarithromycin in penicillin-allergic patients.

The treatment of AOM in the 10% of patients who have perforated their tympanic membrane but have ongoing symptoms is controversial. Topical ciprofloxacin can be used, although the evidence base for this is largely based on its use in grommet-related otorrhoea. Systemic antibiotics are more frequently recommended as more pathogenic organisms, such as group A Streptococcus, are associated with perforation.

Complications of AOM are typically divided into intracranial and extracranial complications. All are rare, although it is interesting to note that adults with AOM are at higher risk of intracranial complications than adults with chronic otitis media. Extracranial complications include facial palsy, acute mastoiditis, purulent labyrinthitis, and abscesses associated with structures connected to the temporal bone, such as the sternocleidomastoid, digastric, or zygoma. Intracranial complications include sigmoid sinus thrombosis, otitic hydrocephalus, subdural empyema, intradural abscesses, Gradenigo's syndrome (middle ear infection complicated by petrous apicitis causing cranial nerve VI palsy and retro-orbital pain), and meningitis. Facial palsy accounts for 30% of these complications, but full recovery occurs in most cases. Treatment of complications is with antibiotics, drainage of any abscess, and urgent mastoidectomy to treat the infection source. Many advocate adding anticoagulants in cases of sigmoid sinus thrombosis.

Recurrent AOM is almost invariably seen in children, but it can occur in adults, and may be treated by grommet insertion, or rarely antibiotic prophylaxis, with modest efficacy. Pneumococcal vaccination has also been shown to be effective in preventing episodes of otitis media in both adults and children.

Proposed treatments for the future include transtympanic or intranasal antibiotics or bacteriophages, probiotics, vaccination against viral pathogens, and treatment directed at *Haemophilus*-associated biofilm. There is limited evidence to support the use of systemic steroids, although they are not used commonly.

Otitis Media with Effusion in Adults

Definition
OME describes a collection of fluid in the middle ear associated with inflammation, but not active infection, of the middle ear cleft.

Incidence
In a very large analysis of U.S. ambulatory medical care attendance with OME, adults >20 years accounted for about one-third of patients for about 1.2 million visits per year (this gives a visit prevalence, and not an incidence). In the United Kingdom, a cross-sectional study found a point prevalence of all ETD diagnoses of about 1% in adults.

Aetiology
The aetiology of otitis media in adults, and the differences in its nature with paediatric disease are incompletely understood. Adult OME is a condition that arises from the interaction of a number of factors, the most important of which are Eustachian tube function and upper respiratory tract inflammation.

Eustachian Tube Function
Objective tests have revealed evidence of abnormal Eustachian tube function in adults with OME. The significance of these tests is uncertain. It is nevertheless well recognised that obstructing lesions in and around the Eustachian tube, such as nasopharyngeal carcinoma, or skull base tumours such as intraosseous meningiomas, may cause OME. Similarly, disorders such as cleft palate that impair ET function can cause OME.

OME may also arise due to acquired dysfunction of the Eustachian tube, most notably, radiotherapy to the head and neck has a strong dose-related relationship with OME. Equally, in patients with prolonged sedation (and consequent lack of swallow), there is a very high incidence of OME. This is also seen in patients with ciliary dysfunction such as smokers and patients with primary ciliary dyskinesia. Barotrauma and hyperbaric oxygen therapy may also cause ETD and consequent OME, but this typically resolves spontaneously. OME has also been associated with sniffing to suppress patulous eustachian tube symptoms.

Upper Respiratory Tract Inflammation
While upper respiratory tract inflammation can a priori cause ETD, it is worthwhile considering it as a different entity, because it may also affect the middle ear mucosa directly. The majority of adults report an URTI prior to episodes of OME, and about two-thirds of aspirates from middle ear effusions are culture positive for pathogens such as *S. pneumoniae, H. influenza* or *Candida* spp. In contrast, pathogens cannot be cultured from irrigation of the middle ear in people without OME. There is also a high incidence of OME in patients with HIV.

There is evidence showing a higher incidence of OME in adults with allergic rhinitis. Furthermore, there is an association with nasal polyposis, which is likely to be mediated by the underlying mucosal inflammation. The role of laryngopharyngeal reflux in the aetiology of OME is controversial, given the high incidence of reflux, and the uncertain significance of the finding of pepsin in middle ear aspirates, but it does seem likely there is a relationship. Other inflammatory conditions associated with OME include granulomatosis with polyangiitis, and polyarteritis nodosa. Eosinophilic otitis media (EOM) is distinct from OME and has a strong association with asthma and allergy. It is characterised by eosinophilic infiltrates in the middle ear mucosa and can be associated with effusion, viscous discharge through a perforation, and/or middle ear granulation.

Diagnosis

History

In a case-control study, symptoms in OME sufferers included the following:

- Hearing loss: 97%
- Aural fullness: 77%
- Pulsatile or crackling tinnitus: 60%

The condition is usually bilateral, but it may be unilateral. Subjects frequently have predisposing factors including smoking, childhood ear infections, and nasal symptoms. A recent URTI, AOM, and/or barotrauma is often a feature.

Examination

Otoscopy reveals a dull tympanic membrane, with a loss of the light reflex. The tympanic membrane may be inflamed, visibly thickened, or retracted. There may be reduced movement of the tympanic membrane to pneumatic otoscopy. A fluid level, or air bubbles, may be seen. Fibreoptic nasoendoscopy is recommended in patients with unilateral symptoms to rule out an obstructing nasopharyngeal lesion.

Differential Diagnosis

Cerebrospinal fluid (CSF) in the middle ear secondary to a skull base defect may be mistaken for OME. EOM and vasculitis-associated otitis media are distinct entities. These require intensive anti-inflammatory treatment in conjunction with respiratory/rheumatological physicians.

Investigations

Audiology and Tympanography

A pure–tone audiogram will show the level of impaired hearing function and typically reveal a conductive hearing loss. Tympanography will commonly show a 'type B' pattern. Experienced clinicians will usually make the diagnosis of OME from tympanic membrane appearance.

Myringotomy

The presence of fluid at surgery confirms the condition of OME, but the absence of fluid does not necessarily refute it, as fluid may still be present in the mastoid. Immediate pre-operative tympanometry has shown that type B and type C2 tympanograms are 92% and 39% predictive of a middle ear effusion, respectively.

Imaging

Unilateral OME may be investigated with contrast magnetic resonance imaging (MRI) of the nasopharynx and skull base, particularly in at-risk populations such as those of Chinese descent. This is in recognition of the potential for skull base tumours or submucosal nasopharyngeal tumours to present in this way with normal endoscopic findings. In addition, certain MRI sequences are useful in differentiating OME from CSF.

Management

There are four management options in adults: (1) nonmedical treatment, (2) medical treatment, (3) hearing aids, and (4) surgical treatment.

Non-Medical Treatment

Autoinflation techniques have a role to play in adults as well as children. Although the benefit is modest, the risks are negligible. Autoinflation is commonly encouraged through the Politzer technique, although mechanical devices such as the Otovent™ balloon and EarPopper™ can be employed to achieve the same effect.

Medical Management

There is limited evidence for topical nasal steroids or decongestants, such as xylometazoline, in the treatment of OME. However, they are likely to be beneficial in patients who have rhinitis. Antibiotics and antihistamines are ineffective, despite being often prescribed. Short courses of oral steroids have been shown to be ineffective in a paediatric population.

Hearing Aids

Hearing aids are highly effective for conductive hearing loss provided there is adequate inner ear function, and they can be offered to adults with long-term OME.

Surgical Treatment

Ventilation Tubes

Ventilation tubes are commonly used for OME in adults for hearing restoration. Several studies have shown evidence for their short-term efficacy. After grommet extrusion, around 25–35% of patients will have recurrent OME depending on the underlying aetiology of the OME. Grommets are not without complications; about 20% of patients will have grommet-related otorrhoea, and persistent perforation rates of 2% with short-term tubes rise to 17% when long-term tubes are used.

Chronic otorrhoea has meant that conservative management is often recommended in patients who have had radiotherapy for nasopharyngeal carcinoma. Actual rates of otorrhoea are relatively low in these patients, so surgery can be offered. Extra-annular tubes may stay in situ for longer periods, and do not cause tympanic membrane perforation, but require a more invasive initial operation.

Laser Myringotomy

The use of a laser to produce fenestration of the tympanic membrane produces a short-term solution. A mean of around 3 weeks for a functioning myringotomy has been reported.

Eustachian Tuboplasty

A meta-analysis including 1155 patients concluded that the balloon Eustachian tuboplasty (BET) offers short-term benefit in the majority of cases and medium to longer term benefit in a smaller number of patients. For that reason it has been proposed as a treatment for patients with recurrent OME after grommet insertion. Laser tuboplasty has also been reported.

KEY POINTS

- AOM, which is symptomatic after tympanic membrane perforation, is more likely to be associated with pathogenic bacteria such as group A streptococcus.
- Vascularity of the normal tympanic membrane should not be confused with the bulging red tympanic membrane seen in AOM.
- Persistent clear fluid during unilateral ventilation tube insertion indicates a CSF leak.
- Complications associated with ventilation tube insertion include otorrhoea (20%) and persistent perforation (2–17% depending on type of tube).
- AOM in adults is usually managed with antipyretics for 72 hours to allow spontaneous resolution.

Unilateral OME requires investigation with nasoendoscopy and/or MRI to exclude a nasopharyngeal lesion.

Further Reading

1. NICE Clinical Knowledge Summary: Acute Otitis Media. https://cks.nice.org.uk/otitis-media-acute#!topicSummary

2. Perera R, Glasziou PP, Heneghan CJ, McLellan J, Williamson I. Autoinflation for hearing loss associated with otitis media with effusion. *Cochrane Database Syst Rev.* 2013;31 (5): CD006285.

3. Fish BM, Banerjee AR, Jennings CR, et al. Effect of anaesthetic agents on tympanometry and middle-ear effusions. *J Laryngol Otol* 2000;114 (5): 336–338.

10. CHRONIC OTITIS MEDIA

Introduction

Chronic otitis media may manifest in a variety of clinical phenotypes, including middle ear effusion (glue ear), cholesteatoma, tympanic membrane retraction, or tympanic membrane perforation (which may be associated with infection). Tympanosclerosis and myringitis are also discussed here, although their relation to chronic otitis media is less clear.

Aetiology

The cause of chronic inflammation of the middle ear is poorly understood. The traditional theory assigning it to a functional abnormality of the Eustachian tube has little evidence to support it (although this mechanism may be important in syndromic cases related to craniofacial malformation).

It seems probable that recurrent bacterial ingress into the middle ear in early childhood triggers inflammation, which in some (genetically) predisposed individuals leads to non-resolving mucosal inflammation (Figure 10.1), with resulting tissue dysfunction and damage.

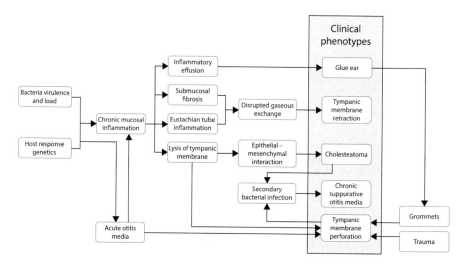

Figure 10.1 Clinical phenotypes of chronic otitis media and presumed aetiology.

Goblet cells in the middle ear mucosa hypertrophy and secrete mucus, leading to middle ear effusion or 'glue ear'.

Mucosal dysfunction can disrupt gaseous exchange and lower middle ear pressure (the relative role of this versus the Eustachian tube in maintaining normal middle ear pressure is debated), and if combined with lysis and weakening of the fibrous layer of the tympanic membrane from chronic inflammation, can lead to tympanic membrane retraction.

Many cases of tympanic membrane perforation are also thought to be caused by lysis from chronic inflammation, although this may also occur secondary to acute otitis media, trauma, or non-healing after grommet extrusion. Some perforations are asymptomatic, whereas others are prone to recurrent infections, and if this occurs, the disease is termed chronic suppurative otitis media (CSOM).

Cholesteatoma can be defined as 'the presence of squamous epithelium in the middle ear cleft'. Aetiology is uncertain, but acquired cholesteatoma has been demonstrated to arise from the squamous epithelium of the tympanic membrane, as a result of active proliferation and medial growth. This seems to occur in response to chronic mucosal inflammation, but the underlying molecular signalling is uncertain. Cholesteatoma is more likely to occur within a retraction pocket. In a few cases cholesteatoma may be iatrogenic, arising from implanted squamous epithelium from previous surgery. Some consider cholesteatoma to be a subtype of CSOM.

Symptoms and Signs

Chronic otitis media typically presents with hearing loss, otorrhoea, and/or otalgia. Hearing loss will be conductive in nature, and it may result from middle ear effusion, tympanic membrane perforation, or erosion of the ossicles (most often the long process of the incus). Recurrent otorrhoea may be seen with tympanic perforation, retraction, or cholesteatoma. Mild otalgia is sometimes a feature in cholesteatoma. Typically, disease has to be present for at least 3 months to be called chronic, but for CSOM some authors use 6 weeks.

Symptoms alone cannot determine diagnosis, and otoscopy is critical to visualise middle ear pathology (using a microscope or endoscope where available), and an audiogram to evaluate hearing loss. A tympanogram can confirm the presence of effusion or perforation.

In some cases, granulation tissue may preclude a full view of the tympanic membrane. Granulation tissue should be treated with topical steroids, but if it fails to settle, surgical exploration is indicated for definitive diagnosis and treatment (including excluding cholesteatoma).

Chronic Otitis Media with Effusion (Come; Glue Ear)

This is covered in more detail in Chapter 9. COME is common in childhood, affecting 5–6% of children at the age of 2, but it becomes rare after the age of 7. Amongst adults who suffer chronic otitis media in some form, the majority will give a history of COME in earlier life.

Tympanic Retraction

This typically affects either the pars flaccida or the posterosuperior pars tensa. The retraction pocket may become adherent to and then erode the ossicles. In more advanced cases there can be bony erosion (typically the scutum) or retraction of the entire membrane, with adhesion to the promontory. Retraction may be graded, and the Sade and Tos systems are most commonly used (Table 10.1). Inter-observer reliability of these systems is poor.

Epidemiological studies suggest that up to 15% of adults have tympanic membrane retraction. Asymptomatic cases may need monitoring for risk of progression, including development of cholesteatoma, although the frequency and duration of monitoring is unclear. Those with recurrent infection or hearing loss (air-bone gap greater than 20 dB) may benefit from cartilage tympanoplasty ± ossiculoplasty. Others advocate grommet insertion or excision of retraction pockets, but there is little evidence on long-term results from such treatment.

Table 10.1   Grading systems for tympanic retraction for the pars flaccida (Tos system) and pars tensa (Sade system)

Grade	Pars flaccida	Pars tensa
1	Retraction to neck of malleus, but airspace visible	Mild retraction
2	Retraction onto neck of malleus, no airspace behind membrane	Retraction onto incudostapedial joint
3	Retraction extends beyond malleus, but full extent visible	Retraction onto promontory (not adherent)
4	Scutum eroded, full extent of retraction not visible	Adhesion of pars tensa to medial wall

Tympanic Perforation and CSOM

Some perforations are asymptomatic (inactive), whereas others will lead to repeated infections (active). Infection (leading to CSOM) may arise from water ingress, an upper respiratory tract infection, or without obvious precipitant. In the United Kingdom, CSOM affects around 1% of adults, but on a global scale it has a high disease burden, affecting around 250 million adults and children. Prevalence is higher in socioeconomically deprived regions and in indigenous populations.

Active infection should be treated with aural toilet (microsuction/ear wicking/iodine washout; Figure 10.2) and topical antibiotics. A mixed bacterial flora is typical of CSOM, including *Proteus*, staphylococci, and *Pseudomonas*. Many advocate quinolone antibiotic drops as first-line treatment, because they are often effective and are not known to be ototoxic. Advice on correct administration of drops is important (head tilted to the side with tragal pumping to push drops medially). Antifungal drops may be indicated if fungal infection is suspected or if spores are seen, and in such cases prolonged therapy may be needed. In low-resource settings human immunodeficiency virus (HIV) infection may be a cause, or tuberculosis (TB; particularly if there are multiple perforations of the tympanic membrane). Failure of initial treatment warrants microbial culture and sensitivity testing, regular aural toilet, and consideration of switching of topical antibiotic class (or considering an antifungal), and possibly addition of oral antibiotics.

Patients with persistent or recurring infection may benefit from tympanoplasty, which typically has a success rate of around 85%. Local anaesthetic tympanoplasty is an option for selected patients, including those not suitable for general anaesthesia. Tympanoplasty is also a treatment for those with hearing loss (air-bone gap greater than 20 dB) from a tympanic perforation or CSOM. Hearing aids are an alternative option but increase the risk of infection. Tympanoplasty is covered in more depth in Chapter 11.

Cholesteatoma

Cholesteatoma affects 1 in 10,000 of the population per year. Once present, cholesteatoma becomes an encapsulated but self-perpetuating mass, typically growing into the mastoid air cells, and eroding surrounding bone. Super-added infection is common, and may increase disease activity and patient symptoms. There is a small risk of death from intracranial spread of infection, estimated at 1 in 10,000 per year.

The only effective treatment for cholesteatoma is surgical excision through mastoidectomy. In patients unfit for surgery, aural toileting to debulk disease may be used, but it is unclear if this is of any benefit. Most surgeons will obtain a computed tomography (CT) scan of the temporal bones prior to operating, to identify anatomical variants and bony erosion.

Mastoidectomy may be performed with either preservation or removal of the bone of the superior and posterior external auditory canal (EAC). Where the EAC is preserved this is termed a 'wall up' procedure, also known as combined approach tympanoplasty. Where the EAC is removed this is a 'wall down' procedure, and it can be classified by the extent of dissection (atticotomy/attico-antrostomy/mastoidectomy).

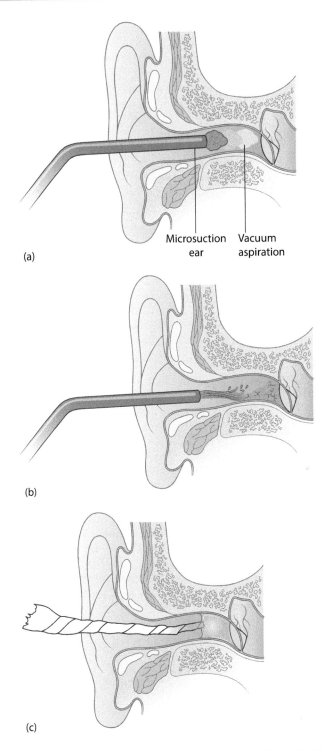

(a)

Microsuction ear   Vacuum aspiration

(b)

(c)

Figure 10.2   Techniques for irrigation in active chronic suppurative otitis media. (a) Suction under microscopic guidance (microsuction). (b) Washout with dilute iodine solution using a syringe. (c) Wicking the ear with spears made of tissue paper (which can be performed by the clinician, patient, or carer.)

The canal wall up procedure risks leaving residual disease hidden in the mastoid, so there needs to be subsequent follow-up with imaging (diffusion weighted magnetic resonance imaging [MRI]) and/or another operation to directly visualise (called a 'second look') the mastoid, typically a year after the first procedure. A wall down procedure leaves a patient with a mastoid cavity, which in some patients can cause problems with wax entrapment (necessitating regular dewaxing) or infection. In the wall down technique, obliteration of the mastoid cavity can reduce the risk of post-operative problems, and meatoplasty will aid clearance of the cavity. In the wall up technique use of an endoscope to aid visualisation and 'painting' the cavity with laser can reduce risk of residual disease.

There is debate about the relative merits of wall up or wall down procedures, and the choice of procedure should be tailored to individual disease and patient factors.

As well as the risk of residual or recurrent disease, mastoidectomy also carries a risk of worse hearing (including a dead ear), persistent otorrhoea (usually from a failure of reconstruction leading to exposed mucosal epithelium), taste disturbance, nausea, vertigo, tinnitus, or facial palsy.

Tympanosclerosis

Tympanosclerosis describes the deposition of calcium or bone at sites of previous middle ear inflammation. Usually it affects only the tympanic membrane (myringosclerosis) and is of no consequence. Rarely it may be found to affect the ossicles, often in an ear undergoing exploration for conductive hearing loss, causing fixation of the ossicular heads (treated with partial ossiculoplasty) or around the stapes footplate (usually causing surgery to be abandoned).

Complications

Complications of chronic otitis media occur from the erosion of surrounding structures. This is most common in cholesteatoma but can also happen in persistent severe CSOM.

Within the temporal bone, erosion can occur of the facial canal (with a risk of facial palsy), or into the labyrinth causing hearing loss or vertigo (typically with a fistula of the lateral semicircular canal). Treatment is by removal of infection/cholesteatoma. If an inner ear fistula is present at surgery, the cholesteatoma sac over the fistula may be marsupialised into a mastoid cavity (associated with a low risk of iatrogenic hearing loss), or removed and the fistula repaired with bone pate (1 in 6 risk of dead ear).

Extra-temporal spread posteriorly or superiorly can lead to intracranial complications of meningitis, sigmoid sinus thrombosis, or temporal lobe or cerebellar brain abscess, which may present with fever and headache, or in advanced cases with altered mental state, seizures, or lateralising neurological signs. Lateral erosion can lead to mastoiditis or a mastoid fistula. Inferior spread can lead to neck abscess. Treatment of complications is with antibiotics, drainage of any abscess (either transcranial or transmastoid for intracranial abscess), and urgent mastoidectomy to treat the infection source. Many advocate adding anticoagulants in cases of sigmoid sinus thrombosis.

KEY POINTS

- Chronic otitis media may manifest as glue ear, cholesteatoma, tympanic membrane retraction, or tympanic membrane perforation (with or without infection).
- Aetiology likely relates to repeated bacterial ingress into the middle ear in early childhood, leading to non-resolving inflammation and tissue dysfunction in predisposed individuals.
- Tympanic retraction or perforation may be treated with tympanoplasty if associated with infection or hearing loss.
- Cholesteatoma is treated by mastoidectomy, with techniques divided by whether the bony EAC is preserved or resected.
- Complications arise from bony erosion and spread of infection, and can be life-threatening.

Further Reading

1. Bhutta MF, Thornton RB, Kirkham LS, Kerschner JE, Cheeseman MT. Understanding the aetiology and resolution of chronic otitis media from animal and human studies. *Disease Models & Mechanisms* 2017: 10, 1289–1300.

2. Bhutta MF, Monono ME, Johnson W. Management of complicated otomastoiditis in resource constrained settings. *Current Opinion in Otolaryngology and Head & Neck Surgery* 2020: 28(3), 174–181.

11. OSSICULOPLASTY AND MYRINGOPLASTY

Myringoplasty

Myringoplasty is defined as surgical repair of the tympanic membrane (TM). This can be performed to rectify a persistent perforation or reinforce a thin or retracted drum. Tympanoplasty is defined as surgical repair of defects of the TM and middle ear ossicles. A type 1 tympanoplasty is synonymous with myringoplasty

Etiology

- Infection
  - Most common cause of acute perforation
  - Follows acute otitis media (AOM)
  - Spontaneously heals (70–80% within 30 days)
  - Negative healing influences: tympanosclerosis, malleus injury, infection, large perforations
- Trauma
  - Direct trauma
    - Foreign bodies (cotton buds, etc.)
    - Barotrauma (air travel or diving)
  - Indirect (temporal bone fracture)
- Iatrogenic
  - Following extrusion of ventilation tube (VT)
    - 2.2% risk with short-term VTs
    - Up to 16% risk with long-term VTs
  - Following middle ear surgery

Presentation

Perforations can be asymptomatic and found incidentally. However, discharge and hearing loss (HL) are the main reasons for presentation.

Hearing Loss

HL is variable depending on the size and location of the perforation. Posterosuperior perforations have larger conductive hearing loss (CHL) than other sites.[2] Lower frequencies tend to be more affected than higher ones but, with increasing size, higher frequencies are affected. More severe HL is associated with coexistent ossicular involvement or discontinuity; complete discontinuity can result in a maximal conductive HL of around 60 dB.

Indications for Myringoplasty

1. *Recurrent otorrhoea*: More likely with hearing aid use.
2. *Hearing loss*: Greater than 25% perforation causes increasing HL as size increases.
3. *Social*: For example, desire to swim.
4. Retraction with risk of developing cholesteatoma.

Contraindications to Myringoplasty

1. *Cholesteatoma*: All squamous epithelium must be excised from the middle ear prior to TM closure.
2. *Contralateral dead ear (relative contraindication)*: The risk of HL is 1.5%.[3]
3. *Severe Eustachian tube (ET) dysfunction*: There is an increased risk of HL and iatrogenic cholesteatoma with elevating Sade grade IV retractions; recurrence of retraction can occur.
4. *Medical comorbidities*: Chronic medical conditions (medications, obesity, smoking, alcohol, etc.) can all negatively influence success rate.
5. *Social*: Varying evidence of influence of smoking on surgical outcomes.

Factors Influencing Treatment Options

- *Timing and age*: Some advocate conservative management until after 7 years of age due to ET maturity. State of the contralateral ear is an important guide to this.
- *Adenoidectomy*: Conflicting information regarding its contribution, with majority of reviews suggesting prior adenoidectomy confers no benefit to success.
- *Infection*: There is a differing opinion as to the influence of infection at time of surgery on outcomes; however, the majority of studies state infection does not confer a negative influence on outcomes.
- *Other ear*: Normal contralateral ear is a positive predictor of success. Conversely, abnormal contralateral ear findings are associated with poorer ipsilateral graft uptake.
- *Mastoid*: Evidence of influence of concurrent mastoidectomy with tympanoplasty is subject to debate.

Graft Materials

- *Paper onlay*: Outpatient procedure; reasonable success for small perforations; may need repeating.
- *Autologous*
  - Temporalis fascia (TF): Most frequently utilised due to availability of abundant tissue and ease of use.
  - Perichondrium (tragus, concha): Easily accessible, long-term reliability, suitable for permeatal approach.
  - Cartilage (tragus, concha): Composite grafts (both cartilage and perichondrium in the same graft) confer practicality and increased graft success, particularly in larger perforations (>50%). Hearing results at 1 year equivalent to fascia/perichondrium.
    - Other: Includes periosteum, fat, and fascia lata.
- *Alloderm*: Human allograft skin rendered immunologically inert for when TF not available; success is 87.5%.
- *Xenogenous*: Equine and bovine pericardium have poorer success rates compared with TF. Basic fibroblast growth factor (FGF) in combination with atelocollagen, on Gelfoam or as drops has shown very encouraging results.

Technique

The 'underlay' technique is briefly described below:

- Local anaesthetic injection into skin incision site (if applicable), ear canal, and graft site.
- Approach may be permeatal, endaural, or post-auricular. The latter is useful in narrow ear canals and for anterior perforations.
- Freshening of perforation edges.
- Elevation of tympanomeatal flap.
- Harvesting of graft and placement medial to TM, supported either by a dissolvable dressing in the middle ear or by using the elevated tympanic annulus to hold the graft in place.
- Replacement of the TM and packing of the ear canal to support the TM.

Other techniques include the following:

- 'Push-through' technique: Variant of the underlay technique, avoids elevation of the TM, and is used for small perforations. A dissolvable dressing is placed through the perforation into the middle ear; the graft is then pushed through the perforation so that it is held laterally against the TM.
- 'Butterfly' technique: Utilises a disc of cartilage with a circumferential groove cut into it; this splays the edges of the cartilage, which 'snaps' into place within the perforation. Suitable for smaller perforations <6 mm in size. Mild myringitis occurs in 11%, resolving within 3 months.
- 'Overlay' technique: Steps similar to the underlay technique, except that the epithelial layer of the TM alone is elevated, with placement of the graft between the collagen (unelevated) and epithelial (elevated) layers. Repair outcomes are similar for overlay and underlay techniques.

Complications

- For reperforation rates, the literature shows success rates 60–99% in adults; 35–94% in children. Success falls over time (85% at 1 year, 78% at 10 years). Most failures are in the early post-operative period.
- Retraction can occur in up to 10%.
- Anterior blunting is a risk for underlay and overlay techniques.
- Iatrogenic cholesteatoma can be as high as 4.4%.
- Myringitis can occur but generally resolves within 3 months with topical treatment.

Ossiculoplasty

Aetiology of Conductive Hearing Loss

- Congenital: 1:15,000 births
  - Minor: Just middle ear (stapes fixation is the most common)
  - Major: Also involve external auditory meatus (EAM) and TM
    - Surgery more challenging
    - Consider bone conduction hearing device or middle ear implant
- Acquired: Secondary to chronic suppurative otitis media

Erosion incudostapedial joint (ISJ)	*More common*
Long process of incus	
Stapes superstructure	
Malleus	*Less common*

Classification of Defects

Table 11.1 Austin Kartush classification of ossicular status

Group	Ossicular status	Abbreviation	Prevalence (%)
A	Malleus handle and stapes superstructure present	M+ S+	60
B	Malleus handle present, stapes superstructure absent	M+ S−	23
C	Malleus handle absent, stapes superstructure present	M− S+	8
D	Malleus handle and stapes superstructure absent	M− S−	8
E	Ossicular head fixation		
O	Intact ossicular chain		
F	Stapes fixation		

Prognostic Factors for Successful Surgery

The Middle Ear Risk Index (MERI) (Table 11.2) provides a measure of severity of middle ear disease and has been correlated with ossiculoplasty hearing outcomes. It includes ossicular status as per the Austin Kartush classification and the Belluci classification of otorrhoea (Table 11.3).

Surgical Materials

- *Autografts*: Incus, cortical bone, cartilage
- *Homograft*: From donor, used widely in Belgium but not in the United Kingdom (Creutzfeldt–Jakob disease [CJD] risk)
- *Alloplastic*: Solid plastics, e.g. polyethylene
  - Porous plastics, e.g. Plasti-pore®(inflammatory reaction risk)
  - Ceramics, e.g. hydroxyapatite
  - Metals, e.g. stainless steel, titanium (newest and most common)

Table 11.2 Middle Ear Risk Index 2001

Otologic factor	Maximum score
Otorrhoea	3
Perforation	1
Cholesteatoma	2
Ossicular status	4
Middle ear granulation	2
Previous surgery	2
Smoking	2

Table 11.3 Belluci classification of otorrhoea

Otorrhoea	Risk value
Dry ear	0
Occasionally wet	1
Persistently wet	2
Persistently wet + cleft palate	

Principles: To try to reconnect inner ear to TM with a piston-like arrangement with rigid material and good coupling at both sides, covered with cartilage if touching TM, low tension, but good stability.

Specific Defects

1 Erosion of LPI
   - Autologous bone: difficult to fashion, may be unstable
   - ISJ prosthesis: fixation difficult as incus remnant tapering
   - Bone cement: easy to use but expensive, and variable results
   - Removal of incus and partial ossicular replacement prosthesis (PORP)
2 M+S+ (see Table 11.1)
   - Refashioned incus interposed between malleus and stapes head
   - Refashioned malleus head interposed between drum and stapes head
   - Cartilage interposed between drum and stapes head
   - PORP - malleus to stapes (stability dependent on anteroposterior relation of malleus and stapes)
     - TM to stapes (Clip-type prostheses to stapes head maybe more stable)
3 M+S−
   - Autologous incus (TM to footplate)
   - Total ossicular replacement prosthesis (TORP)
     - TM to footplate ± footplate shoe for stability, long-term stability and hearing difficult to achieve
4 M−S+
   TM to stapes head assembly as in M+S+, although some advocate neomalleus (metal malleus prosthesis that can be fixed to the attic)
5 M−S−
   TORP as in M+S−

General Considerations

The presence of stapes superstructure is the most important predictor of success. Overlong prosthesis can increase tension, causing inferior results. Two type of cholesteatoma surgery include the following:

- *Primary reconstruction*: May not need second operation, will need diffusion-weighted magnetic resonance imaging (MRI), may need redoing if residual/recurrence.
- *Delayed reconstruction*: Period of poor hearing (concern in children), requires two operations.

KEY POINTS

- Recurrent otorrhoea and HL are main indications for myringoplasty.
- Presence of cholesteatoma is an absolute contraindication to myringoplasty.
- Autologous graft materials are the most commonly used with a success rate of 85% after 1 year.
- Presence of stapes superstructure is the most important predictor of success of ossiculoplasty.
- In cholesteatoma surgery, primary ossicular reconstruction can be achieved, though delayed reconstruction may be appropriate in certain cases.

Further Reading

1. Saliba I, Abela A, Arcand P. Tympanic membrane perforation: size, site and hearing evaluation. *Int J Pediatr Otorhinolaryngol* 2011; 75(4): 527–531.

2. Bellucci RJ. Cochlear hearing loss in tympanoplasty. *Otolaryngol Head Neck Surg* 1985; 93(4): 482–485.

3. Austin DF. Ossicular reconstruction. *Arch Otolaryngol* 1971; 94: 525–535.

12. OTOSCLEROSIS

Definition

Otosclerosis is a localised disorder of bone metabolism of the otic capsule that is characterised by disordered resorption and deposition of bone. It is thought to result from increased pathologic bone remodelling, and the basic lesion consists of areas of bone resorption by osteoclasts and new bone formation by osteoblasts, accompanied by vascular proliferation. Many patients with otosclerosis are asymptomatic and clinical otosclerosis with associated hearing loss only occurs when the lesions involve the stapes footplate, or much more rarely the round window causing a conductive hearing loss. Sensory hearing loss is thought to occur when lesions involve the cochlear endosteum.

The most common site of otosclerosis is the cochlear wall just anterior to the stapes footplate.

Aetiology

The aetiology of otosclerosis remains obscure. There is a clear familial history of hearing loss in approximately half of patients. The measles virus has been suggested as a possible cofactor in the development of otosclerosis, but the available evidence remains conflicting and a number of recent studies have cast doubt on this link.

Genetics

Otosclerosis occurs in familial and non-familial forms. The familial form accounts for 25–50% of cases and has an autosomal dominant inheritance pattern with incomplete penetrance. Whilst a number of gene associations have been noted in affected families, the genetic cause of otosclerosis remains largely unidentified.

Incidence

Histological otosclerosis in a random series of temporal bones harvested in Belgium showed histological evidence of otosclerosis in 3.4% of the bones. The British National Study of Hearing showed the clinical prevalence is around 2% in adults. This increased with age to 3% in the 60- to 80-year-old age group (Table 12.1). Only 10% of those patients had surgery, which explains the lower incidence reported in clinical series. Interestingly this study showed similar prevalence in men and women but that the women had more severe hearing loss, which may account for the finding, commonly reported in clinical series, that otosclerosis is more common in women by approximately 2:1.

Clinical Findings

Otoscopy is usually normal; however, some patients may have dilated arteries on the medial wall of the middle ear due to increased vascularity of the otosclerotic foci. This gives the middle ear seen through the drum a reddish appearance and is known as a flamingo flush or Schwartze's sign. The patients have a conductive hearing loss usually with a negative

Table 12.1 Population prevalence per 100 of the presumptive diagnosis of otosclerosis[1]

	Otosclerosis (%)	95% CI
Overall	**2.1**	**1.5, 2.7**
Age (years)		
18–40	1.6	0.6, 2.6
41–60	2.2	1.3, 3.1
61–80	3.0	1.7, 4.3
Sex		
Women	2.0	1.3, 2.7
Men	2.2	1.2, 3.2
Occupational group		
Non-manual	1.5	0.8, 2.2
Manual	2.7	1.9, 3.5

(bone conduction better than air conduction) Rinne test. Pure-tone audiometry will confirm the conductive hearing loss, which is usually worse at lower frequencies. The bone conduction is frequently reduced at 2 kHz (Carhart's notch), possibly due to the ossicular chain being fixed. If the cochlea is involved patients may have a mixed hearing loss. Pure sensory hearing loss from cochlear otosclerosis with no involvement of the ossicular chain is rare. In cases where there is sensory hearing loss speech audiometry can be useful. If the maximum speech reception score is less than 60% and the other ear is normal, then the benefit of surgery may be limited. Tympanometry may show reduced compliance due to fixation of the ossicular chain but is typically normal. Stapedial reflexes are normally reduced or absent.

History
The classic history is of progressive hearing loss in a young adult. The majority will have bilateral hearing loss, but the loss is often asymmetric and sequential. About half of patients have a positive family history of otosclerosis. Tinnitus is present in two-thirds of cases.

Factors such as onset of hearing loss in childhood, history of ear or head trauma, and associated pain and/or discharge should make the clinician suspicious of other causes, as should extensive tympanosclerosis on the tympanic membrane.

Differential Diagnosis
In a patient with the classic history described above approximately 95% will have otosclerosis. However, superior semicircular canal dehiscence, malleus head fixation, incus erosion, tympanosclerosis, and osteogenesis imperfecta all can on occasion cause difficulties in reaching the correct diagnosis.

Investigations
A high-resolution or cone beam computed tomography (CT) scan can frequently confirm the diagnosis with the appearance of a lucency in the area anterior to the oval window Figure 12.1. It can also show other possible diagnoses such as superior semicircular dehiscence or fixation of the malleus. CT scanning is also useful in predicting possible surgical difficulties such as an obliterative footplate or dehiscence of the facial nerve.

Natural History
Although no perfect studies are available, the average air-bone gap typically deteriorates about 1 dB per year. This is in addition to a sensory hearing deterioration of another 1 dB per year. Clearly in many cases the deterioration is significantly quicker.

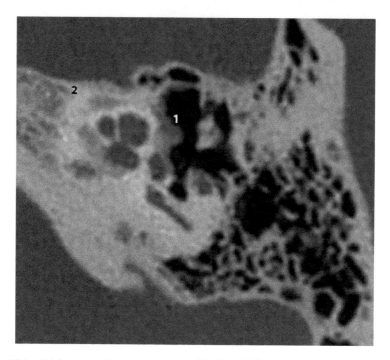

Figure 12.1   Axial computed tomography scan of the left middle ear through the stapes footplate showing lucency anterior to the stapes footplate (1) and around the cochlear (2).

Medical Management

Whilst oral fluoride has been proposed to prevent further deterioration in otosclerosis, the evidence for its use is debated and currently it is not used in the United Kingdom.

The use of bisphosphonates to prevent deterioration is in its infancy and studies show conflicting evidence on benefit. Future studies may show efficacy, but they are currently not used widely.

Hearing Aids

As most patients with otosclerosis have predominantly a conductive hearing loss, conventional hearing aids offer an excellent management option and should always be discussed with the patient. In patients with bilateral hearing loss opting for surgery a hearing aid should be offered for the non-operated ear.

Bone-Anchored Hearing Aids

Bone-anchored hearing aids are a useful method of hearing rehabilitation in patients who are unsuitable for conventional aids and who do not wish to have surgery.

Far Advanced Otosclerosis

Far advanced otosclerosis is defined as average hearing thresholds of over 85 dB with unmeasurable bone conduction. This can occur in patients with conductive hearing loss from otosclerosis combined with sensory hearing loss from ageing, cochlear otosclerosis, or any other cause of sensory loss. These patients are treated either with surgery and a hearing aid or by cochlear implantation. Most clinicians offer surgery and hearing aids in the first instance with cochlear implantation reserved for those who fail the first treatment option. Cochlear implantation in patients with otosclerosis may be challenging due to the presence of otosclerotic plaques obstructing the round window or narrowing of the basal turn of the scala tympani. In addition, facial nerve stimulation from the cochlear implant is more common due to abnormal current spread in the diseased otic capsule.

Controversies in Stapes Surgery

- *Age*: There is no age limit for stapes surgery and, as described above, in patients with severe mixed hearing loss stapedotomy may allow patients to use a hearing aid.
- *Flying after stapes surgery*: Whilst there are no absolute rules, most surgeons recommend not flying after stapes surgery for at least 2 weeks.
- *Scuba diving*: Most surgeons recommend at least a delay to returning to diving with 50% of surgeons recommending a lifelong ban on scuba diving.
- *Unilateral otosclerosis*: When considering surgery for patients with unilateral otosclerosis it is important to consider the chance of achieving symmetry of hearing after surgery. This means looking carefully at the bone conduction thresholds of the proposed ear. Patients need careful counselling on the likely outcomes of surgery for real-world binaural hearing.
- *Second-sided surgery*: Most stapes surgeons will happily operate on the second ear provided the first-side surgery was successful and the appropriate audiometric criteria for the second ear are met. It is prudent to delay the second-side surgery for at least 6 months.
- *Air-bone gap*: Traditionally a minimum average air-bone gap of 20 dB is felt to be a sensible threshold to justify surgery, although in some circumstances experienced surgeons may reduce this required level.

Consent for Surgery

As hearing aids give an excellent outcome for otosclerosis patients they should be offered to all patents. Those contemplating surgery should be aware of the risks. The risks are operator dependent and ideally surgeons should quote their own figures. Total sensory hearing loss is reported to be in the region of 0.4–2%. These dead ears can rarely occur immediately following surgery but more typically are reported as occurring within a week postoperatively and are frequently accompanied by severe rotational vertigo. The cause of such sensory loss is unclear but clearly represents a major insult to the inner ear. Intracochlear bleeding, infection, or perilymph fistulae are all possible causes. Unfortunately there is little evidence that revision surgery is helpful in these unfortunate cases. Most surgeons will give oral steroids and antibiotics. Reparative granuloma where granulation tissue forms around the stapes prosthesis and extends into the inner ear is a potential cause of sensory hearing loss, which was common when total stapedectomy was performed but fortunately is now extremely rare. Closure of the air-bone gap to within 10 dB is achievable in the range of 80% to the high 90%. Some distortion of hearing and discomfort with loud sounds may be reported but typically settles in the first few weeks after surgery. Alteration in taste due to damage to the chorda tympani occurs in up to 30% but in most cases lasts only a few months. Vertigo has become much less common with the move to small fenestra stapedotomy. When vertigo occurs it is usually in the immediate post-operative period and typically settles quickly. Benign positional vertigo presumably from the trauma of surgery is reported in the literature and can be treated with particle repositioning. Facial nerve injury is very rare; however, direct trauma is possible. A delayed facial paresis can occur as with any case of middle ear surgery. Whilst the aetiology of such delayed palsies is debated, they usually recover within 6 weeks.

Surgery

Stapedectomy was first described by John Shea in 1956. This involves removing the fixed stapes and placing a piston from the incus to the vestibule. The basic technique Shea described remains in place. However, refinements have taken place over the last 60 years, and the main modification of the technique is to perform a small stapedotomy rather than removing the whole stapes footplate. This has reduced the risk of total sensory hearing loss and probably improved high-frequency hearing results. There are many piston designs but with little to choose between them. A larger piston diameter should theoretically give better hearing, but the differences are small. Most surgeons use a piston with a diameter between 0.4 and 0.6 mm. There are a variety of methods of removing the stapes superstructure and performing the stapedotomy. Cutting the stapes crura with a laser reduces the risk of stapes dislocation when removing the superstructure. Many surgeons use a laser when performing the stapedotomy, but there is no good evidence to favour laser over microdrill or hand trephine. If the incus is eroded the piston can be secured using bone cement. If the residual incus long process is very short or dislocated a malleostapediopexy can be performed in which a piston is placed from the malleus handle to the stapedotomy. Whilst not as good as standard stapedotomy, excellent results can still be achieved with this technique.

Revision Stapes Surgery

This is usually performed when there is a significant post-operative conductive hearing loss, which may be immediate or come on at a later stage. The most common reasons are erosion of the long process of the incus, displaced prosthesis, too short prosthesis, dislocated incus, or incorrect diagnosis such as malleus head fixation. This surgery should only be performed by experienced stapes surgeons. A laser is very useful in revision surgery to divide soft tissue at the footplate.

KEY POINTS

- Otosclerosis is the presumptive diagnosis in an adult patient with a slow-onset conductive hearing impairment with the presence of a normal mobile tympanic membrane.
- Pre-operative CT scanning is useful in confirming the diagnosis and predicting possible surgical difficulties.
- Conventional hearing aids are effective in managing the hearing loss of otosclerosis.
- Stapedotomy is an effective treatment for the hearing loss and tinnitus of otosclerosis.

Further Reading

1. Browning GG, Gatehouse S. *The prevalence of middle ear disease in the adult British population Clin Otol* 1992; 17: 317–21).

13. BONE CONDUCTION AND MIDDLE EAR IMPLANTS

Some patients are unable to wear, cannot tolerate, or do not gain sufficient benefit from conventional air-conducting hearing aids (ACHAs). Depending on the severity of their hearing loss there are a number of other options. There are non-implantable solutions and implantable options that require surgery. Suitability for a hearing implant requires specialist assessment in one of the United Kingdom's designated hearing implant centres by a multidisciplinary team.

Bone-Conducting Hearing Devices

Due to the efficiency of transcranial transmission, bone-conducting hearing devices (BCHDs) deliver sound energy to both inner ears. Middle ear implants in contrast are ear specific, delivering sound only to the implanted side. There are three main pathways of transmission of bone-conducted sound:

- *Outer*: Down the ear canal transmitting energy to the tympanic membrane.
- *Middle*: Due to the relative inertia of the ossicles and skull, they decouple and cause relative movement.
- *Inner*: Directly through bone exerting inertial or compressive forces on the inner ear fluid.

BCHDs are either percutaneous (an abutment sticks out through the skin) or transcutaneous (the skin is intact). The systems are 'passive' if the vibration occurs within the external processor or 'active' if there is a vibrating component within the implant itself, for example, an internal vibrating actuator or amplification device. Passive transcutaneous devices are affected by skin/scalp attenuation of approximately 10–15 dB of sound energy. Transcranial attenuation is close to 0 dB for frequencies up to 700 Hz and increases with higher frequencies. Higher transcranial transmission is beneficial for patients with single-sided deafness (SSD) where the contralateral cochlea is being stimulated. Lower transcranial transmission is better for binaural cues.

Patient Selection
Candidates
NHS England published commissioning guidelines in 2016.[1] Funding would be considered for the following:

1a Patients with unilateral or bilateral conductive or mixed hearing loss within the manufacturer's fitting criteria

AND

Stable bone conduction (BC) thresholds (<15-dB deterioration in >2 frequencies in a 2-year period)

OR

1b Unilateral sensorineural hearing impairment (including SSD) where the better ear has BC hearing thresholds within the manufacturer's fitting criteria

AND

2 The patient has trialed an ACHA or wireless contralateral routing of sound (CROS)/BiCROS hearing aid for a minimum of 4 weeks, or is anatomically or physiologically unable to undertake a trial of an ACHA

AND

3 Has trialed a BCHD on a headband for a minimum of 14 days and shown benefit in speech tests.

Bone-conducting implants will **not** be commissioned for patients with:

- Bone that is unable to support an implant, e.g. osteoradionecrosis
- Sensitivity or allergy to the materials used (silicone or titanium)
- Physical, emotional, or psychological disorders that, despite suitable treatment and support, would mean significant benefit would be unlikely

Clinical Indications
Conductive and mixed losses are caused by the following:

- Congenital causes such as microtia or atresia
- Acquired causes such as chronic suppurative otitis media, recurrent otitis externa, or ossicular pathology

SSD – sensorineural or severe to profound mixed loss – can be caused by the following:

- Congenital
- Trauma or surgery resulting in hearing loss
- Unsuitable ear canal for a conventional hearing aid and insufficient ipsilateral BC, e.g. radical mastoid cavity, narrow ear canal, or 'blind sac' ear canal closure

Devices
Non-Implantable Solutions

Non-implantable solutions may be indicated for children that are too young for an implant (insufficient skull thickness), as trial devices for patients to gain an understanding of how they would benefit from an implantable solution, and for patients that are not willing to commit to surgical intervention. Devices include the Contact Mini on a Softband, Cochlear Baha 5 Processor or Oticon Ponto 4 Processor on a Softband, MED-EL ADHEAR, Cochlear SoundArc (with Baha 5 processor).

Implantable Solutions

Percutaneous solutions can deliver more power and are therefore suitable for patients with worse hearing levels. Transcutaneous active solutions have more power than transcutaneous passive devices and deliver more gain in the higher frequencies (Table 13.1).

In 2005 an international consensus recommended that BCHD surgery not be undertaken prior to age 2–3 years. This was to allow the skull to reach a sufficient thickness and allow osseointegration. A skin thickness of at least 3 mm is required for Baha Attract to minimise problems with pressure sensitivity from the magnetic attachment. It is, however, important to stimulate hearing as early as possible; therefore in children too young for implantation the use of a BCHD via a Softband is advocated as soon as possible after birth in bilateral cases and around 3 months for unilateral patients.

Percutaneous bone-anchored hearing implant surgery in children can be staged in an attempt to reduce the failure rate in patients with thinner skull bone or developmental/behavioural issues that may predispose them to trauma to the abutment before the implant has osseointegrated.

Table 13.1   Implantable BCHD

Device	Stimulation	BC requirement	SSD CL ear BC	MRI strength
Cochlear Baha Connect	Percutaneous	Up to 65 dB	≤20 dB	Up to 3.0 T
Baha 5				
Baha 5 power				
Baha 5 Superpower				
Oticon Ponto	Percutaneous	Up to 45 dB	≤20 dB	Up to 3.0 T
Ponto 4 Pro				
Pro Power		Up to 55 dB		
Superpower		Up to 65 dB		
Cochlear Baha Attract	Transcutaneous – passive	Greatest benefit up to 25 dB		Up to 1.5 T (without magnet removal)
MED-EL Bonebridge	Transcutaneous – active	Up to 45 dB	≤20 dB	Up to 1.5 T
Cochlear Osia	Transcutaneous – active	TBC	≤20 dB	TBC

Note: BC, bone conduction; CL, contralateral; dB, decibel; MRI, magnetic resonance imaging; SSD, single-sided deafness; T, tesla; TBC, to be confirmed once CE approved.

Traditionally in children a longer time period before loading the sound processor has been recommended to allow more time for osseointegration and to compensate for thinner bone. We load the processor anytime from 4 weeks after the surgery depending on healing at the abutment site, patient factors that may predispose to trauma, and bone quality at the time of surgery. A number of studies in adults have shown that loading at 3 weeks is safe, well tolerated, and does not cause a reduction in stability of the implant/abutment with time.

Surgery

Percutaneous surgery can be carried out through a linear incision or a minimally invasive technique (Figure 13.1). Skin thickness is measured to enable the appropriate choice of abutment length. A hole is drilled in the skull and then widened/finished with a 'countersink' burr. The combined implant abutment is then screwed into the skull hole to a specified tightness (measured with a torque wrench). For Baha Attract surgery the technique is similar to open percutaneous surgery. The same implant/screw that osseointegrates into the skull is used, but the BIM400 implant magnet is attached to the screw rather than an abutment (Figure 13.2). In Bonebridge surgery the implant is embedded and screwed into the skull in an appropriate position behind the ear.

Complications

Skin problems including inflammation, skin overgrowth, and infection occur in up to 10% of patients. Fixture loss can occur in up to 14% of children over 15 years. The linear incision technique and the minimally invasive Ponto surgery (MIPS) technique have significantly reduced rates of localised skin problems with percutaneous devices.

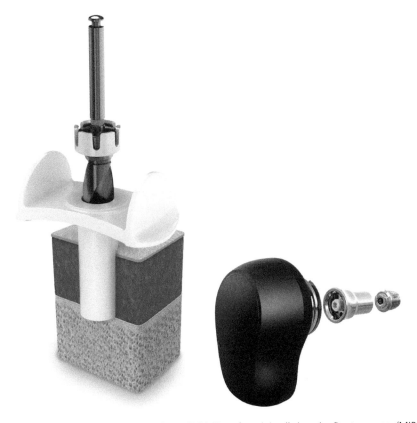

Figure 13.1   Oticon Ponto. (A) Cannula and initial burr for minimally invasive Ponto surgery (MIPS). (B) Ponto 4 processor, abutment. and implant. (Images courtesy Oticon Medical.)

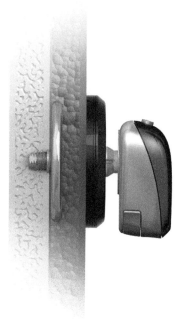

Figure 13.2   Baha Attract. Implant and magnet, external magnet, and Baha 5 processor. (Image courtesy Cochlear Bone Anchored Solutions AB, © 2020.)

Outcomes

Data from systematic reviews of bone-anchored hearing aids (BAHAs) have shown implant survival of 98% and that major complications are very rare. There is improvement in quality of life when measured with the Glasgow Benefit Inventory. Audiological benefits are evident in quiet and in noise as well as for sound localisation.

A 2017 study showed no difference in performance between CROS hearing aids and BAHAs when comparing speech-in-noise and localisation. When CROS aids were initially used by SSD patients, complaints of occlusion in the better ear, poor sound quality, and discomfort reduced uptake. Improvements in hearing aid processor technology mean that CROS aiding provides a more cost-effective, non-invasive solution that is satisfactory for some SSD patients.

Studies comparing unilateral with bilateral BAHAs suggested benefits of bilateral BAHAs in many, but not all, situations.

KEY POINTS

- BCHDs are used for the rehabilitation of hearing loss when conventional acoustic aids cannot be fitted or have been trialed and have failed to improve the hearing.
- Numerous devices are now available, and fitting criteria have expanded up to 65 dB BC on the ipsilateral side for percutaneous devices.
- Non-implantable options enable a thorough trial and/or allow time for children to develop sufficient skull and scalp thickness prior to an implantable solution.

When the hearing thresholds are too poor to enable sufficient benefit with a bone-anchored device or ear-specific stimulation is preferred, a middle ear implant may be possible.

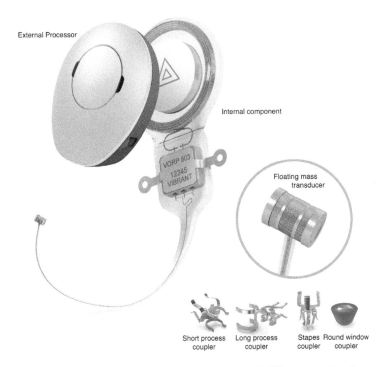

External Processor

Internal component

VORP 503
12345
VIBRANT

Floating mass
transducer

Short process | Long process | Stapes | Round window
coupler | coupler | coupler | coupler

Figure 13.3   Vibrant Sound Bridge System showing implant and different couplers. (Images courtesy MED-EL.)

Middle Ear Implants

Active middle ear implants (AMEIs) are implantable hearing devices that have been developed with the aim of overcoming a number of shortcomings associated with ACHAs, such as distortion, feedback, occlusion effect, discomfort, and ear canal irritation. In some cases, they may also offer the potential for improved sound clarity. All AMEIs utilise a transducer that is coupled to the ossicular chain or inner ear fluid compartment. These devices utilise either an electromagnetic (a coil and magnet) or piezoelectric mode of transmission to drive the ossicles.

The most widely used AMEIs to date are the Vibrant Soundbridge (VSB; MED-EL, Innsbruck, Austria) (Figure 13.3) and the Carina system (Cochlear Ltd, Sydney, Australia), both of which are electromagnetic devices. The VSB is a semi-implantable AMEI (i.e. an implanted internal component and an external audio-processor), whilst the Carina system may be fully implantable (i.e. a subcutaneous microphone, battery, and an electronic receiver connected to a transducer) or used with an external audio-processor. The Carina device has, however, recently been withdrawn from the market.

Patient Selection
Candidates
AMEIs may be an option for adults and children aged 5 years and older with sensorineural, conductive, or mixed hearing loss who are not able to tolerate or benefit from ACHAs or BCHDs. Candidates should not have any skin conditions that may prevent attachment of any external component of the device and should have realistic expectations of outcomes.

Audiological
Current devices are most suitable for mild to severe sensorineural hearing loss (SNHL). More recently, with the application of various couplers, indications have expanded to include patients with moderate-to-severe conductive or mixed hearing loss secondary to, for example, sequelae of chronic otitis media, advanced otosclerosis, and congenital external/middle

ear malformations. In cases of conductive or mixed hearing loss, the main objective of AMEI placement is to raise sound-field thresholds above the residual sensorineural component. Hearing loss should ideally be stable, although very slowly progressive loss may still be considered in some cases.

Audiological assessment includes pure-tone audiometry, tympanometry, and speech perception (e.g. Arthur Boothroyd [AB] word lists) in the best-aided condition to evaluate any retrocochlear loss. In general, there should be no retrocochlear or central element in the hearing loss. The worse hearing ear is usually selected for implantation.

With the VSB, the maximum air-conduction thresholds stated by the manufacturer are 65–85 dB HL for candidates with SNHL, whilst those with mixed hearing loss should have BC thresholds better than 45–65 dB HL (frequency range 0.5–6 kHz). However, clinicians should proceed with caution when assessing candidates with hearing thresholds close to the upper limits of these fitting ranges and counsel carefully with regard to potentially inadequate functional gain from the device.

Surgery

Active middle ear disease should be addressed prior to implantation. In some cases, blind sac closure may be necessary; whether or not AMEI surgery is performed simultaneously or as a staged procedure depends on the assessment by the surgeon of the potential risk of infection in each individual patient. Accurate clinical and radiological evaluation is crucial in determining the optimal site for transducer placement, which may be the incus, stapes superstructure/footplate, or round window.

The surgical approach for AMEI is similar to cochlear implantation (CI). In general, a post-auricular transmastoid route is utilised to access the middle ear via the facial recess or attic. A combined transmastoid/transmeatal approach may be required to gain sufficient access to the middle ear, depending on the device and transducer placement.

Complications

The potential complications of AMEI implantation are similar to that for mastoid surgery (see Chapter 10). Patients should also be warned about the possibility of transducer displacement, extrusion, device malfunction/failure, aural fullness, and insufficient benefit.

Outcomes

Overall and in experienced hands, AMEIs are considered a safe alternative when ACHAs or BCHDs are not suitable. Optimal coupling, be it to the incus, stapes, or round window, is of great importance for good audiological outcomes. Although currently available evidence is somewhat limited and sometimes contradicting, AMEIs appear to have a functional gain at least as good as, if not better than, ACHAs. In general, patients have reported a significant benefit with all current AMEIs in terms of sound quality, ease of communication, reverberation, and listening in background noise compared with the unaided situation.

KEY POINTS

- AMEIs are classically indicated for patients with mild-to-severe SNHL who are not able to tolerate or benefit from other hearing devices.

The indications have expanded to include moderate-to-severe conductive or mixed hearing loss through coupling of the transducer to one of the ossicles or cochlear windows.

Further Reading

1. *NHS England.* Clinical Commissioning Policy: Bone conducting hearing implants (BCHIs) for hearing loss (all ages). *Reference: NHS England: 16041/P. July 2016. Available online https://www.england.nhs.uk/commissioning/wp-content/uploads/sites/ 12/2013/05/16041_FINAL.pdf*

14. SENSORINEURAL HEARING LOSS

Introduction

Sensorineural hearing loss (SNHL) is hearing impairment resulting from damage to the cochlear hair cells and/or impairment of the sensory nerve fibres of the inner ear. An audiogram will show reduction in the bone-conduction thresholds. Several processes can cause such HL as summarised in Table 14.1.

Patient Assessment

Patients may describe hearing loss, or a feeling of blockage or fullness. There is often difficulty with hearing conversation in the presence of background or competing sound. If the hearing deficit is mild, patients may describe a lack of clarity rather than a loss of volume representing impaired discrimination. Recruitment (an abnormal increase in loudness perception between the detection level and maximum comfort level of sound) may also be described. HL may lead to social isolation, depression, and cognitive decline, particularly in elderly populations.

Table 14.1   Causes of sensorineural hearing loss

Degenerative	Age-related hearing loss
Genetic	Syndromic
	Non-syndromic
Toxic	See Table 14.2
Infectious	Meningococcal meningitis
	Encephalitis
	Herpes virus (simplex, zoster, varicella, cytomegalovirus)
	Measles
	Lyme disease
	Rubella
	Syphilis
Traumatic	Barotrauma
	Perilymph fistula
	Intense noise exposure
	Temporal bone fracture
	Ear surgery
	Blast injury
Neoplastic	Cerebellopontine angle tumours, e.g. acoustic neuroma, meningioma
Autoimmune	Granulomatosis with polyangiitis
	Rheumatoid arthritis
	Lupus erythematosus
	Cogan's syndrome
	Sarcoid
Neurologic	Multiple sclerosis
	Migraine
Other	Idiopathic
	Meniere's disease
	Microvascular disease

The main aim in evaluating a patient with SNHL is to identify any treatable causes, and the provision of supportive treatment. The speed of onset of symptoms, laterality, and accompanying otological symptoms should be questioned. Previous otological conditions or surgery, a history of trauma (including barotrauma), or intense noise exposure as well as a recent viral infection may help to identify a cause. A full drug history, particularly aminoglycosides and chemotherapy, is important in considering ototoxicity. A strong family history of early-onset HL (before the age of 40) may indicate a genetic cause.

Examination should include otoscopy, tuning fork tests, cranial nerve examination, and audiometry. Speech testing can help determine the impact of the HL. A magnetic resonance imaging (MRI) scan of the internal auditory meatus should be performed in cases of asymmetrical HL (asymmetry on pure-tone audiometry of 15 dB or more at any two adjacent test frequencies, using test frequencies of 0.5, 1, 2, 4, and 8 kHz; NICE 2020) to exclude a vestibular schwannoma or other intracranial pathology. Blood testing may be helpful to exclude an autoimmune or infective cause.

General Management of Sensorineural Hearing Loss

Guidance should be given to patients to optimise their acoustic environment, and they should be offered psychological counseling if their HL is having a negative impact on their mood. Management may include provision of hearing aids/auditory implants, auditory rehabilitation, and the use of hearing assistance technology (see Chapter 17).

Specific Conditions

Sudden Sensorineural Hearing Loss (SSNHL)

Sudden sensorineural hearing loss (SSNHL) is defined as HL of rapid onset of ≥30 dB over greater than three consecutive frequencies developing over ≤72 hours with a subjective sensation of hearing impairment. The majority of cases are idiopathic, with a cause identified in only 5–10% of cases. Routine laboratory testing is not advised, although one might consider specific blood tests (e.g. Lyme disease serology, autoantibodies, etc.) depending on the clinical history. The possible causes of 'idiopathic' cases include labyrinthine viral infection, vascular insult, intracochlear membrane rupture, and autoimmune inner ear disease. However, epidemiological, serological, and histopathological evidence to support these theories are inconclusive. In general, the shorter the history the better the prognosis. Age >60 years, the presence of vertigo, and a more severe HL with a down-sloping audiogram are all features associated with a poorer prognosis. Spontaneous recovery occurs in 32–65% of cases, typically within 2–6 weeks, even without treatment. Evidence is poor for the various proposed treatments due to the combination of low incidence and high spontaneous recovery rate. Studies using agents other than those detailed below, including antivirals, do not offer any significant benefit.

Specific Management

Steroids

Oral steroids are the standard treatment of SSNHL despite systematic reviews and meta-analyses revealing limited evidence of benefit. Treatment started within 2 weeks of onset is associated with the greatest hearing recovery; there is minimal benefit after 4–6 weeks. A 10- to 14-day course of once-daily oral prednisolone (1 mg/kg [maximum 60 mg]) is associated with better outcomes.

Intratympanic (IT) steroid therapy results in higher inner ear steroid levels than oral therapy. The main advantage is a reduction in systemic side effects; therefore, it can be valuable in diabetics or patients who cannot take systemic corticosteroids. Dexamethasone and methylprednisolone sodium succinate are the most frequently used preparations. There is no evidence on which steroid is superior; however, better hearing outcomes have been associated with higher doses and the cumulative effect of multiple administrations. Commonly this is administered via a grommet or injected intratympanically under local anaesthetic with the patient lying in a supine position and the injected ear facing towards the ceiling for approximately 30 minutes to facilitate diffusion of the drug across the round window membrane. Diffusion across the round window membrane is variable and leads to unpredictable intracochlear bioavailability. Risks of IT administration include pain, dizziness, and persistent tympanic membrane perforation at the site of injection. No comparative trials have shown superiority of primary IT steroid therapy over oral steroids with respect to hearing outcomes; however, combination therapy has been shown to improve overall hearing compared with oral treatment alone.

Hyperbaric Oxygen Therapy (HBOT)

Hyperbaric oxygen therapy (HBOT) delivers 100% oxygen at >1 atm pressure resulting in increased tissue oxygenation and aids the response to infection and ischaemia. Complications of treatment are rare but include barotrauma to ears, sinuses, and lungs; temporary worsening of short-sightedness; claustrophobia; and oxygen poisoning. It is an expensive and time-consuming treatment given over days or weeks and is not widely available. However, some benefit has been shown when initiated within 3 months of the onset of HL; the benefit is potentially greater in cases of severe to profound HL. Studies have shown some benefit of both IT steroids and HBOT as salvage therapies for refractory SSNHL.

Noise-Induced Hearing Loss (NIHL)

The effect of noise exposure on individuals is highly variable. Sound levels <80 dB(A) at any length of exposure will not cause damage to the human ear. Sounds ≥130 dB(A) will definitely cause damage, even if the exposure time is short. Between these levels, the 'safe' period of exposure decreases as the sound level increases, in a logarithmic fashion. Doubling the sound intensity (3-dB increase) effectively 'doubles the noise dose', which means exposure is only safe for half the time period. This is described as the 'equal energy principle'. It only applies approximately in animal experiments.

Initially, excessive noise exposure causes a temporary threshold shift (TTS), resulting in a temporary HL. The high-frequency regions of the cochlea are most sensitive (between 3 and 6 kHz). Recovery of the TTS occurs over hours, days, or weeks following exposure. Expected recovery time is dependent on the loudness and duration of the noise presented. However, a permanent threshold shift (PTS) can occur at the initial insult, or it may evolve where there is continuous or repeated excessive noise exposure at levels that would only have otherwise caused a TTS. It is thought that this may be caused by metabolic factors such as excessive neurotransmitter release, changes in cochlear blood flow, and oxidative stress within the hair cells. Structural factors like depolymerisation of actin filaments in the stereocilia, swelling of the stria vascularis, and damage to afferent nerve endings and supporting cells are also thought to play a part. Synaptic connections between inner hair cells and spiral ganglion cells may also be susceptible to noise damage. Importantly, in animal studies, these synapses can be the first site of damage, even without an HL ('hidden hearing loss', or synaptopathy). Additionally, genetic susceptibility, smoking and cardiovascular disease, and diabetes have been implicated as risk factors.

Patients present with symptoms of HL and tinnitus alongside a history of excessive noise exposure, which may be occupational or recreational. It is more common in men. Hyperacusis may be a feature causing accompanying distress and impaired social functioning. Acoustic shock is a particular subgroup of noise-induced hearing loss (NIHL). It appears more often in women, particularly in call centres, and occurs after exposure to a brief but unexpected loud and unpleasant sound. Acoustic shock appears to cause high levels of psychological distress associated with symptoms of hyperacusis, otalgia, tinnitus, and imbalance. Objective HL is rare.

When assessing a patient with NIHL, volunteered post-exposure tinnitus suggests that TTS was present. It is important to detail all potential sources of noise exposure, typical noise levels and periods of exposure, and any hearing protection used. A high-tone HL with a notch at 3/4/6 kHz may be present, but it may not be obvious and it is not diagnostic. Significant asymmetrical thresholds may be present in military personnel due to the shadow effect from the head when using shoulder-borne weapons.

The main aim in (medicolegal) assessment is to separate the effects of ageing and any other idiopathic or degenerative component from that of the noise exposure. Standardised reference tables provide hearing thresholds at various ages for typical screened and unscreened populations. Comparing the patients' (or claimants') hearing thresholds against expected 'average' values for age-related and idiopathic causes should allow an estimate of any excess HL caused by noise exposure.

Specific Management

NIHL is a preventable health condition. Employers have a statutory duty under the Health and Safety Work Act 1974 to minimise risks to employees from excessive noise exposure. The Noise at Work Regulations 1989 were superseded by the European Control of Noise at Work Regulations 2005 to describe action levels at 80 and 85 dB(A) for daily personal noise exposure, and a peak action level of 135 dB(A). At these levels, the employer has a responsibility to conduct noise surveys and provide employees with hearing protection as well as regular hearing assessments and a programme of employee education. These actions are compulsory when noise levels reach ≥85 dB(A). Personal hearing protection can be in the form of earplugs or earmuffs; earmuffs are more reliable. Electronic active noise reduction (ANR) systems are effective but expensive and are most commonly used in military and aircraft environments.

Age-Related Hearing Loss

Age-related hearing loss (ARHL) is a progressive, bilateral, sensorineural hearing impairment of mid to late adult onset (typically starting between the ages of 40 and 60 years) in the absence of any other cause of HL. Once hearing thresholds have deteriorated to approximately 75–80 dB HL, further progression appears to be slow.

ARHL is associated with male gender. There is likely to be a significant genetic association, and recent gene-mapping studies have identified new and previously unrecognised genetic loci that are relevant to ARHL. Noise exposure, smoking, alcohol consumption, hypertension, blood hyperviscosity, and cardiovascular and cerebrovascular disease have all been suggested as possible contributory factors in developing ARHL.

Other degenerative processes in the central nervous system such as reduced neuronal plasticity, loss of cognitive abilities, and loss of other sensory modalities, particularly vision, can massively increase the impact of HL in the elderly. This also explains why the elderly often require a long acclimatisation period to obtain maximum benefit from hearing rehabilitation and aids. ARHL is associated with cognitive impairment including dementia, depression, and an increased incidence of falls. It has been recognised as one of the most significant of a number of modifiable risk factors active in the development of dementia. Early recognition of the need for, and encouraging the use of, hearing aids may in turn reduce the development of these psychosocial comorbidities.

Most commonly the audiogram shows an HL which tends to be worse at the higher frequencies. In an individual over the age of 60, with normal examination findings and a symmetrical (often predominantly high-tone) HL, a diagnosis of ARHL is fairly secure. However, in younger patients, a diagnosis of genetic, 'non-syndromic' HL should be considered.

Genetic Hearing Loss

Non-syndromic SNHL accounts for approximately 70% of genetic SNHL cases. The remaining 30% are recognised as being part of a syndrome. The inheritance pattern can be autosomal dominant, recessive, X-linked, or mitochondrial. A genetic HL may be recognised when it is observed that several generations of family members have been affected. However, de novo mutation or, a reduced penetrance inheritance pattern, may cause a singleton case. Linkage analysis combined with whole genome/exome sequence analysis enables the identification of novel genes and pathways causing inherited SNHL. To date more than 60 loci for genes causing HL have been mapped, but only just over half of the specific genes have been identified.

The audiometric pattern observed in genetic HL can vary. Some mutations result in a low-frequency HL, whereas others result in a steeply down-sloping HL involving the high frequencies. A 'U-shaped' or 'cookie-bite' audiogram is caused by an HL affecting the mid-frequencies. Although some SNHL loci are associated with particular audiometric patterns or clinical presentations, there is marked variability: the age of onset of HL, progression, and audiometric configuration can vary between individuals even within one family, making distinction between genetic causes difficult. Achieving a molecular genetic diagnosis through genetic testing may help to predict the progress of HL and guide genetic counselling. This is likely to be a more rewarding process in familial clusters rather than isolated singleton cases.

Ototoxicity

Table 14.2 summarises known ototoxic agents and their mechanisms of action. These agents enter the inner ear through various mechanisms where they can cause damage. Entry is predominantly via the blood supply into the perilymph, although the precise mechanism of diffusion across this blood-perilymph barrier is unknown. Endolymph can be accessed via perilymph through selectively permeable membranes and tight junctions between adjacent cells. Diffusion can also occur via the round and oval windows from the middle ear. Any hearing deficit caused by hair cell loss is usually permanent as the organ of Corti cannot spontaneously regenerate hair cells

Temporary Hearing Loss

Agents affecting ion transport across epithelia, such as loop diuretics, cause oedema of the stria vascularis. This alters the endolymph composition, resulting in a reduction in endocochlear potential (EP) leading to a TTS associated with a pan-frequency HL. The effects are completely reversible once administration is stopped, although this may take several days.

When administered in high doses (i.e. 2–5 g/day), salicylates penetrate the blood-perilymph barrier easily and inhibit the activity of outer hair cells (OHCs). The degree of HL is directly proportional to the serum and perilymph drug concentration. Quinines and their derivatives can act as nicotinic acetylcholine receptor antagonists, disrupting synaptic transmission on inner and outer hair cells and/or spiral ganglion neurons. Vestibular hair cells may be affected too, resulting in vertiginous symptoms.

Permanent Hearing Loss and Balance

Aminoglycosides

All aminoglycosides are potentially both cochleo- and vestibulo-toxic, but they vary in their site of maximal effect, for reasons unknown.

Within the inner ear, aminoglycosides specifically target hair cells blocking the mechano-transduction channels at the tips of stereocilia. Apoptosis occurs once a certain concentration of the drug has been reached within the cell. Reactive oxygen free radical production may also play a role. OHC loss occurs first; inner hair cells are relatively spared but can be lost later. Subsequently, the spiral ganglion neurons that supply afferent innervation to the hair cells are lost.

In the vestibule hair cell loss occurs first in the central epithelia of the utricular and saccular maculae, before spreading towards the peripheries.

Toxic effects usually appear after repeated systemic treatment, although even a single topical application to the middle ear cavity can initiate damage. The damage progresses even after administration has ceased and symptoms may not present until after the patient has completed a course of the offending drug. It must be stressed that vestibular symptoms with clinically used drugs such as gentamicin precede HL effects, and should be sought first. Bilateral vestibular damage results in oscillopsia and severe unsteadiness that is worse in the dark. Hearing impairment initially occurs in the high frequencies and progresses to include successively lower frequencies.

Table 14.2   The effects of medication on sensorineural hearing loss

Classification	Compounds	Mechanism of action and notes
Aminoglycoside antibiotics	Most cochleotoxic = neomycin, followed by gentamicin, kanamycin, and tobramycin Least cochleotoxic = amikacin and netilmicin Most vestibulotoxic = streptomycin and gentamicin	Blockade of mechano-transduction channels at stereocilia tips, apoptosis of hair cells, and production of reactive oxygen free radicals Mutations in the gene that encodes 12s ribosomal mitochondrial DNA, including the 'A1555G' mutation (prevalence 0.19–1% prevalence) severely increases cochlear but not vestibular susceptibility to aminoglycoside toxicity Impaired renal function increases susceptibility to damage
Loop diuretics	Bumetanide, ethacrynic acid, frusemide (furosemide), piretanide	Disrupt ion transport across epithelia within the inner ear, resulting in oedema of stria vascularis and reversible TTS and pan-frequency hearing loss Effects are reversible once administration is stopped, although it may take several days
Macrolide antibiotics	Erythromycin, azithromycin, clarithromycin	Similar to that of loop diuretics
Other antibiotics	Ampicillin, capreomycin, chloramphenicol, colistin (polymyxin E), minocycline, polymyxin B, rifampicin, vancomycin, viomycin	Specific mechanism unknown
Antitumor agents	Cisplatin (cis-platinum), carboplatin, oxaliplatin (carboplatin and oxaliplatin are less ototoxic than cisplatin)	Similar to that of aminoglycosides, but has additional effects on spiral ganglion cells and causes atrophy of stria vascularis
	Actinomycin, bleomycin, nitrogen mustards (e.g. mustine), misonidazole	
Anti-inflammatory agents	Salicylate (aspirin)	Direct inhibition of OHCs causes reversible TTS
	Fenoprofen, ibuprofen, indomethacin, naproxen, phenylbutazone,	
Antimalarials	Quinine, chloroquine	Nicotinic acetylcholine receptor antagonism causing disruption of synaptic transmission within inner ear cells and reversible TTS May also cause vertigo
Iron chelators	Desferrioxamine	Specific mechanism unknown
Beta blockers	Practolol, propranolol	Specific mechanism unknown
Contraceptives	Medroxyprogesterone	Specific mechanism unknown
Industrial chemicals	Trimethyltin, toluene, trichloroethylene, styrene, xylene	Loss of OHCs with predilection for middle and apical turns of cochlea

Note: OHC, outer hair cell; TTS, temporary threshold shift.

The dose, drug, route, and duration of administration can influence the degree of impairment. Standard dosing safe levels are not calibrated for vestibular toxicity. Impaired renal function increases susceptibility to damage. Mutations in the gene that encodes 12s ribosomal mitochondrial DNA, including the 'A1555G' mutation (adenosine to guanosine substitution at base position 1555), severely increases cochlear but not vestibular susceptibility to aminoglycoside toxicity. Estimates of the prevalence of A1555G mutation vary from 0.19 to 1% in different ethnic populations, with a carrier rate of 17%.

Cisplatin

A degree of hearing impairment affects >60% of patients treated with current protocols of cisplatin. HL is bilateral, first in the extended high frequencies then progresses with cumulative doses into the speech frequencies. HL can progress after administration has stopped, possibly due to prolonged retention of platinum in the body. The pattern of cochlear hair cell damage greatly resembles that of aminoglycosides, although vestibular hair cells are relatively spared. Cisplatin additionally affects the spiral ganglion cells, causes atrophy of the stria vascularis, and increases the susceptibility to NIHL for several years after treatment has finished.

There are many proposed systems for monitoring hearing during platinum chemotherapy treatment, though adherence is sparse. The minimum requirement (adults) is for a baseline audiogram, retest if complaint of HL arises, and exit audiometry. In children more regular age-appropriate testing is required during treatment. Detection of HL is increased with more frequent testing and when extended high-frequency audiometry (10–16 kHz) is used.

KEY POINTS

- Approximately 50% of idiopathic SSNHL cases will improve spontaneously; oral or IT steroids have limited conclusive evidence of efficacy, but if used should be initiated as soon as possible.
- In the assessment of NIHL one must consider the individual contributions of age and idiopathic and noise-related components that can result in HL.
- AHRL is inevitable, and it can be associated with increased social isolation and impaired cognitive functioning.
- An underlying genetic cause should be considered in younger patients presenting with bilateral SNHL.
- Ototoxic agents exert their effect on the inner ear via different pathways to cause disruption of the EP and damage and apoptosis of hair cells and spiral ganglion cells.
- The mainstay of assessment of SNHL is to identify any potentially reversible causes. The general treatment is with hearing amplification and specific therapy for any accompanying physical or psychosocial symptoms.

15. TINNITUS AND HYPERACUSIS

Definitions and Classification

Tinnitus is defined as the conscious perception of an auditory sensation in the absence of a corresponding external stimulus. Most tinnitus comprises simple sounds like whistling, buzzing, humming, or ringing, but more complex sounds such as distant voices or even music are occasionally reported. Somatosensory tinnitus is a subtype in which the percept can be altered by physical contact or movement, particularly of the cervical spine or jaw. Some tinnitus has a rhythmical nature, which may be synchronous with the heartbeat in which case it is defined as pulsatile tinnitus (Table 15.1) and a vascular origin is

Table 15.1 Pathological causes of pulsatile tinnitus

Type of pathology	Specific pathology
Vascular	Atherosclerotic carotid artery disease
Arterial	Arteriovenous fistula
	Arteriovenous malformation
	Intracranial aneurysm
	Dissection of the carotid artery
Venous	Jugular bulb abnormalities
	Dural venous sinus stenosis
	Abnormal condylar or mastoid emissary veins
Microvascular	Glomus tumour
	Meningioma of middle ear
	Cavernous haemangioma
Circulatory	Increased cardiac output (anaemia, thyrotoxicosis, pregnancy)
	Aortic murmurs
Perceptual	Conductive hearing loss
Other	Idiopathic intracranial hypertension
	Superior semicircular canal dehiscence syndrome

likely. Pulse-asynchronous rhythmical tinnitus may have an underlying muscular origin, arising from myoclonus of palatal or intratympanic muscles. Most tinnitus is subjective in that it can only be detected by the affected person. Occasionally, particularly with some types of rhythmical tinnitus, it is possible for others to hear a sound and in this case the tinnitus is objective. Disorders of sound tolerance are subdivided: hyperacusis is dislike of all sounds above a certain intensity; misophonia is dislike of particular sounds, irrespective of the level of those sounds; and phonophobia is fear of particular sounds. Confusingly, hyperacusis is also used as an umbrella term for all disorders of sound tolerance.

Epidemiology

Estimates of tinnitus prevalence vary from 5.1–42.7% but a large UK study suggested a point prevalence of 10.1% in adults. Approximately 1 in 30 adults have tinnitus that is moderately annoying and 1 in 200 have tinnitus that severely affects their ability to lead a normal life. Prevalence increases with age up to the seventh decade of life: some studies show the prevalence continuing to increase thereafter, whereas others show it plateauing or even dropping. Tinnitus prevalence is similar in men and women. Children are less likely than adults to volunteer that they have tinnitus but when asked directly, the prevalence is not dissimilar to that in adults. Tinnitus is more common in people with hearing loss, but the degree of hearing loss corresponds poorly with the severity of tinnitus. About 1 in 10 people with tinnitus have normal hearing as measured by pure-tone audiometry and conversely, tinnitus can also exist after division of the auditory nerve. There are few longitudinal studies of tinnitus, but those that are available suggest that for most people the natural history is for tinnitus to become less intrusive with time. The prevalence of hyperacusis is unclear.

Pathophysiology

There are multiple theories regarding the underlying cause of tinnitus and it is possible that there are multiple mechanisms. It is suggested that tinnitus emergence is a two-stage process: an initial trigger, which may be in the peripheral or central auditory systems, or even from parts of the brain outside the classical auditory pathways. This is followed by changes in the central auditory system and associated non-auditory areas of the brain, particularly areas involved with emotion and arousal, resulting in the persistence and distress of the symptom. Mechanisms that have been proposed include reorganisation of the brain's tonotopic map following deafferentation, increased spontaneous neuronal firing, increased neuronal synchrony, failure of inhibitory pathways, or errors of predictive coding. The initial trigger can be any form of hearing loss including noise-induced hearing loss, presbycusis, or sensorineural loss secondary to administration of ototoxic drugs. Many patients, however, report that their hearing did not change; instead, they feel that the trigger was a life event such as a bereavement or financial worry. Other triggers that have been suggested are somatosensory triggers such as temporomandibular joint dysfunction.

Associations
Tinnitus is part of the symptom complex in Meniere's disease, otosclerosis, and vestibular schwannoma. Tinnitus and disorders of sound tolerance are frequently comorbid. Tinnitus may be associated with psychological illness, particularly anxiety and depression.

Clinical Assessment
A tinnitus patient should have a detailed neurotological history taken. The character of the tinnitus should be assessed to ascertain whether it is pulsatile or non-pulsatile. Evaluating the impact of the symptom should include questions on mood, sleep, and concentration. Examination is often normal, but it is important to exclude specific neurotological pathologies. With rhythmical tinnitus, auscultation of the head and neck should be performed. If pulsatile tinnitus diminishes with compression of the ipsilateral jugular vein, this points to a venous cause. With pulse-asynchronous pulsatile tinnitus, the pharynx should be checked for myoclonic contractions.

Investigations

Audiometry
Pure-tone audiometry should be conducted and, as many people with tinnitus report that their ears feel full or blocked, tympanometry is useful. Specialist long time-base tympanometry may be helpful in reaching a diagnosis of middle ear myoclonus. Trying to audiometrically match the pitch and tone of tinnitus is difficult, adds little to the subsequent management, and is unnecessary in most cases.

Imaging
For non-pulsatile tinnitus, magnetic resonance imaging (MRI) scanning should be considered if the tinnitus is unilateral, associated with a significantly asymmetric audiogram (asymmetry on pure-tone audiometry of 15 dB or more at any two adjacent test frequencies, using test frequencies of 0.5, 1, 2, 4, and 8 kHz; NICE 2020) or if there are abnormal neurological symptoms or signs. Investigating pulsatile tinnitus is more complex and depends in part on local expertise and availability. Investigative algorithms may include MRI, MR angiography, computed tomography (CT), CT angiography or conventional angiography, and lumbar puncture with cerebrospinal fluid (CSF) pressure measurements.

Haematological Testing
Blood tests rarely add useful information in the tinnitus clinic and should be avoided unless there is good clinical indication. Haemoglobin, pregnancy, and/or thyroid function tests may be needed if the patient has pulsatile tinnitus secondary to a hyperdynamic circulation. There is some weak evidence that tinnitus is more common in people with vitamin B deficiencies, so this should be checked in people with restrictive diets or malabsorption syndromes.

Questionnaires
There is no current objective measure or biomarker for tinnitus. Health care questionnaires are therefore used to estimate tinnitus severity. Tinnitus-specific questionnaires include the Tinnitus Questionnaire, the Tinnitus Handicap Inventory, and the Tinnitus Functional Index. Questionnaires may also be used to assess comorbid conditions including anxiety, depression, and insomnia.

Treatment

If the clinical assessment has revealed that the tinnitus is associated with a specific condition further management may be dictated by that condition. For example, a patient with otosclerosis may need to be counselled regarding the options of watchful waiting, fluoride treatment, hearing aids, or stapes surgery. Surgery for otosclerosis is generally helpful for associated tinnitus, particularly when the hearing is improved. Surgery also has a role for those with tinnitus associated with severe/profound hearing loss: cochlear implantation generally improves the tinnitus though this is not universal and there is a small risk of the procedure triggering tinnitus or worsening pre-existing tinnitus.

Investigation of pulse-synchronous tinnitus may reveal a treatable cause such as a vascular tumor, carotid artery stenosis, arteriovenous fistula, raised intracranial pressure, or venous obstruction or abnormality. Further treatment will then be directed as necessary to rectify that problem.

Investigation of pulse-asynchronous pulsatile tinnitus often draws a blank. If a particular pathology is proven or strongly suspected, specific treatments are available including division of the tensor tympani and stapedius tendons for intratympanic myoclonus or Botox injection of the relevant muscles for palatal myoclonus. These treatments have significant risks attached and in the case of intratympanic tendon division are irreversible. Surgery should therefore probably be best regarded as an option only after careful consideration.

Audiological Management

Most tinnitus is non-pulsatile and not associated with any specific condition. No drug therapy is currently recommended, but helpful management strategies are available. These fall into two broad categories: audiologically based management and psychologically based management.

Audiological management is a combination of addressing any associated hearing loss with hearing aids, assistive listening devices or, if necessary, cochlear implants, using sound therapy, explanation, education and counselling, relaxation training and, if needed, advice regarding sleep. Various protocols have been developed using these principles in a structured way, including tinnitus retraining therapy, progressive tinnitus management and tinnitus activities treatment. There is a modest evidence base supporting these approaches.

Hearing Improvement

The rationale for addressing any hearing loss from the outset is threefold. Firstly, most tinnitus clinicians feel that hearing loss causes people to strain to listen, which makes any tinnitus seem louder. Correcting the hearing loss reverses this process. Secondly, if the person can hear better they pick up more environmental sound, which tends to distract their brains from the tinnitus. Finally, improving the hearing allows people to interact with the education and counselling modules of the therapy more effectively.

Sound Therapy

There are many options for delivering sound therapy: simply opening a bedroom window can allow sound from the outside world into an otherwise quiet domestic environment; sound can be generated by a stand-alone electronic device; there are tinnitus apps for mobile phones or computers; sound from electric fans, fish tank aerators, or indoor water features can be used; and the tinnitus-affected person can wear ear-level devices resembling small hearing aids that produce wideband sound. The consensus is that the sound used should be something that the person finds neither intrusive nor too interesting and should be delivered at a low level that mixes with the tinnitus perception rather than tries to mask it. When used at nighttime, sound therapy can be delivered directly into the bedroom environment or can be delivered more locally via pillow speakers, a small loudspeaker under the pillow, or via Bluetooth headbands. If hyperacusis is the main problem, desensitisation using sound therapy is often helpful.

Combination Devices

All the major hearing aid manufacturers now offer devices that combine hearing aids and sound therapy devices in the same unit with the aim that the device is normally set to the hearing aid setting, but if the person is in a quiet environment they can switch to the sound therapy program.

Psychological Treatments

The treatment with the best evidence base for efficacy in managing tinnitus is cognitive behaviour therapy (CBT). Newer psychological treatment modalities including mindfulness-based cognitive therapy (MBCT), mindfulness-based stress reduction (MBSR), or acceptance and commitment therapy (ACT) also seem helpful. In the United Kingdom there is a dearth of audiologically literate psychologists to deliver such treatments, and alternative care pathways are being investigated including educating audiologists to provide CBT or using the Internet to deliver CBT.

Other Treatments

Although there is no drug approved specifically for the management of tinnitus, drugs have a role in the management of comorbid conditions such as anxiety and depression. Physical therapies may have a role in the management of somatosensory tinnitus. Complementary and alternative medicine treatments do not have any specific anti-tinnitus effect but can improve relaxation and general well-being. Various experimental treatments are being explored, particularly neuromodulation and repetitive transcranial magnetic stimulation (rTMS).

KEY POINTS

- Tinnitus is the conscious perception of an auditory sensation in the absence of a corresponding external stimulus. Hyperacusis is both a dislike of sounds above a certain intensity and a blanket term for several forms of impaired sound tolerance.
- Modern models suggest that tinnitus is due to increased awareness of spontaneous electrical activity in the auditory system. Although changes in the auditory periphery can trigger tinnitus, the processes that cause the symptom to perpetuate and become distressing occur in the central auditory pathways and in associated brain regions, particularly the limbic system.
- Tinnitus is more common in people with a hearing loss, but the degree of hearing impairment correlates poorly with tinnitus severity. About 1 in 10 people presenting with tinnitus have a normal audiogram. Tinnitus can exist after division of the auditory nerve.
- Patients with tinnitus and/or hyperacusis should undergo a basic audiological assessment. Further investigation should be undertaken in the those with pulsatile tinnitus, objectively audible tinnitus, unilateral tinnitus, tinnitus in association with asymmetric hearing loss, and tinnitus in association with neurological symptoms and/or signs.
- Patients are often given negative counselling and being told that nothing can be done for tinnitus. While a cure for tinnitus remains elusive, there are many helpful management strategies, particularly sound-based therapies, counselling, and psychological therapies.

Further Reading

McFerran D, Hoare DJ, Carr S, Ray J, Stockdale D. Tinnitus services in the United Kingdom: a survey of patient experiences. *BMC Health Serv Res.* 2018; 18(1):110. doi:10.1186/s12913-018-2914-3

McFerran DJ, Stockdale D, Holme R, Large CH, Baguley DM. Why is there no cure for tinnitus? *Front Neurosci.* 2019; 13:802. doi:10.3389/fnins.2019.00802

Phillips JS, McFerran DJ, Hall DA, Hoare DJ. The natural history of subjective tinnitus in adults: a systematic review and meta-analysis of no-intervention periods in controlled trials. *Laryngoscope.* 2018; 128(1):217–227. doi:10.1002/lary.26607

16.   AUDITORY NEUROPATHY SPECTRUM DISORDER AND AUDITORY PROCESSING DISORDER

Auditory Neuropathy Spectrum Disorder

Auditory neuropathy spectrum disorder (ANSD) is a phenotypically diverse group of hearing disorders that can affect both children and adults. It is characterised by normal outer hair cell (OHC) function but impaired neural transmission resulting in disruption of coding of acoustic signals in the auditory system.

Clinical Features

One of the key features of ANSD is hearing difficulties greater than would be expected from behavioral audiometry. The hearing difficulties are worse with speech compared with environmental sounds and are particularly affected by background noise. In children, this adversely affects speech and language development.

The test battery for ANSD is shown in Table 16.1. ANSD is typified by the following:

1 Speech tests (in quiet and noise) worse than expected from audiometry
2 Presence of OHC function as measured with cochlear microphonics (CM) and otoacoustic emissions (OAEs)
3 Absence or abnormality of the auditory brainstem response (ABR)

Table 16.1   Audiological test battery for ANSD

Test type		Notes
Behavioral audiometry	Age-appropriate testing of hearing thresholds, e.g. visual response audiometry or PTA	Normal to profound hearing loss
Speech discrimination tests	Speech recognition threshold (SRT) Word recognition score (WRS)	Worse than expected from behavioral audiometry
Speech in noise tests	For example, quick speech in noise test or hearing in noise test	Likely markedly impaired
Objective measure of middle ear function	Tympanogram	Usually normal
Objective measure of cochlear OHC function	CM or OAEs	Normal OHC function, though this can worsen with time
Objective measure of middle ear reflex	Stapedial reflex thresholds	Absent stapedial reflex in ANSD If stapedial reflex is present but ABR is absent, this suggests brainstem neuropathy due to lesion higher than superior olivary complex
Electrophysiological tests	ABR	Absent or grossly abnormal in ANSD
	Auditory late response	May help guide assessment of level of hearing impairment; guide amplification/CI by serving as marker for auditory cortical development

Note: ABR, auditory brainstem response; ANSD, auditory neuropathy spectrum disorder; CI, cochlear implantation, CM, cochlear microphonics; OAE, otoacoustic emission; OHC, outer hair cell; PTA, pure-tone audiogram.

ANSD is therefore differentiated from typical sensorineural hearing loss, in which both OAE and ABR responses are affected, and pure-tone audiogram (PTA) is usually in keeping with the level of functional hearing.

Comorbidities such as developmental delays, attention deficit hyperactivity disorder (ADHD), autism spectrum disorders, visual problems, and motor disorders are reported in up to 54% of children with ANSD.

Epidemiology
ANSD can be congenital or acquired and present at any age. The prevalence of ANSD varies between 1 and 10% in the general hearing-impaired population, and up to 40% in hearing-impaired patients with a history of admission to the neonatal intensive care unit. The prevalence of ANSD in a well-baby population is estimated at 1 in 7000. It is bilateral in 75% of cases.

Pathophysiology
ANSD can arise from abnormalities of electromechanical transduction at the inner hair cell and axons, cell bodies, and myelin sheaths of the auditory nerve.

This results in disruption of temporal synchrony of the auditory neural signals as well as a reduction of amplitude of neural signals.

Risk Factors for ANSD
A wide range of age-dependent risk factors have been implicated in the development of ANSD. Perinatal factors including prematurity, hyperbilirubinaemia, respiratory distress syndrome/neonatal mechanical ventilation, ototoxic drugs, and cerebral palsy are the most common associations of ANSD in children. A number of genetic mutations causing ANSD have been identified. Mutations of the otoferlin, pejvakin, and connexin 26 gene are examples. ANSD can occur in Usher's syndrome and may be associated with hereditary demyelinating neuropathies such as Charcot-Marie-Tooth syndrome and Friedreich's ataxia. Acquired causes of ANSD include multiple sclerosis, autoimmune disease, and hemosiderosis.

Diagnostic Approach
In children, perinatal history and developmental milestone attainment are important considerations, while in adults, family and drug history are key. Clinical examination includes assessment of developmental milestones, peripheral nerve sensation, cerebellar signs, and funduscopy. Vestibular assessment and/or testing should be considered as should referral for formal ophthalmological assessment. The audiological test battery is shown in Table 16.1. Audiometry should be performed on first-degree relatives. Magnetic resonance imaging (MRI) of the internal auditory meati and brain is necessary to identify cochlear nerve hypoplasia/aplasia. Referral to a clinical geneticist should be considered based on clinical picture and patient consent.

Management of ANSD
A multidisciplinary approach, parental counseling, and timely intervention are crucial. Broadly speaking, the main strategies involve (1) improving signal-to-noise ratio and (2) amplification and (3) early language interventions.

Directional microphones, personal frequency modulation (FM) systems, greater support in classroom, reduction in background noise, and workplace adaptations all play a part.

Judicious hearing aid amplification with close monitoring may be considered once reliable behavioral thresholds have been established. However, amplification has been shown to have variable outcomes, since it can amplify the signal but not overcome the neural transmission deficit. Some studies have also shown a detrimental impact on cochlear OHC function.

Cochlear implantation (CI) can be considered in selected cases with good outcomes. Implantation can provide consistent neural firing helping to overcome auditory desynchrony such as in synaptopathy. However, there is some evidence to suggest that CI in patients with

ANSD involving the spiral ganglion and auditory nerve is associated with poorer outcome compared with pre-synaptic ANSD.

Early language intervention is important in young children with ANSD and will involve input from speech and language therapy, teachers of the deaf, and significant parental involvement.

Auditory Processing Disorder

Prevalence and Definition

Approximately 5% of children and 1–10% of adults who present to audiology departments with complaints of significant listening difficulties in noise or in group conversations have normal pure-tone thresholds. In a proportion of these patients, listening symptoms are attributed to functional deficits in sound processing within the extended central auditory nervous system. This clinical presentation is categorised as an auditory processing disorder (APD). APD is a common type of hearing impairment that remains under recognised, despite its high burden on communication, social, and emotional aspects of life. This clinical presentation has attracted considerable debate. A recent European consensus proposes that APD is diagnosed on the basis of the following criteria[3]:

1 Normal audiometric thresholds in both ears
2 Abnormal performance in at least two validated auditory processing tests that assess different processes in at least one ear, including in a non-speech test
3 Presence of listening difficulties (Table 16.2) and/or risk factors associated with APD
4 Normal non-verbal intelligence
5 Good ability to follow test instructions

Etiology

In children, as well as in adults, APD may be diagnosed in the background of neurological disease such as brain tumors, stroke, trauma, prematurity or low birthweight, epilepsy, and brain infections or demyelinating conditions. APD may also overlap with developmental disorders such as language impairment, dyslexia, and attention-deficit hyperactivity disorder. In such cases, the clinician should carefully consider whether the clinical presentation is instead due to deficits in higher order language or cognitive domains. Another subtype of APD is the 'spatial processing disorder (SPD)' that is attributed to a prolonged history of chronic otitis media in childhood, giving rise to deficits in binaural auditory processing

The Diagnostic Approach

The diagnostic process includes history taking, including patient/teacher/parent questionnaires, followed by targeted medical examination. Children and adults with APD have speech in noise, auditory attention, localisation of sound, and other auditory difficulties (see Table 16.2). Children

Table 16.2   Symptoms of APD

Speech understanding difficulties	In background noise, acoustically challenging/complex acoustic environments, when speech quality is degraded
Speech discrimination difficulties	Difficulties to repeat or recall similar sounding words
Auditory memory/attention difficulties	Difficulties recalling instructions; difficulties concentrating in noise
Sound localisation/streaming difficulties	Difficulties identifying the source of a sound; with separation of auditory foreground from auditory background
Relies on multisensory cues	For example, seeking visual/facial cues to better understand
Hyperacusis	With or without a diagnosis of autism spectrum disorder
Disproportionate educational/ cognitive/language difficulties	

Table 16.3   APD test battery (AAA 2010)

Auditory processing domain	What the test assesses
Auditory discrimination	Ability to differentiate similar acoustic stimuli that differ in frequency, intensity, and/or temporal parameters
Auditory temporal processing	Ability to analyse acoustic events over time
Dichotic listening	Ability to separate (i.e. binaural separation) or integrate (i.e. binaural integration) disparate auditory stimuli presented to each ear simultaneously
Low-redundancy speech recognition (monaural)	Recognition of degraded speech stimuli presented to one ear at a time
Binaural interaction	Binaural processes dependent on intensity or time differences of acoustic stimuli
Other tests	
Electro-acoustic measures	Otoacoustic emissions, acoustic reflex thresholds, and acoustic reflex decay usually normal
Electrophysiological measures	Auditory brainstem response usually normal (consider measuring middle latency and auditory late response)

may experience difficulties in the classroom and psychosocial difficulties. History should also ascertain risk factors, educational, and professional history, as well as family history of related disorders (e.g. hearing or neurological disorders). The American Academy of Audiology (2010) proposes that the central auditory processing test battery should include a number of tests in addition to PTA and speech-in-quiet tests, as detailed in Table 16.3.

Assessments of other domains such as language and cognition are of paramount importance as these factors can affect APD test performance. Age-related hearing loss and cognitive decline is such an example. Assessment of cognitive skills, such as working memory, is therefore useful during assessment.

Management Strategies
The goal for APD rehabilitation is to improve the functional deficits of individuals that impact their communication and well-being. A multidisciplinary team approach should be employed and should focus on the following areas:

1 Auditory training (AT) to harness brain plasticity and improve neuro-auditory function (e.g. AT): AT can be a school- or home-based program, as well as therapy conducted by a speech language therapist or audiologist in the clinic. It involves predominantly language-based tasks. Examples of informal AT are discriminating similar sounding notes on a keyboard (temporal or timing skills) and listening to lyrics of songs (speech-in-noise ability). There are also several commercially available computer-based AT programs. Post-training improvements are reported on a range of auditory and non-auditory measures, but long-term benefits are unknown.

2 Signal enhancement strategies including environmental modifications to reduce the deleterious effects of noise and reverberation of the acoustic environment: Remote microphone hearing aids (RMHAs) are personal listening devices that bypass high-level classroom noise and transmit clearer speech to the child's ears. A recent meta-analysis presents moderately strong evidence that use of an FM device (a specific type of RMHA) in the classroom improves children's listening and attention. There is case-control study evidence that these devices improve speech in noise listening in adults.

3 Teaching children and adults compensatory strategies to overcome functional difficulties: These strategies may include 'active listening' where the individual is taught how to take responsibility for their own listening and strategies that aim to enhance auditory memory/attention. Curriculum modifications (e.g. pre-teaching new material, giving breaks to the student during the day) are also widely used.

Further Reading

1. Moser, T. and Starr, A. (2016) 'Auditory neuropathy–neural and synaptic mechanisms', *Nature Reviews. Neurology*, 12(3), pp. 135–149. doi: 10.1038/nrneurol.2016.10.

2. 'Guidelines for Aetiological Investigation into Auditory Neuropathy Spectrum Disorder in Children and Young Adults' (2018). British Association of Audiovestibular Physicians. https://www.baap.org.uk/uploads/1/1/9/7/119752718/guidelines_for_ansd_final_version.pdf.

3. Iliadou, V. V., Ptok, M., Grech, H., Pedersen, E. R., Brechmann, A., Deggouj, N., Bamiou, D. E. (2018). European 17 countries consensus endorses more approaches to APD than reported in Wilson 2018. *International journal of audiology*, 1–2. doi:10.1080/14992027.2018.1442937

17. HEARING AIDS AND AUDITORY REHABILITATION

Introduction

Hearing aids partially overcome the deficits associated with a hearing loss. They make audible sounds, and parts of sounds, that would otherwise be inaudible. They cannot reverse the reduced resolution with which ears with sensorineural hearing loss analyse incoming sounds. However, some signal processing algorithms within hearing aids (directional microphones and noise suppression, see later) help compensate for this reduced resolution and the ensuing reduced understanding of speech in noisy places. Where hearing aids do not fully meet the needs of patients, additional forms of aural rehabilitation should be considered.

Components of a Hearing Aid

The essential components in hearing aids are a microphone, an amplifier with controllable characteristics, a miniature earphone (called a receiver) to output the amplified signal and a battery to power the amplifier. The amplifiers can be controlled so that they amplify signals at different frequencies by different amounts so that they amplify soft sounds more than they amplify loud sounds. Frequency-dependent amplification is needed because the amount of hearing loss usually changes with frequency and because the high-frequency parts of speech are weaker than the low-frequency parts. Intensity-dependent amplification compensates for the reduced dynamic range of sounds between threshold and discomfort that inevitably accompanies sensorineural hearing loss. The rate at which the degree of amplification varies as the input level varies can be very fast (a few milliseconds) or very slow (a few seconds). Fast and slow compression have both advantages and disadvantages relative to each other.

Almost all hearing aids use digital signal processing to amplify as it offers more flexible manipulation of the sound, and it is more easily controlled by the computer used to adjust the hearing aid to an individual patient's needs.

These same basic physical components are used in some multifunction, non-professionally fitted, wearable devices, termed *hearables*. There is a current merging of these device types, as the hearables add amplification to their features, and hearing aids add other features such as fall detection, telephone hands-free operation and step counting.

Most hearing aids also include a wireless receiver so that audio signals can be input to the device from a mobile phone or other streaming device, a remotely located microphone (such as worn by a teacher in a classroom) and/or a hearing aid on the other side of the head. The most common style of hearing aids is behind the ear (BTE), where either the entire hearing aid, or all the components except the receiver, are positioned between the pinna and the head surface. They connect to the ear canal via a sound tube, or via thin wires when the receiver is in the ear canal. The end of the tube or the receiver are held in place in the ear canal by either a custom-shaped ear mould, or a compliant tip that deforms to match the cross-sectional shape of the ear canal. Alternative styles include in the ear, in the canal and completely in the-canal. While the latter two styles have slight cosmetic advantages over BTE devices, BTEs can contain directional microphones, which offer performance in noise that the canal-style devices cannot match. Much less commonly, a contralateral routing of signals (CROS) hearing aid is used to pick up sounds from the side of the head with a completely deaf ear, and play an amplified version of it to the other ear.

Hearing Aid Measurement in Couplers and Real Ears

The amplification characteristics of hearing aids can be measured in a standardised way by placing it in a test box, with the hearing aid output connected to a coupler that very approximately simulates the ear canal acoustic impedance. During fitting, amplification characteristics on an individual are determined by placing a thin probe tube inside the ear canal, and measuring the sound pressure level in the ear canal with and without the hearing aid present. The increase in sound pressure level is called the real ear insertion gain. This gain is affected by the way the hearing aid is coupled to the ear canal, including by how open the fitting in the ear canal is. Open fittings enable the wearer to perceive their own voice as normal, but limit the frequency range over which the hearing aid can amplify sounds, and the effectiveness of the noise reduction strategies in hearing aids. They are most suited for people with mild or moderate loss.

Directional Microphones

Directional microphones provide more amplification for sounds arriving from broadly in front of the wearer than for sounds arriving from the side or behind the wearer. They achieve this by sensing, and then combining the sounds arriving at two closely located sound ports on the hearing aid. Directional microphones are the major means by which hearing aids improve the clarity of the sound, in addition to simply amplifying it. Super-directional microphones, also known as beamformers, achieve a higher level of directivity by wirelessly transmitting signals sensed on one side of the head, to the hearing aid on the other side of the head. Each hearing aid thus has access to signals sensed at four different locations on the head. They can allow people with moderate hearing loss to hear as well in noisy places as people with normal hearing.

Signal Processing

Digital technology makes available several signal processing schemes. These include

- Adaptive noise reduction, which makes sound more comfortable by de-emphasising frequency bands that are dominated by noise, rather than by incoming speech
- Frequency lowering, which moves high-frequency speech information to slightly lower frequencies, where the wearer has less hearing loss, and thus greater ability to use the information

- Feedback canceling, which makes whistling (an oscillation) caused by amplified sound leaking back to the microphone less likely to occur
- Expansion, which lowers the hearing aid gain applied to soft sounds, to make internal hearing aid noise inaudible, even in quiet places

Candidacy

The prime requirements for a person to benefit from hearing aids are that they perceive that they are having difficulty hearing and that they are willing to try hearing aids. These beliefs are much more important than the actual degree of hearing loss present (which of course is only one indicator of the extent to which the hearing and auditory processing system differ from normal).

Prescription

Because hearing loss characteristics vary with hearing loss, so too must the amount of amplification that hearing aids provide. The prescription formula describes how the amplification should vary with frequency and input level to achieve the aim of that formula. The aim of the widely used National Acoustic Laboratories' prescription is to maximise the intelligibility of speech while keeping the loudness to no more than would be perceived by a person with normal hearing thresholds listening to the same speech signal. Prescription formulae also specify the maximum output level that hearing aids should provide at any frequency. Apart from the gain-frequency response and maximum output, other aspects of the fitting that must be considered when choosing the optimal hearing aid for a patient includes the physical style and size of the hearing aid, user controls, wireless connectivity and types or strength of signal processing alternatives. Despite the use of prescription procedures, because of individual differences, there is often a need for fine-tuning of the hearing aids after the user has worn them for a few weeks.

Binaural Hearing

Hearing in two ears enhances our ability to understand speech in noise, and greatly enhances our ability to localise sounds. This occurs because the brain is able to take advantage of differences in the level and timing of sounds at the two ears created by the head. Bilateral fitting is thus increasingly important as hearing loss increases, so that audibility is achieved at all frequencies in both ears. For a minority of people, however, binaural interference causes speech identification ability to be better when unilaterally aided than when bilaterally aided.

Children

The two major ways that hearing aid fitting for babies is different from adults is that the small size of their ear canals must be considered, and protection against ingestion of hearing aid batteries must be provided. More subtle differences are that whereas adults need hearing to use language, children need hearing to *learn* language. The earlier hearing aids are provided, preferably well before 6 months of age, the better the child's language develops. Because children are still learning language throughout childhood, they need a better signal-to-noise ratio than adults to understand speech in challenging situations, like classrooms. The best way to achieve this is when the teacher wears a wireless remote microphone that transmits clear, non-reverberant signals to the child's hearing aids.

More detailed information about the topics above can be found in the book *Hearing Aids.*[1]

Aural Rehabilitation

While some are completely satisfied with the help provided by hearing aids, others have needs which cannot be fully met by them. Support for people with hearing loss may be provided by an aural rehabilitation specialist such as a hearing therapist or specialist clinical psychologist. For many, the experience of losing hearing goes far beyond the frustration of mishearing speech. It can necessitate changes in lifestyle, both at work and at leisure, make conversation effortful and tiring and profoundly alter one's sense of identity. Couples often feel that hearing loss places a strain on their relationship. Those having difficulty adjusting to life with hearing loss may well benefit from an opportunity to discuss their feelings and explore ways of coping with a rehabilitation specialist. A group in particular need of urgent referral to rehabilitation services are those who develop sudden hearing loss; they often report feelings of utter bewilderment and confusion. In a medical emergency, it is easy for emotional needs to be neglected, but timely emotional support is just as important as prompt medical treatment.

Specialist rehabilitative support can also be beneficial to people who feel ambivalent about using hearing aids. There are many reasons for this, including perceived stigma and lack of confidence. An opportunity to spend time discussing one's ambivalence in a supportive environment is likely to be more cost-effective than fitting hearing aids which remain unused.

Aural Rehab Groups and Lipreading Classes
Some audiology clinics run regular aural rehab groups. There are many possible formats, but all have the advantage of bringing people with hearing loss (and sometimes their partners) together to share experiences and ideas.

Outside the healthcare system, other groups and classes exist for people with hearing loss, including lipreading classes. These usually involve a mixture of lipreading exercises and communication tips (such as asking people to face you and moving away from background noise). Although effects of class attendance on lipreading ability are equivocal, qualitative research indicates that people value their classes very highly. Hard-of-hearing groups or clubs are also available in some areas which offer peer support and an opportunity to take part in social activities without being restricted by hearing problems.

Auditory Training
Auditory training attempts to improve speech discrimination by presenting a variety of listening tasks involving phonemes, words and sentences. Several computer-based auditory training programs are available, enabling users to practice regularly at home. A systematic review of 13 computerised auditory training studies[2] found evidence that performance on auditory training tasks improves significantly with practice. Some (but not all) studies also showed generalisation of learning to untrained tasks, which of course has more real-world benefit.

The Voluntary Sector
Additional support for people with hearing loss and related problems (such as tinnitus and balance disorders) is provided by charities and voluntary organisations. These are very often an invaluable source of information; many produce fact sheets about a range of topics and some have telephone and email help lines. There are several forums available via the Internet and social media through which people can share information and offer support.

Technology other than Hearing Aids and Cochlear Implants
There are situations in which many users find their hearing aids or cochlear implants inadequate. Despite recent advances in digital signal processing, interference from background noise is still a primary cause of dissatisfaction. Telephone use can also be problematic. People with more severe hearing loss may find the television unclear, even when using hearing aids, and family disputes over TV volume are a frequent source of irritation. Moreover, there are situations in which most people take their hearing aids or speech processors off (particularly while bathing or in bed) but still need to be aware of signals such as smoke alarms or alarm clocks. Additional technology goes some way towards solving these difficulties, but awareness of it amongst both patients and clinicians tends to be low. Some of the more common types of hearing assistance technology is described in Table 17.1.

Using Personal Listening Equipment without Hearing Aids
Many of the devices described can be used with headphones. These make them accessible to non–hearing-aid users and to people who need or prefer to be without their hearing aids temporarily, perhaps due to an ear infection.

Table 17.1   Common types of hearing assistance technology

Device	Description	Additional information
Frequency-modulated (FM) system	Receiver connects to user's hearing aids by direct audio input or a neckloop. Transmitter with mic placed close to any sound source or clipped to speaker's clothing.	Often used in classrooms and lecture theatres.
Loop system	A looped wire connected to an amplifier creates an electromagnetic field. Signal is picked up by telecoil in hearing aids, which must be activated by audiologist.	Fitted in many theatres, cinemas and service counters. Smaller versions available for home use and travel.
Streamer	A small device worn around the neck enables hearing aids to connect to Bluetooth	Can be used with any Bluetooth-enabled device (mobile phones, MP3 players, tablets, etc.).
Amplified phone	Landline phone with built-in volume control.	Additional features (e.g. extra-large buttons) also available.
Pager	Unit clipped to clothing vibrates to alert wearer to phone, doorbell, alarm, baby monitor, etc.	Under-the pillow vibrating unit available for nighttime.
Visual alert	Bright, flashing light activated by doorbell, phone or alarm.	May be portable or wall-mounted.

A personal amplifier with headphones can be particularly helpful in hospital. Many hearing-impaired patients on a ward will not be wearing their hearing aids. This sometimes results in sensitive information being spoken at high volume by hospital staff and being clearly audible to all those around. Speaking to the patient via a simple amplifier can make all the difference to confidentiality and dignity.

Hearing Dogs
People with severe or profound hearing loss can apply for a hearing dog. Such dogs are trained to alert their owners and lead them to the source of sounds like doorbells, phones and timers. They are also taught a 'danger' signal in response to a smoke alarm. Hearing dogs are identified by a special coat and can accompany their owners in public places. Many deaf people feel more confident with a hearing dog by their side.

Language Service Professionals
Language service professionals (LSPs) are sometimes employed to enable participation in meetings, conferences, training courses or court proceedings. Examples of LSPs are sign language interpreters, speech-to-text transcribers and lip speakers (who repeat what a speaker is saying voicelessly to enable lip reading). However, improvements in voice recognition software mean that it is becoming increasingly easy to provide real-time transcription without the need for a third party.

Conclusion
The consequences of hearing loss are far reaching. Modern hearing aids can provide great benefits, but many people with hearing loss also need additional or alternative rehabilitation services. While it is not the responsibility of otorhinolaryngologists to provide such services, it is important to be aware of what is available in the local area and to be able to make appropriate referrals and recommendations.

KEY POINTS

- Advances in digital technology mean that as well as being able to adjust hearing aids to meet individual hearing loss characteristics, hearing aids now automatically adapt in various helpful ways to the environment in which they are being used.
- Super-directional microphones, and streaming of wireless signals originating from mobile phones, remotely located microphones, televisions and other audio sources are amongst the advances that enable hearing-impaired people to hear well, even in noisy places.
- Despite the huge benefit that hearing aids can provide, they may not completely reverse the negative impact of hearing loss on well-being.
- Emotional and behavioural support for people struggling with hearing loss can be provided individually and in groups by clinicians with specialist training in rehabilitation.
- Hearing assistance technology and LSPs can help in many situations in which hearing aids or cochlear implants do not provide adequate benefit.

Further Reading

1. Dillon, H. 2012. *Hearing Aids*. Thieme, New York.
2. Henshaw, H. & Ferguson, M. A. 2013. *Efficacy of Individual Computer-Based Auditory Training for People with Hearing Loss: A Systematic Review of the Evidence. PLoS One*, 8.

18. COCHLEAR IMPLANTS AND AUDITORY BRAINSTEM IMPLANTS

Cochlear Implants

Cochlear implants (CIs) are neuroprosthetic devices that directly stimulate the auditory nerve. This technology has proven revolutionary in restoring hearing to individuals with severe to profound hearing loss, enabling speech and language development in children, and improving speech perception in adults.

How a CI works

The main components of CI devices are shown in Figure 18.1. The electrode array consists of multiple electrode contacts (between 12 and 22 depending on the manufacturer), each of which is intended to stimulate a distinct population of auditory neurons. CIs attempt to mimic natural tonotopic encoding by representing high frequencies at the basal and low frequencies at the apical end of the array. The array is ideally placed in the lower compartment of the cochlea, the scala tympani, where it lies closer to target auditory neurons. Perimodiolar electrodes are pre-curved and sit closer to target auditory neurons in the modiolus, while lateral wall electrodes are further from these neurons but are associated with less traumatic insertion.

Sound processing refers to how the acoustic signal is transformed into an electrical stimulus and varies between device manufacturers. Most strategies decompose the signal into frequency bands and extract the envelope information (slow amplitude fluctuations) and use this information to modulate electrical pulses at corresponding electrode contacts.

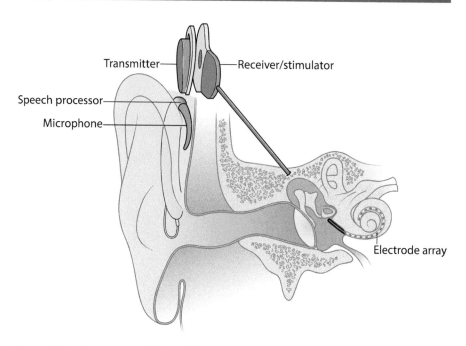

Figure 18.1 Components of the cochlear implant. (1) The microphone picks up the acoustic signal. (2) The sound processor converts the microphone output to an electrical signals (3) head-piece with a transmitting coil held in place by a magnet and uses radio frequency to transmit the signal transcutaneously. (4) The receiver/stimulator decodes information from the transmitter and generates electrical stimuli and (5) the electrode array stimulates auditory neurons.

Criteria for Implantation

Implantation criteria vary between countries. UK criteria were updated by the National Institute of Health and Care Excellence in March 2019:

- Cochlear implantation can be considered for individuals with bilateral severe to profound hearing loss who do not receive adequate benefit from hearing aids.
- Unilateral implantation is recommended in adults.
- Bilateral implantation in children or in adults who are blind or have other disabilities that increase their reliance on auditory stimuli.
- Severe to profound deafness is defined as pure-tone audiometric threshold ≥80dB hearing level (HL) at two or more frequencies (500, 1000, 2000, 3000 and 4000 Hz) bilaterally without hearing aids.
- Trial of hearing aids should occur for at least 3 months. Adequate benefit from hearing aids is defined as the following:
  - For adults, a phoneme score of 50% or greater on the Arthur Boothroyd word test presented at 70dBA
  - For children, speech, language and listening skills appropriate to age, developmental stage and cognitive ability

Prognostic Factors

In children, the most important prognostic factor is age at implantation with earlier age associated with better hearing outcomes. There is growing evidence that CIs should be provided prior to the age of 12 months in congenital deafness. In adults, pre-lingual onset of deafness and later age at implantation are negative prognostic factors. Some studies have shown that longer duration of deafness is associated with poorer outcome in adults. Other factors that may influence outcomes in children and adults include learning disability, communication environment and aetiology of deafness (e.g. better in Meniere's disease but worse in meningitis/temporal bone fracture).

Assessment

Assessment should be performed by a multidisciplinary team including but not limited to surgeons, audiologists and rehabilitationists. It is crucial that patients have realistic expectations of their hearing outcome and adequate pre-operative counselling is necessary. Behavioural audiological assessment involves age appropriate assessment of hearing thresholds and in adults also includes word recognition tests. This can be supplemented with objective measurements including otoacoustic emissions (assessment of auditory neuropathy spectrum disorder; see Chapter 16), auditory brainstem responses (ABRs; for hearing threshold estimation; see Chapter 4) and auditory cortical responses (for assessing benefit from hearing aids; see Chapter 4). This is particularly important in young children and in patients with suspected non-organic hearing loss. Transtympanic electrocochleography is occasionally used in patients in whom there is concern about the presence/function of the cochlear nerve.

Pre-operative imaging may include magnetic resonance imaging (MRI) and/or computed tomography (CT) and should be used to identify inner ear abnormalities and for surgical planning. MRI should be performed in children with congenital deafness to ensure there is a cochlear nerve of normal diameter; additional CT imaging is not required in most cases.

Often the better-hearing/better-aided ear is chosen for implantation in adults due to theoretically better survival of the peripheral and central auditory pathways on this side. Many patients however, will prefer to have their worse ear implanted so that they can continue to wear a hearing aid in their better ear. Vestibular function testing should be considered in patients with imbalance. The ear with poorer peripheral vestibular function is generally preferred for implantation to reduce post-operative vestibular disturbance.

Surgery

Surgery should be performed with strict aseptic technique and a facial nerve monitor should be used. Typically, a postauricular incision is made, an anteriorly/superiorly based periosteal flap is raised and small cortical mastoidectomy is performed. A posterior tympanotomy is then formed to gain access to the round window (RW) and reduce the RW niche. Some surgeons drill a bed for the implant package whilst others place it in a subperiosteal pocket. Electrode insertion is performed through the RW membrane or through a cochleostomy depending on the electrode and surgeon preference. A soft tissue seal is often placed around the electrode at the promontory and the wound is closed in multiple layers. Intraoperatively the implant may be assessed for faults and for correct placement using electrophysiological testing, X-ray or even CT. Chronic middle ear disease should be addressed prior to CI and may necessitate tympanoplasty for perforations and blind sac closure for cholesteatoma/mastoid cavities.

Many surgeons routinely use hearing preservation techniques to conserve inner ear elements. Meaningful preservation of hearing is usually only possible if preoperative low-frequency thresholds are around 70dB or better. This allows electroacoustic stimulation, through a hearing aid for residual hearing and electrical stimulation from the CI. Other advantages to preserving inner ear residual function including reduced post-operative imbalance and opening the possibility of the ear benefiting from future hearing regeneration therapies. 'Soft surgery' techniques include inserting the electrode through steroids or hyaluronate, avoiding suction near the cochlea and performing a slow insertion over minutes. There is some evidence that use of steroids either pre-operatively or post-operatively improves hearing outcome. Recently, intraoperative electrocochleography has been used to provide real-time feedback on basilar membrane trauma during insertion.

Complications

Complications of CI surgery include standard complications of mastoid surgery (see Chapter 10). In addition, patients must be warned of the risk of device failure and of meningitis. For the latter reason, patients should have the 23-valent polysaccharide pneumococcal vaccination (given after the age of 2) in addition to the childhood meningitis immunisation programme. Intraoperative cerebrospinal fluid (CSF) leak can occur when making the cochleostomy or RW opening in patients with inner ear malformations but can be managed by raising the head of the bed and inserting the electrode with a soft tissue seal around it; lumbar drainage is rarely required. Occasionally the electrode cannot be inserted fully due to cochlear fibrosis/ossification, e.g. due to meningitis or otosclerosis. In some cases, it is necessary to drill out the basal turn of the cochlea or even insert a split electrode for which an additional channel is drilled into the middle turn of the cochlea. Tip folds over of the electrode in the cochlea and facial nerve stimulation from the CI are complications that can usually be managed by altering the stimulation settings for the CI. Some patients also experience chronic pain following surgery, which rarely necessitates device explantation. There is a risk of magnet displacement with MRI and the make of implant should always be checked and appropriate precautions taken prior to such imaging.

Post-Operative Rehabilitation and Outcomes

The implant 'switch-on' usually occurs 2–6 weeks after surgery. Patients have several appointments for programming the implant and for auditory rehabilitation in the first few months after surgery. In adults, peak performance is usually reached within 6–12 months. In general, whilst hearing outcomes are usually excellent from CIs allowing 'open set' speech perception, there can be significant variability in outcomes. Speech-in-noise perception is generally limited and adults often struggle with music appreciation. There is evidence that bilateral implantation and bimodal hearing (hearing aid in one ear and CI in the other ear) are associated with better sound localisation and speech-in-noise perception.

Future Developments

Extended criteria for CIs include single-sided deafness and management of tinnitus in patients with severe to profound hearing loss; these indications are currently not funded in the United Kingdom. Research is ongoing into the use of optical stimulation for CI (rather than electrical stimulation) to allow more focused stimulation of auditory neurons, robotic insertion of electrodes to minimise insertion trauma and the use of neurotrophins on electrodes to promote growth of nerve endings. There is also growing interest in the use objective measurements, including electrophysiology and imaging techniques, to guide CI programming.

Auditory Brainstem Implants

Indications

Auditory brainstem implants (ABIs) are used for hearing restoration in patients with severe to profound hearing loss when a CI is not possible. Potential candidates include

- Adults with bilateral vestibular schwannoma due to neurofibromatosis type 2 (NF2), undergoing tumour resection, in whom cochlear nerve preservation is not possible; the function of the cochlear nerve can be checked during surgery with electrically evoked ABR/compound action potential
- Adults with cochlear ossification due to meningitis, labyrinthitis, fractures or otosclerosis
- Children with bilateral cochlear aplasia or bilateral auditory nerve aplasia or dysplasia

Similar to CIs, patients require extensive multidisciplinary assessment and counselling prior to surgery. They also require careful setting up of the device and a rehabilitation programme to help with speech understanding.

Surgery

The ABI has similar components to the CI; the main difference is that the electrode contacts are on a flat paddle. The retrosigmoid or translabyrinthine approaches are typically used for access to the brainstem and the electrode paddle is placed on the lateral recess of the fourth ventricle adjacent to the cochlear nucleus. Paddle position can be optimised based on implant evoked ABRs. The facial and glossopharyngeal nerves are monitored for non-auditory stimulation. Similarly, the vagus nerve can be monitored through the electrocardiogram (ECG). Switch on is typically performed with the patient nil by mouth and with anaesthetic personnel and equipment available in case of nonauditory stimulation causing cardiac rhythm disturbance.

Outcomes

Hearing outcomes from ABI are highly variable and are certainly inferior to CI. In addition, it takes many years for patients to reach peak performance. In most cases, they allow awareness of sounds and an aid to lipreading, with the minority of cases achieving open-set speech perception. Outcomes in adults without tumours are generally superior to that in NF2 patients (see Chapter 22 for further details on outcomes in NF2).

KEY POINTS

- CIs may be considered in patients with severe to profound hearing loss that fulfill NICE 2019[2] guidance.
- In children, an early age at implantation and in adults shorter duration of profound deafness are associated with better-hearing outcomes.
- A positive communication environment is associated with better outcomes.
- ABI may be used for hearing restoration in cases of severe to profound hearing loss where CI is not possible, most commonly in patients with NF2.
- ABI usually enables awareness of sounds, aids lipreading and rarely allows open-set speech perception.

Further Reading

1. Tysome J, Axon P, Donnelly N et al. English consensus protocol evaluating candidacy for auditory brainstem and cochlear implantation in neurofibromatosis type 2. *Otology & Neurotology*: 2013 (34) 1743–1747. doi: 10.1097/MAO.0b013e3182a1a8b4.

2. National Institute for Health and Care Excellence. Cochlear implants for children and adults with severe to profound deafness. 2020. Available from: https://www.nice.org.uk/guidance/ta566. (Accessed 10 July 2020.)

3. Taylor & Francis Online. *Cochlear Implants International*. 2020. Available from: https://www.tandfonline.com/toc/ycii20/17/sup1. (Accessed 10 July 2020.)

19. EAR TRAUMA[1]

Auricular Haematoma and Cauliflower Ear

Auricular haematoma is caused by direct trauma to the pinna. In children there is a strong association with non-accidental injury. Tearing of perforating vessels causes extravasation creating an intracartilaginous space. They are painful, tender and fluctuant.

Haematoma aspiration must be performed within 48 hours and followed by compression. There is a high recurrence rate. A delayed presentation, recurrence or a requirement to return urgently to contact sports mandates a formal procedure. Numerous methods have been described but reliable results are only achieved if granulation tissue is curetted and post drainage compression (e.g. dental rolls or silastic splints) is used.

Inadequate drainage results in new irregular cartilage formation (cauliflower ear) and poor cosmesis.

Caustic Injury – Button Batteries

Caustic injuries to the external canal and drum perforation from button batteries require emergency treatment. Eardrops must not be used. Extensive soft tissue and bone necrosis is possible. Emergency removal, irrigation and debridement should be performed, but repair or grafting should be delayed.

Traumatic Tympanic Membrane Perforation

This is usually caused by slap injuries, penetrating objects and barotrauma.

Careful otomicroscopy with removal of any foreign body is required. A conductive hearing loss is typical.

Antibiotic drops should only be used if there is evidence of infection.

The application of cigarette paper or Gelfoam over the perforation increases the speed but not the incidence of spontaneous healing, which is greater than 80%. Formal repair should be delayed until after 3 months and has a better success rate than for perforations associated with otitis media. Caustic and blast injuries have poorer outcomes, the worst being welding injuries.

Ossicular Trauma

Skull trauma is the most common cause. About two-thirds occur without a concomitant temporal bone fracture. Dislocation of the incus is the most common injury. Isolated malleus fracture may follow sudden pressurisation in the canal.

A high-definition computed tomography (CT) scan is recommended. Three-dimensional (3D) imaging and virtual endoscopy will enable an accurate diagnosis in most cases.

Audiometry will demonstrate a conductive, or mixed, hearing loss in the acute phase. Transmission of force through the ossicular chain to the inner ear may cause a sensorineural component. Both may improve considerably following spontaneous clearance of the haemo-tympanum, healing of the tympanic membrane, scarring around the ossicles and improve-ment of cochlear concussion.

Reparative surgery should be delayed until 3 months. Aiding may be an appropriate alternative.

Inner Ear Trauma (without Fracture)

(Inner Ear Concussion, Cochlear Concussion, Inner Ear Concussive Syndrome, Mild Traumatic Brain Injury)

Minor head injuries are extremely common. Concussion (synonymous with mild traumatic brain injury) is a brief loss of consciousness, or any change in mental state, at the time of the accident. A subjective transient hearing loss occurs in 52% of cases lasting for up to 2 days, but there is little evidence for permanent loss. Tinnitus and hyperacusis are common. True vertigo is the only definite otological symptom occurring in 25% of cases, almost always disappearing within 10 days. Non-specific dizziness, often postural perceptive, occurs in many more cases.

During the first week symptoms include headaches, dizziness, fatigue, memory deficits, anx-iety and depression. Up to 40% of patients have residual symptoms 1 year later. Positional vertigo is common. Multiple repositioning manoeuvres are required in 67% of those with post head injury benign paroxysmal positional vertigo (BPPV) (compared with 14% of those with idiopathic BPPV).

Treatment is supportive; there is no evidence to support the use of steroids. Rare sequelae include perilymphatic fistula (PLF), progressive sensorineural deafness (probably of autoimmune aetiology) and delayed endolymphatic hydrops.

Inner Ear Trauma and Temporal Bone Fracture[2]

Always evaluate for other intracranial and cervical spine injuries in these cases.

Temporal bone fractures are traditionally described as longitudinal or transverse. Otic capsule 'violating' or 'sparing' is a more useful distinction (Figure 19.1) as the serious sequelae of facial nerve paralysis, cerebrospinal fluid (CSF) leak and profound hearing loss are twice, four times and seven times, respectively, more likely in the former.

Any pattern of loss immediate/delayed or transient/permanent/progressive may be seen. A conductive hearing loss is common but usually resolves. A sensorineural loss, usually at and above 4kHz, is often found. The degree of hearing loss is proportional to the degree of head injury; complete loss is common.

Post-traumatic vertigo is usually short-lived in otic capsule–sparing cases. In violating cases resolution is by central adaptation, which may take up to 12 months.

A complete neuro-otological examination should include the conscious level, cranial nerve function (especially facial nerve), clinical testing of hearing (including tuning forks), audiometry, balance, gait and cerebellar function and should be performed as soon as the patient's general state permits. Mastoid bruising (Battle's sign) may indicate an underlying fracture.

The meatus should not be irrigated, and microsuction should be performed only if infection is suspected. Any soft tissue should be left alone. Packing of the meatus is only indicated if there is uncontrollable haemorrhage. Avoid packing material with a radiopaque marker as it may interfere with subsequent imaging.

A high-definition temporal bone scan should be performed. Where hearing loss or vertigo are evident, but with no fracture on CT, T1-weighted magnetic resonance imaging (MRI) may demonstrate a hyperintense signal in the labyrinth indicative of haemorrhage, and it may also identify temporal lobe contusion. Gadolinium-enhanced MRI of the facial nerve, or angiography to exclude vascular injury, more accurately assesses the degree of damage to these structures.

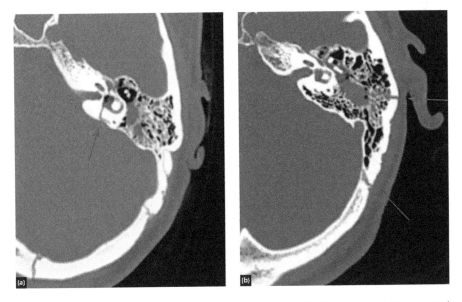

Figure 19.1   Axial CT scan showing (a) otic capsule sparing and (b) otic capsule violating temporal bone fractures.

The use of steroids is associated with increased mortality when there is concomitant traumatic brain injury, so it should not be used routinely.

In rare cases of bilateral temporal bone fracture, urgent hearing evaluation is required as emergency cochlear implantation may be required prior to the onset of reparative cochlear fibrosis.

Facial Palsy[3]

Facial palsy complicates 7% of temporal bone fractures: 66% occur at the geniculate ganglion and 20% at the second genu, 8% in the tympanic and 6% in the mastoid segments. It is important to ascertain whether the onset of a facial palsy was immediate or delayed, and if partial or complete. The implication of an immediate palsy is that the nerve has been directly traumatized, impinged or transected. Delayed onset, even if only by a few minutes, or any residual function, implies neural continuity. Cases where onset cannot be ascertained are best considered as of immediate onset.

The use of steroids is standard practice in those cases without evidence of significant traumatic brain injury; the true benefit is unknown.

The large majority of incomplete and delayed palsies recover to a House-Brackmann grade I or II.

Electrophysiological testing is only necessary in cases of immediate complete palsy, or in those with an uncertain history, where surgical decompression is considered. Without surgery, 50% of complete, and immediate, palsies make a good recovery. The role of surgical decompression remains controversial. Patients with 90% neural degeneration on electroneuronography, performed 14 days post injury are considered for surgery, although 67% of those meeting these criteria still recover well without intervention.

If the trauma is clearly localised to the vertical or horizontal portions then a transmastoid approach provides access from the stylomastoid foramen to the geniculate ganglion. Access to the intralabyrinthine portion while preserving audiovestibular function is best provided by the middle fossa approach, but a translabyrinthine approach gives excellent access in cases where cochlear and vestibular function have been lost.

CSF Leak

CSF leaks complicate 11–33% of temporal bone fractures. Spontaneous closure occurs in 95% within 14 days. The chance of spontaneous closure is proportional to the size of defect. Recurrent late meningitis may occur many years following the apparent spontaneous healing of a CSF leak. Clear fluid found when a grommet is placed for an effusion is a common presentation. The quoted risk of meningitis secondary to ascending infection varies widely but is about 2% when the leak has stopped within a week, increasing to about 7% overall with a persisting leak. This increases to 20% if a concurrent ear infection is present.

Surgical closure is reserved for acute leaks that persist for more than a week, large defects, and herniation of meninges/brain into underlying spaces where there is a risk of infection. The location of a defect on a CT scan is not necessarily the site of the leak. Peri-operative fluorescein cisternography may be useful for locating it.

Small tegmen and posterior dural plate defects may be closed via a transmastoid approach. This approach is familiar to otologists and does not require brain retraction, but it may require disarticulation of the ossicles to obtain access to a medial defect. Large defects and revision cases are best treated via the middle fossa; this approach provides excellent access but requires retraction of the temporal lobe. Repair utilises a multilayered technique with materials such as fascia, cartilage, bone and fibrin glue.

Vascular Injury

The risk of vascular injury is higher in more severe skull base fractures, particularly if there is evidence of otic capsule fracture or cranial nerve palsies. Carotid injury may occur at the junction of the lacerum and cavernous portions or more rarely through the petrous segment. Carotid artery dissection with a carotid–cavernous fistula is a rare consequence as is intimal damage resulting in aseptic sigmoid sinus thrombosis. The jugular and carotid canals should be routinely examined on the CT scan with a low threshold for requesting angiography. A specialist neurosurgical opinion should be sought. Treatment is usually endovascular with a variety of options including detachable balloons, coils and stents.

Otitic Barotrauma

Middle Ear Barotrauma

Injuries include tympanic membrane perforation, ossicular fracture and/or dislocation and are common during flight and scuba diving.

They are caused by an excessive pressure gradient, or a sudden equalization of pressure, across the tympanic membrane. Rapid alterations in ambient pressure increase the risk. The middle ear passively vents during ascent, but the introduction of new air, by active Eustachian tube opening manoeuvres, is required on descent. The more rapid the change in ambient pressure the higher the risk, which is also increased in those whose middle ears asymmetrically equalise, experience an inability to voluntarily equalize at sea level (divers) or have nasal obstruction.

Spontaneous healing, with good hearing outcomes, frequently occurs within the 3 months following trauma. Corrective surgery should therefore not be performed until after this time.

The inability to voluntarily equalise middle ear pressure is the best predictor of susceptibility to diving-related trauma but not for flying-related trauma. Tympanometry is not a useful predictor of susceptibility unless combined with multiple tests.

Proven effective methods of prevention are oral decongestants, regular use of an Otovent™ nasal balloon, Eustachian tube balloon dilation and nasal septal (vomeroethmoidal) surgery. 'Flight earplugs' to decrease the rate of external auditory canal pressure change may improve the ability to 'equalise' middle ear pressures. Topical nasal decongestant sprays are ineffective. Rhinitis should be treated, but individuals should not dive with upper respiratory infections.

Perilymphatic Fistula (PLF)

The most common causes of PLF are barotrauma and head injury, but other causes include head injury, surgery, congenital anomalies and cholesteatoma.

Many PLFs are difficult to diagnose. Controversy continues regarding the existence of spontaneous fistulae. If these do occur, they are rare.

The exact timing of the onset of symptoms relative to an injury is crucial.

A typical history includes difficulty equalizing the middle ear pressure during descent, particularly during an upper respiratory infection. There is a sudden onset of symptoms, usually vertigo, hearing loss and tinnitus, more rarely Tullio's phenomenon (third window effect) and positional vertigo. Muffled hearing and occasional, but persistent, disequilibrium may be the only symptoms. Acute symptoms usually resolve after several days. Mild disequilibrium (which may change to transient vertigo on straining), mild persistent nausea, motion intolerance and a subtle sense of 'not coping', are the most common symptoms of a chronic fistula. Fluctuating hearing may occur, which might be positional due to air in the labyrinth; although a convincing sign, it occurs infrequently.

An expectant approach, bed rest and steroids, is only appropriate for acute presentations if there is minimal hearing loss. Immediate surgery is indicated if there is any significant hearing loss. Chronic fistula symptoms require further evaluation and elective exploration. At tympanotomy, the oval and round windows should be reinforced with fascia/fat/vein adventitia. Surgical results are poor for hearing restoration, usually due to late presentation or delayed surgery, but are excellent for balance control.

Further reading

1. Brodie HA, Thompson TC. Management of complications from 820 temporal bone fractures. *Am J Otol.* 1997;18:188–197.

2. Darrouzet V, Duclos JY, Liguoro D, Truilhe Y, De Bonfils C, Bebear JP. Management of facial paralysis resulting from temporal bone fractures: Our experience in 115 cases. *Otolaryngol Head Neck Surg.* 2001;125:77–84.

3. Hornibrook J. Perilymph fistula: fifty years of controversy. *ISRN Otolaryngol.* 2012; 2012:1–9.

20. METABOLIC BONE DISEASE AND SYSTEMIC DISORDERS OF THE TEMPORAL BONE

Metabolic Bone Disease

Fibrous Dysplasia (FD)

In fibrous dysplasia (FD) normal bone marrow is replaced by proliferating fibro-osseous tissue that expands and thins the overlying cortex. FD accounts for 2–3% of all benign bone tumours and is commonly found in young adults. There are three types[1]:

1 *Monostotic*: single bone disease, craniofacial bones affected in 10–25%
2 *Polyostotic*: involving several ipsilateral bones, craniofacial bones affected in >50%
3 *McCune-Albright syndrome*: cafe-au-lait pigmentation, polyostotic FD and hyper-functioning endocrinopathies

Clinical Features

- Cosmetic deformity or mass.
- Conductive hearing loss (CHL) (stenosis of the external auditory canal [EAC]).
- Sensorineural hearing loss (SNHL) (compression of internal auditory canal [IAC], invasion of the otic capsule, infection).
- Disequilibrium, tinnitus, otorrhea, otalgia, trismus, facial nerve compression (Figure 20.1).
- Alkaline phosphatase (ALP) may be raised.
- Computed tomography (CT) shows 'ground glass appearance', asymmetry of the skull, thickening of the cranial cortex and cystic changes.
- Macroscopically there is gritty/rubbery, grayish-pink material.

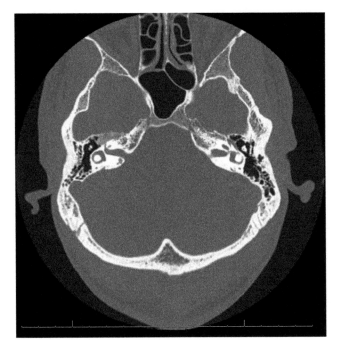

Figure 20.1   Axial computed tomography. Fibrous dysplasia affecting the right petrous temporal bone and facial nerve in its geniculate and tympanic segments.

Treatment

The majority of craniofacial monostotic FD requires no treatment beyond recognition and reassurance. Bisphosphonates can be used to relieve bone pain and reduce fracture risk. Surgical excision can be curative, but risks must be weighed against benefits, and craniofacial monostotic FD often recurs. Radiation has been reported to cause malignant transformation, particularly in polyostotic forms.

Osteitis Deformans/Paget's Disease

Osteitis deformans/Paget's disease is a systemic disease associated with four genetic mutations (the most common mutation is sequestosome 1). There is an increasing risk with age.

Characteristics

- Normal lamellar patterned bone replaced with disorganised woven pattern.
- Disease hallmark is bone expansion and deformity of the axial skeleton.
- Bone pain, pathological fractures.
- 95% have raised ALP.
- 1% undergo malignant transformation.
- Disease can burn out.

Otological Features

- 40% have hearing loss (HL), such as CHL in low frequencies, progressive SNHL starting with high-frequency loss. This is likely as a result of progressive demineralization of the otic capsule.
- 20% have tinnitus and vertigo.[1]
- CT shows 'osteoporosis circumscripta', which is radiolucency of the skull, cotton-wool appearance of bone, demineralization of the otic capsule and loss of the distinct bony contour (Figure 20.2).

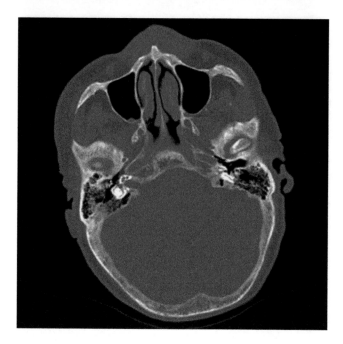

Figure 20.2 Axial computed tomography. Osteitis deformans affecting the occipital and temporal bones. There is loss expansion of the medullary cavity, coarsening of the trabecular pattern and diffuse sclerosis.

Treatment

- Bisphosphonates to prevent bone reabsorption and fractures (may slow hearing decline)
- Non-steroidal anti-inflammatory drugs (NSAIDs) for bone pain
- Hearing aid, cochlear implantation (CI)
- Middle ear surgery usually ineffective

Osteogenesis Imperfecta (Brittle-Bone Disease/Lobstein Disease)

Osteogenesis imperfecta (OI) is a connective tissue disorder caused by defects in type I collagen (>95% caused by dominant mutations in COL1A1/COLI1A2) leading to 'brittle bones'. Severe/lethal forms are associated with the recessive pattern. There are five main subtypes.

Characteristics

- Blue sclerae
- HL (rare in type IV, can be conductive, SNHL or mixed and seen earlier than patients with otosclerosis)
- Defective dentition
- Barrel chest
- Scoliosis
- Pathological fractures, joint laxity
- Growth retardation

Radiology

Radiology shows features similar to otosclerosis (but in OI the bony labyrinths are affected more). These features include demineralization of the otic capsule (halo or double ring on CT), enveloped stapes, obliterated inner ear windows, abnormal bone extension involving semi-circular canals or fallopian canal involvement.

Treatment
Bisphosphonates increase bone density, reduce bone pain and fracture risk. Stapedectomy is generally associated with good outcomes, though surgery can be technically more difficult and outcomes poorer than in otosclerosis. CI is another option.

Osteopetrosis (Albers-Sconberg/Marble Bone Disease)
Osteopetrosis is a rare condition affecting osteoclast activity causing failure of resorption of calcified cartilage and excessive immature bone formation. This leads to cortical thickening of the temporal bone (thick skull) and foramina stenosis/compression of corresponding cranial nerves. The condition is more common in Costa Rica and Saudi Arabia.

Characteristics
There are two types of osteopetrosis:

1 *Benign osteopetrosis (normal life span)*: Often asymptomatic, requiring no medical treatment.
2 *Malignant osteopetrosis*: Often presenting in infancy with bone marrow failure, neurological deficits, pathological fractures, severe anemia, failure to thrive and optic nerve atrophy. It is treated with interferon gamma and steroids.

ENT Manifestations
Ear, nose and throat (ENT) manifestations of osteopetrosis include nasal obstruction, obstructive sleep apnoea, HL (conductive/mixed), otitis media with effusion (OME), thickened tympanic membrane resulting in type B tympanograms (present in 80%), vertigo and facial nerve paresis. Imaging reveals poorly pneumatised mastoid air cells and narrowing of the EAC; middle ear space and Eustachian tube; IAC and petrous carotid canal. Treatment includes regular aural toilet, hearing aids and ventilation tubes.[2]

Infections Affecting the Temporal Bone
Mycobacterium Tuberculosis (TB)

- Mycobacterium tuberculosis (TB) is rare, <1% of all chronic OME
- Hematogenous spread or via Eustachian tube
- Consider if odourless otorrhoea with poor response to antibiotics, multiple perforations/large perforation, pale granulation tissue or patient from TB endemic areas
- Facial nerve palsy and early SNHL
- Send pus/tissue for polymerase chain reaction as microbiology swabs are rarely positive (<20%)
- Consider biopsy (granulomata with caseous necrosis)
- Can cause erosive destruction of the temporal bone

Treatment
Treatment is antituberculous treatment for 6 months, consider surgery for diagnosis or patients failing to respond to medical therapy.

Human Immunodeficiency Virus (HIV)

- RNA virus, preferentially infects neurons and immune cells, particularly CD4+ T cells.
- HL occurs in around one-third of patients; this may be conductive (OME, otitis externa, chronic otitis media) or sensorineural.
- Other features include facial nerve palsy and malignancy.
- Immunodeficiency is a risk factor for necrotising otitis externa.[2]
- Can have successful otological surgery to treat all secondary complications if HIV well controlled.

Lyme Disease

Lyme disease is spread by tick bites (genus *Ixodes*) that cause a localized skin reaction several days after a bite. The ticks that spread the disease are often found in woodland areas. The most common clinical symptoms are painful radiculitis, cranial palsy (43.4%; mostly facial which can be bilateral) and headache. However, there are case reports of stand-alone presentations with only sudden HL ± bilateral vestibular failure, but this is rare. Late stages of the disease can result in severe neurological dysfunction (chronic encephalomyelitis, ataxia, spastic paraparesis).

Investigations include a two-tier approach that include A C6 antigen–based enzyme-linked immunosorbent assay (ELISA; combined IgG and IgM) followed by secondary testing with a confirmatory immunoblot (separate IgG and IgM), if the test was positive or indeterminate.

Treatment is with oral doxycycline for 21 days or intravenous ceftriaxone in Lyme carditis or in unstable patients.

Syphilis

Syphilis is sexually transmitted and is caused by the spirochete *Treponema pallidum*, which can spread through the cerebral spinal fluid and into the endolymph of the inner ear. Otosyphilis is known to mimic Meniere's disease, autoimmune inner ear disease, perilymphatic fistula, sudden HL and bilateral vestibular loss. Secondary syphilis can present with a meningitis.

Radiological findings include inflammatory resorptive osteitis of the temporal bone, and rarely bony erosion of the ossicles. SNHL is reversible in syphilis if treated in time with penicillin antibiotics; consider screening for disease in patients with sudden SNHL (treponemal enzyme immunoassay to detect treponemal IgG and IgM).

Inflammatory Disease Affecting the Temporal Bone

These conditions are treated in conjunction with rheumatologists and/or other specialists. Treatment options may include oral steroids, steroid-sparing immunosuppressants (methotrexate, azathioprine, cyclosporine) or biologics (e.g. rituximab or etanercept).

Autoimmune Hearing Loss

Autoimmune HL is a progressive, bilateral, asymmetric subacute HL that occurs over weeks to months; HL is often steroid responsive. It may be primary (occurring in isolation) or secondary to another autoimmune disease. Vestibular involvement is ~50%. There is no consensus over diagnostic criteria and no clear evidence to suggest that intratympanic medication improves hearing outcomes.[3]

Cogan's Syndrome (CS)

Cogan's syndrome (CS) affects Caucasian adults in the third decade. Typical CS includes SNHL, interstitial keratitis and audiovestibular dysfunction; whereas atypical CS includes inflammatory ocular symptoms (glaucoma, conjunctivitis, episcleritis, uveitis) and SNHL.

CS is associated with systemic vasculitis in 15–21% and can coexist with other autoimmune diseases.

There is no routine laboratory test available for diagnosis. CI is considered for profound SNHL (early ossification of the cochlea).

Vogt-Koyanagi-Harada

Vogt-Koyanagi-Harada is a multisystem, idiopathic, bilateral granulomatous uveitis with neurologic, auditory or dermatologic manifestations.

Otological symptoms include SNHL (high frequency), which is steroid responsive, tinnitus and/or vertigo typically coinciding with the onset of ocular pathology.

ANCA-Associated Vasculitides

Antineutrophil cytoplasmic antibody (ANCA)-associated vasculitides affects small and large vessels. Immunofluorescence testing is done for c-ANCA/p-ANCA and ELISA testing for MPO and PR3 antibodies. Localised tissue biopsies from nose/ear provide low diagnostic yield.

There are three types of ANCA: granulomatosis with polyangiitis (respiratory tract), eosinophilic granulomatosis with polyangiitis (respiratory tract and skin) and microscopic polyangiitis (respiratory tract and kidneys).

Otological symptoms include chronic otitis media, vertigo, polyneuritis causing multiple cranial neuropathies (including facial nerve palsy) and SNHL. These symptoms (serous otitis media/HL) can be the first presentation of the disease.

Relapsing Polychondritis

Relapsing polychondritis is systemic, but episodic inflammatory disease primarily affects the cartilaginous structures of the ears, nose and tracheobronchial tree joints; inner ear; eyes and the cardiovascular system. It has an unknown aetiology but is often associated with rheumatoid arthritis (RA) and systemic lupus erythematosus. Cartilage biopsy is not recommended. Mortality is double that of the normal population.

Sarcoid

Sarcoid diseases are characterized by non-caseating granulomata mainly developing in the lungs. The skin, lymph nodes and joints may also be affected. Facial nerve palsy is the most common otologic manifestation and can develop either in isolation or with uveitis and parotitis as a component of Heerfordt's disease (uveoparotid fever). Raised angiotensin-converting enzyme titre helps to confirm the diagnosis and hypercalcaemia may also be present. Management is in conjunction with respiratory physicians and usually involves systemic corticosteroids/immunosuppressants.

Idiopathic

Langerhans Cell Histiocytosis (LCH)

The aetiology of Langerhans cell histiocytosis (LCH) is unknown, and the accumulation of clonal Langerhans cells occur within any part of the body. It can be single system or multisystem. Isolated pulmonary histiocytosis is common in adults. LCH can develop into malignant histiocytosis.

LCH is diagnosed based on positive immunohistochemistry (Langer CD 207 or CD1a) and histological examination demonstrating Birbeck granules on electron microscopy. Otologic symptoms are rare (<4%) but include otorrhea, soft tissue or postauricular swelling and often bilateral disease.

Imaging shows punched out lesions. LCH of the temporal bone rarely violates the otic capsule. It can mimic otitis media but mastoid disease sparing the middle ear, or outside-in osseous erosion.

On magnetic resonance imaging (MRI), LCH lesions are hypointense on T1-weighted images, isointense to hyperintense on T2-weighted images and avid with gadolinium. Positron emission topography is used to diagnose multisystem disease. LCT is treated with chemotherapy, radiotherapy and surgery for unifocal disease.

KEY POINTS

- There is a limited role for surgery in FD and Paget's disease of the temporal bone.
- Lyme disease can cause facial palsy particularly in children.
- TB of the temporal bone can present with odourless otorrhoea, middle ear granulation, facial palsy and HL.
- Autoimmune HL is typically subacute, bilateral, fluctuating and steroid responsive.

Further Reading

1. Xie C, Mathew R, Adam J, Patel PM. Metabolic bone diseases of the temporal bone: Part 2. *The Otorhinolargologist.* 2018;11(3).

2. Cohen BE, Durstenfeld A, Roehm PC. Viral causes of hearing loss: a review for hearing health professionals. *Trends Hear.* 2014;18:2331216514541361. doi:10.1177/2331216514541361

3. Strum D, Kim S, Shim T, Monfared A. An update on autoimmune inner ear disease: a systematic review of pharmacotherapy. *Am J Otolaryngol.* 2020; 41(1):102310.

21. THE FACIAL NERVE

Anatomy of the Facial Nerve

The key functions of the facial nerve include:

- Primarily motor nerve supplying muscles of facial expression
- Parasympathetic secretomotor supply to lacrimal and salivary glands
- Sensory supply from external auditory canal
- Special sensory (taste) from anterior two-thirds of tongue

The course of the facial nerve is shown in Figure 21.1 and can be divided into intracranial, intratemporal and extratemporal portions. The intracranial portion is approximately 24 mm

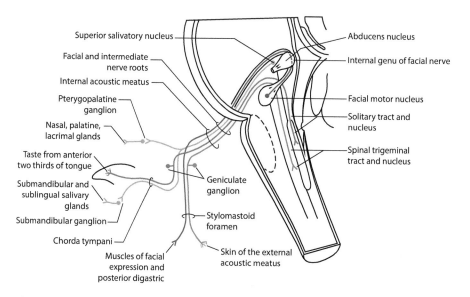

Figure 21.1 General visceral afferent axons (nasopharynx, palate, submandibular and sublingual salivary glands) not shown. Cell bodies of origin in the geniculate ganglion project to more caudal regions of the solitary nucleus. (With permission from Haines DE. Fundamental Neuroscience for Basic and Clinical Applications. London: Elsevier Health Sciences, 2012.)

long and courses through the cerebellopontine angle (CPA) cistern to the porus of the internal auditory meatus (IAM). The intratemporal portion is 28–30 mm long. This includes the meatal segment, which runs in the IAM. The labyrinthine segment then runs laterally to the first genu and the geniculate ganglion, the tympanic segment runs posteriorly from the geniculate ganglion to the second genu and the vertical segment runs from the second genu to the stylomastoid foramen. The extratemporal segment runs forward into the parotid gland where it divides into upper and lower branches.

Pathophysiology of Nerve Injury

Peripheral nerves may be injured in a variety of ways, with local or systemic causes. Ischaemia induced by mild pressure may produce transient paraesthesia with no obvious structural changes, and recovery is rapid. Prolonged ischaemia or immune-mediated attack may cause loss of myelin without loss of axonal integrity. In trauma, if the compressing force, such as a spicule of bone or a haematoma, is removed, remyelination typically takes place within 2–4 months, usually with little residual loss of function.

An injury that physically separates axons from their cell bodies triggers cellular events at the site of the lesion and in distant parts of the injured neurons and their target organs, which has a significant impact on outcome. Wallerian degeneration refers to the degeneration of a nerve distal to the site of injury. Peripherally, atrophy of chronically denervated muscles may preclude their reinnervation. Table 21.1 shows the Seddon and Sunderland classifications of nerve injury.

Table 21.1   Nerve injury classification and electrophysiological correlates

Seddon	Sunderland	Pathology	Electrophysiological correlate
Neurapraxia	Grade 1	A transient light compression causing endoneurial edema but no significant morphological changes. A more substantial and prolonged mechanical compression or stretch is most likely to cause a focal demyelination that may be paranodal or affect whole internodes. Anoxia plays a role in the pathogenesis	Conduction block ± conduction slowing. Never distal to 'lesion' shows normal conduction
Axonotmesis	Grade 2	Axons degenerate distal to the site of the 'lesion', irrespective of calibre or modality Endoneurium, perineurium and epineurium remain intact. Schwann cell basal lamina tuubes either remain continuous across the 'lesion' or are minimally separated within a morphologically intact perineurium and epineurium	Fibrillation Mild diminution to complete absence of SNAP and CMAP responses, in proportion to degree of axonal loss ± varying degrees of conduction block and slowing associated with demyelination
Axonotmesis	Grade 3	Endoneurium disrupted, axons degenerate distal to the site of the 'lesion'	Fibrillations, absent SNAP and CMAP responses
Axonotmesis	Grade 4	Perineurium disrupted, axons degenerate distal to the site pf 'lesion'	Fibrillations, absent SNAP and CMAP responses
Neurotmesis	Grade 5	Epineurium disrupted, axons degenerate distal to the site of the 'lesion'	Fibrillations, absent SNAP and CMAP responses

Source: Modified from Birch. Surgical disorders of the peripheral nerves. 2nd ed. Springer; London; 2011.
Note: SNAP, sensory nerve action potential; CMAP, compound muscle action potential.

Clinical Evaluation of Patients with Facial Palsy

History

Most patients with acute-onset facial palsy will be assumed to have an idiopathic (Bell's) palsy. Progressive palsy, or an incomplete facial nerve palsy that does not start to recover after 3 to 6 weeks, should prompt suspicion of neoplasm and further investigation. Ipsilateral recurrent facial nerve palsy is occasionally seen in patients with idiopathic palsy, Melkersson-Rosenthal syndrome (a condition characterised by facial oedema, familial history and fissured tongue) and tumours. Bilateral concurrent facial nerve paralysis is most commonly associated with severe head trauma or systemic conditions including Guillain-Barré syndrome, sarcoidosis, Lyme disease, rabies and Moebius syndrome.

Physical Examination

A thorough head, neck, otologic and cranial nerve examination is required when evaluating facial nerve dysfunction. The degree of facial weakness must be recorded and an attempt made to localise the site of the cause.

The House-Brackmann Staging System is the most widely used of several grading scales (Table 21.2).

Facial nerve dysfunction includes secondary effects which usually result from aberrant neural regeneration and include synkinesis, hemifacial spasm, contracture, crocodile tears, epiphora, dysgeusia, pain and hyperacusis. The Sunnybrook Facial Grading scale attempts to include some of these secondary effects in the overall score.

Functional and psychological impairments that include difficulties in eating, drinking, speaking and conveying emotion are not captured in any of the clinician-ranked scales and would be better measured by patient-reported outcome measures.

Table 21.2   House-Brackmann staging system

Degree of injury	Grade	Definition
Normal	I	Normal symmetrical function in all areas
Mild dysfunction (barely noticeable)	II	Slight weakness noticeable only on close inspection
		Complete eye closure with minimum effort
		Slight asymmetry of smile with maximal effort
		Synkinesis barely noticeable, contracture or spasm absent
Moderate dysfunction (obvious difference)	III	Obvious weakness, but not disfiguring
		May not be able to lift eyebrow
		Complete eye closure and strong but asymmetric mouth movement with maximal effort
		Obvious, but not disfiguring synkinesis, mass movement or spasm
Moderately severe dysfunction)	IV	Obvious disfiguring weakness
		Inability to lift eyebrow
		Incomplete eye closure and asymmetry of the mouth with maximal effort
		Severe synkinesis, mass movement, spasm
Severe dysfunction	V	Motion barely perceptible
		Incomplete eye closure, slight movement of the corner of the mouth
		Synkinesis, contracture and spasm usually absent
Total paralysis	VI	No movement, loss of tone, no synkinesis, contracture or spasm

Investigation and Nerve Monitoring

Electrophysiological Tests

Electrophysiological tests provide prognostic information to guide management in complete paralysis.

Electroneuronography (ENoG)

During electroneuronography (ENoG), a supramaximal stimulus is delivered to the facial nerve trunk as it exits the stylomastoid foramen and the evoked biphasic compound muscle action potential (CMAP) is recorded using surface electrodes. The response of the paralysed side is expressed as a percentage of the normal contralateral side. If the CMAP amplitude on the affected side is 10% of the normal side, then it is assumed that 90% axonal loss has been sustained. ENoG is said not to be useful until the fourth day of facial nerve paralysis, which is when axonal degeneration associated with injury occurs.

Electromyography (EMG)

Electromyography (EMG) records active motor unit potentials of the orbicularis oculi and orbicularis oris muscles during rest and voluntary contraction. EMG has a role in decision making, as seen in Table 21.3.

Table 21.3   ENoG and EMG

Study	Measurement	When to measure	Use in acute-onset paralysis	Use in long-standing paralysis	Long-term paralysis management decision
ENoG	Evoked CMAP compared with normal site	Between 3 days and 3 weeks	>90% of degenerated fibres suggests poor prognosis	Not useful because of desynchronisation	N/A
EMG Acute paralysis	Active motor unit potentials after voluntary forceful contraction	Complementary to ENoG, after 2 weeks	Presence of active motor potentials in response to voluntary contractions indicates good prognosis		
EMG Prolonged paralysis		In long-standing paralysis		Fibrillation potentials suggest Wallerian degeneration (arise 2–3 weeks after injury) Polyphasic potentials suggest reinnervation (may precede clinical recovery by 6–12 weeks) 'Silence' on EMG (no electrical output) indicates long-term denervation and suggests that muscle has been replaced by fibrous tissue.	Surgical exploration is indicated with a view to achieving nerve continuity Surgical intervention not indicated Static or dynamic facial reanimation is indicated.

Blood Investigations

In patients who present with an atypical history or who fail to recover within 6 weeks, the authors practice is to arrange the following blood tests:

- Angiotensin-converting enzyme: elevated in sarcoidosis
- Anti-neutrophil cytoplasmic antibody: elevated in granulomatosis with polyangiitis (GPA)
- Human immunodeficiency virus (HIV), Lyme and syphilis serology

Radiological Imaging

The optimal imaging modality for facial nerve disorders may include:

- Computed tomography (CT) if ear abnormality present or history of trauma
- Magnetic resonance imaging (MRI) with pre- and post-contrast of whole facial nerve course (cortex to neck) for tumours
- Scan at 3/12 in cases of presumed idiopathic if incomplete recovery

Management of the Patient with a Facial Nerve Disorder

Acute Facial Palsy

Eye Care

Appropriate eye care, including advice regarding corneal protection with lubrication and patching should be instituted immediately in cases where eye closure is impaired. Patients should be instructed in the use of drops (day) and ointment (night) and in manually closing their eyes and stretching the upper lid to prevent shortening. Upper eyelid weighting with external adhesive skin-tone coloured weights (Blinkeze™) can be advised.

Idiopathic (Bell's) Palsy

Patients present with a prodromal illness, which may include periauricular pain and general malaise. Within 72 hours they rapidly develop lower motor neuron facial weakness. In up to 70% of cases this weakness is complete (House-Brackmann VI).

The aetiology of idiopathic palsy remains unclear, but evidence suggests an infectious origin, which triggers an immunologic response resulting in damage to the facial nerve. Pathogens implicated include herpes simplex virus type 1 (HSV-1), herpes simplex virus type 2 (HSV-2), human herpesvirus and varicella zoster virus (VZV). Idiopathic palsy is more common in pregnancy and has a poorer prognosis with the majority of cases being in the third trimester.

Normal function is usually regained within 6 months in about two-thirds of all patients, but a significant proportion have long-term issues with facial asymmetry, tightness and synkinesis. Poor prognosis has been related to complete paralysis at onset.

The pharmacological management of idiopathic palsy primarily involves oral corticosteroid medication with benefit if instigated within 72 hours. In addition, the most recent evidence from a Cochrane review[1] concludes that the addition of antiviral medication likely improves the rate of recovery and reduces the long-term after effects of idiopathic palsy. A typical treatment regimen is prednisolone 1 mg/kg/day for 10 days and oral acyclovir (400 mg five times daily) for 10 days.

Inflammatory Disorders

For inflammatory conditions that cause facial palsy, including GPA, sarcoid and Lyme disease, see Chapter 20.

Iatrogenic Injury

If facial palsy is observed immediately after tympanomastoid surgery and the nerve was not injured/not at risk, a few hours of observation will allow local anaesthetic-induced weakness to clear. The possibility of a tight mastoid dressing over an exposed nerve should prompt consideration of pack removal. If the paralysis is incomplete or delayed, the patient should be started on oral steroids and observed. In cases where re-exploration is needed, this should be performed with an expert colleague. In rare cases, a delayed palsy is observed a few days after uneventful middle ear surgery. Use of systemic steroids should be considered and prognosis appears to be good.

Cerebellopontine Angle Tumour Surgery

Postoperative facial nerve function in CPA tumour surgery mainly depends on tumour size and surgical experience. When the facial nerve is lost during dissection, it may be possible to achieve an end-to-end anastomosis or place a cable interposition graft.

Facial Nerve Trauma

Management of facial nerve paralysis following trauma is often deferred until the patient is medically stable. Facial nerve paralysis can result from stab wounds to the face or mandibular fractures. If possible, it is advisable to explore the region within 3 days as a nerve stimulator may be used to identify the distal nerve branches. With gunshot wounds care must be taken when assessing facial nerve function as there is often significant facial oedema and both muscle tone and eye closure appear adequate when in fact they are not. For temporal bone fractures see Chapter 19.

Tumours of the Facial Nerve

Facial nerve tumours are rare. The most common histological type are facial nerve schwannomas (FNS); however, facial nerve haemangiomas, malignant nerve sheath tumours and 'skip' lesions from parotid malignancies, amongst others, can also occur. As with other schwannomas, FNS are benign, slow-growing tumours arising from Schwann cells within the nerve sheath.

Clinical Presentation of Facial Schwannomas

FNS can arise from anywhere along the course of the facial nerve from the CPA to the ramifications within the parotid. FNS are commonly found to involve multiple segments with the most common sites being the geniculate ganglion (68%), labyrinthine (52%) and tympanic (43%) segments. Symptoms vary according to the segment involved. Whilst presentation can be with sudden-onset facial weakness, progressive weakness or hemifacial spasm, particularly the combination of synkinesis and partial paralysis are more suggestive of FNS. In addition, many patients preserve normal facial nerve function and may present with hearing loss, tinnitus, imbalance or a neck lump. Hearing loss may be sensorineural with IAM/CPA involvement or conductive if the horizontal portion of the facial nerve is affected.

Investigations

Diagnosis is with high-resolution cross-sectional imaging including T1-weighted MRI with gadolinium. FNS that are limited to the IAM/CPA can be difficult to differentiate from vestibular schwannomas, but involvement of the geniculate ganglion with extension along the greater superficial petrosal nerve is indicative of FNS (Figure 21.2). CT of the temporal bones may demonstrate smooth bony expansion at the site of the FNS.

Management of Facial Nerve Schwannomas

The primary aim of management is preservation of optimal facial function for as long as possible. For most patients this is achieved through conservative management with observation and serial scanning. For tumours that grow and/or develop loss of facial function, treatment options will include stereotactic radiosurgery (SRS), bony decompression of the IAM/facial canal, surgical debulking or excision with grafting/reanimation. Facial nerve resection with grafting is unlikely to achieve better than House-Brackman grade III, therefore, for patients with growing tumours but normal facial function, SRS is usually preferred.

Multidisciplinary Management of Established Facial Palsy

Facial palsy has a huge negative impact on quality of life and is best managed by a multidisciplinary facial nerve clinic comprising surgeons from otolaryngology and plastic surgery and

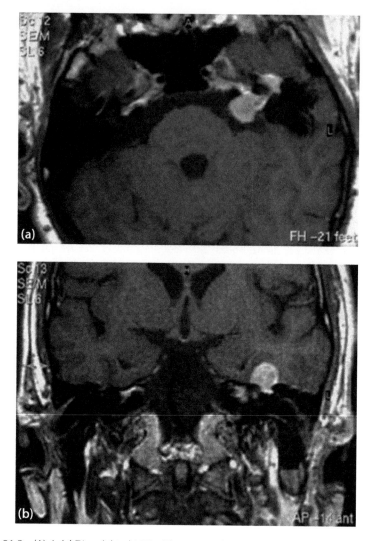

Figure 21.2 (A) Axial T1-weighted MRI with contrast showing enhancing nerve facial schwannoma filling the internal auditory meatus and extending along the greater superficial petrosal nerve into the middle fossa. (B) Coronal MRI showing a facial schwannoma arising from the geniculate ganglion and extending through the petrosal foramen into the middle fossa, pushing upwards into the temporal lobe.

highly specialised facial therapists. Additional support from an oculoplastic surgeon, expert radiologist, clinical photography and psychological services is advised. The development of support networks and groups has enabled patients to benefit from the experience of others.

Physiotherapy
Tightness and shortening of the muscle fibres can result in a 'frozen face'. Specific guidance regarding muscle stretches allows the muscles to relax and facial symmetry to improve. Once the muscle length is restored, more active movement is usually achieved.

Chemodenervation with Botulinum Toxin
Botulinum toxin can be used to release the over-tightened facial muscles. In patients with synkinesis (unwanted muscle contractions resulting from aberrant reinnervation)

chemodenervation is helpful in reducing these unwanted movements. Chemodenervation can be employed to weaken the more active 'normal' facial muscles to achieve a more balanced facial appearance.

FACIAL REANIMATION

Reinnervation
Lack of recovery of facial function by 12 months is considered a permanent deficit as loss of motor end-plate units likely means that reinnervation techniques will have no beneficial effect. Prior to this point, nerve transfers including contralateral facial nerve, nerve to masseter and the hypoglossal nerve can be employed.

Static Reanimation
Periocular surgery, including lower-lid tightening, lateral canthopexy, brow lift and upper eyelid positioning/weighting surgery may be performed under local anaesthesia and can provide benefit for the patient with troublesome eye symptoms. Various face-lifting techniques can improve the static position of the face.

Dynamic Reanimation
In those patients in whom active movement is desired, particularly in terms of smile, it is usually necessary to bring new tissue to the area. This may be in the form of muscle transfer, for example, a temporalis transfer or free muscle graft. In the latter case, innervation of the muscle graft may be from the facial nerve stump (e.g. in a cancer case) or more commonly the nerve to masseter or cross face nerve graft.

KEY POINTS

- Most common cause is idiopathic (Bell's palsy).
- Slowly progressing weakness suggests space-occupying lesion (anywhere along the course of the nerve).
- Corticosteroids are the mainstay of acute management (antivirals indicated in complete palsy).
- Two-thirds of patients with Bell's palsy recover completely by 6 months.
- Established weakness should be managed in specialist multidisciplinary treatment.

Further Reading

1. Gagyor I, Madhok VB, Daly F, Sullivan F. Antiviral treatment for Bell's palsy (idiopathic facial paralysis). *Cochrane Database Syst Rev.* 2019; 9(9):CD001869. doi: 10.1002/14651858.CD001869.pub9.
2. Peitersen E. The natural history of Bell's palsy. *Am J Otol.* 1982; 4(2):107–111.

22. VESTIBULAR SCHWANNOMA

Overview
Vestibular schwannomas (VS) are the most common tumours of the cerebellopontine angle (CPA) although, with an incidence of 33.8 tumours per 1,000,000 person-years, they remain rare clinical entities. They are benign lesions that arise from abnormal proliferation of Schwann cells along the vestibular divisions of the vestibulocochlear nerve (cranial nerve [CN] VIII).

Table 22.1   Classification of VS according to size[a]

Classification	Grade	Size (mm)
Grade 0	Intrameatal	0
Grade 1	Small	1–10
Grade 2	Medium	11–20
Grade 3	Moderately large	21–30
Grade 4	Large	31–40
Grade 5	Giant	>40

[a]   Consensus Meeting on Reporting Systems on Vestibular Schwannomas (Kanzaki et al., 2003).

VS may be confined to the internal auditory canal (IAC) or extend into the CPA. Uncommonly they can be entirely medial. Rarely, they can also invade the labyrinth. Current consensus is that the largest extrameatal dimension should be used to report tumour size (Table 22.1).

The diagnosis of VS relies mainly on magnetic resonance imaging (MRI) scanning. VS are iso/hypointense on T1- and T2-weighted sequences and they enhance avidly with contrast (gadolinium). T2-weighted imaging is adequate for diagnosis and monitoring, but a contrast-enhanced scan can help distinguish VS from other lesions, and fat suppression can diagnose lipomas. It is generally accepted that every patient with unilateral audiovestibular symptoms of unknown aetiology should undergo an MRI scan of the IACs. This is also true for patients presenting with sudden sensorineural hearing loss (SSNHL), where an underlying VS is found in 1.9–4.9% of cases.

At diagnosis, the average tumour size is 10 mm but 33% are confined to the IAC. Approximately 30% of tumours demonstrate growth after diagnosis (>2mm) with approximately 10% showing regression and approximately 60% remaining stable. Tumour growth can, but rarely does, occur after 5 years of radiological stability.

Those VS that demonstrate growth have a mean annual growth rate of 1.6–4.7mm. Over a 5-year period, 23% of purely intrameatal tumours will extend into the CPA.

Most tumours are solid, but cystic changes are seen in around 10% of tumours. Cystic changes are associated with more unpredictable tumour behaviour and some authors have reported that radiotherapy is less effective in these cases. Growing cystic tumours may therefore be considered earlier for surgery.

Overall, 95% of VS patients will suffer from hearing loss, either at presentation or subsequently (Table 22.2). It is usually progressive but it may be of sudden onset in up to 10% of neurofibromatosis type 2 (NF2)-related tumours and 20% of sporadic tumours. Seventy percent of patients have tinnitus, usually not disturbing, and 50% have balance disturbance at presentation. There is no association between audiological symptoms and tumour size. Non-audiovestibular symptoms such as facial numbness, ataxia or headache may also develop but usually only occur with larger tumours. The most widely used hearing classification systems for VS patients are the American Academy of Otolaryngology-Head and Neck Surgery classification (AAO-HNS) and the Word Recognition Scale (WRS).

Over a 10-year period of observation, 54% lose their AAO-HNS class A hearing level. Over the same period, those who had WRS class 0 hearing at presentation will deteriorate to class 2 or worse in 31% of patients.

Tumour Treatment

There are three main treatment options: wait and rescan, radiotherapy and surgery.

Based on the current literature, a few general management principles can be established:

- An initial wait and rescan approach is indicated for tumours below 20mm as long as there is no significant brainstem compression.

Table 22.2   Classification of hearing levels

AAO-HNS (1995)		
Class[a]	Pure-tone average (dB)[b]	Speech discrimination scores (%)
A	≤30	>70
B	>30 and ≤50	≥50
C	>50	≥50
D	Any level	<50
Word Recognition Scale		
Class[c]	Speech discrimination scores (%)	
0	100	
I	70–99	
II	50–69	
III	1–49	
IV	0	

a   Class A and B hearing are referred to as 'serviceable', while class C and D are 'non-serviceable'.
b   Pure-tone average: average thresholds (dB) at 500, 1000, 2000 and 4000 Hz.
c   Class 0 and I hearing are considered 'good'.

- If significant tumour growth occurs (>2 mm), active treatment (radiotherapy or surgery) must be considered although it may be deferred if growth is slow and tumour size is small, or if there are medical contraindications or limited life expectancy, as around 20% of tumours stop growing after a period of growth.
- Growing tumours up to around 25 mm may be treated with radiotherapy, although surgery is an option depending on the patients risk preferences.
- Tumours larger than 25 mm are generally treated with surgical resection.

Radiotherapy

Two different types of radiotherapy treatment are currently available, stereotactic radiosurgery (SRS) and fractionated radiotherapy (FRT). SRS is generally given as a single dose of treatment. Two main types of radiotherapy are used: gamma radiation or electrons. The former is delivered by the Gamma Knife. The latter is delivered via a linear accelerator (LINAC) with several types of machines available that vary with regards to their method of targeting (e.g. Novalis and CyberKnife). A dose of 12–14Gy at the tumour margins is the usual dose used, which balances tumour control with risk of complication. In FRT, multiple treatment sessions are required (1.8–2Gy/day over 5–6 weeks or 5–7Gy/day over 3–5 fractions) and treatment is usually delivered using a LINAC. Accuracy is sub-millimetric with the head fixed by a tight mask for LINAC and by a frame fixed to the head in Gamma Knife.

The main objective of radiotherapy in VS is to stop tumour growth and avoid further need for surgical intervention. Tumours may transiently enlarge up to 24 months post-treatment, after which they usually stabilise or regress. When a tumour begins or continues to enlarge after that period, treatment failure is confirmed and surgery is generally indicated. The reported tumour-control rate following radiotherapy ranges from 92–98% over a 3- to 10-year follow-up period. Patients may experience various complications after treatment, including:

- Trigeminal neuropathy (0, 3–27%)
- Facial nerve palsy and/or facial hemispasm (<2%)
- Hydrocephalus (<1%; increased risk if CPA component >2.5cm)
- Brain radionecrosis and/or stroke
- Hearing loss
- Induction of new tumours
- Conversion of a benign tumour to a malignant one

A recent meta-analysis found that of those that had serviceable hearing (AAO-HNS class A or B), only 25% of patients retain serviceable hearing after 10 years of follow-up. Induction of new tumours and malignant transformation in the existing tumour are very rare, occurring in much less than 1% of patients per decade after treatment. These latter risks are less relevant to the older patient and make radiotherapy, with its relatively low morbidity, particularly attractive to this group.

Surgery

Surgery is the treatment of choice for tumours >25 mm and may be offered instead of radiotherapy for smaller growing tumours, particularly in the younger age group. Three surgical approaches are widely used to resect VS: translabyrinthine, retrosigmoid and middle fossa (Table 22.3). The retrolabyrinthine, transcochlear and endoscopic transpromontorial approaches have also been described.

Table 22.3 Surgical approaches to the CPA

Surgical approach	Key surgical steps	Advantages	Disadvantages
Translabyrinthine	1 Skin and periosteal flap 2 Extended cortical mastoidectomy 3 Bony labyrinthectomy 4 Jugular bulb and facial nerve skeletonisation 5 IAM skeletonisation 6 Identification of the facial nerve (lateral portion of the IAM) 7 Opening of the posterior fossa dura 8 Tumour removal 9 Closure (with abdominal fat graft)	1 Extradural drilling 2 No cerebellar retraction 3 Early identification of the facial nerve (lateral end of the IAC) 4 VS of any size can be removed 5 Immediate repair of facial nerve possible	1 No hearing preservation 2 Increased incidence of postop CSF leaks
Middle fossa	1 Skin incision and division of temporalis muscle 2 Middle fossa craniectomy 3 Extradural approach to the middle fossa floor and posterior fossa 4 IAM skeletonisation 5 Identification of facial and vestibular nerves 6 Tumour removal 7 Closure	1 Hearing preservation (possible) 2 No cerebellar retraction 3 Extradural drilling 4 Good access to the lateral end of the IAM compared with retrosigmoid	1 Facial nerve between the surgeon and the tumour (unfavorable position) 2 Temporal lobe retraction with risk of epilepsy 3 Removal of tumour with a maximal CPA dimension of 10–15 mm
Retrosigmoid	1 Skin and soft tissue incisions 2 Retrosigmoid craniectomy 3 Dural opening and CSF decompression 4 Intradural approach to the tumour 5 Tumour removal (± IAC drilling) 6 Closure	1 Hearing preservation (possible) 2 Excellent visualisation of the CPA	1 Intradural drilling 2 Cerebellar retraction 3 Increased incidence of postoperative headache 4 Limited access to the lateral portion of the IAM

Both the middle fossa and retrosigmoid approaches offer the potential benefit of hearing preservation. This is also true for the retrolabyrinthine approach. To preserve hearing, the tumour must be small (maximal CPA component of <10 mm) and not extend up to the fundus of the IAC. Approximately 50% of patients retain serviceable hearing 10 years after surgery. However, hearing preservation rates vary widely depending on the surgical approach used.

There are two main factors affecting surgical outcomes and postoperative complication rates: tumour size (most important) and experience/surgical skills of the skull base unit. While mortality is rare (≤1%), surgical excision of a VS is a major surgical intervention that has a wide range of potential complications, the most common of which is cerebrospinal fluid (CSF) leakage. The leak may occur through the wound, from the external ear canal or from the nose via the Eustachian tube. Minor leaks may be managed conservatively with a lumbar drain. More severe CSF leaks are managed with blind sac closure and Eustachian tube obliteration, with or without CSF lumbar drainage. Refractory leaks will rarely require permanent CSF diversion (<1%).

The facial nerve is in close proximity to the tumour and its preservation is a key aim of surgery. Most series report the following facial nerve outcomes, using the House-Brackmann (HB) classification:

- *0–15 mm*: 80–95% HB grade I–II with 100% anatomical preservation
- *>15–25 mm*: 80–90% HB grade I–II with 90% anatomical preservation
- *>25 mm*: 50–70% HB grade I–II with 65–80% anatomical preservation

Recurrence rate after surgery is mainly influenced by the completeness of resection. Following gross total excision, recurrence is observed in 1–3% of cases. For near-total (linear remnant of tumour adherent to the facial nerve) and subtotal resections (solid mass of tumour left behind), regrowth rates can reach up to 21% and 22%, respectively. The tumour residuum may necessitate further treatment by radiotherapy or surgery depending on its size and whether or not it is growing on radiological follow-up.

Neurofibromatosis Type 2 (NF2)

NF2 is a genetic condition associated with the development of numerous tumours involving the nervous system. The disorder is inherited in an autosomal dominant fashion. In around 50% of cases, patients do not have any positive family history and present with a *de novo* mutation. Among *de novo* cases, up to 60% display somatic mosaicism, where one cell lineage with a mutated NF2 gene and one without any mutation develop throughout the body. In the presence of mosaicism, mutation is postzygotic and patients have more localised manifestations with less severe phenotypes. Because of mosaicism, the transmission rate in *de novo* cases is below 50%. In the second generation and beyond, transmission is 50%, as children inheriting NF2 from a mosaic parent will have the NF2 mutation in their germline.

The NF2 gene is located on chromosome 22q12.2 and encodes the NF2 protein, also known as merlin or schwannomin. This cell cytoskeleton–associated protein is involved in cell growth inhibition. The loss of these tumour-suppressor functions is believed to be the main factor in the formation of all schwannomas and meningiomas. A range of mutation types has been identified in NF2 including missense, truncating and splice site mutations and deletions. There is a strong genotype/phenotype relationship with missense mutations being associated with milder disease compared with truncating mutations.

The birth incidence of NF2 in the United Kingdom is estimated at 1 in 33,000 live births. By 60 years of age, almost every NF2 patient will be symptomatic. Bilateral VS are almost pathognomonic in NF2 and 95% of patients will develop bilateral tumours by the age of 30. Schwannomas may also affect other cranial, spinal and peripheral nerves. Approximately 50% of patients have intracranial or spinal meningiomas. Less frequently, they can develop other low-grade intracranial tumours, such as ependymomas. Ophthalmic abnormalities are also frequently encountered (e.g. 60–80% cataracts). Over the years, different clinical diagnostic criteria have been proposed, among which the 'Revised Manchester criteria' is the most widely used.

When NF2 is suspected, contrast-enhanced MRI scanning of the head and whole spine must be performed. At-risk individuals requiring further investigations must meet one of the following criteria:

- Positive family history of NF2
- <30 years old presenting with unilateral VS and/or meningioma
- Multiple spinal tumours (schwannomas and/or meningiomas)
- Cutaneous schwannomas

The screening protocol for VS in asymptomatic at-risk patients is as follows:

- Genetic screening
- Start MRI screening from age 10
  - 10–20 years: MRI every 2 years
  - 21–40 years: MRI every 3–5 years (because this group have slower growing tumours)
- If genetic screening negative and no tumour by age 40 then discharge

NF2 can also be diagnosed by identifying pathological mutations in patients' blood, with a success rate of 93% in non-mosaic cases. The presence of the NF2 mutation in blood is much lower in mosaic cases.

Overall, 60% of patients with NF2 have bilateral VS at their initial assessment. VS in NF2 tend to be more aggressive than sporadic tumours, but behavior is influenced by genotype/mosaicism. Overall 65% of NF2 VS demonstrate growth over time, with an average growth rate of 2mm/year. Over the course of their disease, most patients will develop bilateral profound deafness either as a result of the tumour or treatment.

Historically, VS treatment in NF2 has been mainly surgical. A conservative approach is, however, indicated for small- or medium-sized stable or very slow growing tumours. New systemic therapies such as bevacizumab, a monoclonal antibody of vascular endothelial growth factor A, have demonstrated considerable efficacy in controlling VS growth and may also preserve audiological function. In a limited number of cases, radiotherapy may be considered, although control is less effective compared with sporadic tumours. There is also a greater risk of inducing new tumours within the radiotherapy field and of inducing malignant change in previously treated tumours (malignant peripheral nerve sheath tumours) compared with sporadic tumours, especially if treated at a young age.

Optimising hearing rehabilitation in NF2 is critical as bilateral hearing loss has a very significant impact on quality of life. In those who develop profound hearing loss in an ear with a stable tumour (whether through its natural behaviour or through treatment with radiotherapy/bevacizumab) there is now good evidence for the effectiveness of cochlear implantation. Similarly, there is good evidence that, in selected cases, tumour removal with preservation of the cochlear nerve together with cochlear implantation offers reasonable hearing outcomes. Outcomes are, however, less good in NF2 than the average non-NF2 cochlear implant user, with untreated ears having the best outcome and those having had radiotherapy or nerve-preserving surgery having poorer outcomes. For most patients having surgery, cochlear nerve preservation is not possible and the only way to provide some audition is through auditory brainstem implantation (ABI). These provide environmental sound awareness and act as an aid to lipreading in most cases. Only 10% of recipients achieve open-set speech discrimination. Both cochlear implantation and ABI have a non-user rate of around 20% in NF2.

KEY POINTS

- Sporadic and NF2-related VS are rare benign slow-growing tumours originating from the vestibular divisions of CN VIII.
- They most often present with hearing loss, tinnitus or balance disturbance.
- While there is no correlation between tumour size and hearing loss at presentation, other non-audiological symptoms are associated with larger tumour size.
- MRI scan with contrast is the diagnostic modality of choice for VS and must be performed in the presence of unilateral or asymmetric audiovestibular symptoms of unknown aetiology.
- NF2 is an autosomal dominant disorder associated with a mutation on chromosome 22q12.2. Bilateral VS is almost pathognomonic of this condition.
- Small- or medium-sized VS may be managed conservatively (watch and wait) with only 30% demonstrating growth. Growing small- or medium-sized tumours may be managed with surgical resection or with radiotherapy. Large tumours (>3cm) are generally managed with surgical resection. In NF2, systemic drug therapies, such as bevacizumab, have demonstrated significant efficacy in controlling tumour growth.
- Radiotherapy has a high tumour control rate (92–98%) and low short-term complication rates. Hearing loss increases greater than it would otherwise do following treatment and there is a small risk of inducing new tumours or inducing malignant change in the treated tumour in the long run.
- Surgery is the treatment of choice for large tumours or following radiotherapy failure. It is also a viable option for growing small- and medium-sized VS. There is a risk of facial palsy, which increases with increasing tumour size.

Further Reading

Borsetto D., Faccioli C., and Zanoletti E., Sporadic acoustic neuroma: current treatment options with focus on hearing outcome. *Hearing, Balance and Communication*, 2018. 16(4): p. 248–254.

Carlson M.L. (Ed.), *Comprehensive Management of Vestibular Schwannoma*, New York: Thieme, 2019.

Kanzaki J, Tos M, Sanna M, et al. New and modified reporting systems from the consensus meeting on systems for reporting results in vestibular schwannoma. *Otol Neurotol* 2003; 24(4): 642–648.

23. LESIONS OF THE CEREBELLOPONTINE ANGLE, PETROUS APEX AND JUGULAR FORAMEN

Introduction

Most conditions of the petrous apex (PA), cerebellopontine angle (CPA) and jugular foramen (JF) can be distinguished by using a combination of computed tomography (CT) and magnetic resonance (MR) without the need for biopsy (Table 23.1). Bony destruction in the CT is suggestive of a malignant process, whereas well-defined expansion is indicative of a benign process.

Petrous Apex Lesions
Anatomy

- The PA is the anteromedial pyramid-shaped portion of the petrous temporal bone.
- It is divided into two compartments by the internal auditory meatus: an anterior portion, principally consisting of bone marrow/air cells and a posterior portion, from the dense bone of the otic capsule (Figure 23.1).

Table 23.1 Conditions of the PA, CPA and JF with characteristic radiological findings

Pathology	Location	CT	T1	T2	Contrast	Peculiarity
					MRI	
Cholesterol Granuloma	PA	Expansile	↑	↑	No	Peripheral low-signal hemosiderin ring (T2) Consistency on T2 can be variable reflecting contents
Asymmetric marrow	PA	No expansile changes	↑	↑	No	Saturation on T1 fat sequences
Epidermoid cyst	PA/CPA	Expansile	↓	↑	No	High signal on DWI
Mucocele	PA	Expansile	↓	↑	No	DWI with no restricted diffusion
Meningioma	PA/CPA/JF	Hyperostosis	→/↑	→/↓	Yes	Dural tail, calcification
Arachnoid cyst	CPA	CSF density	↓	↑	No	Same signal as CSF
Schwannoma	CPA/JF	Isodense to the brain	→/↓	↑	Yes	Can contain cystic areas
Paraganglioma	JF	Expansile	→	↑	Yes	'Salt and pepper' appearance in larger lesions
Lipoma	CPA	Fat density	↑	↑	No	Saturation on T1 fat sequences
Chordoma	Clivus					
Chondrosarcoma	PA/petro-occipital fissure		→/↓	↑	Yes	Honeycomb enhancement
Metastasis, myeloma	PA/CPA	Aggressive Bony destruction	→/↓	→/↑	Yes	↑ age
Sarcoma, Langerhans cell histiocytosis	PA					↓ age
Petrositis	PA		→/↓	↑	Rim-enhancing	Meningeal thickening, enhancing Meckel cave, cranial nerves (especially cranial nerves V and VI)

- The tentorium inserts onto the petrous ridge to separate the middle and posterior cranial fossae.
- Relations of the PA include the petro-occipital fissure and clivus (medial), the inner ear (lateral), the petrous carotid artery as it exits the foramen lacerum (anterior), the CPA (posterior), the jugular bulb and inferior petrosal sinus (inferior), the middle cranial fossa and Meckel's cave (superior).
- Dorello's canal carries the sixth cranial nerve and is found at the medial end of petrous ridge at the confluence of the inferior petrosal and cavernous sinus.

Clinical Conditions

- Cholesterol granulomas and epidermoids: Cholesterol cysts or granulomas are thought to arise from haemorrhage into the air cell system causing an inflammatory reaction. Causative theories for this bleeding include Eustachian tube dysfunction and marrow exposed to the air cell system. Epidermoid lesions are thought to originate from transplantation of epithelial cell rests by the laterally migrating optic and

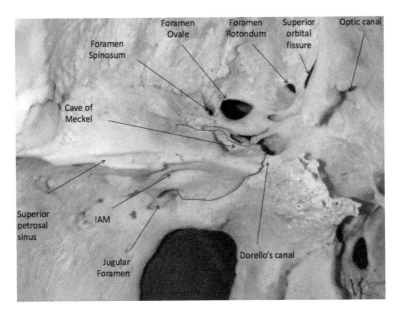

Figure 23.1 Anatomy of the petrous apex. IAM, internal auditory meatus.

otic capsules or developing neurovasculature. While cholesterol granulomas often present with fluctuating conductive hearing loss (presumably related to Eustachian tube dysfunction or cyst content leakage), epidermoids are more likely to present with progressive sensorineural hearing loss. Epidermoids may present with progressive facial nerve palsy while cholesterol granulomas rarely do. Trigeminal neuralgia, otalgia and ear pain can feature in cholesterol granulomas but this is unusual for epidermoids. Epidermoids show low signal on Tl-weighted images, while cholesterol granulomas exhibit high signal. Both types of cyst give high signal on T2-weighted images, but they can exhibit signal inhomogeneity depending on the nature and amount of cyst content.

Factors that must be considered when considering treatment approach include patient's symptoms, life expectancy and surgical anatomy. Neural deficits are rarely reversed by surgery. Figure 23.2 shows a proposed approach to management. Most cholesterol cysts can be drained into the mastoid or sphenoid system, allowing hearing to be retained. Approaches include the infra-labyrinthine and infra-cochlear approach (both limited by the height of the jugular bulb) and the trans-sphenoidal approach (limited by the position of the carotid). Drainage is associated with higher recurrence rate. For patients with facial palsy, pain, recurrent cysts and without serviceable hearing, resection may be favoured. A middle fossa, or subtotal petrosectomy + cochlear drill out may be used for small cysts, whilst an infratemporal fossa type B approach can be used for larger lesions.

- *Infection*: Petrous apicitis may present with middle ear infection, retro-orbital pain and sixth nerve palsy.
- *Tumours*: Chordomas arise from notochord remnants and are locally malignant (regional metastasis rare) and have a high tendency to recur. Chordomas almost always arise in the midline, and spread to the PA is common. They can present indolently with headache, visual disturbance or lower cranial nerve palsies. Chondrosarcomas likely develop from cartilaginous remnants from development. They too present insidiously and can cause various cranial nerve palsies. Surgery is considered the standard of care in the treatment of skull base chordomas and chondrosarcomas. Radiation therapy, in the form of proton beam therapy, stereotactic radiosurgery (SRS) or conventional fractionated radiation, is often used as adjuvant therapy.

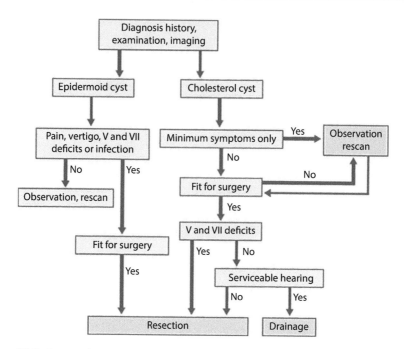

Figure 23.2   Proposed management scheme for epidermoid and cholesterol cysts.

Non-Vestibular Schwannoma Tumours of the Cerebellopontine Angle
Anatomy

- The CPA is an inverted, triangular subarachnoid space containing cranial nerves (V–XI) and blood vessels bathed in cerebrospinal fluid (CSF).
- Relations include pons (medial), cerebellum (posterior), tentorium (superior) and posterior temporal bone (lateral).
- Extends into the petrous bone as the internal auditory canal (IAC); its medial aperture is known as the porus acousticus.

Clinical Conditions

Vestibular schwannomas (VS) represent 80–90% of CPA tumours with the remaining 10–20% a mixture of predominantly benign pathologies. The symptoms at presentation are normally sensorineural hearing loss, tinnitus or vertigo. Other cranial nerves may be affected, causing altered facial sensation, facial weakness/spasm and lower cranial nerve compromise. Larger tumours may also cause brainstem compression.

The most common non-VS CPA lesions include:

- *Meningioma*: They form from clusters of epithelial cells at the tips of arachnoid villi. They may be well circumscribed or, more rarely, en plaque when their growth pattern results in a flat lesion. Bony infiltration may result in hyperostosis. Typically they displace or surround neurovascular structures. Histologically, meningiomas may be graded from 1 to 3 according to the World Health Organization (WHO) grading system (grade 1 and 2 benign, grade 3 malignant). Meningiomas occur in neurofibromatosis and are associated with radiotherapy and hormone therapy. Watchful waiting is less effective for meningiomas compared with VS due to tumour growth. The treatment of choice for large or symptomatic tumours is surgery with removal of the tumour, affected dura and bone. Surgical approaches are similar to that for VS. Fractionated stereotactic radiotherapy and SRS have a high success rate in controlling tumour progression for small low-grade tumours.

- *Epidermoid cyst*: Epidermoids can occur in CPA as well as the PA. Surgery is the treatment of choice for large or symptomatic cysts, and the aim of surgery is decompression of the cysts and removal of the lining if possible. Subtotal removal is advocated to preserve neurovascular structures. Recurrence rate is high and revision surgery may be required periodically. The retrosigmoid approach is the standard surgical approach. Post-operative aseptic meningitis is not uncommon and is almost unique to this condition.
- *Arachnoid cyst*: These are congenital malformations of the arachnoid histologically characterised by a cyst wall that resembles arachnoid and a cystic space filled with CSF. Eighty-five percent of these cysts are asymptomatic and require neither treatment nor ongoing surveillance. For symptomatic cysts, microsurgical decompression and fenestration via the retrosigmoid approach is the most commonly recommended procedure.
- *Lipoma*: These are congenital malformations, which rarely grow. Almost always managed conservatively, they often do not need follow-up, but subtotal removal may be considered for symptomatic lesions.
- *Facial nerve and lower cranial nerve schwannomas*: These are covered elsewhere.
- *Inflammatory conditions*: The CPA can be affected by autoimmune or idiopathic pachymeningitis, tuberculosis and sarcoidosis.
- *Malignant lesions*: These are usually metastatic lesions from either intra-cranial or extra-cranial sources (e.g. breast, prostate or lung). Diagnosis may be aided by lumbar puncture and CSF cytology. Solitary metastases may be treated with surgical resection or with SRS. Melanomas and lymphoma can also occur at the CPA. Intra-axial or intraventricular tumours may also invade the CPA and these include medulloblastomas, astrocytomas, ependymomas and gliomas.

Jugular Foramen Lesions and Their Management
Anatomy

- The JF is divided by intrajugular processes into a lateral compartment that contains the sigmoid-jugular complex and a medial compartment that contains the inferior petrosal sinus and cranial nerves IX, X and XI (Figure 23.3).
- The superior and inferior petrosal sinuses, the occipital sinus and the mastoid and condylar emissary veins drain into the sigmoid-jugular complex.

Clinical Conditions

Symptoms of JF lesions include paralysis of cranial nerves IX, X and XI (Vernet's syndrome). Cranial nerves VII and VIII may also be affected by pathology at the JF and venous involvement may rarely cause cavernous sinus syndrome or raised intracranial pressure. Pulsatile tinnitus may be a feature of paragangliomas or jugular vein diverticulum. Otoscopy may reveal a red lesion behind the eardrum in paragangliomas (rising sun sign) and a bluish discolouration behind the eardrum may signify a high jugular bulb. Brown's sign designates blanching of the lesion with pneumatic otoscopy.

The most common conditions affecting the JF are paragangliomas, schwannomas and meningiomas. Other conditions that affect this area include infections (e.g. complications of otitis media or necrotising otitis externa) and malignancy (e.g. distant metastases).

The three most common tumours are briefly described below and their management is considered together:

Temporal bone paragangliomas: Paraganglia are present in the adventitia of the jugular bulb, along cranial nerves IX and X, and in the middle ear in association with Jacobsen's plexus. Up to 40% of patients with head and neck paragangliomas have a mutation of the succinate dehydrogenase gene that makes them prone to developing multiple paragangliomas, including intra-abdominal tumours with a higher propensity to

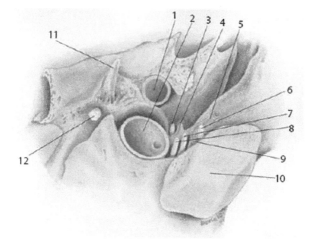

Figure 23.3   Basal view of the jugular foramen. View of the jugular foramen (right side) as shown from below. 1, internal carotid artery; 2, internal jugular vein; 3, glossopharyngeal nerve; 4, inferior petrosal sinus; 5, pha- ryngeal vein; 6, hypoglossal nerve; 7, vagus nerve; 8, spinal accessory nerve; 9, condylar emissary vein; 10, occipital con- dyle; 11, styloid process; 12, facial nerve.

secrete catecholamines. Patients should have their blood pressure checked and either 24-hour urinary catecholamine collection or an assay of plasma free metanephrines. In addition to magnetic resonance imaging (MRI)/CT of the neck, assessment with MR angiography, CT angiography or conventional angiography should be performed as these tumours are highly vascular. Staging should be done with positron emission tomography (PET) or MRI from the head to the pelvis. Fluorodeoxyglucose (FDG) PET imaging can be used to indicate metabolic activity as evidenced by standardised uptake value (SUV) max, which correlates with tendency to growth.

The Fisch classification of paragangliomas is as follows:

- *Class A*: limited to the middle ear (mesotympanum)
- *Class B*: middle ear (meso-and hypotympanum) and mastoid
- *Class C*: involvement of infra-labyrinthine and apical compartments of temporal bone; subclassification by degree of carotid canal erosion
- *Class D*: tumours with intracranial extension; subclassification by presence and extent of intradural extension

Schwannomas: These develop from the Schwann cells in the perineurium affecting cranial nerves IX, X or XI in the medial part of the JF. The biological behaviour of schwanno-mas in the JF is similar to that in the CPA and is often slow growing or apparently static.

Meningiomas: Basal meningiomas can penetrate the skull base through the JF. Management includes:

- *Wait and see policy*: Intervention in this area is fraught with danger to important neu-rovascular structures. Therefore conservative management is appropriate in patients with minimal symptoms and non-growing tumours.
- *SRS and fractionated radiotherapy (FRT)*: These are associated with high rates of tumour control and lower rates of cranial nerve palsy compared with surgery. SRS has the advantage of being delivered in a single sitting. Consider this for small vol-ume (<3cm) progressive disease and minimal symptoms, residual disease after sur-gery, inoperable tumours and in patients of advanced age/poor physical condition. Recovery of compromised nerves has been reported.

- *Surgery*: Considered in patients with significant symptoms, large tumours and growing tumours. Pre-operative embolisation of feeding vessels 48 hours before surgery is recommended for paragangliomas as well as vascular meningiomas (risk of stroke <1%). Permanent balloon occlusion of the petrous carotid artery should be performed if the artery is not salvageable. If carotid occlusion is not tolerated, the artery can be reinforced with a covered stent or vascular bypass may be performed. The lateral transtemporal approach is commonly utilised. Transposition of the facial nerve may be required depending on its relationship with the tumuor.

KEY POINTS

- The diagnosis for most PA lesions can be made radiologically (CT + MRI): active treatment is not always required and 'watchful waiting' is often most appropriate.
- Paragangliomas, schwannomas and meningiomas are by far the most common lesions found in the JF. There is no uniformity of opinion on the best therapeutic approach, and the need for surgical treatment should be balanced with the considerable risk of functional loss.
- Twenty percent of CPA tumours are not VS.

24. TEMPORAL BONE TUMOURS

Introduction

Primary temporal bone tumours are rare, with squamous cell carcinoma (SCC) representing the most common subtype. However, a myriad of less common benign and malignant tumours can occur with varying biological behaviour and prognosis. This chapter provides an overview of the presentation and management of temporal bone tumours.

Pathology and Epidemiology

The reported incidence of temporal bone SCC is fewer than six cases per million per year, accounting for approximately 0.3% of all head and neck cancer. There is a slight male sex preponderance and a median age of presentation in the seventh decade. The epidemiological features of the rarer primary temporal bone tumours are difficult to establish given their scarcity.

Risk Factors

- *Genetic*: Some temporal bone tumours already have a known genetic predisposition, such as Von Hippel-Lindau (VHL) disease and endolymphatic sac tumours (ESTs). Additionally, genetic syndromes predisposing patients to skin malignancies have increased risk of cutaneous head and neck lesions with direct temporal bone invasion.
- *Chronic suppurative otitis media (CSOM) and cholesteatoma*: An aetiopathological relationship has been postulated between SCC of the petrous temporal bone and CSOM and cholesteatoma. In some series, up to 68% of SCC patients have a prior history of either CSOM or cholesteatoma. The association between these two conditions is poorly understood. The current assumption is that chronic inflammation and cellular trauma can result in malignant transformation of the temporal bone epithelium.

Table 24.1   Presenting symptoms in temporal bone tumours

LE 115.1 Frequency of presenting symptoms (%)	
Presenting symptoms in temporal bone tumours	Frequency
Otalgia	(52–74%)
Otorrhoea	(45–84%)
Hearing loss	(25–69%)
Headache and localised pain	(23–42%)
Facial nerve palsy	(13–30%)
Lower cranial nerve palsies (CNs IX–XII)	(6–24%)
Cervical metastases	(4–8%)
Trismus/temporomandibular joint dysfunction	(16–31%)

- *Radiation*: Radiation-induced malignancies are a known complication of both frac-
  tionated radiation and radiosurgery. Differentiating between primary, second pri-
  mary, recurrent and radiation-induced malignancies is often clinically challenging.
  Lustig et al. 1997 developed a diagnostic criterion for defining radiation-induced
  temporal bone tumours as follows:
  - Second neoplasm in irradiated field
  - Latent period between radiation and malignancy diagnosis of several years
  - Previous histological and radiological confirmation of malignancy
  - Second neoplasm of differing histological subtype to primary malignancy
- *Ultraviolet (UV) light exposure*: UV light exposure increases the risk of cutaneous skin
  malignancies. Temporal bone involvement may occur due to direct infiltration via
  primary disease of the lateral external auditory canal (EAC) or pinna, or as a result
  of advanced metastatic deposits within the parotid gland, which is the primary lymphatic drainage of much of the cutaneous head and neck.

Clinical Presentation and Examination Findings

The presentation of temporal bone tumours can often be non-specific, therefore a clinician should look to exclude temporal bone tumours in any patients with recalcitrant
symptoms (Table 24.1). Tumour can extend via anatomical deficiencies such as the foramen of Huschke, fissures of Santorini, tympanomastoid fissure and Eustachian tube into
the parotid, temporomandibular joint, skull base and nasopharynx. Cervical metastasis
may occur with malignancy; however, it is relatively uncommon. Unexplained lower cranial nerve (CN) dysfunction (CNs VII–XII) should always warrant a complete head and
neck and otological examination, in addition to imaging of the skull base and petrous
temporal bone.

Diagnostic Workup

- *Biopsy for histopathological examination*: Biopsy can usually be performed trans-canal
  under local anaesthetic. Tumours situated deep in the temporal bone, or patients who
  have had previous non-diagnostic biopsies, may require biopsy under general anaesthetic.
- *Audiometry*: Pure-tone audiometry should be performed in all patients and vestibular
  assessment may be required depending on clinical presentation.
- *Multi-modality cross-sectional imaging*: Physical examination alone is insufficient to
  characterise the extent of a patient's disease, particularly in malignant conditions.
  High-resolution computed tomography (CT) (axial and coronal) and gadolinium-
  enhanced magnetic resonance imaging (MRI) are complementary studies, allowing
  assessment of the disease burden. Additionally, in malignant conditions, staging of
  the neck and chest is often appropriate to assess for metastatic disease.

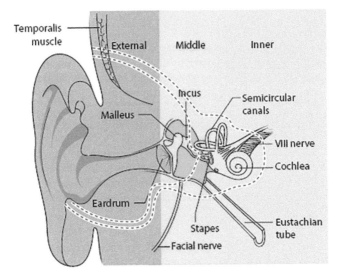

Figure 24.1   Anatomy of the left temporal bone in the coronal plane, showing the extent of a lateral temporal bone resection (outlined in red) and an extended temporal bone resection (outlined in green).

- *Staging and multi-disciplinary team (MDT) discussion*: Malignant tumours of the EAC are often classified via the modified Pittsburgh staging system (Figure 24.2). Whilst several systems have been described, there is no established staging system for primary malignancy of the middle ear or petrous apex, likely due to the rare and varied nature of the disease. Malignancies infiltrating the temporal bone from a cutaneous source are staged via the non-melanoma skin cancer (NMSC) AJCC TNM criterion (Table 24.2). All malignant disease should be discussed within an MDT with expertise in skull base surgery.

Table 24.2   Comparison of AJCC cutaneous malignancy tumour staging to modified Pittsburgh staging system

Stage		Pittsburgh tumour staging system	AJCC 8th edition for cutaneous malignancy of the head and neck
T classification	T1	Limited to the EAC without bony erosion or evidence of soft tissue involvement	<2 cm
	T2	Limited to the EAC with bone erosion (not full thickness) or limited soft tissue involvement (<0.5 cm)	≥2 cm but <4 cm
	T3	Erosion through the osseous EAC (full thickness) with limited soft tissue involvement (<0.5 cm), or tumour involvement in the middle ear and/or mastoid	≥4 cm or any size with deep invasion or perineural invasion or minor bone erosion
	T4	Erosion of the cochlea, petrous apex, medial wall of the middle ear, carotid canal, jugular foramen or dura; with extensive soft tissue involvement (>0.5 cm, such as involvement of the TMJ or styloid process) or evidence of facial paresis	T4a gross cortical bone/marrow invasion T4b skull base invasion and/or skull base foramen involvement

Management
Benign Disease

A comprehensive discussion of the management of all benign tumours of the temporal bone is beyond the scope of this chapter. The general treatment consensus in benign disease is complete surgical resection with narrow surgical margins, unless the morbidity of resection is unacceptable.

Middle Ear Adenomas (MEAs)

- Middle ear adenomas (MEAs) represent a rare benign primary middle ear tumour, thought to be derived from the middle ear mucosa. These tumours lack the aggressive features of malignancy such as bone erosion and are generally accepted to have a good prognosis. Histologically and immunohistochemically, these tumours can display both epithelial and neuroendocrine differentiation. Surgical resection, without adjuvant treatment, is the management of choice, although they have a high recurrence rate.

Endolymphatic SAC Tumours (ESTs)

- ESTs are a primary tumour originating from the endolymphatic sac. Patients classically present similar to cerebellopontine angle (CPA) pathology with sensorineural hearing loss, tinnitus and vertigo. Classically, they are associated with VHL disease. Generally, surgical removal is recommended; however, similar to other CPA pathology, radiation or observation may be appropriate if resection confers significant morbidity.

Malignant Disease

The general management consensus for temporal bone malignancy is en bloc surgical resection followed by post-operative radiation therapy as described in Table 24.3.

Sleeve Resection

Sleeve resection, isolated resection of the soft tissue of the EAC, can be appropriate for very carefully selected small T1 tumours, which are laterally based in the EAC. Typically the soft tissue defect is reconstructed with a split-thickness skin graft.

Lateral Temporal Bone Resection

Tumours lateral to the tympanic membrane (T1 and T2) can be appropriately managed with lateral temporal resection. A wide cortical mastoidectomy is performed, following the tegmen anteriorly into the zygoma towards and up to the mandibular condyle. The facial nerve is identified in the mastoid segment and traced through to the stylomastoid foramen. An extended posterior tympanotomy is performed to isolate the bony EAC, sacrificing the chorda tympani. The incudostapedial joint is divided under direct vision. An osteotomy is introduced through the posterior tympanotomy, and the bony EAC is fractured anteriorly off the bony carotid canal to allow for en bloc delivery of the EAC. The tympanic membrane, middle ear mucosa, incus and malleus are removed and the Eustachian tube is obliterated (Figure 24.1).

Table 24.3 Summary of management of malignant EAC lesions based on modified Pittsburgh staging

Stage	Management	Adjuvant therapy
T1	• Consider sleeve resection if very lateralised and no aggressive features • LTBR + parotidectomy	• Consider PORT
T2	• LTBR + parotidectomy	• PORT
T3/T4	• ETBR + parotidectomy	• PORT
N0	• Neck dissection if necessary for reconstruction	• PORT if indicated for T stage
N+	• Neck dissection	• PORT

Note: ETBR, extended temporal bone resection; LTBR, lateral temporal bone resection; PORT, post-operative radiotherapy.

Extended Temporal Bone Resection

Disease extending medially to the tympanic membrane (T3 or T4) mandates an extended temporal bone resection. The specimen includes a lateral temporal bone resection, as described previously, with extension to resect the inner ear, exposing the air cell of the petrous apex. The facial nerve is resected at the internal auditory meatus. The procedure is often combined with resection of the head of the mandible.

Treatment of the Adjacent Nodal Basins

Parotidectomy

Superficial parotidectomy is often performed for SCC, given it is the primary lymphatic basin and in proximity to disease. For disease with more indolent behaviour, such as basal cell carcinoma (BCC), parotidectomy is not necessary unless required for surgical margins.

Cervical Nodal Disease

Cervical nodal metastasis is uncommon in early tumours. In the absence of clinical neck disease, surgical neck dissection may still be performed in selected cases, e.g. to facilitate free flap reconstruction or to enable accurate neck staging in high-risk patients, such as those who are immunosuppressed. The presence of clinical nodal disease mandates a comprehensive neck dissection.

Adjuvant Treatment

Post-operative radiotherapy (PORT), usually commencing 6–8 weeks after surgery, is the accepted gold standard of management for temporal bone malignancy. The literature suggests PORT improves disease-specific survival (DSS) and locoregional control (LRC). In patients with tumour in an already radiated field, re-irradiation may be considered if free vascularised tissue has been used to reconstruct the field. Palliative radiotherapy may be offered to patients with non-resectable disease, or in patients whose comorbidities preclude surgery.

Chemotherapy

There is little evidence to support the use of pre- or post-operative chemotherapy in temporal bone tumours. Palliative systemic therapies, including chemotherapy, may be given in advanced or metastatic disease.

Immunotherapy

Whilst there is no evidence supporting immunotherapy in primary temporal bone tumours, there is emerging evidence supporting checkpoint inhibitor therapy for advanced cutaneous tumours. These therapies include hedgehog signalling pathway inhibitors in BCC, and PD-1/PD-L1 inhibitors in SCC. These are currently used primarily on a trial basis in unresectable or metastatic disease.

Treatment Outcomes and Prognosis

Benign Disease

Collectively, benign disease often has a good prognosis when amenable to complete surgical resection. Adjuvant treatment is usually not necessary.

Malignant Disease

The prognosis of malignant disease depends on its biological behaviour. Given that SCC is the most common tumour of the temporal bone it will form the focus of this section. Prognosis is favourable in early (T1/T2) tumours with 5-year survival rates between 80 and 100% in most series. Survival with advanced disease (T3/T4) is variable but generally confers a worse prognosis, with 5-year survival rates between 28 and 86% reported in the literature.

Poor prognostic factors include facial nerve, internal carotid or dural/brain parenchymal infiltration, poorly differentiated tumours, positive surgical margins and advanced disease.

Further Reading

Arriaga, M., et al. Staging proposal for external auditory meatus carcinoma based on pre-operative clinical examination and computed tomography findings. *Ann Otol Rhinol Laryngol.* 1990; 99(9 Pt 1):714–721.

Lustig LR, Jackler RK, Lanser MJ. Radiation-induced tumors of the temporal bone. *Am J Otol.* 1997; 18(2):230–235.

Masterson L, Rouhani M, Donnelly NP, et al. Squamous cell carcinoma of the temporal bone: clinical outcomes from radical surgery and postoperative radiotherapy. *Otol Neurotol.* 2014; 35(3):501–508. doi:10.1097/MAO.0000000000000265.

RHINOLOGY AND FACIAL PLASTIC SURGERY

25. ANATOMY OF THE NOSE AND PARANASAL SINUSES

Introduction

This chapter outlines paranasal sinus development, neurovascular and anatomical structures of the external nose, nasal cavity and nasal septum. A surgically relevant approach to sinus anatomy is discussed.

Development of the Nose and Paranasal Sinus

Maxillary Sinus

The maxillary sinus appears between the 7th and 10th weeks of gestation with rapid growth until the age of 7, and reaches final size by 17–18 years. Any disruption in development may result in maxillary sinus aplasia or hypoplasia.

Ethmoid Sinus

The ethmoid sinus is present at birth and develops from four to five folds called ethmoturbinals. These define a series of lamella that must be removed to pass from the anterior sinonasal cavity to the sphenoid sinus. These include the following:

1 Agger nasi (ascending portion) and uncinate process (descending portion)
2 Bulla ethmoidalis
3 Basal lamella of the middle turbinate
4 Superior turbinate
5 Supreme turbinate if present

The furrows between ethmoturbinals develop into nasal meatuses. The first furrow (between the first and second ethmoturbinal) becomes the middle meatus (hiatus semilunaris), while the second furrow becomes the superior meatus.

Sphenoid and Frontal Sinus

Pneumatisation of sphenoid sinus begins at the age of 3 with three described patterns:

- Sellar (pneumatisation posterior to the sella turcica, 90%)
- Pre-sellar (pneumatisation up to the anterior sella, 9%)
- Conchal (shallow bowl with minimal sphenoid pneumatisation, 1%)

The sphenoid sinuses can also pneumatise laterally into the pterygoid root resulting in the presence of a lateral sphenoid recess and exposure of the neurovascular structures surrounding the sphenoid sinus.

At birth, the frontal sinus is a small pocket. It is the last sinus to develop, and only seen in most radiological studies by the age of 8 years, with significant pneumatisation occurring in early adolescence. It remains hypoplastic or aplastic in approximately 10% of the population

Anatomy of the Nose and Paranasal Sinuses

Skin and Muscles of the External Nose

The thickness of the skin and soft tissues of the nasal bridge vary according to individual skin type and anatomical location. Over the dorsum and sides of the nose, the nasal skin is thin and loosely adherent to the underlying framework. The nasal skin becomes thicker and more adherent toward the nasal tip and alar cartilages where it contains numerous sebaceous glands. The elasticity and mobility of the skin over the nose also varies according to the quality of the collagen fibers anchoring the skin to the underlying structures.

The superficial musculoaponeurotic system (SMAS) provides a vascular rich covering to the underlying skeleton from superior labial and facial artery branches and corresponding venous and lymphatic vessels. Its function is to compress, dilate, depress or elevate the nostrils and nasal tip. These muscles are all supplied by branches of the facial nerve. The nasal elevators include the procerus, levator labii superioris alaeque nasi and anomalous nasi muscles. The depressors include the alar nasalis and depressor septi nasi muscles. Compressor muscles include the transverse nasalis and compressor narium minor. The dilator naris anterior muscle acts as a minor dilator.

The subcutaneous tissue of the nose is made up of four layers: superficial fatty, fibromuscular, deep fatty and periosteal layers. The superficial fatty layer is directly connected to the dermis. The fibromuscular layer comprises the nasal SMAS. The deep fatty layer lies deep to the SMAS and contains the neurovascular system. The deepest layer is the periosteum and perichondrium. During external approach rhinoplasty, dissection deep to the third layer (deep fatty tissue) minimises post-operative scarring and retraction because the neurovascular and SMAS structures are preserved.

Anatomical subunits of the nose are divided into thirds (Figure 25.1):

- Upper (nasal bones, articulating the frontal processes of maxilla and bony septum)
- Middle ('vault') (paired upper lateral cartilages (ULCs) inserting under the caudal end of the nasal bones and their fusion with the midline cartilaginous septum)
- Lower (from caudal edges of the ULCs to cephalic edge of lower lateral cartilages [LLCs])

Vestibule

The nasal vestibule is the anterior most aspect of the nasal cavity and serves as the entry point from the external nares into the nasal cavity. The vestibule is demarcated by the limen nasi located at the caudal border of the LLC. The limen nasi is the location where the marginal incision is made during external approach rhinoplasty. It is important to note that only a small part of the alar rim is composed of cartilage from the lateral crus of the LLC; the majority is composed of fibrofatty tissue.

Nasal Cartilages

The LLC is divided into medial, intermediate and lateral crus that form the nasal ala arch. Medial crural footplates extend to the lower columella, anterior to the caudal septum. The nasal tip consists of paired LLCs. Within the intermediate crus lie the domes and tip-defining points.

The ULCs attach to the dorsal septum in the midline, nasal bones cranially at the rhinion and LLCs caudally via the scroll area.

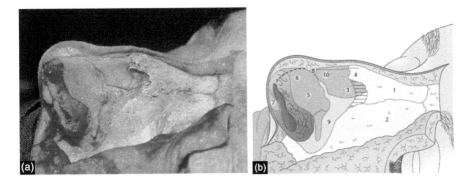

Figure 25.1   (a) Lateral view demonstrating the constituents of the anatomical subunits of the nose. (b) 1. Nasal bone. 2. Frontal process of the maxillary bone. 3. Upper lateral cartilage. 4. Area of overlap of upper lateral cartilage by nasal bone. 5. Lateral crus of the lower lateral cartilage. 6. Dome area within intermediate crus. 7. Medial crus of the lower lateral cartilage. 8. Quadrilateral cartilage. 9. Connective tissue. 10. Scroll region. 11. Shaded area showing removed nasal bone. (Reproduced with permission from Anatomy. RML Poublon In Rhinoplasty; A Practical Guide to Functional and Aesthetic Surgery of the Nose. 1993 Amsterdam/New York. Kugler publications.)

The LLCs and their combined support contribute to the concept of the 'tripod'. The fibrous connection between the medial crura of the LLC are considered one leg of the tripod, with the lateral crura of the LLC forming the other two legs (Figure 25.2). The tripod mechanism plays a dynamic role in the cantilevering of the nasal tip in cosmetic rhinoplasty.

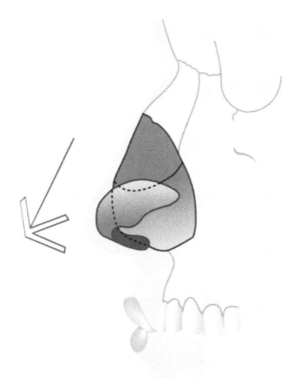

Figure 25.2   Tripod complex of the lower third of the nose. The conjoint medial crura comprise one leg of the tripod, while the lateral crura comprise the other two legs.

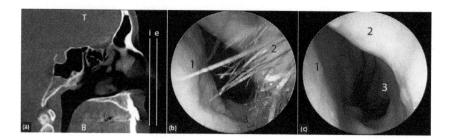

Figure 25.3   Nasal valves. (A) Midline sagittal computed tomography scan with green line indicating the relative positions of the external (e) and internal (i) nasal valves. (T) represents brain parenchyma and (B) base of tongue.(B) Endoscopic view of the left external nasal valve comprised of the (1) septum medially, (2) alar rim laterally (comprised of lower lateral crus, sesamoid complex and fibrofatty tissue) and (3) nasal sill inferiorly. (C) Endoscopic view of the left internal nasal valve comprised of the (1) septum medially, (2) caudal edge of upper lateral cartilage and (3) head of inferior turbinate laterally and nasal floor inferiorly.

Nasal Valve

The LLC and ULC form the external and internal nasal valves, which are critical to nasal airflow. Boundaries of both external and internal valve are depicted in Figure 25.3. Anatomical abnormalities of external nasal valve or compromise in its structural integrity can cause narrowing, stenosis or dynamic valve collapse that is exacerbated during inspiration.

The internal nasal valve is the narrowest portion of the nasal cavity. The apex of the internal nasal valve is approximately 10–15 degrees in Caucasians and wider in non-Caucasian populations. Changes in the relationship of any structure within this space can cause symptoms of nasal obstruction.

Nasal Septum

The nasal septum consists of the following structures (Figure 25.4):

- Bone (comprised of the perpendicular plate of the ethmoid bone, vomer, maxillary crest and palatine bone)
- Cartilage (composed of the quadrilateral cartilage)
- Membranous portions (segment of connective tissue between the caudal septal cartilage and columella)

The inferior attachment of the cartilaginous portion sits within the nasal crest of the maxilla and is bound by looser connective tissue creating a pseudoarthrosis, reducing risk of traumatic fracture or dislocation.

Lateral Nasal Wall and Turbinates

The middle and superior turbinate arise from the ethmoid bone. The inferior turbinate is an embryologically independent osseus structure. The space between the turbinates is the meatus, which is associated with well-defined drainage pathways. This three-dimensional area is often referred to as the hiatus semilunaris, which is a crescent-shaped groove in the lateral wall of the nasal cavity just inferior to the ethmoidal bulla. It is the location of the openings for the frontal sinus, maxillary sinus and anterior ethmoidal sinus (Figure 25.5).

The lacrimal duct drains into the inferior meatus approximately 1cm posterior to the inferior turbinate head by an opening called Hasner's valve. The middle and superior meatuses and sphenoethmoid recess will be discussed later.

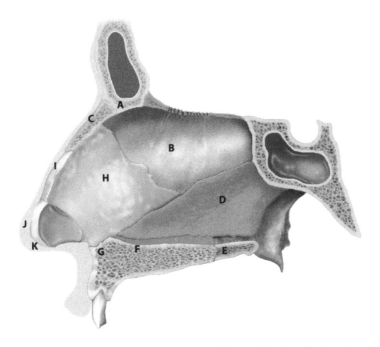

Figure 25.4   The cartilaginous and bony components of the nasal septum. Nasal septum. A – Nasal process of frontal bone. B – Perpendicular plate of ethmoid. C – Nasal bones. D – Vomer. E – Horizontal plate of palatine bone. F – Palatine process of maxillary bone. G – Anterior nasal spine. H – Quadrangular cartilage. I – Upper lateral cartilage. J – membranous part of septum. K – Alar cartilage.

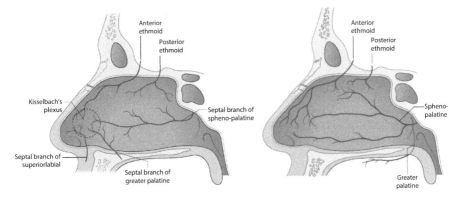

Figure 25.5   Vascular supply of (A) nasal septum and (B) lateral nasal wall.

Blood Supply of External Nose

Branches of the facial artery (angular and superior labial arteries) supply the alar region. The nasal side wall and dorsum also receive supply from the ophthalmic, infra-orbital and external branch of the anterior ethmoid arteries.

Venous networks do not parallel the arterial supply but correspond to territories. The upper lip and nose are considered the danger area of the face because infections in this region may be transmitted retrograde to the cavernous sinus through the valveless ophthalmic vein.

Blood Supply of Nasal Cavity

The sphenopalatine artery is the major contributing artery (Figure 25.3). It enters through the sphenopalatine foramen inferior to the middle turbinate horizontal attachment. The crista ethmoidalis is a small crest of palatine bone located anterior to sphenopalatine foramen serving as a consistent surgical landmark.

The anterior ethmoid artery, posterior septal artery (branch of sphenopalatine artery) and septal branch of superior labial artery contribute to Kiesselbach's plexus along the anterior septum at Little's area (Figure 25.3). This is a common location of epistaxis due to its rich vascular supply, and it is susceptible to injury from turbulent airflow and digital trauma.

Internal carotid artery contribution occurs via anterior and posterior ethmoid arteries (branches of ophthalmic artery). The anterior ethmoid artery traverses three compartments of the head during its course from the orbit between the superior oblique and medial rectus muscle, through the ethmoid cavity either within skull base bone or a mucosal mesentery, and enters through the lateral lamella of the lamina cribrosa into the olfactory fossa intracranially.

Functional Anatomy of the Paranasal Sinuses

The paranasal sinuses are divided into functional units based on drainage pathways:

- Anterior unit (maxillary, anterior ethmoid and frontal sinuses draining into ostiomeatal complex, lateral to the middle turbinate)
- Posterior unit (posterior ethmoid and sphenoid sinus drain into superior meatus)
- Sphenoid compartments (sphenoid sinus draining into sphenoethmoid recess)

Details of anatomy for each unit are depicted in Figure 25.5.

Anterior Functional Unit

Uncinate Process and Maxillary Sinus

The uncinate process is a sickle-shaped bone which attaches inferiorly to the inferior turbinate and palatine bone, and anterosuperiorly to the lacrimal bone. The uncinate, together with a fold of mucosa called the anterior and posterior fontanelle, cover the opening to the maxillary sinus. Accessory ostia may be present in the fontanelle that can be mistaken for the true maxillary ostium. Failure to correctly identify the true ostia and connect it with the common sinus cavity may result in a phenomenon known as mucous recirculation. During recirculation, mucuus is directed towards the natural opening along the mucociliary drainage pathway and re-enters the sinus through the accessory ostium.

Ethmoid Bulla

The ethmoid bulla is the largest and most consistent anterior ethmoid air cell. It attaches to the lamina papyracea laterally and has variable attachments to the skull base and basal lamella creating a series of clefts and spaces that are well described.[1] An infra-orbital anterior ethmoid cell can pneumatise into the maxillary sinus as a normal variant called a Haller cell.

Middle Turbinate

The complex shape of the middle turbinate is divided into three segments:

- Sagittal (attaches to the skull base at the lateral lamella)
- Coronal (basal lamella which separates anterior and posterior ethmoid cavities)
- Axial (attaches to the lateral nasal wall at the sphenopalatine artery terminal branch point)

Frontal Sinus

To define the limits of the frontal sinus recess, one must consider structures that may encroach this space:

- Anteriorly (agger nasi, posterosuperior uncinate process and frontal ethmoid cells)
- Posteriorly (supraorbital ethmoid and suprabulla cells)
- Medially and lateral directions (intersinus septal cells and a medially inserting uncinate)

Agger nasi is the anterior-most ethmoid cell and its medial border is formed by the uncinate process. The degree of agger pneumatisation influences the superior uncinate position and nasofrontal beak thickness.

The uncinate process can insert into the medial orbital wall, skull base or middle turbinate and has multiple attachments in more than 50% of cases. The uncinate inserts into the medial orbital wall in 85% of cases resulting in a frontal recess drainage pathway medial to the uncinate. An uncinate with an isolated attachment to the skull base or middle turbinate occurs in 15% of cases leading to drainage lateral to the uncinate.

Frontal ethmoid cells pneumatise above the agger towards the frontal sinus. The Wormald classification describes four configurations:

- Type 1 (single frontal ethmoidal cell above the agger nasi and below the frontal sinus floor)
- Type 2 (tier of cells above the agger nasi)
- Type 3 (cells that fill less than 50% of the frontal sinus)
- Type 4 (cells fill greater than 50% of the frontal sinus)

Supraorbital ethmoid cells are anterior ethmoid cells extending superiorly and laterally over the orbital roof. Suprabulla cells are pneumatised extensions above the ethmoid bulla up the skull base and frontal sinus posterior table.

Medial structures encroaching on the frontal recess include intersinus septal cells and a medially inserting uncinate. Intersinus septal cells represent pneumatisation of the frontal sinus septum. Lateral encroaching structures include frontal cells, agger nasi and a lateral uncinate attachment.

Posterior Functional Unit

The posterior functional unit is comprised of the posterior ethmoid cells which drain into the superior meatus. An Onodi cell is a posterior ethmoid cell that pneumatises laterally and posteriorly over the optic nerve exposing it to injury during surgery.

Sphenoid Functional Unit

The sphenoid functional unit is comprised of the sphenoid sinus which drains into the sphenoethmoid recess between the superior meatus and septum. The supreme turbinate may be seen here. The sphenoid ostium opens behind the superior turbinate. Structures associated with the sphenoid sinus include the optic nerve, carotid artery and sella turcica.

KEY POINTS

- Identify key fixed anatomical landmarks to delineate the limits of dissection of the paranasal sinus surgical cavity (box) for safe and complete endoscopic sinus surgery.
- The main structures are the orbit and skull base. These are defined by the (1) maxillary sinus roof (orbital floor), (2) medial orbital wall, (3) sphenoid sinus roof (skull base) and (4) the lateral sphenoid wall (orbital apex).
- Paranasal sinuses are divided into anterior, posterior and sphenoid compartments that serve as functional units based on mucociliary drainage pathways. Once a compartment is surgically entered, all mucosal cells within the compartment must be completely dissected to create a new functional neo-sinus cavity.

Further Reading

1. Stammberger HR, Kennedy DW, Anatomic terminology group. Paranasal sinuses: anatomic terminology and nomenclature. *Ann Otol Rhinol Laryngol Suppl* 1995; 167: 7–16.
2. Kew J, Rees GL, Close D, et al. Multiplanar reconstructed computed tomography images improves depiction and understanding of the anatomy of the frontal sinus and recess. *Am J Rhinol* 2002; 16(2): 119–23.

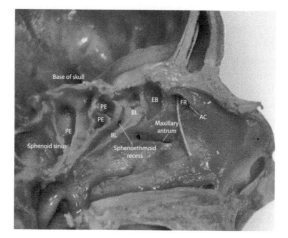

Lateral nasal wall.

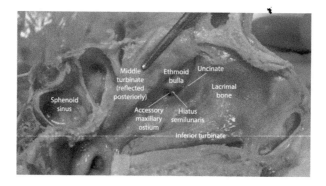

Lateral nasal wall with middle turbinate reflected posteriorly exposing the middle meatal complex.

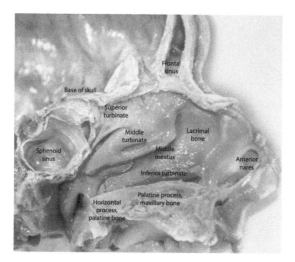

Lateral nasal wall with middle turbinate removed illustrating the basal lamella (BL) separating the ethmoid bulla (EB) from the posterior ethmoid cells (PE). FR – to frontal recess. AC – Agger nasi cell.

26. PHYSIOLOGY OF THE NOSE AND PARANASAL SINUSES

Introduction
The nose is a complex organ that forms an important part of the face and has multiple functions.

Respiratory functions include heat exchange, filtration, humidification, nasal neurovascular reflexes and voice modification. The nose also serves as a sense organ, housing the olfactory apparatus that allows individuals to smell substances for pleasure and defence purposes.

The physiological role of the paranasal sinuses is uncertain, but several possible functions have been suggested including:

- Physical buffer against injury to face
- Vocal resonance
- Reduction of skull weight
- Heat insulation
- Humidification
- Air conditioning

Nasal Blood Flow
The nasal mucosa is very vascular containing arterioles, arteriovenous anastomoses and venous sinusoids, with a large surface area of 150 cm². They can expand and shrink, which has an impact on the nasal resistance and nasal airflow. Inferior turbinate has erectile tissue and a rich blood supply, increasing interaction of inspired air with nasal mucosa. If the mucosal thickness increases by 1–2 mm, nasal flow velocity significantly decreases, from 0.89–0.42 m/s in the normal nose.

Autonomic Nervous System
The autonomic nervous system controls the activity of smooth muscle found in the walls of the arteriovenous anastomoses leading to changes in nasal blood flow. Parasympathetic fibres travel via the maxillary branch of the trigeminal nerve (CN V_2) to provide secretomotor supply to the mucous glands in the nasal cavity. Sympathetic fibres predominantly innervate smooth muscle in the walls of arterioles and sinusoids. Drugs may mimic the effects of the sympathetic and parasympathetic nerve supply (Table 26.1).

Epithelium-Ciliary Function
There are three types of epithelium in the nose:

1 Stratified squamous epithelium covering nasal vestibule containing vibrissae, sweat glands.
2 Pseudostratified ciliated columnar epithelium covers the majority of the nasal cavity and contains ciliated and non-ciliated columnar cells, mucin-secreting goblet cells and basal cells.
3 Olfactory neuroepithelium is located along the upper one-third of septum, medial superior/supreme turbinates and roof of nasal cavity.

Defence Mechanisms of the Nasal Mucosa
The nose has a role in protective mechanisms to prevent noxious substances from entering the lower respiratory tract, which can be divided into mechanical and immunological defence.

Table 26.1   Drugs acting on the nasal mucosa

Drug group	Mode of action	Example
Sympathomimetics	Compounds act on alpha-1 receptors and cause vasoconstriction, reducing nasal congestion	Adrenaline, noradrenaline, xylometazoline (Otrivine)
		Cocaine blocks uptake of noradrenaline in nerve endings; also acts as a local anaesthetic
		Antagonist: Alpha blockers e.g. doxazosin for hypertension
Parasympathomimetics	Compounds act to cause vasodilation and increase nasal secretions	Pilocarpine causes vasodilation and watery secretions
		Antagonists: Ipratropium bromide blocks muscarinic receptors, thus preventing acetylcholine from binding
Antihistamines	Predominantly block H1 receptors Histamine is found mainly in mast cells and causes vasodilation and increases plasma leaking from capillaries	Antihistamines
Local anaesthetics	Inhibit Na channel influx therefore reduce the rate of depolarisation/repolarisation	Lignocaine

Mechanical Defence   The nose can protect the lower airway by removing particles of approximately 30 µm or upward such as pollen in inspired air (mechanical defence). The velocity of the inspired air drops significantly after the nasal valve. Superficial viscous layer produced by goblet cells traps particles. The columnar epithelial cells with specialised ciliary modifications produce a rowing-like action and push particles entrapped in mucous backwards into the nasopharynx.

Each cilium is composed of a bundle of interconnected microtubules beating 10–20 times per second. Dry conditions, hyper- (>5%) or hypotonic (<2%) saline solutions, temperatures below 10°C and temperatures above 45°C can stop ciliary movements. Infections in the upper respiratory tract can cause damage to the epithelium, and the function of cilia also deteriorate with age. Smoking causes a reduction in the number of cilia and change in mucous viscosity.

Immunological Defence   Mucous consists of compounds that can neutralise antigens through innate mechanisms and learned and adaptive immunological responses. Immunoglobulin A (IgA) and IgE are found on the surface, and they act whenever the mucosa is breached.

Nasal Aerodynamics

Nasal flow is laminar as it enters the vestibule. Increased resistance at the nasal valve area, the narrowest part of the upper respiratory tract, leads to a drop of airflow velocity.

The velocity of air increases as it passes the nasal valve, the narrowest part of the upper respiratory tract (Figure 26.1). With change of velocity, laminar flow turns into a turbulent flow, which results in reduced air velocity and prolonged contact of inspired air with the nasal mucosa, allowing the nose to perform its vital functions. Normally, 50% of air flows via the middle meatus. Septal deviations and turbinate hypertrophy may increase resistance and cause nasal obstruction. However, when resistance is too low, patients may suffer with paradoxical obstruction known as 'empty nose syndrome'.

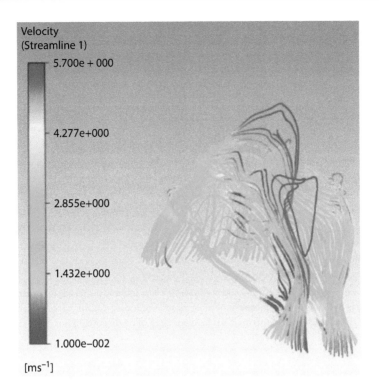

Velocity
(Streamline 1)

5.700e + 000

4.277e+000

2.855e+000

1.432e+000

1.000e−002

[ms⁻¹]

Figure 26.1   Velocity streamlines. Fluid dynamic experiments of the nose have shown that nasal flow is laminar as it enters the vestibule, with no mixing of the different air layers at low velocity.

Nasal Cycle

The nasal cycle is a physiological process during which each side of the nose alternates between congestion and decongestion. Changes are cyclical, occurring every 4–12 hours and are present in 80% of adults, although difficult to demonstrate in children. Nasal cycle is operated by the autonomic nervous system, which regulates constriction of the arterioles, precapillary sphincters and venous sinusoids within the erectile mucosa. Amplitude of nasal cycle may be influenced by exercise, pregnancy, hormones, congestion, allergy, fear, emotions and sexual activity.

KEY POINTS

- The principal physiological function of the nose is to
  - humidify and warm inspired air
  - remove noxious particles from the air
  - serves as a sense organ
- The nose has an abundant blood supply, from branches of both the internal and external carotid arteries.
- The venous sinuses form the erectile tissue that is located on the anterior nasal septum and the inferior turbinates.
- Smoking causes a reduction in the number of cilia and change in mucous viscosity.
- The nasal cycle is a well-recognised physiological activity whereby each side of the nose alternates the phases of congestion and decongestion.
- Nasal resistance plays a crucial role in preventing the collapse of the lower respiratory tract, notably the lungs, with nasal resistance contributing to up to 50% of the total airway resistance.

27. NASAL AIRWAY MEASUREMENT

Nasal obstruction is one of the most common complaints presenting to ear, nose and throat (ENT) surgeons, but treatment is usually initiated without any objective measurement of nasal airflow.

Establishing a normal range of nasal patency is confounded by several factors related to nasal physiology:

- Direct exposure to the external environment where the nose acts as an air conditioner to protect the lungs from infection and variations in environmental conditions.
- The nose is subject to spontaneous changes in nasal patency associated with the 'nasal cycle'.

'Anatomical' nasal patency is the nasal patency measured after decongestion of the nasal blood vessels by application of a topical nasal decongestant or by standard exercise. Anatomical nasal patency is a useful measure for the nasal surgeon, as it is determined solely by the hard tissues of the nose such as cartilage and bone.

Rhinomanometry provides a functional measure of nasal patency, whereas acoustic rhinometry provides an anatomical measurement of cross-sectional area or nasal volume. Nasal peak inspiratory flow can also provide useful measures of nasal patency.

Rhinomanometry

Rhinomanometry provides a measure of nasal resistance to airflow, which is calculated from two measurements: nasal airflow and trans-nasal pressure.

Active rhinomanometry involves the generation of nasal airflow and pressure with normal breathing.

Passive rhinomanometry involves the generation of nasal airflow and pressure from an external source, such as a fan or pump, to drive air through the nose. Passive rhinomanometry involves the direction of an external flow of air through the nose and out of the mouth.

Acoustic Rhinometry

Acoustic rhinometry consists of generating an acoustic pulse from a spark source or speaker, and the sound pulse is transmitted along a tube into the nose. The sound pulse is reflected back from inside the nose according to changes in the local acoustic impedance which are related to the cross-sectional area of the nasal cavity. The reflected sound is detected by a microphone, which transmits the sound signal to an amplifier and computer system for processing into an area distance graph.

Acoustic rhinometry cross-sectional measurements correlate very well with computed tomography (CT) scans, and nasal airway resistance measured by rhinomanometry, but the accuracy is unreliable in the posterior part of the nose, especially when the nasal passage is congested.

Peak Nasal Flow

The peak inspiratory or expiratory airflow through the nose associated with maximal respiratory effort can be used as a measure of nasal conductance. The measurement is effort dependent and is less sensitive than rhinomanometry or acoustic rhinometry in determining small changes in conductance. Expiratory measurements are likely to cause expulsion of nasal secretions into the measuring instrument, and inspiratory flow measurements are likely to cause nasal alar collapse and flow limitation. Simple peak flow instruments are used to measure peak nasal inspiratory flow (PNIF) with the use of a face mask.

Subjective Measurements

Nasal sensations are important in the study of nasal disease, as it is the patient's perception of nasal sensations (symptoms) that is of primary concern to the patient. Objective measures of nasal function such as rhinomanometry and acoustic rhinometry do not always correlate with the patient's own assessment of the sensation of nasal airflow. The reason for the lack of correlation between the perception of nasal airflow and nasal resistance may be because the resistance to nasal airflow is primarily determined by the nasal valve area, whereas the symptoms of nasal obstruction may be influenced by other areas of the nose as well as the nasal valve area, as illustrated in Figure 27.2.

Congestion in the ethmoid region may cause a sensation of pressure and obstruction that has no relationship to nasal airway resistance. Similarly, pressure changes in the middle ear and paranasal sinuses may cause a sensation of nasal obstruction and pressure without any effect on nasal airway resistance. Another factor that may explain the lack of correlation between objective and subjective measures of nasal obstruction is that the nasal airway consists of two parallel airways and the total nasal conductance may be near normal even if one nasal passage is completely obstructed. Objective and subjective unilateral measures of nasal obstruction have been shown to have a much better correlation than combined bilateral measures for the two nasal passages indicating that the nose should be assessed as two separate organs rather than a single combined airway.

Studies on the effects of menthol on nasal sensation of airflow clearly demonstrate the lack of any correlation between objective measures of nasal airway resistance and subjective measures of airflow. In patients with nasal obstruction associated with the common cold, ingestion of a menthol lozenge causes a great improvement in the sensation of nasal airflow without any change in nasal airway resistance

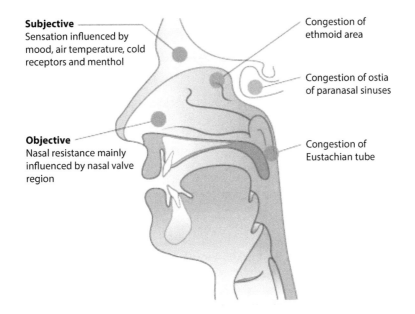

Subjective — Sensation influenced by mood, air temperature, cold receptors and menthol

Congestion of ethmoid area

Congestion of ostia of paranasal sinuses

Objective — Nasal resistance mainly influenced by nasal valve region

Congestion of Eustachian tube

Figure 27.2 Factors that influence the patient's perception of nasal airflow and relationship to objective and subjective measures of nasal obstruction. *Objective measurements* are mainly determined by the cross-sectional area of the nasal valve region at the tip of the inferior turbinate. *Subjective measurements* are influenced by the stimulation of cold receptors in the airway. Congestion in the ethmoid area, ostia of paranasal sinuses and Eustachian tube cause a perception of congestion and pressure that is unrelated to any change in nasal airway resistance as these areas are distant from the nasal valve.

KEY POINTS

- Objective and subjective measurements of nasal conductance do not correlate well for bilateral measures but do correlate for unilateral measures.
- The spontaneous changes in unilateral nasal resistance associated with the nasal cycle cause great variability in physiological nasal airflow.
- Subjective measurements are important as they relate directly to symptoms.
- Decongestion of the nose eliminates the effects of the nasal cycle and allows the measurement of anatomical nasal airflow.
- Acoustic rhinometry provides anatomical rather than functional measurements of the nasal airway.
- Rhinomanometry is generally accepted as the 'gold standard' for measurement of nasal airway resistance.

Acoustic rhinometry and rhinomanometry in their current forms have not found a routine place in the day-to-day assessment of patients in the rhinology clinic.

28. OUTPATIENT ASSESSMENT

This chapter covers history taking, clinical examination, nasendoscopy and patient-reported outcome measures (PROMs).

History Taking

This is best initiated by characterising the index nasal symptoms such as obstruction, rhinorrhoea (anterior or posterior), olfactory dysfunction and pain. Secondary symptoms such as sneezing, itch, epiphora, taste disturbance and dry mouth should also be elicited, and characteristics such as duration, periodicity, nocturnal variation, seasonal effects, laterality, association with trauma or prior surgery and any alleviating or provoking factors may help to further characterise the problem.

Understanding nasal symptoms and their associations not only helps diagnostically, but also creates a picture of the quality-of-life (QOL) impairment suffered, and recognition of psychological aspects (prior injury, pain, sleep) that commonly exacerbate perceived nasal symptoms.

The character of the nasal mucosa, nasal discharge or crusting gives clues to infective (mucopurulent), chronic (rhinosinusitis) or inflammatory origins. Increasing unilateral obstruction associated with epistaxis (often minor) or facial pain and swelling suggests neoplasia and indicates the need for urgent assessment.

Specific triggers may be recognised, or at least known to the patient in some other form, so do inquire about allergies, hay fever, exposure to animal dander, asthma (or more general respiratory symptoms), and nonsteroidal anti-inflammatory drug (NSAID) hypersensitivity (in Samter's triad: nasal polyposis, asthma and NSAID intolerance).

A history of nasal trauma or surgery (e.g. rhinoplasty, cleft palate repair) may suggest obstruction secondary to septal fracture, dislocation, or failure of support to the internal nasal valve.

Many systemic diseases have nasal manifestations. Granulomatous polyangiitis (GPA) is associated with diffuse inflammation, crusting or necrosis of the nasal mucosa and structure.

Table 28.1   Selected examples of the more prevalent and well-validated patient-reported outcome measures that may be useful in a rhinology clinic

Instrument	Validation
The Short Form-36 (SF-36), EQ-5D	Generic quality of life
Sinonasal Outcomes Test (SNOT-22)	Chronic rhinosinusitis
Rhinoconjunctivitis Quality of Life Questionnaire (RQLQ)	Allergic rhinitis, non-allergic rhinitis
Nasal Obstruction Septoplasty Effectiveness (NOSE)	Septoplasty, functional septorhinoplasty, nasal valve surgery
Rhinoplasty Outcomes Evaluation (ROE)	Rhinoplasty

Sarcoidosis, eosinophilic GPA (EGPA), Behçet's syndrome, cocaine abuse and excessive nose picking may have a similar presentation. Cocaine abuse and habitual nose picking can cause septal crusting, septal perforation and saddle deformity, all of which have the potential to cause nasal impairments. Immunodeficiencies, ciliary defects and smoking are commonly associated with nasal pathology and symptoms.

Many drugs have common nasal side effects, especially those with anti-muscarinic effects, such as medications for prostatism, epilepsy, hypertension, sedatives, depression, psychiatric illness and Parkinson's disease. Nasal obstruction (with vasomotor rhinitis) is a side effect of many of these drugs as well as oral contraceptives and medicines used to treat erectile dysfunction. Overuse of sympathomimetic decongestant nasal sprays can cause rhinitis medicamentosa.

Patient-Reported Outcome Measures (PROMs)

Sinonasal disease has a significant and varied impact on patients' QOL, which doctors should measure to evaluate the success of their medical or surgical interventions. This process is simplified by the routine use of PROMs, such as questionnaires that capture and quantify the bulk of symptomatology and disease impact (Table 28.1). Unfortunately, 'simpler' outcomes like overall patient satisfaction are influenced by many variables, such as the availability and convenience of health care, the 'bedside manner' of the doctor, affability of the extended team and perceived cleanliness of the hospital that can bias the evaluation. QOL questionnaires require the patient to rate the impact of their disease across several specified 'domains' or areas of interest; reducing this bias. Overall scores can be used to follow patients with chronic disease, or to compare symptoms/scores before and after an intervention at an individual patient level.

Examination

Nasal Structure/Aesthetics

Examination of the external nose should begin with careful inspection and palpation of the nasal bones, alar cartilages and septum, noting skin type, scars, soft tissue envelope thickness, integrity of the upper and lower lateral cartilages, nasal tip support and configuration, nares shape and integrity of the external and internal nasal valves. These factors can elicit more subtle causes of dysfunction such as nasal valve insufficiency. Saddle deformity, septal deviation and deficiencies of the lateral cartilages are relevant to both cosmesis and nasal patency.

Functional Assessment/Anterior Rhinoscopy

Nasal patency is assessed through anterior rhinoscopy, which is the examination of the anterior nose using a Thudicum's speculum and headlight illumination. The patient is asked to breathe normally through his or her nose, noting any difficulty or noise. A thumb is used to gently occlude each nostril in turn and assess unilateral patency, remembering that many normal subjects are unable to breathe comfortably through a single nasal airway

Any septal deformity should be noted, and the degree of alar margin (external nasal valve) collapse is observed on normal and on forced inspiration, again noting that some dynamic

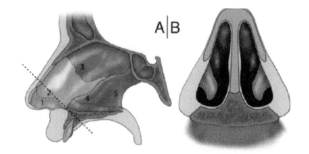

Figure 28.1 Cottle's areas of the nasal septum and the internal nasal valve region (dotted line). Deviations of the nasal septum can be classified by location and by severity. 1. Caudal septum. 2. Internal nasal valve. 3. High mid septum. 4. Low mid septum. 5. Posterior septum. Severity is graded: 0, no deviation; 1, minimal; 2, less than 50% lateralized; 3, more than 50% lateralised and 4, fully lateralised (mucosal contact with lateral wall). (This figure is available free of charge, with certain provisos; from www.surgtech.net)

narrowing is normal (Figure 28.1). The inferior turbinates should be evaluated for congestion, mucosal thickening and the presence of exudate.

Nasendoscopy

Nasendoscopy is best performed after the use of a decongestant (often combined with a local anaesthetic). The appearances of the nasal mucosa and turbinates should be noted before and after application since decongestion will mask some pathological signs (erythema, congestion).

Endoscopic evaluation using a three-pass technique (Table 28.2). Narrow diameter (2.5–3.0 mm) angled endoscopes (30–45°) confer greater opportunity to look laterally into each nasal meatus. Examples of the endoscopic anatomy, and common pathologic findings, are provided in Figure 28.2.

Endoscopic Nasal Biopsy

Any nasal masses should be evaluated for colour, consistency, vascularity and origin. In the absence of unusual appearance, bilateral nasal polyps may not need be biopsied.

Table 28.2 Nasendoscopy technique

First pass: front to back
The endoscope is passed along the nasal floor, visualising the septum and inferior turbinate.
In the post-nasal space, the Eustachian cushion and orifice, and the fossa of Rosenmüller are seen. Any mucopurulent post-nasal drainage can be noted. On withdrawal, the inferior meatus and, where possible, Hasner's valve are inspected.
Second pass: medial to the middle turbinate
Passing the endoscope medial to the middle turbinate, the sphenoethmoidal recess, superior turbinate, and slit-like opening of the sphenoid ostium are often visualised.
The olfactory cleft is seen more anteriorly. Head repositioning may be required, and an angled endoscope is recommended.
Third pass: the middle meatus
Retracting, rotating the view laterally, and rolling the endoscope into the middle meatus will medialize the turbinate to expose any middle meatal mucopurulence (sometimes subtle), accessory ostia or other pathology. The hiatus semilunaris bounded by the uncinate and ethmoid bulla can be seen, as well as the membranous fontanelles and any associated accessory ostia. An angled endoscope is recommended.

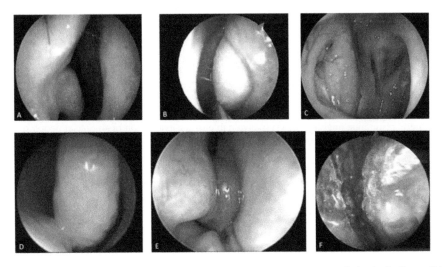

Figure 28.2 Examples of the endoscopic anatomy, and common pathologic findings. (A) Endoscopic view of the right internal nasal valve. (B) Endoscopic view of right middle meatus. (C) Endoscopic view of the right side of the nasopharynx. (D) Left inferior turbinate hypertrophy in allergic rhinitis. (E) Right nasal polyp. (F) Severe crusting of the left inferior turbinate and septum in granulomatous polyangiitis (GPA).

Sinonasal tumours and unusual polyps should be imaged prior to biopsy. In-office biopsy can be considered but the possibility of a vascular nature (e.g. juvenile angiofibroma) or meningo(encephalo)coele must be excluded. In such cases, a computed tomography with contrast or magnetic resonance imaging scan may prevent significant complications.

KEY POINTS

- Well-developed skills in clinical history and examination are key to correct diagnosis and management.
- Nasal endoscopy is a necessary investigation for all patients referred for a specialist rhinologic assessment.PROMs have become an integral component of patient assessment.

29. IMAGING IN RHINOLOGY

Imaging Modalities: Technical Aspects

Computed Tomography (CT)

The mainstay of routine sinus imaging is multidetector row computed tomography (MDCT). In most instances, intravenous contrast administration is not required.

Advantages

- Excellent definition of osseous anatomy and anatomic variants
- Multiplanar reformatting
- Depicts calcifications and high-density secretions
- Guidance of stereotactic surgery

Disadvantages

- Ionising radiation. Routine MDCT paranasal sinuses results in a radiation doses of approximately 0.3–0.6mSV (corresponding to 1–2 months of background radiation) although low-dose approaches and systems may now achieve <0.1mSV.
- Inability to reliably distinguish between inflamed mucosa and other tissue types.

Magnetic Resonance Imaging (MRI)

Magnetic resonance imaging (MRI) is invaluable in the evaluation of sinonasal neoplasms, complex infections and rarer inflammatory disorders.

Advantages

Excellent soft tissue/fluid contrast resolution aids differentiation of inflammatory from neoplastic conditions, cerebrospinal fluid (CSF) from secretions and helps detection of perineural spread and intracranial extension.

Disadvantages

- Higher cost (2–4 time) and reduced availability.
- Unsuitable for claustrophobic patients and those with incompatible metallic implants.
- Long scanning times.

Cone Beam CT (CBCT)

Cone beam CT (CBCT) has well-established uses in dental imaging, but its use can be extended to image other anatomical regions including the paranasal sinuses.

Advantages

- Low cost and compact (can be performed in clinics or intraoperatively).
- Potentially reduced radiation dose. There is a 40–80% reduction compared with routine MDCT paranasal sinuses, although now low-dose MDCT may achieve doses comparable to CBCT.
- Excellent depiction of osseous detail.

Disadvantages

- Longer scanning time (motion artefact)
- Poor definition of soft tissues
- Limited field of view

18F-fluorodeoxyglucose (FDG) Positron-Emission Tomography/Computed Tomography (PET-CT)

The 18F-FDG PET-CT provides functional information, based on metabolic activity, in addition to anatomical detail, but it lacks specificity (uptake can be seen in both malignant and inflammatory conditions). Nevertheless, it can be useful in staging (distant disease in particular) and in detecting disease recurrence (in combination with other modalities).

Imaging: Applications

Depicting Anatomy

Sinonasal anatomy is subject to tremendous variation and can be well delineated on CT (Figure 29.1). In particular, the components of the ostiomeatal complexes (Figure 1A) and frontal sinus drainage pathways (Figure 1B), along with clinically relevant anatomical variants, can be depicted.

Notable variants in the nasal cavities include septal deviation and concha bullosa. In the maxillary antra they include infra-orbital (Haller) cells, which can increase the risk of orbital injury.

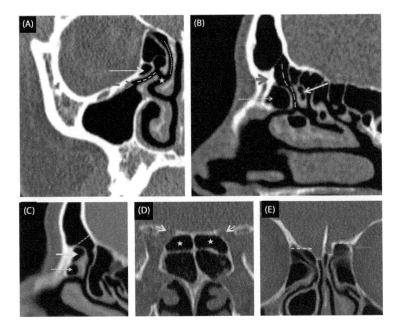

Figure 29.1   Imaging anatomy. CT images depicting anatomical details. (A) Components of the ostiomeatal complex on a coronal image (red dashed arrow, maxillary sinus ostium; yellow arrow, ethmoid bulla; dashed line, ethmoid infundibulum; star, middle meatus; dotted line, frontal recess). (B) Frontal sinus drainage pathway on a sagittal image (dotted line, frontal ostium; red dashed arrow, frontonasal beak; small yellow arrow, agger nasi cell; large yellow arrow, ethmoid bulla). (C) Variant frontal sinus drainage pathway with a supra agger cell (large yellow arrow). (D) Coronal image demonstrating bilateral Onodi (sphenoethmoidal) cells (stars) and their close relationship with the optic nerve canals (arrows). (E) Coronal image of the anterior skull base demonstrating asymmetry in the heights of the fovea ethmoidalis (dashed lines) and cribriform plates (dotted lines); note the left anterior ethmoidal artery ostium (red arrow).

In the frontal sinus drainage pathway variants include:

- Agger nasi, supra agger (Figure 1C) and supra agger frontal cells
- Bulla ethmoidalis, suprabulla and suprabulla frontal cells
- Other frontoethmoidal cells (e.g. supraorbital and frontal septal cells)

In the sphenoethmoidal region, Onodi (sphenoethmoidal) cells (Figure 1D), projecting posteriorly and lateral/above the sphenoid sinus, can put the optic nerves at risk (Keros classification). Variation in the heights of the structures of the anterior skull base (Figure 1E) can increase the risk of CSF leakage, and variation in the position and dehiscence of the canals for the carotid and ethmoidal arteries can risk inadvertent vascular injury.

Sinus Inflammatory Disease
Incidental

- Minor mucosal thickening and retention cysts are common findings in asymptomatic patients imaged for other reasons.
- Incidental mucosal thickening up to 3 mm is usually of no clinical significance and that in the ethmoid sinuses 1–2 mm of mucosal thickening (related to the nasal cycle) occurs in most asymptomatic patients.
- Retention cysts are common findings and are recognised as dome shaped, smoothly marginated opacities on CT with high (fluid) signal on T2-weighted MRI.

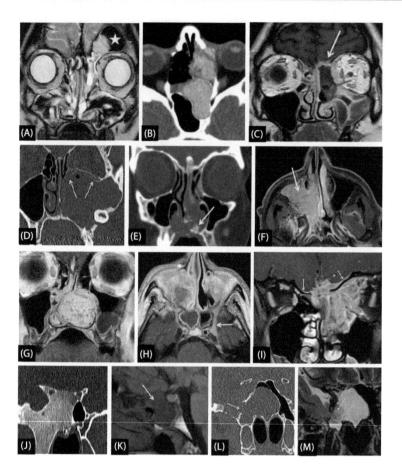

Figure 29.2 Depicting pathology. Examples of the utility of imaging in the depiction of a range of pathologies. (A) Coronal T2W image demonstrating hyperintense inflammatory thickening of the paranasal sinus mucosa; the signal dropout within the left frontal sinus corresponds with desiccated secretions (star). (B) Axial computed tomography (CT) image demonstrating the utility of CT in depicting high-density fungal material within the left ethmoid labyrinth and sphenoid hemi-sinus. (C) Coronal T1W + contrast image of a patient with invasive fungal sinusitis demonstrating intracranial extension (yellow arrow) and turbinate necrosis (red arrow). (D) Coronal CT demonstrating a dentigerous cyst, expanding into the left maxillary antrum (yellow arrows). (E) Coronal CT revealing calcified matrix (yellow arrow) within a chondrosarcoma of the nasal septum. (F) Axial fat-saturated T1W + contrast image revealing the 'cerebriform' enhancement pattern (yellow arrow) of a right maxillary antral inverted papilloma. (G) Coronal T1W + contrast sequence demonstrating an enhancing mass within the left nasal cavity with flow voids, compatible with a juvenile angiofibroma. (H) Axial T1 + contrast sequence demonstrating perineural spread of tumour along the maxillary division of the left trigeminal nerve (yellow arrow). (I), Coronal T1W + contrast at-saturated sequence demonstrating thin linear dural enhancement (yellow arrows) representing reactive inflammation interrupted by nodular tumour tissue (red arrow), in keeping with intracranial invasion by alveolar rhabdomyosarcoma. (J) Coronal CT demonstrating expansile ground-glass density within the medial and right lateral aspects of the sphenoid, in keeping with fibrous dysplasia. (K) Sagittal T1W sequence from the same case, where the fibrous dysplasia manifests as low signal (yellow arrow) (L) Coronal CT demonstrating an osseous defect (yellow arrow) within the sphenoid adjacent to the right foramen rotundum. (M) An accompanying coronal T2W sequence from the same case demonstrates the intermediate signal brain tissue (yellow arrow) extending through the sphenoid defect, surrounded by high signal cerebrospinal fluid, compatible with an encephalocele.

Rhinosinusitis

- The diagnosis of rhinosinusitis is largely a clinical and endoscopic with CT performed to corroborate the diagnosis.
- CT has a role in defining the bony anatomy and providing a surgical roadmap, in identifying significant anatomic variants and in demonstrating patterns of disease and sinonasal obstruction.
- Disease extent can be quantified using one of several staging systems, of which the Lund-Mackay system is perhaps the best known.
- CT acquisition is also needed for complex surgical approaches requiring a surgical navigation system.
- CT or MRI with contrast is required to assess intraorbital or intracranial complications of rhinosinusitis.

Fungal Sinus Disease

Fungal sinus disease is classified into invasive and non-invasive forms as follows.

Invasive

- Acute invasive fungal sinusitis (AIFS) usually occurs in immunocompromised patients and is a rapidly progressive, potentially fatal condition.
- In the appropriate clinical setting, unilateral, nasoethmoid mucosal inflammatory changes should raise suspicion; however, bony erosion and extrasinus soft tissue extension is more specific.
- Chronic (granulomatous) invasive fungal sinusitis (CIFS) affects immunocompetent or mildly immunocompromised patients.

Non-Invasive

- Allergic fungal rhinosinusitis (AFRS) typically effects immunocompetent patients with a history of atopy. CT shows unilateral or bilateral opacification of multiple sinuses, with sinus expansion and bony erosion.
- Intrasinus high attenuation is typical in AFRS (due to heavy metals, calcium and inspissated secretions). Although this may also be seen in chronic rhinosinusitis, it will be associated with wall thickening and sclerosis.
- Fungal ball/mycetoma tends to effect older immunocompetent individuals. Usually a single sinus is involved in fungal ball, and on CT, a hyper-attenuating soft tissue mass is seen, often containing punctate or nodular calcifications.
- The sinus contents are typically low to signal void on T2-weighted MRI in both forms of non-invasive fungal sinus disease.

Midline Destructive Infectious and Non-Infectious Sinonasal Disease

- The differential diagnosis for septal perforation and midline sinonasal destruction includes granulomatous disorders (e.g. sarcoid, granulomatous polyangiitis [GPA], neoplasia (e.g. natural killer [NK]-cell/T-cell lymphoma), infection (e.g. syphilis, tuberculosis) and cocaine misuse.
- GPA (Wegener's granulomatosis) may be marked neo-osteogenesis and have an 'auto-rhinectomy' appearance on CT.
- Sarcoidosis is suggested by the finding of soft tissue nodules on the septum or turbinates. Palatal erosion is more suggestive of cocaine misuse, although there is overlap in appearances with GPA, particularly when a cocaine-induced vasculitis results from the mixing agent levamisole.

Miscellaneous Benign Sinonasal Entities

- Antrochoanal polyps are usually isolated lesions which fill the maxillary antrum and extend through the (usually accessory) ostium into the middle meatus.
- Inflammatory sinonasal polyps are usually multiple and are seen to be crowded in the nasal vault with potential bony remodelling and demineralisation. They are associated with atopy and aspirin intolerance.
- Silent sinus syndrome is due to obstruction of the ostiomeatal complex with opacification of the sinus and retraction of the walls (as opposed to sinus hypoplasia where the walls are straight). There is a characteristic clinical presentation of hypoglobus.
- Mucoceles are most frequently demonstrated in the frontal sinus with complete opacification and expansion or wall thinning.
- An odontogenic cause may be present in 20% of maxillary sinusitis. Odontogenic cysts or tumours should be considered in the context of the opacified maxillary sinus when a 'double line' of calcification is seen at its periphery.

Sinonasal Neoplasms

- Whilst biopsy will usually be required for definitive diagnosis, imaging plays a role in alerting the clinician to those occasions when biopsy would be ill advised (e.g. cephalocele, highly vascularised tumours, aneurysm).
- All efforts should be made to perform biopsy after imaging as bleeding or inflammation may confound findings.
- Diagnostics should include CT and MRI.

Benign Sinonasal Tumours
Inverting Papilloma

- A unilateral mass most commonly originating in the lateral nasal wall and involving middle meatus and maxillary sinus.
- CT features include internal calcification, and bony erosion or bowing. A focal bony spur may correlate with the origin of this neoplasm and its identification is important for surgical planning.
- On MRI there is a characteristic convoluted, cerebriform pattern.

Vascular Lesions

- These include haemangioma, haemangiopericytoma, angiomatous polyp and the juvenile nasal angiofibroma (JNA). Vascular nature may be indicated by the finding of flow voids and avid enhancement.
- The location of the lesion is an important feature of the JNA, which characteristically expands and erodes the sphenopalatine foramen.

Bone and Cartilage Tumours

- Osteomas are typically found in the frontoethmoid region, and they appear as dense cortical bone but may have lower density elements. Fibro-osseous lesions (fibrous dysplasia or ossifying fibroma) are usually recognisable on CT due to typical ground-glass elements.

Malignant Sinonasal Tumours
Imaging Appearances

- The more aggressive malignant sinonasal tumours, such as the common sinonasal carcinoma and aggressive neuroendocrine tumours (e.g. SNUC- Sinonasal Undifferentiated Cancer and SNEC- Sinonasal Neuroendocrine Carcinoma), demonstrate frank bony erosion without bony remodelling or displacement on CT.
- Adenoid cystic carcinoma has a propensity for perineural spread.

- Sinonasal melanoma is rare but melanotic forms may demonstrate high signal on T1-weighted images.
- T-cell lymphomas characteristically affect the nasal septum whilst B-cell lymphomas arise more laterally and may demonstrate tumour on either side of the maxillary sinus wall.
- Olfactory neuroblastomas tend to arise in the superior nasal fossa and may be associated with peritumoural cysts when extending into the anterior cranial fossa.

Staging

- MRI is particularly useful to delineate the intrasinus extent of tumour relative to (increased T2w signal) inflammatory change and obstructed secretions. Extrasinus extension to the intracranial compartment, orbit and infratemporal fossa is defined.
- In particular, pial enhancement, nodular dural enhancement and dural thickening of more than 5mm have been found to be predictive of dural invasion whilst brain parenchymal signal abnormality suggests brain invasion.

Table 29.1 Approach to analysing a CT scan for inflammatory disease and anatomical variants

		Comment	Variants
Coronal	Maxillary sinus	-Extent of soft tissue thickening and density -Bony thickening/thinning -Mucoperiosteal calcification	Hypoplasia
	Ostiomeatal complex	-Soft tissue obstruction	Lateralised uncinate Patterns of uncinate attachment Infra-orbital air (Haller) cell
	Nasal cavity	-Polyps -Diffuse soft tissue thickening (note nasal cycle)	Deviated nasal septum and spurs Concha bullosa Paradoxical turbinate
	Anterior skull base	-Skull base defect	Low skull base or asymmetric (Keros classification) Anterior ethmoidal artery canal position and dehiscence
	Sphenoid sinus	-Extent of disease and density -Degree of pneumatisation	Optic nerve canal and carotid dehiscence Onodi (sphenoethmoid) cells
Sagittal	Frontal sinus	-Extent of soft tissue thickening and density and obstruction of frontal sinus drainage	Frontoethmoid cells and agger nasi cells
	Sphenoethmoid junction	-Extent of soft tissue thickening and density and obstruction of sphenoethmoid recess	Onodi (sphenoethmoid) cells
Axial	Ethmoid sinuses	-Extent of soft tissue thickening and density -Medial orbital wall defects	
	Sphenoid sinus	-Extent of disease and density	
	Extrasinus soft tissues	-Dental disease	
		-Nasopharynx	
		-Intracranial/skull base/orbital/ deep face	

Table 29.2   Pearls and pitfalls

CT		
Isolated sinus opacification	Consider a neoplasm, fungal disease or (in the maxillary sinus) an odontogenic source	Correlate with endoscopic appearances and possibly MRI
Isolated nasal polyp	Consider a cephalocele if extending to anterior skull base	Consider MRI prior to biopsy
Bony attenuation of sinonasal structures	Maybe due to pressure de-ossification from benign disease or bony erosion from aggressive disease	Look for any evidence of bony remodelling or expansion which indicates benign process such as mucocele or polyps. Some thin structures (such as the anterior skull base) may be poorly seen if there is adjacent soft tissue
MRI		
T1w high signal	Usually due to proteinaceous secretions (e.g. in a mucocele). Also, due to haemorrhage (or rarely melanoma)	Always look at pre and post gadolinium sequences to distinguish high T1w proteinaceous secretions from enhancement
T2w high signal	Usually inflammatory although occasionally can be seen in tumours (e.g. salivary gland tumours or chondroid tumours)	T2w is a useful sequence to distinguish high T2 signal inflammation from the extent of intermediate T2w signal (cellular) tumours. Note that very low T2w signal is seen in benign fungal disease
Gadolinium enhancement	Useful to delineate extent of tumours and to assess intracranial and perineural spread	Note that enhancement due to dural inflammation or physiological perineural enhancement should not be confused with tumour invasion

- Post-contrast MRI sequences are particularly helpful to evaluate for perineural spread.
- High-resolution T2w signal coronal images are useful to define invasion since they delineate the periosteum and periorbita.

CSF Leaks

- CSF rhinorrhoea may be traumatic (including post-surgical), or non-traumatic (tumours, infections or congenital lesions and in the setting of intracranial hypertension).
- In most cases, non-contrast CT of the skull base is the only imaging investigation required to identify a skull base defect.
- MRI may demonstrate associated pathologies such as tumours. Heavily T2-weighted thin section imaging (e.g. Constructive Interference in Steady State (CISS), Fast Imaging Employing Steady-state Acquisition (FIESTA) may demonstrate dural defects and associated cephaloceles.
- CT cisternography may be helpful if there are multiple bony defects, to define the dural breach, however, it is rarely successful in the absence of active leakage.
- MR cisternography using intrathecal gadolinium is not widely available (partly due to a lack of FDA approval).

30. ABNORMALITIES OF SMELL

Introduction
Although commonly overlooked by medical professionals and laypersons alike, the sense of smell is critical for quality of life, as well as safety from such environmental hazards as leaking natural gas, pollution and spoiled foods. Importantly, decreased smell function is common in later life and can be an early sign of such neurodegenerative conditions such as Alzheimer's and Parkinson's disease. Independent of such diseases, older persons who cannot smell are three times more likely than their normosmic counterparts to die over the course of the ensuing half decade.

This chapter briefly summarises important aspects of olfactory anatomy and physiology, common olfactory disorders encountered in clinical practice and practical techniques for the evaluation and management of smell disturbances.

Anatomy and Physiology
The pseudostratified olfactory neuroepithelium harbours the 6–10 million ciliated olfactory receptor cells critical for smell function. It lines the cribriform plate and sectors of the superior turbinate, middle turbinate and septum in the upper recesses of the nose. The olfactory receptor cell axons traverse the cribriform plate and pia matter via 30–50 fascicles, termed the olfactory fila. Because of their direct projection into the olfactory cleft without an intervening synapse, the receptor cells can serve as a conduit for the movement of viruses and other exogenous agents from the environment into the brain. This was recognised many years ago for the poliovirus, leading to public health programs to chemically cauterise the olfactory epithelium of school children with zinc sulfate to avert contracting polio during epidemics in the 1930s.

The incoming olfactory receptor cell axons synapse with second-order neurons within distinct spherical olfactory bulb structures termed glomeruli. A considerable amount of convergence of information occurs within the glomeruli, from which projection neurons, the mitral and tufted cells, send processes directly to higher structures such as the anterior olfactory nucleus, the piriform cortex, the entorhinal cortex and amygdala without first synapsing within the thalamus. Reciprocal interactions occur among such structures.

Clinical Evaluation of Smell Function
Proper assessment of a patient's smell function requires a detailed clinical history and a thorough physical examination including appropriate brain and sinonasal imaging. The latter may include a computed tomography (CT) or of the paranasal sinuses to evaluate conductive smell disturbance such as nasal polyps or a lesion, and a magnetic resonance imaging (MRI) of the paranasal sinuses and brain to examine sensorineural impairment. Other tests include objective olfactory, and in some cases, taste testing. It is important to recognise that patients frequently confuse 'taste problems' with true smell loss, and that many deny any olfactory disturbance until formal testing proves otherwise. Self-administered olfactory tests are commercially available, making accurate testing practical without having to otherwise tie up clinic resources. The most popular of these tests is the 40-item University of Pennsylvania Smell Identification Test (UPSIT; Figure 30.1), which is a test that provides an accurate indication of not only absolute dysfunction (e.g. anosmia or mild, moderate or severe microsmia), but a percentile rank relative to a patient's age and sex and an index of probable malingering (Figure 30.1).

A number of questions should be made during a patient's evaluation. What is the timing of onset, duration of impairment and pattern of occurrence? *Sudden olfactory loss* can be consistent with possible head trauma, ischaemia, infection or a psychiatric condition. *Gradual*

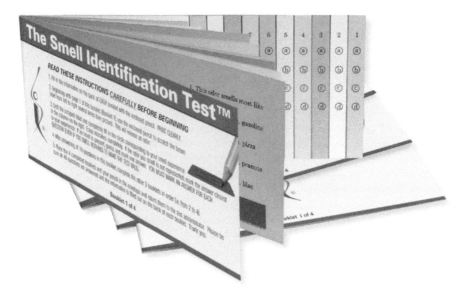

Figure 30.1   The four booklets of the 40-odorant University of Pennsylvania Smell Identification Test (UPSIT; commercially known as the Smell Identification Test™). Each page contains a micro-encapsulated odorant that is released by means of a pencil tip. This test, which has been administered to ˜1,000,000 patients since its development, is the most widely used olfactory test in the world, with multiple language versions available. The UPSIT is considered to be the 'eye chart for the nose.' (Photo courtesy Sensonics International, Haddon Heights, NJ 08035 USA. Copyright © 2000 by Sensonics International.)

loss may indicate a progressive and obstructive lesion in or around the sinonasal region, particularly if the loss is unilateral. *Intermittent loss* may suggest an inflammatory process in association with nasal and sinus disease. Is there a history of precipitating antecedent events, such as head trauma, viral upper respiratory infections, chemical or toxin exposures or sinonasal surgery? Does the patient have any nasal discharge that is mucous appearing (e.g. allergy), purulent (e.g. infection) or clear (cerebrospinal fluid [CSF] rhinorrhoea after trauma)? Does the patient use drugs, such as intranasal cocaine, ethanol or tobacco? Each of these substances has been associated with some form of olfactory impairment. Cigarette smoking results in a loss of olfactory ability that is proportional to the cumulative smoking dose. Cessation of smoking can result in improvement in olfactory function over time. Are there any medications that the patient is taking that might compromise function? Awareness of pending litigation and the possibility of malingering should be considered since olfactory loss is a compensable injury.

Causes of Smell Disturbance

In general, loss of olfactory function can be subdivided into two classes:

- *Conductive or transport impairments* from obstruction of the nasal passages (e.g. chronic nasal inflammation, polyposis, etc.)
- *Sensorineural impairment* from damage to the olfactory neuroepithelium, central tracts and connections (e.g. viruses, airborne toxins, tumours, seizures, etc.)

In some circumstances, both can be involved. Chronic rhinosinusitis, for example, can produce damage to the olfactory membrane in addition to blocking airflow, and altered membrane function can, over time, lead to degeneration within the olfactory bulb, which is a central structure. Although many causes of olfactory disturbance due to conductive factors

Table 30.1 Reported agents, diseases, drugs, interventions and other etiologic categories associated in the medical or toxicologic literature with olfactory dysfunction

Air pollutants and industrial dusts	Lesions of the nose/airway blockage
Acetone, benzol, chlorine, formaldehyde, silicone dioxide	Inflammatory diseases, structural abnormalities, nasal masses
Drugs	**Medical Interventions**
Adrenal steroids (chronic use)	Intracranial/sinonasal procedures, radiotherapy
Analgesics (antipyrine)	
Anaesthetics, local (cocaine HCl, procaine HCl, tetracaine HCl)	**Neurologic**
	Alzheimer's disease, Down's syndrome, head trauma, meningitis, Parkinson's disease, syphilis
Anticancer agents (e.g. methotrexate)	
Antihistamines (e.g. chlorpheniramine malate)	
Antimicrobials (lincomycin, macrolides, penicillin, tetracyclines)	**Nutritional/metabolic**
	Chronic alcoholism, gout, vitamin deficiency
Antirheumatics (e.g. mercury/gold salts)	**Endocrine/metabolic**
Antithyroids	Addison's disease, Cushing's syndrome, diabetes mellitus, Kallmann's syndrome Pregnancy, panhypopituitarism, pseudohypoparathyroidism
Antivirals	
Cardiovascular/hypertensives	
Gastric medications (e.g. cimetidine)	
Hyperlipoproteinemia medications (e.g. cholestyramine)	**Psychiatric**
Psychopharmaceuticals (e.g. LSD, psilocybin)	Anorexia nervosa, depressive disorder, schizophrenia
Sympathomimetics (e.g. amphetamine sulfate)	

Note: This is a shortened table with examples per category. Full table can be found in the Scott-Brown Textbook.

or inflammation of the olfactory epithelium can be treated, most olfactory disorders due to sensorineural factors remain untreatable.

A listing of the causes of olfactory dysfunction that have been reported in the medical literature is presented in Table 30.1. The three most more common disorders or entities associated with olfactory impairment are head trauma, chronic rhinosinusitis and upper respiratory infections, such as those due to the common cold, influenza, bacterial infections and, more recently, infection with the SARS-CoV-2 (COVID-19) virus. Cumulative damage over time can occur, such that persons are predisposed for significant loss later in life as a result of prior nasal infections and exposures to air pollutants that induce subclinical damage.

Treatment of Smell Disorders

The most effective treatments available are those for *conductive* anosmia, where inflammation and other factors obstruct movement of molecules to olfactory receptors. Conductive and sensorineural olfactory loss are often distinguishable using a brief course of systemic steroid therapy since patients with conductive impairment often respond positively to the treatment, although long-term systemic steroid therapy is not advised. Increased topical efficacy can occur when the nasal drops or spray are administered in the head-down Moffett position. Proper allergy management is essential and may require the use of an antihistamine. When a bacterial infection is suspected (e.g. infectious sinusitis), a course of antibiotics should be used. Importantly, pre- and post-intervention olfactory testing should be performed to establish intervention efficacy, as well as to screen for subsequent slow relapse that is characteristic of most conductive disorders.

Sensorineural impairment of olfaction is typically more difficult to manage, and the prognosis for patients suffering from long-standing total loss due to upper respiratory illness or head trauma is poor. The majority of patients who recover smell function subsequent to trauma do so within 12 weeks of injury, although in rare cases return can occur over a several year period. Patients who quit smoking typically have dose-related improvement in olfactory function and flavour sensation over time. Central lesions, such as central nervous system (CNS) tumours that impinge on olfactory bulbs and tracts can often be resected with significant improvement in olfactory function. Patients with neurological conditions such as epilepsy, migraine or multiple sclerosis should be treated appropriately with specialist input. If there is depression or psychosis a psychiatric referral is indicated.

Practicing smelling odours (olfactory training) before and after sleeping may be helpful in returning function, but careful double-blind studies with adequate controls are lacking. There is some evidence to support administration of antioxidants such as alpha-lipoic acid. Spontaneous recovery depends on severity of disturbance. Literature reports that only 11% of anosmic and 23% of microsmic patients regain normal age-related function over time. Olfactory training involves at least four odours of separate categories (typically floral, rose; fruity, lemon; aromatic, eucalyptus and resinous, clove; patients are advised to sniff these for 15 seconds at least twice a day, for up to 6 months.

In patients with complete anosmia, supportive measures are necessary to protect them from further harm:

- Smoke and carbon monoxide detectors need to be installed and properly working.
- Electric stoves should be used instead of gas.
- Expirations dates for food products should be checked.
- Balanced diet to prevent weight loss and malnutrition (particularly in the elderly).
- Adding flavour enhancers (e.g. monosodium glutamate, food colouring, chicken or beef stock) to foods can also help with their appeal.

31. ALLERGIC RHINITIS

Introduction

Allergic rhinitis (AR) is characterised by inflammatory changes in the nasal mucosa caused by exposure to an inhaled allergen to which an individual has become sensitised (a type I hypersensitivity reaction in the Gell and Coombs classification).

In the preparation phase (sensitisation), the allergen is processed by dendritic cells and presented to T-helper 2 cells (TH2). TH2 cells release interleukins (IL-4, IL-5, IL-13 and others) that promote B-cell differentiation into plasma cells producing immunoglobulin E (IgE), which binds to mast cells receptors. Memory B cells are formed from activated B cells and are specific to the antigen encountered during the sensitisation.

On subsequent interaction with the antigen (primary phase), cross-linking of IgE results in degranulation of mast cells. This triggers the release of inflammatory mediators, including histamine and leukotrienes, resulting in the classic symptoms of AR.

During the late phase, inflammatory cells (mast cells, eosinophils, T cells and others) infiltrate mucosa, resulting in increased and persistent symptoms. Repeated interaction with the same allergen stimulates mast cells more quickly.

AR is part of a systemic disease process termed the unified allergic airway that involves other organs such as the lungs with allergic asthma and the eyes with allergic conjunctivitis.

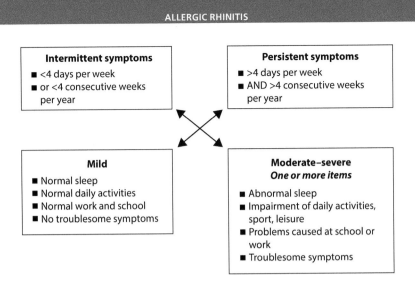

Figure 31.1   Classification of allergic rhinitis. (Reproduced with permission of authors, Bousquet et al., 2008.)

Definition

AR is subdivided into intermittent AR (IAR) and persistent AR (PER), and the severity into mild, moderate or severe (Figure 31.1).

Other causes of rhinitis may have similar symptoms, but allergic disease can be diagnosed by correlating typical symptoms with diagnostic tests such as skin prick tests or measurement of specific IgE levels in the blood.

Prevalence

The prevalence of allergic disease varies around the world from 0.8–39.7% of the population. Disease prevalence has increased significantly in western society over the last 50 years to 23%, possibly caused by reduced exposure to infectious microbes or to reduced infestation with worms in the gut, which appear to exert a regulatory effect on the immune system.

Natural History

Having parents who are atopic increases the risk of atopy in their children by 3- to 6-fold, but exposure to allergens also plays a role. The term 'atopic march' refers to the sequential development of allergic disease, starting with infantile atopic eczema, then the development of AR and finally allergic asthma. Conversely, AR often becomes less severe with age and skin prick testing shows reduced reactivity in the elderly.

Presentation and Diagnosis

AR typically presents with two or more of the following symptoms: anterior or posterior rhinorrhoea, sneezing and nasal block and/or itching. Other symptoms include itchy eyes, pharyngeal itch, reduced smell, cough and sore throat.

Nasal blockage may also result in a reduced quality of life, sleep disorders, learning and attention impairment, mouth breathing and malocclusion.

Unilateral symptoms, purulent discharge, epistaxis and pain are not typical of AR and should prompt further investigation.

The timing of symptoms and their severity will allow the disease to be classified. For example, symptoms worse in the morning may suggest house dust mite sensitivity from exposure in bed or symptoms that occur in the spring may indicate tree pollen sensitivity. If the allergen driving the AR is unclear from the history, then skin prick testing or measurement of specific IgE levels can be undertaken to clarify this.

Treatment

Allergen Avoidance

Allergen avoidance can be difficult to achieve or may be relatively ineffective, but measures such as using anti-allergy covers on mattresses and pillows can be tried in patients with house dust mite sensitivity. Keeping pets out of the bedroom is also advised in patients with dog or cat allergy.

Pharmacological Treatments

The mainstay of drug treatment in AR involves the use of oral and topical antihistamines and topical corticosteroids. The basic summary of recommendations for treatment according to the Allergic Rhinitis and its Impact on Asthma (ARIA) guidelines[1] is shown in Figure 31.2.

Oral and topical antihistamines are rapid acting and reduce symptoms of sneezing and itch but are less effective at improving the airway. Topical (and occasionally systemic) corticosteroids are slower acting but have a greater effect on reducing blockage. Combined intra-nasal fluticasone propionate and azelastine hydrochloride in a single device is more effective than

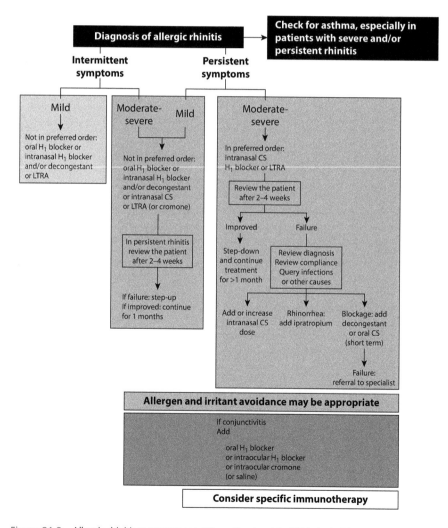

Figure 31.2   Allergic rhinitis management. CS, corticosteroids; LTRA, leukotriene receptor antagonist. (Reproduced with permission of authors, Bousquet et al., 2008.)

Table 31.1 Pharmacological treatments and their effects in allergic rhinitis

	Itch/sneezing	Discharge	Blockage	Impaired smell
Sodium cromoglicate	+	+	+/–	–
Oral antihistamines	+++	++	+/–	–
Ipratropium bromide	–	+++	–	–
Topical decongestants	–	–	+++	–
Topical corticosteroids	+++	+++	++	+
Oral corticosteroids	+++	+++	+++	++
Antileukotrienes	–	++	+	+/–
Combined topical steroid and antihistamine	+++	+++	+++	++

Note: – No effect; + marginal effect; +++ substantial effect.

monotherapy and is indicated for patients when monotherapy with either an intra-nasal H1-antihistamine or glucocorticoid is considered inadequate.

Leukotriene receptor antagonists such as montelukast can be useful in some patients, particularly those with asthma or who develop wheeze at the peak of the pollen season.

Ipratropium topical spray can be useful if rhinorrhoea is a particular problem and can be used as an adjunct to a steroid spray.

Nasal douching with saline may be effective in physically removing allergens from the nose and is safe and easy to perform.

A summary of the effects of the common drugs used to treat AR is noted in Table 31.1.

Anti-IgE humanised monoclonal antibodies may increasingly play a role in allergic disease modification. Licensed drugs such as omalizumab bind to and reduce levels of active circulating IgE and therefore reduce symptoms, but they are expensive and must be given by injection. Newer drugs such as dupilumab (an IL-4 receptor antagonist) are being developed that can target specific cytokines and may allow a more patient-specific therapy with fewer side effects than current treatment options.

Immunotherapy (desensitisation) is a method of inducing tolerance to an allergen and therefore a reduction in symptoms with exposure. Treatment may be given by injection (subcutaneous immunotherapy [SCIT]) or sublingually (sublingual immunotherapy [SLIT]). Therapy involves exposing the patient to the allergen to which they have become sensitised, usually in gradually increasing doses. Immunotherapy is usually reserved for patients who have had poor symptom control with standard treatment and in carefully selected patients can be very effective. Treatment is normally continued over 3 years, which causes a modification of the immune system, and long-lasting symptom control may be achieved following cessation of treatment. It has a risk, however, of causing anaphylaxis and patients should be monitored for 30–60 minutes following each injection (SCIT). SLIT can safely be taken by the patient at home if the first dose has been monitored and a minimal reaction has occurred.

Children with AR

AR is the most prevalent allergic disease in children and may have significant effects on their quality of life. The treatment algorithm for children is broadly similar to that for adults. Avoidance measures then, if necessary, and an oral non-sedating antihistamine are the first-line therapies, but a trial of a leukotriene receptor antagonist may be considered in children who are already using an inhaled steroid for asthma, or if a topical steroid is not tolerated. Fluticasone (licensed from age 4 years) or mometasone (licensed from 6 years) have low systemic bioavailability and are the topical corticosteroids of choice.

Pregnancy

Rhinitis of pregnancy is relatively common and probably caused by high levels of oestrogen. It may occur in women without any past history of rhinitis, allergic or otherwise. Symptoms of AR may also be exacerbated during pregnancy, probably by the same cause. Although topical nasal steroids with low bioavailability are relatively safe, hypertonic saline douches or occasional use of topical decongestants may be preferable. The condition is self-limiting and resolves rapidly following childbirth.

KEY POINTS

- AR is an IgE-mediated disease.
- In western society it is common (>20%).
- It may have significant negative effects on sleep, work and study.
- History and patient symptoms are crucial to making a diagnosis.
- Patients may have other systemic diseases such as asthma.
- Treatment strategies are mainly allergen avoidance, topical or systemic antihistamines and topical corticosteroids.
- Immunotherapy and humanised monoclonal antibodies have an increasing role in disease modification.

Further Reading

1. Bousquet J, Khaltaev N, Cruz AA, et al. Allergic Rhinitis and its Impact on Asthma (ARIA) 2008 update (in collaboration with the World Health Organization, GA(2) LEN and AllerGen). *Allergy* 2008; 63: S8–160.

32. NON-ALLERGIC RHINITIS

Introduction

Rhinitis causes widespread morbidity, treatment costs, reduced productivity and lost school days. It is defined as a symptomatic inflammation of the inner lining of the nose, leading to nasal obstruction, rhinorrhea (anteriorly or posteriorly), sneezing or nasal/ocular itch. Two nasal symptoms should be present for at least 1 hour daily for a minimum of 12 weeks per year to define chronic rhinitis.

Non-infectious rhinitis can be divided into allergic rhinitis (AR; see Chapter 31) and non-allergic rhinitis (NAR). Unlike AR there are no specific diagnostic tests for NAR, and the diagnosis is made on the basis of rhinitis symptoms in the absence of identifiable allergy (by allergy testing), structural abnormality, immune deficiency, sinus disease or other cause.

Subgroups of NAR are as follows: drug-induced rhinitis, rhinitis of the elderly, hormonal rhinitis including pregnancy-induced rhinitis, nonallergic occupational rhinitis, gustatory rhinitis and idiopathic rhinitis.[1]

Types of Non-Allergic Rhinitis
Idiopathic Rhinitis

Idiopathic rhinitis is present in up to 50% of patients with NAR and is characterised by nasal blockage, rhinorrhoea and sneezing, although sneezing, conjunctival symptoms and pruritis is lower than that in AR. The aetiology is unknown in most cases and the disease is thought to be triggered mainly by irritants and changes in atmospheric conditions.

Rhinitis of the Elderly

Among patients with chronic symptoms, the percentage with a non-allergic aetiology increases progressively with age and reaches >60% beyond the age of 50 years. Neurogenic dysregulation is considered the cause of the symptoms. The dominant symptom is bilateral watery rhinorrhoea without mucosal and/or anatomic abnormality.

Occupational Rhinitis

Occupational rhinitis is defined as rhinitis caused by exposure to airborne agents present in the work place. These agents elicit predominantly sneezing, nasal discharge and/or blockage and may act via both immunologic (IgE-mediated) and non-immunologic mechanisms. The non-immunologic triggers are often irritant or toxic small-molecular-weight compounds such as aldehydes, isocyanates, aircraft fuel and jet stream exhaust, solvents and so forth, or they may be physical (long-term exposure to cold air).

Hormonal Rhinitis

Hormonal rhinitis is typically associated with pregnancy, although puberty is also known to induce the symptoms of rhinitis. The cumulative incidence of pregnancy rhinitis is 22%, and in women who smoke there is a relative risk enhancement of 69%. Oestrogens cause vascular engorgement, not only in the female genital tract, but also in the nose, leading to nasal obstruction and/or nasal hypersecretion. Beta-oestradiol and progesterone have been shown to increase the expression of histamine H1 receptors on human nasal epithelial cells and mucosal microvascular endothelial cells, and to induce eosinophil migration and/or degranulation, in marked contrast to testosterone, which decreases eosinophil activation and viability.

Drug-Induced Rhinitis

Common medications, including non-steroidal anti-inflammatory drugs (NSAIDs), beta blockers, angiotensin-converting enzyme (ACE) inhibitors, methyldopa, oral contraceptives, psychotropic agents and nasal topical decongestants (e.g. xylometazoline) may induce symptoms of rhinitis. They may be predictable, as would be the case for known side effects of particular drugs, or unpredictable, based on individual hypersensitivity to certain drugs. Intolerance to aspirin and/or NSAIDs predominantly produces rhinorrhoea, which may be either isolated or part of a complex involving hypertrophic rhinosinusitis, nasal polyps and asthma. In contrast, intolerance to ACE inhibitors, methyldopa or oral contraceptives, which is less common than aspirin intolerance, leads predominantly to nasal blockage. Persistent overuse of topical nasal vasoconstrictors also causes nasal hyper-reactivity and hypertrophy of the nasal mucosa, a condition known as 'rhinitis medicamentosa'.

Other Forms

Other forms include gustatory rhinitis, which presents as watery discharge after ingestion of hot or spicy food.

Mixed Rhinitis

In reality, a significant portion of chronic rhinitis patients have more than one known/unknown aetiologic factor. Therefore, the precise diagnostic process is paramount.

Diagnosis as a Stepwise Approach

Diagnosis of NAR and its subgroups is mainly based on a comprehensive clinical history and rhinologic examination, followed by the stepwise exclusion of possible differential diagnoses (Figure 32.1).

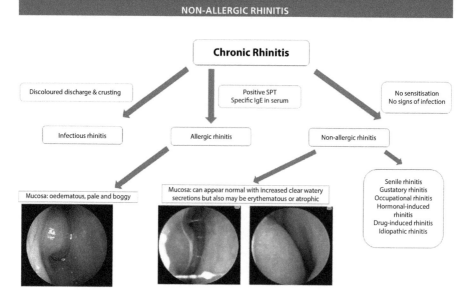

Figure 32.1 Diagnosis as a stepwise approach. SPT, skin prick test. (Adapted from Hellings PW, Klimek L, Cingi C, et al. Non-allergic rhinitis: position paper of the European Academy of Allergy and Clinical Immunology. Allergy. 2017;72(11):1657–1665).

If the case history is suggestive of clinically relevant non-infectious rhinitis then

- Check possible stimuli, severity and duration of disease
- Check drug use (systemic and topical), exposure at workplace, hormonal status (pregnancy, hypothyroidism, acromegaly) and involvement of other organs (asthma, hormonal status)
- Exclude other nasal disease (nasal endoscopy)
- Exclude allergy by using skin prick test (SPT) or serum IgE-antibodies for the most frequent inhalant allergens
- Exclude chronic rhinosinusitis (nasendoscopy ± computed tomography [CT] scan of the paranasal sinuses)

Up until now, allergen provocation testing, microbiological analysis, nasal cytology and nasal hyperreactivity is not recommend due to low clinical value.

Local Allergic Rhinitis (LAR)
Local AR (LAR) or entopy is a localised nasal allergic response with negative SPT and undetectable specific IgE to inhalant allergens. The diagnosis is made by the detection of nasal-specific IgE and/or a positive nasal allergen provocation test. As in AR, patients with LAR respond well to nasal corticosteroids. Due to unavailability of diagnostic testing for LAR, patients are still frequently classified as having NAR.

Treatment for Non-Allergic Perennial Rhinitis
In case of drug-induced, food-induced or occupational rhinitis, avoidance is employed as first-line therapy. Aspirin-intolerant individuals may benefit from aspirin desensitisation (Figure 32.2).

Several treatments (pharmaceutical and surgical) have been employed for idiopathic NAR. Intra-nasal anticholinergics (ipratropium bromide) may be useful in patients with nasal hypersecretion as the predominant symptom, especially those suffering with senile rhinitis. Topical nasal glucocorticoids and antihistamines (e.g. azelastine) form the mainstay of treatment. Two randomised control trials (RCTs) found azelastine nasal spray to be more

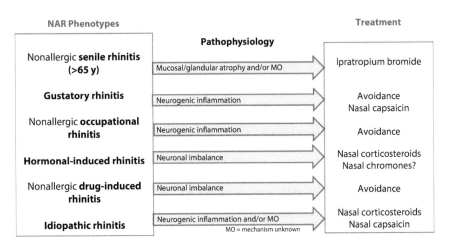

Figure 32.2   Overview of non-allergic rhinitis (NAR) management. (From Hellings PW, Klimek L, Cingi C, et al. Non-allergic rhinitis: position paper of the European Academy of Allergy and Clinical Immunology. Allergy. 2017;72(11):1657-1665. doi:10.1111/all.13200.)

effective than placebo for control of rhinorrhoea, post-nasal drip, sneezing and nasal congestion. The precise mode of action remains to be elucidated. The efficacy of intra-nasal steroids in patients with vasomotor rhinitis has been inconsistent.

Furthermore, whilst topical nasal steroids are more frequently used for treatment of more severe symptoms, they are mostly useful in patients in whom an inflammatory pathogenesis is a prominent feature of their disease (occupational rhinitis and drug-induced rhinitis). In patients with idiopathic rhinitis who do not respond to treatment with nasal steroids, treatment with non-conventional therapies, particularly intra-nasal capsaicin, may be beneficial.

In cases where nasal obstruction is resistant to medical treatment and/or the inferior turbinate is hypertrophic, turbinate reduction has been shown to be useful. Endoscopic transnasal vidian neurectomies (excision, diathermy and cryotherapy) produced results with varying degrees and duration of success.

KEY POINTS

- Approximately half of rhinitis patients may suffer from NAR.
- NAR is diagnosed on the basis of rhinitis symptoms in the absence of identifiable allergy, structural abnormality, immune deficiency, sinus disease or other cause.
- A thorough clinical history is the best diagnostic tool available and should focus on drugs, occupational exposure and hormonal status to subdivide the condition into subgroups.
- Surgery is an option in patients with persistent nasal obstruction not improved by medication.
- LAR entails a negative SPT and undetectable specific IgE to inhalant allergens, but positive nasal-specific IgE and/or nasal allergen provocation test. Patients with respond well to nasal corticosteroids.

Further Reading

1. Hellings PW, Klimek L, Cingi C, et al. Non-allergic rhinitis: position paper of the European Academy of Allergy and Clinical Immunology. *Allergy.* 2017; 72(11):1657–1665. doi:10.1111/all.13200.

33. RHINOSINUSITIS

Rhinosinusitis Definition

International guidelines have provided current definitions of rhinosinusitis. EPOS2020 maintains the criteria laid out in Table 33.1.[1] Making a diagnosis therefore relies on the history and clinical examination with radiological confirmation if required. Rhinosinusitis can then be further defined as acute or chronic based on duration of symptoms: acute <12 weeks duration; chronic ≥12 weeks. Within acute rhinosinusitis (ARS), further distinctions can be made on a timeline basis such that a common cold (acute viral rhinosinusitis) will last for less than 10 days and acute post-viral rhinosinusitis will last between 10 days and 12 weeks in duration.

For a diagnosis of recurrent acute rhinosinusitis (RARS), there must be symptom-free episodes between the clinical events. RARS is defined as four episodes per year with symptom-free intervals. Some patients may experience acute exacerbations of chronic rhinosinusitis (AECRS) with worsening of symptoms for short periods, which may be triggered by viral upper respiratory tract infections (URTIs).

Epidemiology and Socioeconomic Impact

ARS is a very common condition with reported prevalence rates varying from 6–15% with a prevalence of recurrent ARS estimated at 0.035%. It is estimated that 5.5% of the population consult their primary care physician for an acute respiratory tract infection each year. This high volume of patients then receives a variable response from medical practitioners in terms of treatment. Only 0.5–2.0% of all cases of ARS are thought to be bacterial with over prescribing of antibiotics based on symptoms and limited examination.

Chronic rhinosinusitis (CRS) represents a significant disease burden worldwide, affecting at least 11% of the population with a higher prevalence in the United Kingdom than ischaemic heart disease (3.7%), diabetes (4%), chronic obstructive pulmonary disease (1.5%), heart failure (<1%) and stroke (<1%) and equivalent to that of peripheral vascular disease, arthritis and back pain, several of which have been shown to have a lesser impact on patients' quality of life than CRS. Patients with CRS also have a 5–17% prevalence of asthma as shown by a recent European study; when broken down into phenotypes the prevalence of asthma is 21%

Table 33.1   EPOS2020 clinical definition of rhinosinusitis[1]

Diagnostic criteria for rhinosinusitis	Symptoms should be correlated by either endoscopic and/or radiological findings
Primary symptoms (requires at least one to be present, but if both present is sufficient to make diagnosis on basis of symptoms)	Nasal blockage/obstruction/congestion Nasal discharge (anterior/posterior)
Additional symptoms *(may also be present and at least one is needed if only one of the primary symptoms is present)*	Facial pain/pressure Olfactory dysfunction (Hyposmia/anosmia)
Duration	>10 days, <3 months = acute >3 months = chronic
Endoscopy *(any of these)*	Nasal polyps Mucopurulent discharge (middle meatus) Oedema/mucosal obstruction in middle meatus
CT scan findings *(as well as or instead of endoscopic findings)*	Mucosal changes within the ostiomeatal complex and/or sinuses

in CRS without nasal polyps (CRSsNPs), 47% in CRS with nasal polyps (CRSwNPs) and 73% in allergic fungal rhinosinusitis (AFRS).

A recent UK study has shown that CRS affects the social spectrum equally and that poor socioeconomic status does not appear to be a risk factor for CRS, but there remains a need for larger scale studies that may also examine the natural history of the disease. Two European studies have reported direct costs of CRS. In CRSwNP, it was estimated that yearly costs were €1501. In a mixed group of CRS, individual costs for primary and secondary care amounted to £2974 compared with £555 for controls and £304 versus £51 for out-of-pocket expenses. In England and Wales, CRS is thought to account for at least 120,000 outpatient visits per year and leads to over 30,000 polypectomies or sinus operations being performed. With data suggesting 1 in 5 are undergoing revision surgery within 5 years, the specific cost of this revision surgery is estimated at £15 million per year. Surgical treatment for CRS certainly appears to influence drug costs, and there is increasing evidence that earlier surgical intervention may reduce the prevalence of late-onset asthma.

Acute Rhinosinusitis

The viruses most commonly implicated in ARS include rhinoviruses (50%), influenza and parainfluenza viruses, adenovirus, respiratory syncytial virus and enterovirus. If bacteria do become implicated the organisms, those most commonly seen are *Streptococcus pneumoniae* (27%), *Haemophilus influenzae* (44%) and *Moraxella catarrhalis* (14%) with other organisms sometimes seen including *S. pyogenes* and *Staphylococcus aureus*. The proportion of these organisms has changed in recent years with vaccination schemes. Diagnosis of ARS is typically the domain of primary care and therefore endoscopy and computed tomography (CT) are rarely available in this setting. Key determinants of whether a case of ARS appears more likely to be bacterial are listed in Table 33.2. Most cases will be self-limiting with complications of ARS exceedingly rare; there is an estimated 2–4 cases per million of the population per year. This was perhaps thought to be due to the high rate of antibiotic use, but there is evidence to suggest that in cases where complications have occurred, this has not been prevented by prior use of oral antibiotics.

Chronic Rhinosinusitis

To date, CRS has been largely subcategorised into cases with polyps (CRSwNPs) or without polyps (CRSsNPs) based on pathophysiology.

CRSwNPs is characterised by an intense oedematous stroma in the sinonasal epithelium, with albumin deposition, pseudocyst formation and subepithelial/perivascular inflammatory cell infiltration. It appears to be associated with a typical T-helper 2 cell (TH2) skewed eosinophilic inflammation, with high interleukin (IL)-5 and eosinophil cationic protein (ECP) concentrations in the polyps.

In comparison, CRSsNPs is characterised by fibrosis, basement membrane thickening, goblet cell hyperplasia, subepithelial oedema, and mononuclear cell infiltration. It exhibits a T-helper 1 cell (TH1) milieu, with increased levels of interferon gamma (IFN-γ) in inflamed sinus mucosa and low ECP/myeloperoxidase ratios. Also, Asian studies have identified a predominantly TH1 cell and TH17 pattern within polyp tissue.

This basic division into the two subgroups does, however, represent an oversimplification of a heterogeneous disease. The various aetiological mechanisms that have been proposed for

Table 33.2 Additional symptoms or signs for acute bacterial rhinosinusitis

At least three of the following should be present:
• Discoloured discharge (unilateral predominance) • Severe local pain (unilateral predominance) • Fever (>38°C) • 'Double sickening' – deterioration after initial milder phase of illness

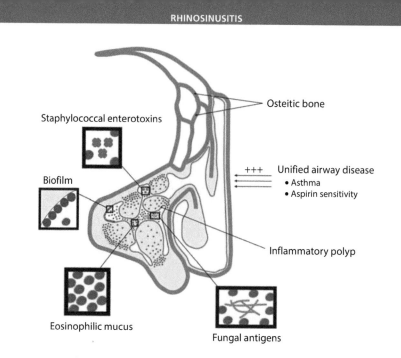

Figure 33.1   Aetiological mechanisms proposed for CRS[1].

CRS are summarised in Figure 33.1. EPOS 2020[1] has sought to introduce a new classification for CRS separating out primary and secondary cases and anatomical cases (Figure 33.2).

This classification helps to guide the clinician to the appropriate management. Anatomical causes, be they primary or secondary, ultimately need a surgical solution, whereas primary diffuse cases lend themselves to appropriate medical treatment prior to consideration of surgical management. In a similar vein, diffuse secondary cases require appropriate management of the underlying systemic disorder which may often be medical. With the advent of biologics this classification may also help to focus these new therapeutic agents on the correct patient cohort.

Anatomical variation may predispose a patient to isolated inflammation in only one of the sinuses as a post-obstructive phenomenon. CT scanning may identify anatomic variants such as an infra-orbital ethmoid cell, concha bullosa and narrow nasal cavity secondary to deviated nasal septum. Microbiology sampling of mucopus should be performed in conjunction with surgical drainage and aeration as medical therapy typically fails but these patients tend not to need any sustained post-operative medical treatment. In approximately 10% of these cases the cause will be odontogenic, and in unilateral cases an oral examination and a careful review of the maxillary sinus floor should be undertaken to look for signs of an oro-antral fistula. Involvement of oral maxillofacial surgery colleagues will be beneficial at an early stage where odontogenic aetiology is suspected to enable optimisation of management. In CRSwNP, ostiomeatal complex (OMC) obstruction may be a 'barometer' of overall disease burden, in that increasing Lund-Mackay scoring is associated with OMC involvement overall.

The new classification also helps to remind the clinician that 'nasal polyposis' is not a diagnosis; it is merely a description of a pathological endpoint of sinonasal disease, and localised examples of nasal polyps include antrochoanal polyps and reactive polyps as may be seen around other inflammatory foci such as a fungal ball or inverted papilloma. A unilateral nasal polyp should always be viewed with suspicion, especially in older patients and in anyone exposed to wood dust. CT scanning and biopsy of a unilateral polyp are needed to decide on the medical and surgical treatment strategy to pursue. Caution should be advised with

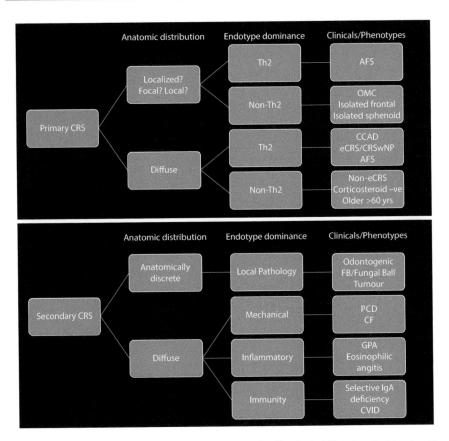

Figure 33.2   Primary and secondary CRS – EPOS2020 classification[1]. CRS = chronic rhinosinusitis, AFS = allergic fungal sinusitis, OMC = ostiomeatal complex, CCAD = central compartment atopic disease, eCRS = eosinophilic chronic rhinosinusitis, CRSwNP = chronic rhinosinusitis without nasal polyps, FB = fungal ball, PCD = primary ciliary dyskinesia, CF = cystic fibrosis, GPA = granulomatosis with polyangiitis, IgA = immunoglobulin A, CVID = common variable immune deficiency

performing a biopsy of any polyp that arises superiorly within the nose, or from the back of the nose in a juvenile male patient. Magnetic resonance imaging (MRI) scanning may be appropriate in select cases where extra-sinus involvement is identified or suspected.

Given the insidious nature of CRS, some cases may appear as CRSsNP at first presentation but eventually develop nasal polyps. A number of recognised mechanisms appear to have a role in polyp formation, including bacterial (super-antigen response), fungal sensitisation and atopy. These may be associated with biofilm formation or frank eosinophilia, both exacerbating and propagating the inflammatory process.

A proportion of patients with CRSwNP also fall into a unique subset, characterised by coexistent asthma and aspirin sensitivity known as Samter's triad or aspirin/non-steroidal anti-inflammatory exacerbated respiratory disease (NERD). NERD is believed to account for approximately 15% of CRSwNPs, classically manifest by severe nasal and/or respiratory symptoms following ingestion of salicylates.

When severe bilateral nasal polyposis is the possibility, NERD should be considered as well as AFRS, another smaller subgroup, believed to represent 10% of those with CRSwNP. CT scanning may elucidate a pansinus opacification typical of AFRS/NERD (double density signs), with thick granular (eosinophilic) mucin usually found at initial presentation, during

Table 33.3 Systemic conditions causing rhinosinusitis or possible differential diagnosis

Category	Diagnosis	Key features
Congenital	Cystic fibrosis	Abnormal sweat test CFTR gene mutation on chromosome 7
	Primary ciliary dyskinesia	Abnormal mucociliary clearance and cilial ultrastructure
	Primary immunodeficiencies (CVID, SCID, hypo/dysgammaglobulinaemias	Low/absent antibodies
Infectious/ inflammatory	HIV	Positive ELISA for HIV
	Sarcoidosis	Non-caseating granulomata Elevated ACE CXR signs (hilar lymphadenopathy)
	Tuberculosis	Acid-fast bacilli Mantoux test positive
	Granulomatosis with polyangiitis (Wegener's syndrome)	cANCA positive Leukocytoclastic vasculitis on biopsy
	Eosinophilic granulomatosis with polyangiitis (Churg-Strauss Syndrome)	pANCA positive
Neoplastic	Haematological malignancies	Abnormal FBC/bone marrow
	Sinonasal malignancies	Biopsy positive Radiological changes
Iatrogenic	Atrophic rhinitis	Excessive crusting following radical nasal surgery
	Chemotherapy/immunosuppression	Relevant dug history
Metabolic	Malnutrition	Low BMI

Note: CFTR = cystic fibrosis transmembrane conductance regulator, CVID = common variable immune deficiency, SCID = severe combined Immunodeficiency, HIV = human immunodeficiency virus, ELISA = enzyme-linked immunoassay, ACE = angiotensin converting enzyme, CXR=chest X-ray, cANCA = cytoplasmic antineutrophil cytoplasmic antibody, pANCA = perinuclear antineutrophil cytoplasmic antibodies, FBC = full blood cell count, BMI = body mass index

surgery or sometimes in the post-operative period. The role and significance of osteitis in CRS is currently unclear, although it may explain why some cases are resistant to standard oral treatment regimens. In CRSwNPs, osteitis may act as a marker of severity and has been shown to occur significantly more often in revision cases.

Systemic Conditions Causing Rhinosinusitis

Ciliary Dyskinesia

Although newborn screening for cystic fibrosis (CF) will pick up most cases, any doubt in a child presenting with diffuse nasal polyposis in conjunction with total opacification of the sinuses as well as hypoplastic sinuses (typically frontal and sphenoid) should be followed up with a sweat test. Nasal endoscopy demonstrates polyp formation in up to 45% of adults with CF, although most will show radiological evidence of disease. Polyps from children with CF have a significantly lower eosinophil count than patients with 'typical' adult-onset CRSwNPs. However, there have also been studies to demonstrate significant overlap in eosinophil concentrations between groups.

Primary ciliary dyskinesia is often associated with situs inversus and known in this circumstance as Kartagener's syndrome. Patients often present in adolescence and may have a prior history of otitis media with effusion; they may also suffer with bronchiectasis. Ciliary dyskinesias will show delayed mucociliary clearance times and require investigation at specialist centres, of which there are three in the United Kingdom. Absent mucociliary clearance exhibited in primary ciliary dyskinesia results in recurrent bacterial infections and CRSwNP in approximately 40% of patients.

Other systemic conditions such eosinophilic granulomatosis with polyangiitis, granulomatosis with polyangiitis and sarcoidosis are described in detail in Chapter 44.

Other Differential Diagnoses to Consider

Clear rhinorrhoea, especially unilaterally, should always prompt investigation for a cerebrospinal fluid (CSF) leak. Tumours will typically present with unilateral symptoms such as blockage or bleeding, but inverted papillomas may sometimes be found amongst bilateral CRSwNPs; hence, this is why it is important to send material for histology during any surgery to remove polyps, especially the first time, if there is any index of suspicion.

Rhinosinusitis may also be a presenting or secondary feature of patients with immunodeficiencies (e.g. HIV) or who are immunocompromised by systemic treatment for other disorders (e.g. receiving immunosuppressive drugs for organ transplantation). In those cases, patients require endoscopic retrieval of mucopus where possible, as unusual organisms may be found.

Immunodeficiency should always be considered a possibility in patients who appear not to respond to standard medical and surgical care for CRS and in cases of recurrent ARS. Common variable immune deficiency (CVID), selective IgA deficiency, IgG subclass deficiency, and specific antibody deficiency are all possible immunodeficiencies that can be detected in cases of CRS. Certainly there is a role for screening for immunodeficiency in CRS patients refractory to standard treatment.

In all secondary cases, involvement of relevant physicians is likely to be needed for their global management.

KEY POINTS

Rhinosinusitis is a common disease with CRS affecting an estimated 10% of the population worldwide
- Most ARS is not bacterial and requires symptomatic relief only.
- CRS is a heterogeneous disease with differing phenotypes and endotypes; the latter have yet to be clearly determined.
- CRS presents a significant burden on health care resources, but guidelines exist for its medical and surgical management.
- Where other clues are present, consideration must be given to other systemic causes for sinonasal disease.

Further Reading

1. Fokkens WJ, Lund VJ, Hopkins C, et al. European Position Paper on Rhinosinusitis and Nasal Polyps 2020. *Rhinology.* 2020;58(Suppl S29):1–464. Published 2020 Feb 20. doi:10.4193/Rhin20.600.

34. NASAL POLYPOSIS

Nasal polyps (NPs) are oedematous protrusions of sinonasal mucosa on a background of chronic inflammation. They are a pathological endpoint of sinonasal disease, phenotypically described as chronic rhinosinusitis with nasal polyposis (CRSwNP). Based on the up-to-date EPOS2020 classification described in the Chapter 33, CRSwNP falls mainly into the category of bilateral diffuse CRS with type 2 endotype dominance.[1] However, polyps can also accompany localised CRS such as allergic fungal rhinosinusitis (AFRS).

Incidence and Prevalance

The annual incidence of CRSwNP is 1–20 per 1000 population. This incidence declines after 60 years of age. Prevalence is 1–4% in adults and 0.1% in children. NPs are more common in males (2–4:1). There is no racial predilection.

Clinical Presentation

Clinical presentation is variable and depends on the extent of polyp disease. Small polyps may be asymptomatic whilst larger polyps can cause significant nasal obstruction, congestion, hyposmia, rhinorrhoea, postnasal discharge and facial pain. Rarely, proptosis, hypertelorism and diplopia can result from alterations in the craniofacial structure.

Pathogenesis

Factors causing CRS are complex, individual to the patient and usually unknown, hence the interest now is centred on the resulting inflammation that develops in the sinus tissue. When the mucosal barrier is breached, a self-limited immunodefensive response is generated, characterised by a cellular and cytokine repertoire targeting one of the three classes of pathogens: type 1 immune responses target viruses; type 2 responses target parasites and type 3 responses target extracellular bacteria and fungi, all of which resolve with elimination of the pathogens and restoration of barrier integrity.

In cases of CRS, barrier penetration results in a chronic inflammatory response that fails to resolve, but still typically utilises the type 1, 2 or 3 pathways alone, or in combinations. Approximately 80% of NPs in Western countries are associated with a type 2 eosinophilic inflammatory response, characterised by activation of T-helper 2 cells and innate lymphocytes to produce the key cytokines interleukin (IL)-4, IL-5 and IL-13. These cytokines upregulate the expression of vascular cell adhesion molecule 1 (VCAM-1) on endothelial cells allowing selective adhesion and migration of eosinophils into sinonasal tissue. Furthermore, IL-4 facilitates B-cell maturation into IgE producing plasma cells that release specific IgE and trigger mast cell degranulation and activation. IL-5 can stimulate synthesis and release of eosinophils aiding in their propagation and survival in the bloodstream. The overall effect of this type 2 inflammatory response is an eosinophilic-mediated mucosal injury and chronic inflammation, which results in nasal polyposis.

Allergy

The role of allergy is unclear and varies with phenotype. NPs are found in 25.6% of patients with allergy compared with 3.9% in a control population.

Bacteria

The link between bacterial colonisation and NPs has been postulated but remains unproven. *Staphylococcus aureus* enterotoxin is thought to be the main species involved. The secreted enterotoxins behave as super-antigens, directly activating T cells stimulating a massive cytokine response resulting in eosinophilic inflammation and formation of IgE antibodies.

Histologically, NPs consists of loose connective tissue, goblet cell hyperplasia, inflammatory cells and fluid and are usually covered by pseudostratified, columnar, ciliated epithelium.

Associated Diseases

Asthma

There is a strong correlation between NPs and asthma. In 25% of patients, NPs coexist with asthma out of which up to 45% will develop asthma within 10 years of NP diagnosis. Patients with asthma are more likely to suffer treatment failure and need repeated surgeries.

Non-Steroidal Anti-Inflammatory Drugs Exacerbated Respiratory Disease (NERD)

NERD is a chronic eosinophilic inflammatory disorder of the respiratory tract in patients with asthma and/or CRSwNP. It has also described as aspirin exacerbated respiratory disease (AERD) or Samter's triad.

Its prevalence is 0.9% in normal population, 10–20% in asthmatics and 30–40% among asthmatics with NP.

It is related to cyclo-oxygenase inhibition resulting in increased leukotriene synthesis leading to mast cell instability with histamine release, causing increased vascular permeability, oedema and eosinophilic inflammation of sinonasal membranes resulting in NP formation. NPs tend to be extensive with a higher recurrence rate post-surgery (90% recurrence at 5 years).

Allergic Fungal Rhinosinusitis

AFRS is subset of CRSwNP characterised by a type I mediated hypersensitivity reaction to fungi with the presence of eosinophilic mucin and non-invasive fungal hyphae within the sinuses. The Bent and Kuhn diagnostic major and minor criteria is used to make the diagnosis of AFRS.

Medical therapy alone is inadequate and surgery is the mainstay treatment for AFRS. Oral steroids have been shown to reduce recurrence. Little evidence exists for use of antifungals in AFRS.

The five major Bent and Kuhn criteria which must be met for diagnosis are:

1 Type 1 hypersensitivity to fungi (demonstrated by skin allergy test, fungal IgE in sinus mucin, or PCR)
2 Positive fungal staining of an intranasal surgical specimen
3 Eosinophilic mucin
4 Nasal polyposis
5 Characteristic CT findings – central hyperdense allergic mucin, peripheral hypodense.

Other Diseases Associated with Nasal Polyposis

Cystic fibrosis, primary ciliary dyskinesia (Chapter 33), and eosinophilic granulomatosis with polyangiitis (Chapter 44) are also frequently associated with NPs.

Diagnosis

Anterior rhinoscopy and nasendoscopy are required for assessment and identification of NPs, discharge, crusting or scarring. Blood tests including eosinophil count, specific serum IgE levels for allergens and other serological tests aimed at underlying associated systemic causes should be performed. Computed tomography (CT) scanning with coronal sections is used to assess the extent of disease and detail the anatomy before surgery. In cases of extensive disease with attenuation of anterior skull base, magnetic resonance can be helpful to differentiate from tumour.

Imaging Studies and Staging Systems

Endoscopic and CT-based staging systems are used to determine the extent of disease and evaluate efficacy of therapeutic responses (Table 34.1).

Management

The primary objective is to eliminate symptoms, re-establish nasal breathing and olfaction, prevent recurrence and improve quality of life.

Medical (Further Described in Chapter 35)

Patients should have a trial of medical therapy first unless histology is required. Medical management includes:

- Intra-nasal corticosteroids (INCS).
- Short courses of systemic corticosteroids in more extensive polyposis.
- Antihistamines help only if allergy is present.
- Leukotriene inhibitors may help patients with coexisting asthma and/or aspirin sensitivity.

Table 34.1   Endoscopic staging of nasal polyps in CRSwNP

Lund-Kennedy Endoscopic staging of nasal polyps in CRSwNP		The Lund-McKay Score Radiological staging CRS	
Polyp	0 = Absence of polyp 1 = Polyps in middle meatus only 2 = Beyond middle meatus	0 = No abnormalities 1 = Partial opacification 2 = Complete opacification	Maxillary sinus
Oedema	0 = Absent 1 = Mild 2 = Severe		Anterior ethmoid sinus
Discharge	0 = No discharge 1 = Clear, thin discharge 2 = Thick, purulent discharge		Posterior ethmoid sinus
Scarring	0 = Absent 1 = Mild 2 = Severe		Sphenoid sinus Frontal Sinus
Crusting	0 = Absent 1 = Mild 2 = Severe	0 = Not occluded 2 = Occluded	Ostiomeatal complex

Note: The Lund-McKay Score: each side is scored separately and the total score is calculated.
Source: Lund VJ, Kennedy DW. Quantification for staging sinusitis. In: Kennedy DW. International Conference on Sinus Disease: Terminology, Staging, Therapy. Annals of Otology Rhinology and Laryngology. 1995;104(Suppl 167):17–21; Lund VJ, Mackay IS. Staging in rhinosinusitis. Rhinology. 1993;31(4):183–184.

Recent advances in biological treatments have resulted in availability of therapeutic monoclonal antibodies (mAbs) targeting several key mediators of NP pathogenesis that can potentially improve treatment of nasal polyposis in the setting of type 2 CRS:

1 Omalizumab binds free circulating IgE, downregulates the expression of IgE receptors on mast cells/basophils and reduces release of inflammatory mediators ([IL-4).
2 Dupilumab is an mAb to IL-4 receptor that inhibits the signaling of IL-4/IL-13 and reduces Th2-mediated inflammation. It is the only biological therapy approved for use in CRSwNP.
3 Mepolizumab prevents activation of IL-5 receptors by binding to IL-5, which is important for differentiation/maturation/survival of eosinophils in tissue.

The EPOS2020 guidelines have highlighted specific criteria for their application in NP[1] (Table 34.2).

Recent trials using these biological treatments in NP and comorbid asthma as well as CRSwNP refractory to standard therapy have shown encouraging results with decrease in total polyp and symptoms scores.

Surgical (Further Described in Chapter 36)

Surgical management is considered for patients who have failed to respond to adequate medical treatment. Endoscopic sinus surgery (ESS) aims to improve sinus ventilation and drainage and facilitate topical INCS delivery. Patients with NPs derive the greatest benefit from ESS, and those whose main pre-operative symptom is nasal obstruction or headache report higher benefit.

Post-operatively, patients should be treated with nasal irrigation and intra-nasal or systemic corticosteroids. Compliance influences the long-term efficacy of surgery. There is good evidence that post-operative use of topical nasal steroids reduces the rate of polyp recurrence.

Table 34.2   EPOS2020 criteria for biological treatments in CRS[1]

Presence of **bilateral nasal polyps** in a patient who has had **endoscopic sinus surgery**	
+	
Three criteria required	
Criteria	Cutoff points
Evidence of **type 2 inflammation**	*Tissue eosinophil count ≥10/hpf, OR* *Blood eosinophil count ≥250, OR* *Total IgE ≥100*
Need for **systemic corticosteroids** OR Contraindication to systemic steroids	*≥2 courses per year, OR* *Long term (>3 months) low-dose steroids*
Significantly impaired **quality of life**	*SNOT-22 ≥40*
Significant loss of **smell**	*Anosmic on smell test (score depending on test)*
Diagnosis of comorbid **asthma**	*Asthma needing regular inhaled corticosteroids*

Source: Adapted from Fokkens WJ, Lund VJ, Hopkins C, et al. *European Position Paper on Rhinosinusitis and Nasal Polyposis 2020.* Rhinology. 2020;58(Suppl S29):1–464.

KEY POINTS

- Nasal polyps are the end result of chronic inflammation.
- The pathophysiology remains unclear but is the result of type 2 eosinophilic inflammatory response, characterised by activation of T-helper 2 cells and innate lymphocytes to produce the key cytokines IL-4, IL-5 and IL-13.
- Certain systemic diseases are associated with a much higher incidence of CRSwNP with a prevalence of around 7% in patients with asthma and up to 30–60% in patients with NERD.
- Adequate medical therapy with intranasal corticosteroids, nasal irrigations and oral steroids are first-line treatment for NPs.
- Surgery is indicated where there is failure to respond to adequate medical therapy. ESS aims to improve sinus ventilation and drainage and facilitate topical intranasal corticosteroids delivery.

Further Reading

1. Fokkens WJ, Lund VJ, Hopkins C, et al. European Position Paper on Rhinosinusitis and Nasal Polyps 2020. *Rhinology.* 2020;58(Suppl S29):1–464. Published 2020 Feb 20. doi:10.4193/Rhin20.600.

---

35.   MEDICAL MANAGEMENT OF CRS

Introduction

Acute rhinosinusitis (ARS) is common, affecting 6–15% of the population each year. Most cases are viral, with acute bacterial rhinosinusitis (ABRS) estimated in less than 2% of cases. Nearly all cases of ARS resolve spontaneously within 10 days, and the incidence of complications is very low. Medical treatment may be antimicrobial or anti-inflammatory (Figure 35.1).

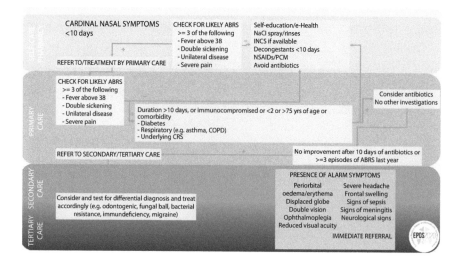

Figure 35.1 ARS management chart (EPOS2020).[1] ABRS, acute bacterial rhinosinusitis; COPD, chronic obstructive pulmonary disease; CRS, chronic rhinosinusitis; INCS, intra-nasal corticosteroid; NSAIDS, non-steroidal anti-inflammatory drugs.

Reduction of Infective Load

Although the majority of ARS is viral, antibiotics are often expected by patients. Most studies have shown little benefit from antibiotics in most patients with ARS and should be restricted in uncomplicated ARS.

Differentiating Bacterial from Viral ARS

ABRS is suggested by the presence of three out of four symptoms including nasal purulence, purulence in the post-nasal space, high fever (>39°C) and raised erythrocyte sedimentation rate (ESR). A description of 'double-sickening', unilateral disease and severe pain may also be helpful. In ABRS or due to the presence of complications the choice of antibiotics is preferably based on culture results. If treatment is empiric, a short course of narrow-spectrum agents is recommended.

Reduction of Inflammation

Studies of intra-nasal glucocorticoids have demonstrated benefit for the relief of symptoms in both viral and ABRS; as the risk of harm is low, these can be offered to all patients. Similarly, meta-analysis supports a role for systemic steroid treatment as adjunctive treatment to antibiotics. Patients treated with oral corticosteroids were more likely to have short-term resolution or improvement of symptoms than those receiving antibiotics alone. However, given the risks of systemic steroids, these should only be considered in severe cases.

Symptomatic Improvement

Nasal decongestants may have a small symptomatic effect in reducing nasal congestion but not overall duration of ARS. There is little evidence that saline therapies assist in symptom relief. Low-volume saline sprays may assist in removing mucus and crusts, but high-volume irrigations are often poorly tolerated during acute inflammation.

Management of ARS complications is described in Chapter 37.

MEDICAL MANAGEMENT OF CHRONIC RHINOSINUSITIS

Introduction

The treatment of chronic rhinosinusitis (CRS) is primarily medical, with surgery reserved for those who fail a trial of maximal medical therapy (Figure 35.2). However, there are important exceptions.

Overview of the Pathophysiology of CRS

As described in chapter 33, the EPOS 2020 group has chosen to look at CRS as primary and secondary[1]:

- *Primary* CRS refers to most patients with unexplained inflammation of the upper airway. It is common to find lower airway disease as part of a broader respiratory condition.

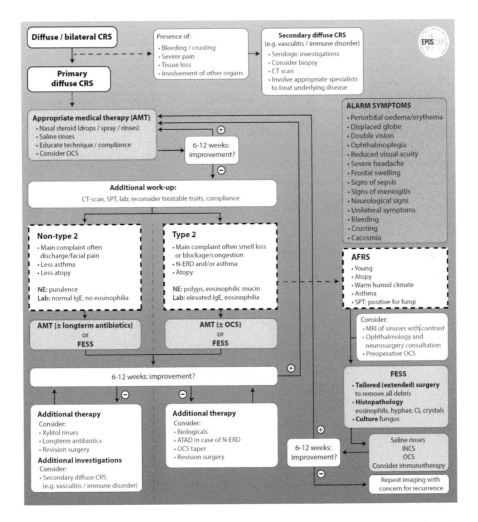

Figure 35.2 Management of Rhinosinusitis (EPOS2020).[1] ATAD, aspirin treatment after desensitisation; CRS, chronic rhinosinusitis; CT, computed tomography; FESS, functional endoscopic sinus surgery; INCS, intra-nasal corticosteroid; MRI, magnetic resonance imaging; N-ERD, non-steroidal anti-inflammatory exacerbated respiratory disease; OCS, oral corticosteroids; SPT, skin prick test.

- *Secondary* CRS refers to sinonasal disease with a manifestation of systemic disease; examples include vasculitis, cystic fibrosis, sarcoidosis and ciliary motility disorders. CRS may also occur as a direct result of focal abnormalities including a foreign body, fungal ball, odontogenic infection or an anatomical obstruction. Medical management plays no significant role in first-line management in this group.

Primary CRS may be subcategorised phenotypically by the presence or absence of polyps: *CRS with* polyps (CRSwNP) or CRS *sine* (*without*) polyps (CRSsNP). It is acknowledged that there is a move away from phenotyping the disease and increasing focus on endotyping of the mucosal inflammatory pattern to identify those with eosinophil-dominated (eCRS or T-helper 2 cell (Th2) skewed) inflammation.

Treatment Targeting Intrinsic Mucosal Inflammation
Mucosal inflammation is the defining feature of CRS. Glucocorticoids have formed the mainstay of medical therapy for CRS, whereas long-term macrolides, doxycycline and monoclonal antibodies also target the inflammatory pathway.

Intra-Nasal Corticosteroids
It has been shown in many studies that topical corticosteroids improve symptoms, decrease the polyp score and size and prevent polyp recurrence after surgery. Intra-nasal corticosteroids have an excellent safety profile with low systemic bioavailability and are also safe for long-term use in children. Instruction in correct delivery techniques is essential (Figure 35.3).

Systemic Corticosteroids
In contrast, there is a relative paucity of data for the efficacy of systemic corticosteroids. In CRSsNP, there are no studies evaluating systemic steroids alone. In CRSwNP, a systematic review showed a short-term benefit of a short (2-to 4-week) course of oral steroids of variable doses and duration when compared with placebo. There was a reduction of polyp size and improvement of nasal symptoms and quality of life; however, by 3 months there was no difference between groups. Therefore, short courses of systemic steroids can be recommended

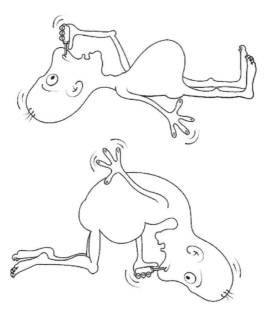

Figure 35.3   Correct application for nasal drops. (A) Head-back position. (B) Head-down position.

for the treatment of CRSwNP, although the risk of side effects must be considered with repeated courses.

Immunomodulatory Antibiotics

Long-term (often 12 weeks) macrolide antibiotics are used for their anti-inflammatory effects, especially on neutrophil-mediated inflammation.

There are two prospective randomised controlled trials. The first study included only CRSsNP and showed a significant effect of roxithromycin on symptom scores and with greater efficacy in patients with normal IgE levels. A subsequent study has found no effect; however, this study included both CRSwNP and CRSsNP, and therefore it is likely that this study included more patients with elevated IgE than the first.

Long-term use of macrolide antibiotics is associated with macrolide resistance, and gastrointestinal side effects are relatively common. Therefore, use should be directed at those patients most likely to benefit (i.e. CRSsNP, normal IgE levels). Macrolides interact with many other drugs and may prolong the QT interval; a careful medical history should be taken prior to usage.

A 20-day course of doxycycline has been shown to have a moderate and sustained effect on polyp size over a 12-week period, and doxycycline may be an adjunct in patients with CRSwNP.

Novel Immunoregulation

Direct targeting of the inflammatory pathway is possible using monoclonal antibodies such as omalizumab (anti-IgE), mepolizumab (anti-IL-5) and dupilumab (anti-IL-4 and 13). They can significantly reduce symptom scores and polyp size. However, high cost, risk of anaphylaxis, and need for subcutaneous injection are limiting factors that likely to restrict use to those failing more established treatment regimens. EPOS2020 suggested criteria for biological treatment that are described in Chapter 34.

Aspirin Desensitisation

Aspirin sensitivity is usually associated with nasal polyposis and asthma (Samter's triad). Patients often have extensive polyposis, with high rates of recurrence after treatment. A placebo-controlled randomised control trial has shown a reduction in polyp recurrence when tolerance is achieved by aspirin desensitisation and ongoing daily aspirin maintenance. This must be performed under medical supervision, with optimum results achieved in the early post-operative period.

Treatment Aimed at Reducing Microbial Load

Treatment aimed at reducing microbial load or eradicating pathogens from the sinuses assumes that these play a role in causing or propagating CRS. Bacteria may play a role in acute infective exacerbations where culture-directed short-term antibiotics may be indicated, but there are no studies evaluating long-term symptom control.

Treatment Aimed to Improve Mucociliary Clearance

Saline irrigation can improve mucociliary clearance by the removal of mucus, infected crusts and pro-inflammatory agents. A Cochrane meta-analysis demonstrated benefit from saline irrigation both when used as the sole modality treatment and as an adjunct.

As irrigation is generally well tolerated, and it can be recommended for use in patients with CRS. Again, patients should be instructed in their use (Figure 35.4).

Mucoactive Agents

Johnson & Johnson Baby Shampoo® has been shown to have both antibiofilm-forming properties at 1% solution and is useful for treating crusting, thick mucus and chronic bacterial mucosal colonisation.

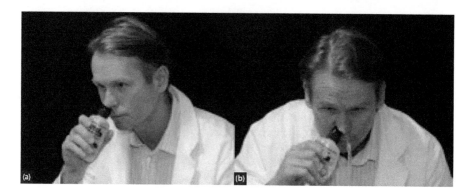

Figure 35.4 Technique for nasal irrigation (A) Stand over a sink or in the shower/bath, keep your head straight and put the nozzle of the bottle in one nostril. (B) Squirt half the bottle into one nostril and then repeat on the other side. Following irrigation, blow your nose gently.

Delivery of Medical Therapy

Studies have documented poor penetration of topical therapies into the sinuses in the pre-operative state. Consequently, systemic therapy is necessary to treat the sinus mucosa. Endoscopic sinus surgery (ESS) can improve delivery and in the post-operative state, topical therapy is paramount in managing disease. Delivery of topical steroid by high-volume irrigation has been shown to achieve better control of the sinus cavity on endoscopy than an equivalent dose of steroid delivered by conventional spray.

The delivery device is important, and the most effective devices are the positive-pressure, high-volume irrigation bottles (Figure 35.4).

Assessment of the Response to Medical Treatment

The aim of treatment for CRS is to reduce symptoms and improve quality of life. Subjective symptoms need to be quantified using disease-specific quality-of-life measures. The SNOT-22 questionnaire is most used but many others exists.

Response to treatment should be considered and if not achieved, the history and examination should be reviewed. It may be necessary with more aggressive medical therapy or consider combination with surgery. More than two courses of systemic corticosteroid per year (of 2–3 weeks' duration and less than 40 mg maximal daily dose) indicates failure.

Any patient with unilateral polypoid disease, where there is a suspicion of malignancy, the presence of associated neurological or orbital symptoms or atypical features should not be considered for medical therapy. They require urgent radiological imaging, followed by surgery and histological examination where indicated.

KEY POINTS

- Medical therapy should have a three-way goal of reducing inflammatory load, normalising microbial community and restoration of mucociliary function.
- Medical therapy to the paranasal sinus is primarily via the systemic route in the unoperated patient.
- Systemic corticosteroid is effective in CRSwNP, but use is usually limited to two courses a year.
- Surgery, while potentially curative for some, is more commonly utilised to enable long-term local or topical therapy to control disease.
- Intra-nasal corticosteroid irrigations are a common effective delivery mechanism in the post-surgical patient. Their use is similar to that of a prophylactic inhaler for asthma patients.

Further Reading

1. Fokkens WJ, Lund VJ, Hopkins C, et al. European Position Paper on Rhinosinusitis and Nasal Polyps 2020. *Rhinology*. 2020;58(Suppl S29):1–464. Published 2020 Feb 20. doi:10.4193/Rhin20.600.

36. SURGICAL MANAGEMENT OF CRS

Introduction

The aims of functional endoscopic sinus surgery (FESS) are the restitution of physiology and should fulfill the following criteria:

- Creating a sinus cavity that incorporates the natural ostium
- Allows adequate sinus ventilation
- Facilitates mucociliary clearance
- Facilitates instillation of topical therapies

Several acronyms are used to describe the extent of FESS:

- *'Mini FESS'*: approach involving simple ventilation of the lower sinuses (less aggressive endotypes)
- *'Full-house FESS'*: complete sinus opening including anterior and posterior ethmoidectomy, middle meatal antrostomies, sphenoidotomy and frontal opening
- *Extended endoscopic surgery*: Draf III and other extended frontal sinus approaches, pre-lacrimal approach to maxilla and radical sphenoidotomy
- *Mucosal 'reset'*: includes significant removal of inflamed/dysfunctional mucosa

Surgical Procedures

Anaesthesia for Sinus Surgery

- Usually performed under general anaesthetic with a laryngeal mask.
- Hypotensive anaesthesia for optimal surgical field; Desflurane (at low concentration only) and remifentanil combined probably provides just as good a surgical field as total intravenous anaesthesia (TIVA) and avoids the need for bispectral index (BIS) monitoring.
- A systolic mean arterial pressure (MAP) of approximately 90 mmHg is recommended and best achieved with a heart rate (HR) ≤60 beats/min. Volatile agents, which achieve hypotension by reducing systemic vascular resistance (SVR), can cause a deterioration of the surgical field from vasodilatation of the microvasculature.

$$MAP = HR \times stroke\ volume(SV) \times SVR$$

Surgical Position and Intranasal Preparation

- Reverse Trendelenburg position (up to 15° angle), produces a 35–40% reduction in nasal blood flow.
- Eyes can be left open with lubrication or taped to provide better corneal protection whilst still allowing rapid access to the globe.

Table 36.1   CLOSE mnemonic is widely used to facilitate systematic preoperative interpretation of the CT images

Mnemonic	Evaluated anatomical structures
C	Cribriform niche: depth and asymmetry should be evaluated
L	Lamina papyracea: examined for dehiscence
O	(Onodi) sphenoethmoidal cells
S	Sphenoid sinus: examined for dehiscence of bone overlying the optic nerve and carotid artery
E	Ethmoidal arteries: the position of the anterior and posterior

- Cocaine and adrenaline, ± sodium bicarbonate ('Moffat's solution'), soaked on neuro-patties are used for topical decongestion.
- Lignocaine 5% and phenylephrine 0.5% (co-phenylcaine) or oxymetazoline can be used if cocaine is not available.
- Infiltration (2.2 mL 1% lignocaine with 1:80,000 adrenaline) of the middle turbinate, nasal septum and frontal process of the maxilla (optional).
- Allow time for topical and injected vasoconstrictors to establish their local effect, whilst allowing their systemic effect to dissipate.

Fess for Rhinosinusitis

General Principles

Recent sinus computed tomography (CT) scans are mandatory and need to be available to the surgeon throughout the operation (Table 36.1).

Surgical Techniques

Uncinectomy

The use of a sickle knife on the inferior portion of the uncinate is to be discouraged as orbital penetration can easily occur. Back-biting forceps allow for safer uncinate incision (Figure 36.1).

The uncinate process can be removed using angled through-biting forceps or can be dislocated forward using a double right-angled ball probe and cautiously removed with the micro-debrider or through-biting forceps. The bone of the horizontal portion can be dissected free from the mucosa and the natural ostium stretched open with an angled probe or sucker, without removing any mucosa. For more advanced disease (or in revision cases), it may be necessary to create a large middle meatal antrostomy.

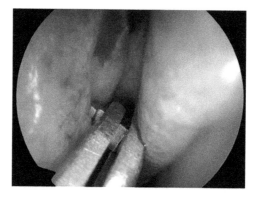

Figure 36.1   A paediatric back-biting forceps is used to perform the inferior uncinectomy incision.

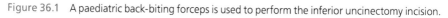

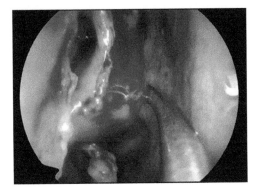

Figure 36.2 A double right-angle ball probe is inserted into the natural ostium of the bulla ethmoidalis (medial) and then the anterior face is fractured anteriorly.

Removal of the Ethmoidal Bulla
The anterior face of the bulla can be fractured forwards (Figure 36.2) then removed with a microdebrider. Other anterior ethmoidal cells can be removed in a similar manner. The use of through-biting instruments is preferred to minimise the risk of exposing bone.

Posterior Ethmoidectomy
The ground lamella of the middle turbinate should be perforated in its inferomedial quadrant. The roof of the maxillary sinus can be used as a guide to the superior limit of dissection within the posterior ethmoid. The optic nerve may traverse through an Onodi cell.

Sphenoidotomy
The natural sphenoid ostium is located medial to the superior turbinate at the height of the antral roof. Part of the middle turbinate can be resected with a back-biting forceps, entering the superior meatus. The inferior third of the superior turbinate can then be resected to access the sphenoethmoidal recess. As an alternative, an artificial opening into the sphenoid can be made through the posterior ethmoid and then extended medially to incorporate the natural sphenoid ostium.

Frontal Sinus Surgery
Using a Kerrison's punch in the axilla of the middle turbinate (Figure 36.3), the anterior portion of the agger nasi can be removed.

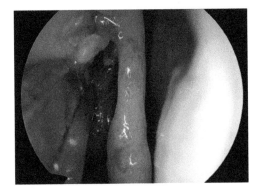

Figure 36.3 A 2-mm 450 forward-angled Kerrison's punch is used to raise the axilla of the middle turbinate and improve access to the agger nasi and the frontal recess.

Curettes and angled instruments can then be used to remove the posterior wall and roof of the agger nasi to expose the frontal recess. Axillary mucosal flaps are not required as adhesions can easily be prevented using other methods. Once the agger nasi has been removed, any remaining frontoethmoidal cells can be removed, after identification of the anterior ethmoidal artery. Advanced frontal instrumentation such as a giraffe forceps or 3.5-mm Hosemann punch may greatly facilitate surgery in this area.

Post-Operative Management

- In severe disease (and most of chronic rhinosinusitis with polyps [CRSwNP]), a 10-day course of 25mg of oral prednisolone can be given without tapering.
- In extensive eosinophilic disease, a 3-week course of steroids (or longer) may be required (with tapering to avoid an Addisonian crisis).
- There is no evidence that prophylactic antibiotics improve outcomes.
- Routine nasal steroids; it is important to emphasise to patients with severe disease that they may need to be on topical steroid sprays or irrigations for some time (and in some cases of eosinophilic chronic rhinosinusitis (CRS), for an indefinite period) to prevent disease recurrence.
- Initially large-volume saline irrigations are used to clean the nose of mucopus, blood clot and other tissue.
- Following first review at 7–10 days, less frequent irrigations can be continued until review at 6 weeks or 3 months.

Surgical Complications

Analysis of the literature reveals a range of significant complications between 0.3 and 22.4% (median 7.0%). Excessive bleeding and poor visualisation are associated with an increase in complication rates. High-level evidence has demonstrated that intraoperative image guidance significantly reduces the incidence of complications.

Avoiding Complications

Anti-coagulation drugs, non-steroidal anti-inflammatory drugs (NSAIDS) and homeopathic preparations (e.g. fish oil and multivitamins) that can affect bleeding should be stopped pre-operatively. The CT scans will identify dehiscence of the lamina papyracea, angulation of the vertical lamella of the cribriform plate and congenital defects in the skull base and over the carotid artery, which all carry higher risk.

Orbital Injury

The orbit can be damaged with the first incision of a sickle knife through the inferior portion of the uncinate process or when performing a middle meatal antrostomy with a long thin infundibulum. If just orbital fat is exposed, no repair of the defect is usually necessary and the eye should be routinely checked to identify any intra-orbital haemorrhage. Any proptosis should be regarded as significant and decompression of the orbit by removing the lamina papyracea and incising the orbital periosteum may be required, with or without a lateral canthotomy and/or cantholysis. If damage to the ocular muscles is suspected (increased with microdebrider injury), an ophthalmological opinion should be obtained, although there is usually little that can be done to repair a transected muscle and late oculoplastic surgery may never restore normal movement to the damaged eye.

Optic Nerve Injury

The optic nerve can be damaged due to intra-orbital haematoma or direct injury. It is most at risk if the optic nerve is on a mesentery within an Onodi cell. If injury to the optic nerve is suspected, steroids should be given and an urgent ophthalmological consultation should be obtained.

CSF Leak

The estimated prevalence of intra-operative cerebrospinal fluid (CSF) leak is 0.5% of cases, usually at the vertical lamella of the cribriform plate. Often a CSF leak can be identified immediately and repaired using fat plugs, artificial materials or homografts with or without covering mucosal grafts and fibrin glue.

Carotid Artery Injury

Pre-operative CT identification of carotid dehiscence will reduce risk. A carotid injury can be extremely difficult to manage due to the high volume of blood, which will obscure the operative field. The sphenoid needs to be packed and the anaesthetist must commence immediate haemostatic resuscitation. Although direct carotid artery repair (with either a J-suture or muscle pack) has been advocated, placement of an endovascular stent is an effective alternate treatment option.

Outcomes

The limited randomised controlled trial (RCT) evidence does demonstrate more benefit for patients with CRSwNP than CRS without nasal polyps (CRSsNP). Other non-RCT data provide more support for surgery. The Royal College of Surgeons of England (RCSEng) comparative audit also found that patients with CRSwNP did better following surgery than patients with CRSsNP. Total revision rates were 3.6%, 11.8% and 19% at 1, 3 and 5 years, respectively.

Balloon Sinuplasty

Balloon dilatation of either the maxillary, frontal and/or the sphenoid sinus ostia is an alternative technique that is increasingly being performed. It is expensive and highly controversial, but there is evidence that balloon dilatation can maintain 91.6% patency of the sinus ostia at 2 years. Small RCTs have shown balloon dilatation to be non-inferior to FESS and a non-RCT has shown balloon dilatation to produce lower sinonasal outcome test (SNOT-20) scores compared with conventional FESS at 3 months.

Rhinosinusitis in Children

Adenoidectomy alone is recommended as a first-line treatment of acute rhinosinusitis (ARS; 50–80% improvement), reserving endoscopic sinus surgery for rare and resistant cases. In CRS, there may be a role for surgery in patients with cystic fibrosis and immune deficiencies to provide better access for topical irrigations and medications.

KEY POINTS

- FESS is an effective technique for patients with both CRSwNP and CRSsNP when medical management has failed.
- Revision rates for FESS are generally between 10 and 20% over a 5-year period, more so in patients with CRSwNP.
- Good pre-operative planning, surgical technique and post-operative follow-up have been demonstrated to produce optimal outcomes.
- FESS has been demonstrated to improve the effective medical management of patients with eosinophilic CRS.
- CRS remains a mucosal disease, and ongoing medical management is typically required to prevent recurrent symptoms despite adequate FESS.

37. COMPLICATIONS OF RHINOSINUSITIS

Complications of rhinosinusitis result from progression of infection beyond the sinuses, causing significant morbidity from local or distant spread. Complications are more accentuated in children and adolescents because of their thinner, more porous bony septa and sinus walls, open suture lines and larger vascular foramina.

Classification

Complications may be caused by either local progression or distant spread via the bloodstream (Table 37.1). Local progression is typically through areas where the surrounding bone is thin such as the porous lamina papyracea, where there is a direct anatomical connection or through osteitic bone. Direct routes of spread occur through neurovascular foramina such as the infra-orbital canal, or via the valveless diploic veins of Breschet. The venous drainage of the sinus mucosa is via these diploic veins, which communicate with the dural venous plexus. Local complications can be specific for the individual sinus groups and may be discussed relating to their presumed anatomical sinus of origin.

Frontal

Anterior spread of frontal sinusitis may cause a subperiosteal abscess and osteomyelitis (Pott's puffy tumour [PPT]). Posterior spread of infection can cause intra-cranial complications.

Ethmoid

Orbital cellulitis is the most frequent complication of ethmoid sinusitis.

Maxillary

Isolated maxillary rhinosinusitis rarely gives rise to acute complications. Acute cheek swelling usually results from dental disease, though there may be an associated secondary maxillary rhinosinusitis.

Sphenoid

Isolated sphenoid sinusitis is rare, but complications can result in meningitis or cavernous sinus thrombosis. In cavernous sinus thrombosis infection may spread through veins from the paranasal sinuses and orbit to the cavernous sinuses as thrombophlebitis or by septic emboli.

Table 37.1 Complications of rhinosinusitis (figures in brackets indicate relative frequency)

Orbital (60%)	Intracranial (15–20%)	Bony (5–10%)	Chronic
Preseptal cellulitis (50%)	Subdural empyema (38%)	Osteomyelitis and Pott's puffy tumour	Mucocoele and pyocoele
Postseptal cellulitis or orbital cellulitis without abscess (35%)	Intra-cranial abscess (30%)		
Subperiosteal abscess (15%)	Extradural abscess (23%)		
Orbital abscess (<1%)	Meningitis (2%)		
Cavernous sinus thrombosis*	Cavernous* or superior sagittal sinus thrombosis (2%)		

* Cavernous sinus thrombosis is classified as an intracranial complication but is also often included among orbital complications due to its relation to the orbit.

Clinical Presentation

Any of the complications described above may present with symptoms or signs of rhinosinusitis. The rhinosinusitis can also be asymptomatic.

Orbital Complications

Up to 3% of sinusitis cases will progress to orbital cellulitis with 60–85% of orbital cellulitis cases secondary to sinusitis. The remainder of cases are caused by processes such as dacryocystitis or facial infection.

Figure 37.1 illustrates the management algorithm. Onset is noted by swelling around the eye. Oedema results from congestion of veins draining the eyelid and can be present when the infection is still confined to the sinus. Orbital cellulitis is far more common in children and young adults. Visual problems are a late sign. Initially signs may be unilateral, bilateral disease propagates via the intercavernous sinuses. According to Chandler's classification, orbital complications may be divided into five stages based on their clinical and radiological findings (Table 37.2).

Investigations

Examination

- Nasendoscopy
- Eye assessment for chemosis, eye movements, proptosis, relative afferent pupillary defect, visual acuity (Snellen chart), colour vision (Ishihara plates) and fundoscopy
- Neurological examination for signs of intra-cranial complications (cavernous sinus thrombosis): progressive ophthalmoplegia, visual impairment, headaches and trigeminal paraesthesia
- A neurological examination for intracranial complications

The aim of these investigations is to:

- Confirm diagnosis
- Define the extent and site
- Plan treatment including surgical approach
- Identify covert complications
- Monitor response to treatment

Contrast-enhanced computed tomography (CT) is advised first-line imaging. As CT scanning can miss up to 50% of intra-cranial complications, magnetic resonance imaging (MRI) is advised for suspected intracranial complications.

Other Investigations

- Blood cultures
- Sinonasal/abscess pus culture, ideally from initial nasal endoscopy

Treatment

Most patients with complications require admission. Non-surgical management of rhinosinusitis complications is often first choice unless abscess formation is demonstrated. The exception is when vision is affected by pressure on the optic nerve from inflammation without abscess.

Antibiotics form the mainstay of medical treatment. Expert opinion suggests decongestants aid resolution by reducing mucosal oedema, though evidence is inconclusive. Selection of antibiotics is empirical (broad spectrum) followed by culture-specific sensitivities. Polymicrobial and anaerobic isolates are more common in patients over 15 and with intracranial complications.

Evidence of an abscess on the CT scan or lack of clinical improvement after 24–48 hours of intravenous (IV) antibiotics are indications for orbital exploration and drainage.

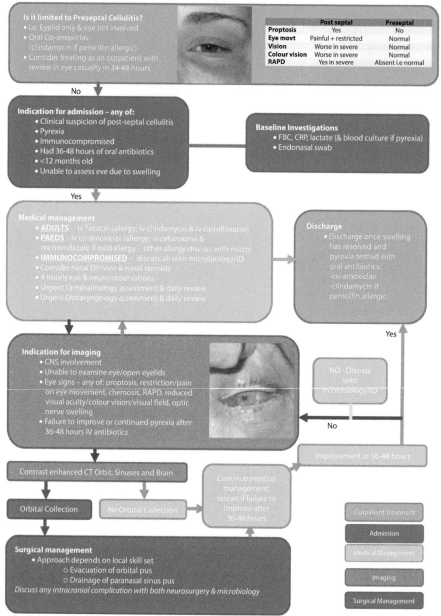

Orbital cellulitis management guideline – For Adults & Paediatrics

Is it limited to Preseptal Cellulitis?
- i.e. Eyelid only & eye not involved
- Oral Co-amoxiclav (clindamycin if penicillin allergic)
- Consider treating as an outpatient with review in eye casualty in 24-48 hours

	Post septal	Preseptal
Proptosis	Yes	No
Eye movt	Painful + restricted	Normal
Vision	Worse in severe	Normal
Colour vision	Worse in severe	Normal
RAPD	Yes in severe	Absent i.e normal

No

Indication for admission – any of:
- Clinical suspicion of post-septal cellulitis
- Pyrexia
- Immunocompromised
- Had 36-48 hours of oral antibiotics
- <12 months old
- Unable to assess eye due to swelling

Baseline Investigations
- FBC, CRP, lactate (& blood culture if pyrexia)
- Endonasal swab

Yes

Medical management
- **ADULTS** – Iv Tazocin (allergy; Iv clindamycin & iv ciprofloxacin)
- **PAEDS** – iv co-amoxiclav (allergy; iv cefuroxime & metronidazole if mild allergy – other allergy discuss with micro)
- **IMMUNOCOMPROMISED** – discuss all with microbiology/ID
- Consider nasal Otrivine & nasal steroids
- 4 hourly eye & neuro-observations
- Urgent Ophthalmology assessment & daily review
- Urgent Otolaryngology assessment & daily review

Discharge
- Discharge once swelling has resolved and pyrexia settled with oral antibiotics:
  - co-amoxiclav
  - clindamycin if penicillin allergic

Yes

Indication for imaging
- CNS involvement
- Unable to examine eye/open eyelids
- Eye signs – any of: proptosis, restriction/pain on eye movement, chemosis, RAPD, reduced visual acuity/colour vision/visual field, optic nerve swelling
- Failure to improve or continued pyrexia after 36-48 hours IV antibiotics

NO - Discuss with microbiology/ID

No

Improvement in 36-48 hours

Contrast enhanced CT Orbit, Sinuses and Brain

Continue medical management, rescan if failure to improve after 36-48 hours

Orbital Collection | No Orbital Collection

Outpatient Treatment

Admission

Surgical management
- Approach depends on local skill set
  - Evacuation of orbital pus
  - Drainage of paranasal sinus pus
Discuss any intracranial complication with both neurosurgery & microbiology

Medical Management

Imaging

Surgical Management

Figure 37.1 Management algorithm for orbital complications. FBC = full blood cell count, CRP = c-reactive protein, CNS=central nervous system, RAPD=relative afferent pupillary defect (From Okonkwo ACO, Powell S, Carrie S, Ball SL. A review of periorbital cellulitis guidelines in Fifty-One Acute Admitting Units in the United Kingdom. *Clin Otolaryngol.* 2018;43(2):718–721.)

There have been a few studies showing good outcomes with IV antibiotics in children with subperiosteal abscesses. In such cases, and provided there is clear clinical improvement within 24–48 hours, no decrease in visual acuity, small size (<0.5–1 mL in volume), medially located and no significant systemic involvement, the decision might be to withhold surgical drainage and closely monitor the patient.

Table 37.2   Chandler classification

Stage 1	Stage 2	Stage 3	Stage 4	Stage 5
Preseptal cellulitis	Postseptal cellulitis or orbital cellulitis without abscess	Subperiosteal abscess	Orbital abscess	Cavernous sinus thrombosis/ abscess
Inflammation does not extend beyond the orbital septum*	Inflammation extends into the tissues of the orbit beyond orbital septum*	Abscess formation deep to the periosteum of the orbital bones, typically at the lamina papyracea from ethmoid sinusitis	Abscess formation within the orbit, which has breached the periosteum	Cavernous sinus thrombosis after posterior extension of the infection through the superior ophthalmic veins

* Medial orbital periosteal reflection that is attached to the medial eyelid at the tarsal plate.

An endoscopic approach involves an ethmoidectomy followed by opening the lamina papyracea and draining the abscess. External approaches to lateral and medial orbital abscesses can also be used if necessary.

Cavernous Sinus Thrombosis

Prolonged broad-spectrum antibiotics must be given for at least two weeks beyond clinical resolution as bacteria sequestered within the thrombus may not be eradicated until the dural sinuses recanalise. Surgery is indicated for non-draining sinus infection or abscess. There remains no consensus for anti-coagulation; proponents suggest anti-coagulants prevent thrombus propagation and are anti-inflammatory. Those against hypothesise thrombus formation walls off infection and prevents spread, with anticoagulants increasing the risk of intra-cranial bleeding.

Prognosis of Orbital Complications

If prompt treatment is carried out with adequate monitoring, the prognosis for normal vision is excellent. However, there is a small risk of diplopia following surgery.

Intracranial Complications

Brain Abscess

Estimates suggest 40–60% of brain abscesses arise from rhinosinusitis. Reported incidence of intra-cranial complications from acute rhinosinusitis is between 3 and 17% of hospitalised sinusitis patients.

Subdural Empyema

Subdural empyema is one of the most common intracranial complications. The brain is more exposed as the infection is beyond the dura mater and allows thrombosis of the local venous network. Serious neurological injury can occur if not treated rapidly and aggressively with combined medical treatment and neurosurgical drainage to decompress the brain and evacuate empyema. Subdural empyemas present with meningeal irritation and neurological signs such as seizures or focal deficits.

Extradural Empyema

Extradural empyemas tend to be less symptomatic as the brain is protected by the dura mater. The signs are less marked and specific and are often only present when the collection reaches a size to cause mass effect.

Brain Infarction

Cerebral ischaemia and infarction are rare vascular complications of sinusitis from either dural venous thrombosis secondary to adjacent empyema, or cavernous carotid artery occlusion.

Clinical Presentation

Early symptoms are often non-specific such as headache, fever, seizure, drowsiness, diplopia (cranial nerve VI palsy), eye pain and nausea. There may not be symptoms and signs of acute rhinosinusitis. Adolescent males are most affected, which may be due to the vascularity of the diploic system. There may be specific neurological symptoms with a well-defined intracranial abscess including acute pain or possible loss of consciousness associated with meningitis.

Investigations

MRI is more sensitive than CT for intracranial complications. CT is desirable to demonstrate bony anatomy of the paranasal sinuses. Intracranial complications may be relatively silent and a high index of suspicion should be maintained. Intracranial complications may also develop after the initial presentation and any change in neurological status should merit consideration for repeat imaging.

Treatment

As soon as an intracranial complication is detected, joint management of the case with neurological or neurosurgical colleagues is mandatory. If possible, surgery to drain affected paranasal sinuses should be undertaken synchronously with neurosurgery. The rationale is to evacuate the intracranial collection and manage the source of infection using a rhinological approach, which will provide microbiological samples.

Prognosis from Intracranial Complications

Published mortality rates vary between 0 and 25% according to the complication, increases with age and decreased level of consciousness on presentation. Early recognition of complications and multidisciplinary treatment is essential.

Bony Complications

Pott's Puffy Tumour (PPT)

PPT is subperiosteal cellulitis or abscess of the frontal bone associated with frontal osteomyelitis. The reported rate of coexistent intracranial complications is high, but not all are present on initial imaging, suggesting prompt imaging and treatment are paramount.

There is a growing body of evidence that uncomplicated PPT can be managed successfully via an endoscopic approach/minimal external drainage, combined with long-term antibiotics. Once the acute phase has subsided the patient should be re-evaluated to determine whether a frontal sinus drainage procedure is required for long-term management.

Associated intracranial complications necessitate prompt neurosurgical intervention. This is typically performed through a bifrontal craniotomy enabling drainage of intracranial pus and removal of necrotic bone. Complete removal of the posterior table will require frontal sinus cranialisation. Extensive osteomyelitis of the anterior table may necessitate a Riedel's procedure with removal of the anterior wall and floor of the frontal sinus allowing the forehead skin to collapse onto the posterior table. The cosmetic deformity can be reconstructed when all infection has resolved.

Chronic Complications

Chronic complications usually result from chronic rhinosinusitis. The nature of the complication depends on the sinus or group of sinuses involved. Mucoceles are chronic, slowly expanding lesions in any of the sinuses that may result in bony erosion and can extend beyond the sinus. It is unusual for chronic rhinosinusitis to cause orbital cellulitis or intracranial complications unless there is an infective exacerbation.

38. NASAL AIRWAY SURGERY: MANAGEMENT OF SEPTAL DEFORMITIES

Nasal Septum

The nasal septum is divided into bony, cartilaginous and membranous parts. The bony septum is mainly formed by the perpendicular plate of ethmoid and vomer. The palatine bones and maxillary crest form the most posterior parts of the bony septum. The cartilaginous septum (i.e. quadrilateral cartilage) is not an isolated cartilage and is in unison with the upper lateral cartilages (ULCs). An L-shaped strut of septum (forming the dorsal and caudal segments) measuring approximately 1 cm in width is required to support the external nasal skeleton (Figure 38.1).

Septal examination should include inspection as well as palpation. During inspection, the position of deviation should be mapped in relation to the L-strut. Nasendoscopy will allow inspection of the anatomy in the neutral position; it also shows more posterior elements in the nasal cavity (e.g. adenoidal tissue).

Nasal airflow can be demonstrated by misting of the examination mirror or metal tongue spatula. Absence or reduction of the misting indicates a structural blockage but a satisfactory amount of misting does not indicate a patent nasal airway as perceived by the patient during inspiration.

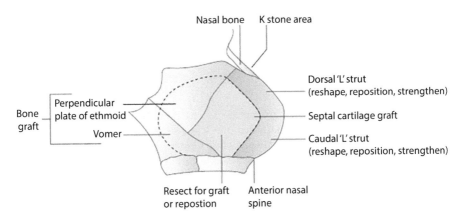

Figure 38.1 Septal cartilaginous L-strut with a minimum 10-mm width is preserved for structural support. The body of the bony and cartilaginous septum can be used as grafts.

Table 38.1 Special considerations in septoplasty approaches

Endoscopic septoplasty	• Used for limited septal excision • Good visualisation • Requires minimal access • Can be performed at the same time of sinus surgery to improve access
External (open) septoplasty	• Mostly used when the dorsal L-strut deformity requires correction • It can improve surgical access • It is favourable in complex septal reconstructive cases such as extracorporeal septoplasty

Septal Surgery

Submucosal Resection (SMR)

This technique addresses deviation at the body of the septum (not the L-strut). A Killian incision is placed about 1 cm from the caudal septal edge and the flap is raised. The deviated part of the septum is excised after being freed from its peripheral attachments. The harvested bony or cartilaginous septum can then be used as a graft or it can be straightened and reinserted in its place.

Septoplasty

A number of studies have shown septoplasty to have a good effect on nasal blockage and to be cost-effective compared with non-surgical management. In most cases of septal deviation, the septal L-strut is involved and the approach should allow adequate exposure. The surgical approach is often through an endonasal route; however, other approaches are available (Table 38.1):

1 Hemitransfixion incision is placed at the caudal edge of the septum.
2 Mucosal flap is raised on the concave side.
3 In certain deformities (e.g. S-shaped deformity), both mucosal flaps are raised.
4 When the osseocartilaginous junction is reached, depending on type of deformity, this junction can be disarticulated, and a segment of bone or cartilage removed.
5 Disarticulation of the septal cartilage from the maxillary crest allows the septum to move to midline (the 1 cm of bony-cartilaginous junction at the L-strut is left undisturbed if possible).

The deviated septum can be addressed by a variety of techniques. Here, the most commonly employed techniques are described:

- **Scoring** of the septal cartilage on the concave side allows the septum to become straight. This technique is not reliable as under-scoring or over-scoring can occur; splinting the septum against a batten graft adds security. (Figure 38.2)
- **Septal batten grafts** (harvested from the septal cartilage or bone) can be used to keep the deviated septum in a straight line. Spreader grafts can be used as batten grafts to straighten the deviation of the dorsal L-strut.

Paediatric Septoplasty

Controversy remains regarding the optimal age and extent of septal surgery in the paediatric population. Studies have demonstrated that septal surgery performed in children as young as 6 years old provides long-term satisfactory outcomes. Delaying surgery in children with bilateral nasal blockage and septal deformities may adversely affect nasofacial growth. Conservative cartilage resection with preservation is essential to avoid disruption of important endochondral ossification plates.

Nasal Valve

Nasal valve is the area caudal to the nasal bones and it contains the narrowest section of the nasal airway (i.e. internal nasal valve) as well as a mobile collapsible lateral nasal sidewall

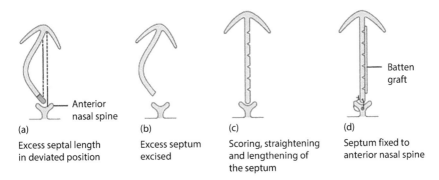

(a) Excess septal length in deviated position

(b) Excess septum excised

(c) Scoring, straightening and lengthening of the septum

(d) Septum fixed to anterior nasal spine

Anterior nasal spine

Batten graft

Figure 38.2 'Swinging door technique' is a reliable method in dealing with caudal septal deviations. (a) Septal convexity to the right has resulted in excess caudal septal length. (b) The excess length of the septum is excised. (c) The height of septum is restored after scoring of the concave side. (d) The weakened septum is splinted against a batten graft and secured to the midline.

The nasal valve has traditionally been divided into two three-dimensional (3D) areas: (1) internal valve and (2) external valve. This division is arbitrary as there is no clear line between them. Nasal valve angle refers to the angle between the ULC caudal edge and the septum, and it is measured at 10–15° in Caucasian noses.

Obstruction at the nasal valve can occur due to either **static narrowing** (the airway is constantly restricted due to deformed anatomy) or **dynamic collapse** (the nasal airway gets blocked on inspiration due to collapse of the nasal sidewall).

A thorough nasal examination is essential in diagnosing the cause of nasal blockage. The misting test is not a reliable way to assess nasal blockage secondary to nasal valve collapse as it relies on nasal expiratory flow, whereas dynamic collapse occurs on inspiration. A nasal speculum can be used to examine the anterior nasal cavity; however, the nasal airway and the valve area should be examined by an endoscope in its neutral position. Cottle's manoeuvre (i.e. gently pulling the cheek laterally) has little specificity. However, a modified version of Cottle's manoeuvre where the ULC is gently lifted by a probe is a more reliable way to detect the structural cause of nasal valve collapse.

Nasal Valve Surgery

The two commonly employed grafting techniques are described here.

- **Spreader grafts** are used to reconstruct the dorsal 'T' junction between the ULC and septum. (Figure 38.3) Their use is both for functional and aesthetic purposes (some argue the magnitude of their functional advantage).
- **Strut/batten grafts** are usually taken from the septal or conchal cartilage and attached to the lateral crus of the lower lateral cartilage (LLC) to strengthen the collapsing lateral nasal sidewall.

Dressing and Splints

Postoperative nasal packing remains a varied practice. Some surgeons use septal splints to prevent adhesions or to provide extra support for the septum. Most surgeons apply an external splint after external (open) septoplasty.

Complications

The rate of complications varies in different studies and it depends on the operator and whether turbinate surgery is performed at the same time of septoplasty. These complications include the following:

- Bleeding (5–10%)
- Infection (2–3%)
- Septal perforation (1–7%)

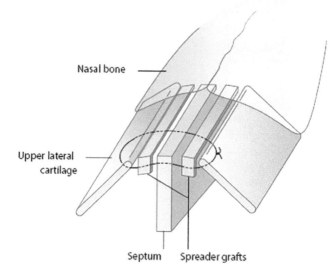

Nasal bone

Upper lateral cartilage

Septum   Spreader grafts

Figure 38.3 Spreader grafts are placed between the upper lateral cartilages and the septum to reconstruct the dorsal septal 'T' segment.

- Adhesion (1–7%)
- Adverse nasal shape, e.g. saddle deformity, nasal tip depression (4–8%)
- Septal haematoma and septal abscess (1–2%)
- Hyposmia (1–2%)
- Upper middle incisors anaesthesia and discolouration (0.1%)

KEY POINTS

- Nasal obstruction can be caused by septal deflection, which can be developmental or secondary to trauma.
- The misting test assesses the nasal airway in expiration; it does not test the dynamic elements of nasal obstruction which occur in inspiration.
- The nasal airway should be examined before and after topical decongestion to assess the effect of mucosal swelling.
- The patient's nasal airway should be examined in the neutral position using an endoscope.
- Nasal airway surgery requires attention to the nasal septum as well as nasal valve areas.
- Nasal valve dilator devices and nasal steroid medications play a part in the non-surgical management of nasal valve obstruction.
- In septoplasty, the attention is more on reconstruction rather than excision.
- When septal deviation involves the L-strut, SMR is not effective as it cannot address the caudal and dorsal struts; septoplasty techniques are needed in these circumstances.
- In certain situations, especially where the dorsal L-strut deformity is concerned, external approach septoplasty can improve surgical access (with the septum in situ or through extracorporeal techniques in severely distorted cases).
- Most nasal valve procedures will have an aesthetic effect and the patient should be warned of these prior to the operation.
- There remains controversy about the optimal age and extent of septal surgery in the paediatric population.

The most important aspect of paediatric septal surgery is to resect the cartilage conservatively and to avoid disrupting the endochondral ossification plates.

39. NASAL AIRWAY SURGERY: MANAGEMENT OF ENLARGED TURBINATES

Introduction
The inferior turbinates are dynamic structures that form a crucial part of the normal functional nose but being relatively easy to access, they have been subject to numerous operative techniques in attempts to alleviate nasal obstruction. Inferior turbinate surgery is a frequently performed ear, nose and throat (ENT) procedure for nasal obstruction. The evidence base for surgery is weak and there is currently no ideal surgical procedure.

Pathogenesis of Inferior Turbinate Enlargement
Rhinitis and rhinosinusitis will accentuate the effect of the nasal cycle and nasal reflexes, inducing a sensation of nasal obstruction. Severe allergic rhinitis causes marked large, pale oedematous inferior turbinates.

Frequent self-medication with xylometazoline may induce rhinitis medicamentosa with increased nasal congestion that persists after vasoconstriction.

Compensatory hypertrophy of the inferior turbinate is associated with deviation of the nasal septum to the opposite side.

Hyperplasia generally affects the whole structure, but enlargement can sometimes be localised to the anterior head or posterior section of the turbinate.

Clinical Assessment
Patients with enlarged inferior turbinates require a full rhinological history and nasal endoscopy to determine the cause:

1 Nasal examination (before and after mucosal vasoconstriction to differentiate between hyperplastic or just congested turbinate)
2 Assessment of impact on quality of life (QoL) using validated the questionnaire Nasal Obstruction Symptom Evaluation (NOSE) prior instigating any treatment
3 If available, objective assessment of nasal obstruction including acoustic rhinometry, anterior rhinomanometry, rhinospirometry and the peak nasal inspiratory

Management of the Enlarged Inferior Turbinate
The primary treatment of enlarged inferior turbinates is medication. This will generally include topical nasal steroids for a minimum period of 3 months. Surgery should be considered if symptoms persist.

Informed consent should include a discussion of possible outcomes and warn patients that symptom relief may be short-lived, but reduction surgery can be repeated.

There is much diversity in opinion and practice of inferior turbinate surgery and the terminology of surgery lacks standardisation: turbinectomy refers to any degree of resection but turbinoplasty strictly means changing the shape of the turbinate. It can also refer to a specific procedure that includes resection of the conchal bone. A simple system of classifying turbinate operations is shown in Table 39.1.

Turbinate Surgery in Various Clinical Situations
Rhinosinusitis and Endoscopic Sinus Surgery
Mucosal congestion from chronic rhinosinusitis (CRS) may induce enlargement of the inferior turbinates. Mucosal inflammation within the sinuses should improve significantly after endoscopic sinus surgery and continued medication, which should reduce congestion of the turbinates. Should inferior turbinate surgery still be deemed necessary, the authors would suggest submucosal turbinoplasty.

Table 39.1   Simple system of classifying inferior turbinate operations

Category of surgery	Technique	
Mucosal preservation	Submucosal diathermy	The diathermy needle is advanced submucosally from the anterior end to the posterior section of the inferior turbinate (IT). It is then slowly withdrawn over several seconds. Two to three different passes are often performed.
	Mini-microdebrider surgery	The tiny blade is inserted submucosally and passed to the posterior section of the IT. The blade is used in oscillation mode to reduce the submucosal erectile tissue and steadily withdrawn. A couple of passes may be needed.
	Radiofrequency	The radiofrequency needle is advanced submucosally from the anterior end to the posterior section of the IT. It is then slowly withdrawn over several seconds. Two to three different passes are often performed.
	Coblation	The Coblation wand is inserted submucosally and advanced posteriorly. It is activated in bursts of about 12 seconds in three to four sites along the IT.
	Turbinoplasty	The mucosa is lifted off the IT laterally and the conchal bone removed. The mucosa is laid down against the reduced IT.
	Lateralization by outfracture	A suitable elevator is used initially to infracture and then gently outfracture the IT.
Mucosal destructive reduction	Superficial electrocautery	The diathermy needle is applied to the surface of the IT.
	Chemocautery with chromic acid or trichloroacetic acid	Application of chemicals is now rarely performed.
	Cryosurgery	The cryoprobe is activated along sections of the IT, forming an ice ball at each site.
	Laser surgery	Superficial lesions are induced by the laser, either directly with a flexible KTP laser or indirectly by mirror for CO_2.
	Direct microdebrider mucosal reduction	The standard microdebrider blade is used to remove redundant mucosa from the IT.
Turbinate excision procedures*	Partial	The anterior third of the IT is divided by scissors and removed. The tissue if often crushed initially to limit bleeding.
	Subtotal*	Angled scissors are used to excise a length of the IT. It is advisable to leave some tissue posteriorly.
	Posterior end	

* Complete or subtotal of the inferior turbinate is not recommended and risks causing prolonged nasal crusting or inducing an empty nose syndrome.

Septoplasty and Septorhinoplasty

Compensatory enlargement of the inferior turbinate is often observed on the opposite side to a septal deflection. Histological studies of the inferior turbinate have shown that the enlargement of the turbinate on the contralateral side to the septal deviation may be due to an increase in the conchal bone as well as increased mucosal thickness. Recent findings favour turbinoplasty in patients with clinically confirmed unilateral inferior turbinate hypertrophy.

Some surgeons will routinely excise the inferior turbinates at the time of doing septorhinoplasty to maximise the chance of improving nasal obstruction. However, this will increase the potential for post-operative epistaxis and nasal adhesions, but it is unlikely to result in any significant long-term advantage.

Sleep Disordered Breathing

There is a cogent argument to maximise the nasal airway in patients with sleep disordered breathing, particularly when there may be a problem of compliance with continuous positive airway pressure (CPAP) due to nasal obstruction. This is an instance where there may be a tendency for surgeons to be radical in their approach to the inferior turbinate and to excise the turbinates whilst correcting septal deformity. However, there is a lack of evidence to support radical excision in this situation and a conservative approach is recommended.

Inferior Turbinate Surgery in Children

Most children with nasal obstruction have rhinitis or adenoid enlargement. Rhinitis is mostly allergic and generally improves following treatment with anti-allergic medication, allergen avoidance and in some cases, immunotherapy. Turbinate reduction surgery would be indicated where there is significant nasal obstruction and large inferior turbinates. Children with sleep disordered breathing or obstructive sleep apnoea may also benefit from inferior turbinate surgery

Complications

The most common complications include

1 Severe haemorrhage (particularly after turbinate resection)
2 Prolonged nasal crust formation
3 Adhesions or synechiae between the turbinate and the septum

The incidence of individual complications in clinical practice is typically not analysed or published, so actual figures are generally unavailable.

Visual change and temporary blindness after monopolar diathermy is reported but extremely rare. Hypothesised mechanisms are excessive use of monopolar diathermy to reduce the posterior end of the turbinate and/or epinephrine injected under pressure into the mucosa causing a retrograde flow through the anterior ethmoidal artery into the ophthalmic artery, vasospasm, hypoperfusion and optic nerve neuropathy.

Total or excessive resection of the inferior turbinate carries a risk of inducing 'empty nose syndrome', which induces a sense of nasal obstruction.

Outcomes

There is overwhelming data supporting the efficacy of turbinate surgery but few studies have reported on both subjective and objective results, or compared different surgical techniques. Recent studies (e.g. The Nasal AIRway Obstruction Study [NAIROS]) have focused on the efficacy of septoplasty with or without turbinate reduction surgery for nasal airflow obstruction. There is a deficit of published randomized controlled trial (RCT) research or controlled studies in the literature, and the evidence base for the efficacy of turbinate surgery as a standalone procedure for nasal airflow obstruction remains low.

KEY POINTS

1. Carefully consider the need for turbinate surgery (especially in children), and defer surgery until following suitable medication has been trialed.
2. Look for underlying causes of enlarged inferior turbinates such as nasal allergy or CRS.
3. Use minimal intervention if possible and ideally preserve mucosa.
4. Warn patients about bleeding, recurrent obstruction and the possibility of revision surgery.
5. Avoid excessive bilateral resection that may lead to persistent crusting and/or a sense of nasal obstruction (the empty nose syndrome).

40. EPISTAXIS

Background
Epistaxis is one of otolaryngology's most common and most difficult to treat emergencies.

Key Anatomical Areas

- Ninety percent of epistaxis occurs from Little's area (anastomoses of vessels at the anterior nasal septum).
- Two-thirds of adult bleeds originate from the septum and remaining one-third from the lateral wall.
- Posterior bleeding is predominantly from nasal septum.
- Anterior ethmoidal artery runs between ethmoid fovea and lamina papyracea where iatrogenic damage/trauma can result in retraction of the bleeding end into the orbit with subsequent pressure haematoma and risk of visual loss. Open approach is often indicated (Figures 40.1 and 40.2).
- U-shaped notch in the palatine bone, the sphenopalatine foramen, is the entry portal for major arterial supply located lateral to pterygopalatine space and is key to endonasal endoscopic sphenopalatine artery ligation (ESPAL)

Classification of Epistaxis

Clinical Classification

- Adult or childhood epistaxis: bimodal distribution in the age of onset of epistaxis
  - Childhood (>16 years) or adult (<16 years)
- Primary or secondary
  - Primary: 80% of all cases of epistaxis are idiopathic
  - Secondary: caused by clear and definite causes such as trauma, surgery or anticoagulant overdose

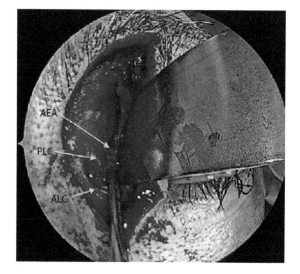

Figure 40.1   Open approach to ligate left anterior ethmoidal artery (AEA). ALC, anterior lacrimal crest; PLC, posterior lacrimal crest.

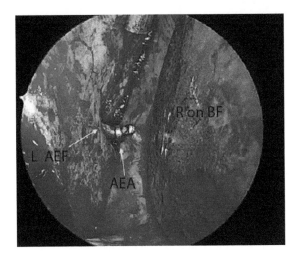

Figure 40.2 Operative field in ligation of anterior ethmoidal artery (AEA; left). AEA, anterior ethmoidal artery with titanium clips applied; L AEF, lamina papyracea and anterior ethmoidal foramen; R on BF, retractor on bulbar fascia.

The distinction between primary and secondary epistaxis is important as the management of each type is different, e.g. bipolar cautery is unlikely to be successful in warfarin overdose.

Classification Based on Site of Bleeding

This classification includes terms anterior and posterior epistaxis, which are imprecise, inconsistent and less useful.

- *Anterior epistaxis*: easy to identify bleeding source located anterior to the plane of the piriform aperture (anterior septum, rarely the vestibular skin and mucocutaneous junction)
- *Posterior epistaxis*: challenging epistaxis situated posterior to the piriform aperture

Adult Primary Epistaxis

Demography

- Occurs at any age but is mainly a disease of the elderly.
- Seven to 14% of adults have epistaxis at some time, but only 6% of cases are seen by otorhinolaryngologists.
- Peak presentation is the sixth decade, and there is a slight male predominance.

Most cases are minor, self-limiting or easily managed anterior bleeds. However, a significant number require admission to the hospital. After head and neck cancer, epistaxis stands out as a prominent cause of mortality in ear, nose and throat (ENT) patients

Aetiological Factors

- Greatest frequency of admissions in the autumn and winter months (environmental temperature and humidity)
- A circadian rhythm: hospital admissions are peaking in the morning and late evening
- Non-steroidal anti-inflammatory drug (NSAID) use (mechanism via an anti-platelet aggregation effect)
- Alcohol consumption (especially within 24 hours of admission): prolonged bleeding time despite normal platelet counts and coagulation factor activity

Population studies have failed to show a causal relationship between hypertension and epistaxis. Elevated blood pressure is observed in almost all epistaxis admissions, but this may be a result of anxiety associated with hospital admission and the invasive techniques used to control the bleeding.

Secondary Epistaxis

The following causes of secondary epistaxis deserve special mention:

- *Trauma*: Its origin and severity are almost infinitely variable. Severe haemorrhage refractory to packing should be managed by open ligation. (Figures 40.1 and 40.2).
- *Post-surgical*: Minor epistaxis requiring observation is common, severe haemorrhage occurs in between 3 and 9% of turbinate surgery where re-exploration and ESPAL is often required.
- Nasal tumours present with recurrent blood-stained discharge, which should be distinguished from epistaxis per se (rare).
- Hereditary haemorrhagic telangiectasia:
  - Autosomal dominant condition affecting blood vessels in skin, mucous membranes and viscera.
  - Recurrent epistaxis occurs in 93% of cases.
  - Management involves packing, cautery, anti-fibrinolytics, systemic or topical oestrogens, coagulative lasers, septal dermoplasty, ligation and embolization and as a last resort permanent surgical closure of the nostrils (Young's operation).
- *Drug related*:
  - Warfarin-related bleeding constitutes 9–17% of epistaxis admissions.
  - Packing may be required as bleeding is often from multiple sites.
  - If international normalized ratio (INR) is within the therapeutic range and bleeding is controlled, it may be safe to continue the warfarin, otherwise consult haematology.
  - New oral anti-coagulants (target-specific oral anti-coagulants [TSOACs] rivaroxiban, dabigatran): Reversal is difficult and can be incomplete, hence liaison with haematology team is required.
  - Aspirin should not be discontinued if there is a history of cardiovascular disease or vascular graft surgery; otherwise temporary cessation of aspirin may be required to allow the recurrent bleeding to settle.
  - Patients using topical nasal medications frequently report minor recurrent bleeds which are mainly caused by damage to septal mucosa induced by the nozzle.

Management

Effective management follows an incremental sequence of interventions (Figure 40.3). Ideal treatment identifies the bleeding point and directly controls the bleeding, at source. First, the patient is resuscitated, bleeding slowed, the nasal cavity examined and a treatment plan established.

Resuscitation

- Sixty-five percent of cases had already some form of therapy by an accident and emergency team.
- First aid is performed by pinching ala nasi in anterior bleed.
- Intravenous access and baseline blood estimations are taken.
- Detailed history should be taken with a focus on predisposing factors.
- Routine coagulation studies in the absence of a positive history are not indicated.

Assessment

- Performed in semi-recumbent position and nursing assistance is mandatory.
- Protective visors and clothing should be worn.

Management strategy

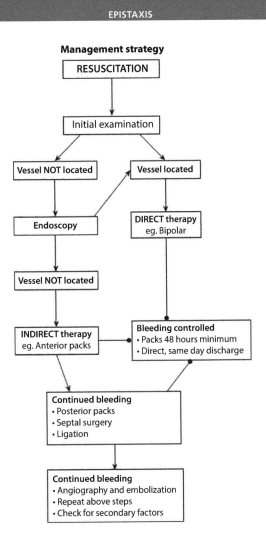

Figure 40.3 Management algorithm for epistaxis.

- Basic equipment includes couch or reclining chair, headlight, suction, vasoconstrictor solutions (lignocaine and pseudoephedrine) and a selection of packs, tampons and cautery apparatus.
- Nasal endoscopy equipment and bipolar electrodiathermy is recommended.

Direct or Indirect Therapies

- Indirect treatments do not require identification of the bleeding point.
- Direct treatments are superior, and a committed search for the bleeding vessel should always be undertaken.

Direct Management

There has been a slow but steady uptake of direct strategies throughout the United Kingdom. Despite this, a minority of cases there are managed by direct control of the bleeding point. Reluctance to use direct approaches reflects the fact that over 70% of cases are managed by the most junior members of the specialty. Anterior epistaxis is usually very straightforward to treat and over 90% can be controlled with silver nitrate cautery or bipolar. The use of packing for primary anterior epistaxis should be strongly discouraged.

Endoscopic Control

Failure to locate the bleeding point is an indication for rod lens endoscopy and targeted haemostasis using modern single fibre bipolar electrodes. Endoscopy identifies the source of posterior epistaxis in over 80% of cases. Success rates for immediate control by endoscopic guidance are consistently reported in the 90% range.

Indirect Therapies

Lack of specialist skills is an indication for use of one of many of the following traditional indirect strategies:

- *Anterior nasal packing*:
  - Ribbon gauze impregnated with petroleum jelly or bismuth iodoform paraffin paste (**BIPP**), tampons, resorbable packing and inflatable balloon packs are used.
  - Removal after 24–72 hours; antibiotic cover is required.
  - Persistent bleeding with packs in situ is observed in up to 40% of cases requiring further examination of the nasal cavity.
  - Complications of packing include sinusitis, septal perforation, alar necrosis, hypoxia and myocardial infarction.
- *Posterior nasal packing*:
  - Largely obsolete as packing causes considerable pain, but it is indicated in extreme cases or where no specialist rhinologist is available.
  - Posterior tamponade is achieved by endonasal insertion of Foley urethral catheter, which is inflated with water once it reached nasopharynx.
  - Removal after 24–72 hours or at least until rhinologist can attend; antibiotic cover is required.
  - Complications include hypoxia secondary to soft palate oedema, sinusitis, middle ear effusions and necrosis of the septum and columella.

Medical Therapy

- *Systemic medical therapy*:
  - Tranexamic acid reduces the severity and risk of re-bleeding (oral, 1.5g, 3x/day).
  - Topical thrombin compounds (e.g. Floseal) are an additional tool for the management of difficult bleeds (especially secondary).

Surgical Management

If the techniques described above fail, surgical intervention is required. Endoscopic diathermy of the bleeding point under anaesthesia may control the bleeding, but if the vessel still cannot be controlled (or even located) indirect surgical therapy is indicated. Surgical management for continued epistaxis consists of the following:

- *Ligation techniques*:
  - Sphenopalatine artery
  - External carotid artery
  - Internal maxillary artery
  - Anterior/posterior ethmoidal artery
- Embolization techniques

Endonasal Endoscopic Sphenopalatine Artery Ligation (ESPAL)

- ESPAL has now largely replaced all other ligation procedures.
- Under general anesthesia, incision is made 8 mm anterior to and below the posterior end of the middle turbinate.
- Once the artery is identified (posterior to the crista ethmoidalis), it is ligated using haemostatic clips and divided/coagulated using bipolar diathermy.

Table 40.1   Classification of epistaxis

Primary: no proven causal factor	
Secondary: proven causal factor	
Childhood: <16 years	
Adult: >16 years	
Anterior: bleeding anterior to piriform aperture	
Posterior: bleeding point posterior to piriform aperture	

- Success rate is almost 100%.
- Complications include re-bleeding (anastomoses), infection and nasal adhesions (less common than with other procedures).

Anterior/Posterior Ethmoidal Artery Ligation (EAL)

Given the minimal contribution of these arteries to the nasal blood supply, this is best reserved as an adjuvant to one of the procedures described above or in cases of confirmed ethmoidal bleeding (e.g. ethmoidal fracture, iatrogenic tear). The arteries are approached by a medial canthal incision (Figures 40.1 and 40.2).

Embolisation

- Success rate to control severe epistaxis is 82–97%.
- Particles (polyvinyl alcohol, tungsten or steel microcoils) are used.
- Complication frequency depends on local expertise and includes skin necrosis, paraesthesia, cerebrovascular accident, blindness and groin haematomas.

KEY POINTS

- Direct bleeding point–specific approaches are superior to indirect nasal packing strategies.
- Epistaxis secondary to drugs or coagulopathy requires management of the underlying cause.
- Endoscopic ligation of the sphenopalatine artery is the ligation of choice.
- The endoscope has revolutionized the treatment of epistaxis.

41. NASAL FRACTURES

Introduction

The treatment of nasal fractures was first recorded 5000 years ago. An isolated nasal pyramid fracture accounts for about 40% of all facial fractures. It is essential to exclude concurrent facial fracture and neurological injury in patients presenting with nasal trauma. Delays in management can result in significant cosmetic and functional deformity that may result in medicolegal action.

Young men are twice as likely to sustain a fractured nose as women. Fractures in younger children tend to be greenstick in nature. Compound and comminuted fractures are more common in the elderly who are prone to falls.

Relatively little force is required to fracture the nasal bones. Most fractures result from laterally applied forces (>66%). Greater force is required to fracture the nose with a blow directed from the front as the nasal cartilages behave like shock absorbers.

Clinical Presentation

History

Key issues include the following:

- How and when the injury was sustained
- Nasal obstruction (with persisting pain may indicate a septal haematoma)
- Change in appearance (based on the patient's own assessment)
- Anosmia, hyposmia, watery rhinorrhoea → skull base injury
- Visual disturbance, diplopia, ecchymosis, epiphora → orbital trauma
- Altered bite, loose teeth, trismus, cheek paraesthesia → damage to temporomandibular joint (TMJ), mandible or zygomaticomaxillary complex

Examination

Key issues to consider when examining a patient include

- Deviation, depression, step deformities
- Mobility, crepitus, specific areas of point tenderness
- Generalised swelling and focal bruising
- Skin and mucosal lacerations
- Septal fracture/haematoma/abscess

Investigations

Plain facial X-rays are not required to make the diagnosis or aid subsequent reduction. If there is clinical evidence of a more extensive facial injury, computed tomography (CT) scan of the facial bones and brain should be acquired. Samples of any watery rhinorrhoea must be collected and tested for beta-2 transferring.

Treatment

Timing of Initial Assessment

- Ideal window for assessment is either within the first 3 hours, or 4–7 days post-injury (due to significant swelling between these times).
- In cases of septal haematoma, surgical drainage is required. Associated facial fractures or neurological injury (uncommon) may also indicate surgical intervention.
- Delayed intervention beyond 2–3 weeks post-injury makes effective reduction less likely, and sometimes impossible without making osteotomies.
- In children, healing can take place even more quickly and earlier intervention is indicated.

Some patients will have a pre-existing nasal deformity. These patients should be advised that, at best, their nose will only return it to its most recent appearance.

Timing of Reduction

- <3 hours after injury in adults and children has the potential for optimal results (if minimal oedema is present).

OR

- 7–10 days after injury in adults (after oedema has resolved and before the setting of fracture fragments)
- 3–7 days after injury in children (after oedema has resolved and before the setting of fracture fragments)

Anaesthesia

- It can be performed under local or general anaesthesia.
- *Local anaesthesia*:
  - Suitable for simple fractures of nasal bones/naso-septal complex.
  - External infiltration along the nasomaxillary groove, infraorbital nerve in its foramen and around the infra-trochlear nerve.

- Intra-nasal local anaesthesia is also acceptable, using combinations of cocaine, lignocaine, adrenaline and phenylephrine (caution in hypertension or cardiovascular disease).

There are easily identifiable groups of patients who are not suitable for reduction under local anaesthesia. Children and patients with low pain tolerance or significant anxiety are better admitted for general anaesthesia. Extensive fracture-dislocation of nasal bones and septum and open fractures are not suitable for local anaesthesia.

Technique

Closed and open technique can be utilised in reduction of nasal fractures. This nasal trauma classification can be used to determine the optimal technique:

- *Injury restricted to soft tissue (type I)*: no fracture
- *Simple, unilateral nondisplaced fracture (type IIa)*: no reduction
- *Simple, bilateral nondisplaced fracture (type IIb)*: no reduction
- *Simple, displaced fracture (type III)*: closed reduction
- *Closed comminuted fracture (type IV)*: open reduction
- *Open comminuted fracture or complicated fracture (type V)*: open reduction with use of septorhinoplasty reconstruction techniques

Closed nasal reduction involves first increasing and then decreasing the degree of deformity, i.e. an initial slight increase in deformity away from the side of the blow to disimpact the fragments, followed by steady movement back toward and often slightly beyond the midline. Generally, this can be achieved by firm digital pressure but sometimes instruments are necessary, particularly in those where there has been delay in treatment. Various elevators and forceps can be used including the Freer, Hills and Howarth elevators and Ashe and Walsham forceps (Figure 41.1). Closed reduction alone may not achieve a satisfactory result when the final position of the nasal dorsum reflects the deformity of the underlying septum. Segments of the fractured perpendicular plate of the ethmoid or septal cartilage may overlap, requiring repositioning by open reduction. If the bones are fixed, especially if the fracture is old, then osteotomies are necessary to release the fragments before manipulation.

It is advisable to refrain from contact sports for at least 6 weeks.

Occasionally, open reduction or rhinoplasty techniques may be desirable or required to provide optimal results, despite the increased time and effort involved. In indicated cases, open

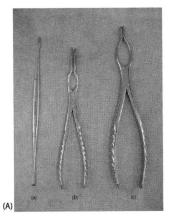
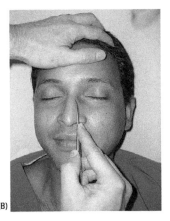

(A) (B)

Figure 41.1 (A) Instruments used in nasal fracture manipulation. (a) Howarth's elevator, (b) Ashe's forceps (septum) and (c) Walsham's forceps (nasal bones). (B) Determining depth of insertion of instrument into nasal cavity. The instrument is held so that the index finger of the dominant hand is placed along the instrument in the line of the nose.

technique offers better exposure and precise approximation of dislocated structures. Open technique is further described in Chapter 47.

Management of the Nasal Septum

Septal fracture is seen in almost half of nasal fractures. This is often missed and is a major reason for poor functional and cosmetic results. A satisfactory reduction of nasal bones is often not possible without improving the position of the septum.

Septal reduction can sometimes be performed with Ashe's forceps, but often requires a Killian or hemitransfixion incision, elevation of mucosal flaps to expose the cartilage and bone fragments and replacement and/or removal of cartilaginous and bony fragments, as in an endonasal septoplasty. Quilting sutures may reduce the risk of haematoma.

Complications

Attempts to reduce deformity or improve obstruction are not always successful. This is multifactorial, and influenced by pre-existing nasal injury, surgical technique, under-recognition of concurrent septal fractures and post-operative scarring. Some patients inevitably require a septorhinoplasty, which should be delayed by 6–12 months to allow the fractures to heal, oedema to settle completely so the underlying nasal skeleton is evident and for any fibrosis to develop. Other complications include epistaxis and septal haematoma.

Management of Septal Haematoma

Septal haematoma presents with acute unilateral or bilateral nasal obstruction and, on inspection, a reddish-purple, fluctuant swelling of the caudal septum. A deviated septum can be confused with a septal haematoma. Gentle pressure on the bulging area will ascertain that it is fluctuant if a collection is present. Untreated, an abscess may develop and the patient becomes very unwell with a fluctuating fever and severe facial and cranial pain.

The haematoma or abscess must be drained as soon as possible. This can be performed under local or general anaesthetic. Incision and drainage is preferable to needle aspiration; often the collection will have become organised and impossible to aspirate fully. Once drained, through-and-through quilting sutures are inserted to eliminate the dead space. Packs or splints can be used to provide gentle pressure on the septum. The patient must be re-examined within 48 hours to establish that the collection has not recurred. The management of a septal abscess is similar, but with the addition of intravenous antibiotic therapy. If left untreated, there is significant risk of cartilage necrosis and/or abscess and subsequent saddle nose deformity, columellar retraction and broadened septum, as well as a risk of intracranial infection.

KEY POINTS

- Timing of initial assessment is critical and dictates optimal outcome:
  - Within first 3 hours or 4–7 days post-injury (due to significant swelling in between)
- Timing of reduction:
  - <3 hours after injury in adults and children has potential for optimal results

    OR

  - 7–10 days after injury in adults
  - 3–7 days after injury in children
- Exclusion of septal haematoma, related injuries to face, orbit, jaws and central nervous system at initial assessment.
- Most cases can be reduced adequately with closed techniques, unless the fractures are complex or a significant septal fracture-dislocation is present.
- If tolerated, local anaesthesia has comparable results with general anaesthesia in indicated cases.
- Patients should be advised that residual cosmetic deformity and nasal obstruction are relatively common.

42. SINONASAL TUMOURS

Introduction

Evidence now supports endoscopic approaches as a suitable treatment option for the management of benign sinonasal tumours. The role of such approaches for malignant sinonasal tumours has been more controversial with early concerns raised regarding the lack of en bloc resection, difficulty in addressing vascular complications and challenges in defect reconstruction. Recent studies refute these concerns with demonstrated reductions in morbidity, improved vascular control and equivalent survival outcomes to open approaches. The endoscopic approach for sinonasal tumours is now supported by European and American societal position papers.

Sinonasal Tumour Epidemiology

- Sinonasal tumours are a rare and diverse group of lesions arising from any of the structures comprising the paranasal sinuses (Table 42.1).
- Sinonasal osteoma is the most reported benign lesion (radiological incidence 1%).
- Ossifying fibroma, fibrous dysplasia and inverted papilloma are the next most reported benign lesions of the paranasal sinuses.

Table 42.1 Summary of sinonasal tumours by tissue of origin

Tissue of origin	Benign lesions	Malignant lesions
Epithelial	• Inverted papilloma • Oncocytic papilloma • Exophytic papilloma • Respiratory epithelial adenomatoid hamartoma (REAH) • Salivary gland adenomas	• Squamous cell carcinoma • Sinonasal undifferentiated carcinoma (SNUC) • Lymphoepithelial carcinoma • Adenocarcinoma • Salivary gland carcinomas • Mucoepidermoid • Adenoid cystic carcinoma • Acinic cell carcinoma
Neuroendocrine		• Carcinoid
Soft tissue	• Myxoma • Leiomyoma • Haemangioma • Schwannoma • Meningioma • Neurofibroma • Angiofibroma • Haemangiopericytoma	• Fibrosarcoma • Rhabdomyosarcoma • Angiosarcoma • Malignant peripheral nerve sheath tumour
Bone and cartilage	• Fibrous dysplasia • Osteoma • Osteoblastoma • Chondroma • Ameloblastoma	• Chondrosarcoma • Osteosarcoma • Chordoma
Haematological and lymphatic		• Lymphoma • Langerhans cell Histiocytosis
Germ cell tumours	• Dermoid cyst	• Teratoma sinonasal yolk sac tumour
Neuroectodermal tumours		• Aesthesioneuroblastoma

Table 42.2 Concerning features on clinical examination

Clinical finding	Reason for concern
Conductive hearing loss/middle ear effusion	Obstruction/invasion of eustachian tube
Visual change/loss Visual field change diplopia/ophthalmoplegia Pain on eye movement Chemosis/orbital displacement	Optic nerve involvement Intra-cranial extension, optic chiasm compression Involvement of intra-orbital contents
Clear rhinorrhoea	Dural/intra-cranial involvement with CSF leak
Facial paraesthesia	Compression/invasion of the maxillary or infraorbital nerve
Loose teeth dental paresthesia	Invasion of the alveolar process and dental roots
Facial asymmetry	Possible involvement of facial soft tissues
Oronasal or oroantral fistula	Erosion of the nasal floor or maxillary sinus floor
Palpable cervical nodal disease	Possible metastatic spread
Reduced neck range of motion	Paraspinal muscle involvement

- Sinonasal malignancies are less common (incidence 0.5–1/100 000):
  - 1% of all malignancies and 3–5% of all head and neck cancers
- Squamous cell carcinoma is the most common subtype followed by adenoid cystic carcinoma and adenocarcinoma.

Diagnosis and Pre-Operative Planning

A thorough history, examination and cranial nerve assessment should be performed in all patients with sinonasal masses. Table 42.2 highlights concerning features that should be looked for on clinical examination.

Endoscopy

Nasal endoscopy is important in pre-operative planning. Visualizing the likely site of origin, along with involvement or destruction of the local anatomic structures, guides surgical planning. Decisions regarding the likely pathology, lesion resectability, endoscopic access and approach can also be made. Endoscopy can facilitate biopsy following review of the relevant radiology.

Radiology

High-resolution computed tomography (CT) and magnetic resonance imaging (MRI) are critical to the management of sinonasal tumours and provide complimentary information regarding the tumour's nature, extent and involvement of local structures (Table 42.3):

- CT is excellent for osseous margins of the skull base and sinus walls.
- MRI is superior for soft tissue resolution permitting the differentiation of tumour from retained secretions and hemorrhage. Allows appreciation of soft tissue tumour margins and their interface with local structures (Figure 42.1).
- Positron emission tomography (PET) is indicated for the detection of distant metastases.

Biopsy

Tumour histopathology directs intra-operative decision making and adjuvant management.

- Multiple representative endoscopic-guided biopsies should be taken before the definitive surgical procedure.
- Tissue should be sent both fresh and in formalin fixative, for histopathology and flow cytometry.
- Biopsies should always be performed after reviewing the relevant radiology to exclude vascular lesions or prolapsed meningo-encephaloceles.

Table 42.3   Radiological features on CT/MRI and their possible implications

Feature	Potential clinical implication
Orbit	
Breech of lamina papyracea Loss of orbital fat planes Involvement of extra-ocular muscles	May indicate involvement of orbit and the need for orbital exenteration.
Septum	
Erosion of septum	Important implications for surgical access and repair. Lesions crossing midline will require a septectomy and binasal approach. Gross septal involvement may preclude the use of the nasoseptal flap.
Skull base	
Asymmetrical or low lying Position of anterior ethmoid arteries Skull base defect	Increase risk of inadvertent entry and CSF leak during surgery Mesentery suspended arteries are at increased risk of injury Suggestive of intra-cranial extension of sinonasal pathology or intranasal extension of intra-cranial pathology
Sphenoid sinus	
Extent of pneumatization Onodi cells Location of sphenoid septations	Laterally pneumatized sinuses may place the carotid at risk May contain optic nerve and be confused with sphenoid sinus Septations may be closely related to carotid artery and optic nerve, requiring great care when removing.
Paranasal sinus	
Osteitic changes	Possible site of tumour origin
Widened bony foramina	Perineural invasion of tumour Nerve sheath tumour
Tumour calcification	See to varying degrees with aesthesioneuroblastoma, chondroma, chondrosarcoma, osteoma, ossifying fibroma and osteosarcoma
Expansion of paranasal sinus/fossae	Tends to indicate the presence of a mass within the space

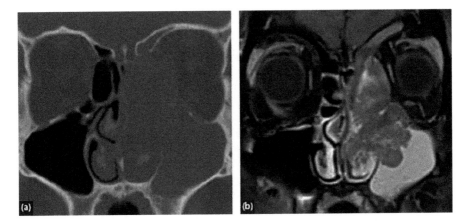

Figure 42.1   Coronal CT and MRI of a sinonasal tumour. Although the CT would suggest involvement of the extra-ocular muscles (a), the MRI demonstrates clear preservation of the fat plane. (b) The MRI also facilitates a differentiation of tumour from retained secretions seen in the maxillary sinus. These images highlight the importance of obtaining both a CT and MRI for skull base tumours.

Multidisciplinary Planning Meetings

All patients with malignant and complex pathology should be presented to a multidisciplinary team, comprising surgeons, radiologists, medical and radiation oncologists and allied health professionals. Treatment recommendations should not only consider the pathology of the tumour but also the age, health, functional status and wishes of the patient. Patients and families should be informed of all available treatment options along with the risks, benefits and likelihood of success to enable an informed consent.

Principles of Endoscopic Management of Sinonasal Tumours

Case Selection

Appropriate case selection is critical to the success of endoscopic skull base surgery. To minimize complications and improve outcomes, surgeons should first become proficient in the surgical management of sinonasal inflammatory disease, before progressing to benign and eventually malignant tumours.

The anatomic and technical limits of endoscopic resectability have continued to evolve as experience builds.

Endoscopically resectable anatomical areas include the following:

- Entire anterior cranial base from cribriform plate to planum sphenoidale.
- Dura, olfactory bulbs and lamina papyracea.
- Nasopharynx, clivus and odontoid process can now be reached, limited inferiorly at the nasopalatine line.
- Laterally, the pterygopalatine and infratemporal fossa can be reached, with the transpterygoid approach affording additional access to the petrous temporal bone, Meckel's cave and middle cranial fossa.

Relative contraindications to an entirely endoscopic approach include involvement of

- Skin and subcutaneous tissue
- Nasolacrimal sac
- Carotid artery
- Anterior table of the frontal sinus
- Dural and brain

Image Guidance Technology

Image guidance technology aids endoscopic skull base surgery, providing the surgeon with enhanced anatomical localization. It may decrease surgical disorientation, improve surgical completeness and potentially lower complication rates.

Principles of Oncologic Resection

Complete resection of a tumour with minimal morbidity is the primary goal of any oncological surgery. The anatomical confines of the nasal cavity prevent en bloc resection for the vast majority of sinonasal tumours. Fortunately, many sinonasal tumours have a well-defined area of origin or tissue invasion. Provided en bloc excision of the origin is performed, ideally with a cuff of normal surrounding tissue, the remainder of the tumour can be selectively debulked down to attachment points, without compromising the completeness of resection.

Surgical Access Techniques

Prior to resection or debulking the tumour, the surgeon needs to obtain maximal access. This allows room for instrumentation and improves the approach to the peripheral aspects of the tumour. It also facilitates early identification of tumour-free zones and aids in defining the tumour extent.

Improving Lateral Access

Endonasal endoscopic techniques can access tumours extending laterally as far as the infra-temporal fossa. Tumours within the nasal cavity without extension beyond the infra-orbital nerve can usually be managed through the ipsilateral nostril. Those extending further laterally may require a transeptal approach along with removal of part or all the medial maxillary wall.

Transeptal Approach

Non-opposing septal incisions permit use of the contralateral nostril to pass instruments or endoscopes, increasing lateral access and allowing a second surgeons' involvement.

Transmaxillary Approaches

Stepwise increases in maxillary sinus access allow a tailored approach to sinonasal tumours in this region. Initially, an uncinectomy to identify the natural maxillary ostium should be performed and enlarged accordingly. Posterior lesions medial to the infra-orbital nerve can usually be accessed with a mega-antrostomy. Further lateral extension requires enhanced lateral access via a modified medial maxillectomy, allowing preservation of the lacrimal duct.

Access for more superiorly based lesions may require a total medial maxillectomy with transection of the nasolacrimal duct. Anterolateral maxillary sinus tumours can be approached with a pre-lacrimal approach, which preserves the structure and function of the lateral nasal wall.

Improving Posterior Access

Binasal access is useful for tumours involving the nasopharynx, sphenoid sinus, pituitary fossa and the infra-temporal and pterygopalatine fossae. This access is facilitated by posterior septectomy.

Posterior Septectomy

A pedicled nasoseptal flap may be raised before performing the septectomy and used for later reconstruction. A bilateral, wide sphenoidotomy to maximize visualization should extend to the skull base superiorly and lamina papyracea laterally, helping avoid inadvertent injury of critical neurovascular structures. The extent of the septectomy can be tailored to the extent of access required. The septal window should extend anteriorly enough to enable complete visualization of the entire surgical field and limit contralateral instrument clash. Where possible, surgeons should preserve at least 1.5 cm of posterosuperior septal mucosa within the olfactory cleft for olfaction provided oncologic outcome is not compromised.

Improving Superior Access

The entire anterior skull base can be accessed endoscopically. When the intra-cranial component lies posterior to the anterior ethmoidal artery, targeted resection of the posterior skull base is usually sufficient for access. If the intra-cranial extent of the tumour lies anterior to the anterior ethmoid arteries, an endoscopic modified Lothrop procedure (EMLP) will typically be required to access the anterior aspect of the tumour. The EMLP also improves lateral access to lesions within the frontal sinus.

Tumour Resection

With appropriate access obtained, the tumour can be debulked down to its site of attachment. Where possible, all tumour removed from the patient should be sent for histopathological analysis. Following debulking, the attachment site can be resected, with attainment of clear surgical margins the goal. Frozen sections may aid intra-operative margin assessment; however, all surgical margin specimens should undergo formal histopathological analysis.

While the ultimate goal of surgery is a complete oncological resection of the tumour, the tumour nature and patient characteristics may, on occasion, necessitate compromise. Benign tumours may be appropriate for subtotal resections with post-operative surveillance where there is significant risk to critical structures or in the elderly, frail population. Malignant tumours may also be palliated in this fashion while limiting morbidity from the resection.

Reconstruction and complications are discussed in Chapter 43.

Post-Operative Care and Tumour Surveillance

Surveillance is performed with regular endoscopic examinations and serial imaging. An early post-operative CT or MRI scan within 3–6 months post-surgery provides a baseline that can be referenced, should the patient develop clinical features suggestive of recurrence.

KEY POINTS

- Current evidence supports endoscopic endonasal approaches for many sinonasal tumours.
- Thorough patient assessment and pre-operative planning is critical to success.
- Multiple approaches are available to enhance surgical visualization and tumour access.
- Safe and effective surgical plans can be formulated for the endoscopic approach to many sinonasal tumours.

---

43. EXTENDED ANTERIOR SKULL BASE APPROACHES

Endonasal approaches to the ventral skull base are classified based on their orientation in sagittal and coronal radiological planes relative to the sphenoid sinus. For large intra-cranial tumours or malignant sinonasal tumours that involve the skull base, transfrontal, transcribriform and transplanum approaches can be combined to provide complete access to the anterior cranial fossa (Table 43.1). Lateral margins of the anterior cranial base may be extended to the midline of the orbits by removal of the medial orbital roofs.

Sinonasal neoplasms suitable for endoscopic endonasal surgery (EES) include olfactory neuroblastoma (aesthesioneuroblastoma), neuroendocrine carcinoma, sinonasal undifferentiated carcinoma (SNUC), squamous cell carcinoma, adenocarcinoma, adenoid cystic carcinoma and melanoma. Surgery is generally preferred as the first treatment option for resectable tumours that do not have a high risk of distant metastases. For tumours with aggressive biological behaviour and increased risk of metastases (SNUC, melanoma), systemic therapy (chemotherapy, immunotherapy) is considered first.

Table 43.1   Indications for endoscopic endonasal surgery of anterior cranial base (by surgical approach)

Transfrontal	Chronic sinusitis, mucocele, osteoma, nasal dermoid
Transcribriform	Meningoencephalocele, olfactory groove meningioma, olfactory schwannoma, olfactory neuroblastoma, sinonasal malignancy
Transplanum (suprasellar)	Pituitary adenoma, craniopharyngioma, meningioma
Transsellar	Pituitary adenoma, Rathke's cleft cyst, craniopharyngioma
Supra-orbital	Osteoma, meningioma, sinonasal malignancy

Surgical Approaches

Transfrontal Approach

Table 43.2 Key landmarks and limits of the transfrontal approach

Key landmarks
Foramen cecum
Crista galli
Frontal sinus
Limits
Anterior: anterior table frontal sinus
Posterior: posterior table frontal sinus
Medial: crista galli
Lateral: lacrimal fossa
Superior: posterior table midpoint

Transcribriform Approach

Table 43.3 Key landmarks and limits of the transcribriform approach

Key landmarks
Crista galli
Olfactory filia, olfactory bulbs
Lateral lamella
Limits
Anterior: frontal sinus
Posterior: planum, posterior ethmoid artery
Medial: crista galli
Lateral: orbit

Transplanum Approach

Table 43.4 Key landmarks and limits of the transplanum approach

Key landmarks
Posterior ethmoid artery
Olfactory tracts
Limits
Anterior: cribriform plate
Posterior: superior intercavernous sinus
Posterolateral: optic canals
Lateral: orbital apex

Supra-Orbital Approach

Table 43.5 Key landmarks and limitations of the supra-orbital approach

Key landmarks
Anterior and posterior ethmoid arteries
Limits
Anterior: frontal sinus
Posterior: optic canal
Superolateral: midplane of orbit

SUPRASELLAR APPROACH

Table 43.6 Key landmarks and limitations of the suprasellar approach

Key landmarks
Optic canals
Tuberculum
Ophthalmic arteries
Limits
Anterior: planum sphenoidale
Lateral: optic canals, paraclinoid internal carotid artery

Reconstruction

Reconstruction of dural defects of the anterior cranial base is ideally performed using vascularized tissue. Local vascularized flaps include middle turbinate, inferior turbinate and nasal septal flaps, all of which are based on terminal branches of the sphenopalatine artery. Regional vascularized flaps include peri-cranial and temporoparietal fascial flaps. Of these, the nasal septal flap and extra-cranial peri-cranial flap offer the best coverage and are preferred for reconstruction of large defects of the anterior cranial base.

Dura defects (<1cm) are typically amenable to a 'bath plug' type repair using fat or overlay autologous or synthetic grafts. Larger defects will usually require multilayer closure often incorporating a free-mucosal graft or vascularized flap. Very large defects (>3cm) usually require rigid reinforcement via septal cartilage or titanium mesh to minimize the risk of encephalocele formation.

Complications

Post-operatively, the most common complication is cerebrospinal fluid (CSF) leak. Potential risk factors include the size and location of the dural defect, patient factors (prior treatment, obesity), reconstructive technique (materials, vascularized flap, packing) and peri-operative care (patient activity, lumbar drain, debridement). In most cases, endoscopic repair supplemented by a lumbar spinal drain is successful. Intra-cranial infection is rare and is usually associated with a post-operative CSF leak. Prompt repair of CSF leaks and limited use of lumbar spinal drains is encouraged to limit the risk of infection.

Sinonasal complications include sinusitis, epistaxis, synechiae, chronic crusting, cosmetic deformity and loss of olfaction. Delayed epistaxis is usually due to a branch of the sphenopalatine artery. A saddle-nose deformity can result from loss of septal support. Even if the olfactory nerves are preserved, some loss of olfaction is common and may be due to altered airflow patterns, mucosal oedema and crusting, post-operative irradiation or direct damage to the olfactory epithelium or olfactory tracts. Fortunately, quality of life (QoL) studies demonstrate that overall sinonasal morbidity is low.

KEY POINTS

- The anterior cranial base from the frontal sinus to the sella and from orbit to orbit is accessible using EES.
- These techniques can be applied to a wide variety of lesions including meningoencephaloceles, benign tumours (nasal dermoids, meningiomas, craniopharyngiomas, pituitary adenomas) and malignant tumours (sinonasal malignancy) with preservation of microsurgical and oncological principles.
- Many of the challenges of endonasal surgery have been solved, and large dural defects can be reconstructed effectively using vascularized flaps.

Oncological and functional outcomes are comparable or superior to other approaches with the potential for decreased morbidity.

44. GRANULOMATOUS CONDITIONS OF THE NOSE

Introduction

A granuloma is an organized collection of macrophages which fuse to form multinucleated giant cells. This histologic configuration is encountered in a number of infective, inflammatory and neoplastic conditions of the nose and sinuses (Table 44.1) and is also seen in vasculitides.

There are often systemic manifestations, but these conditions may present with otorhinolaryngological symptoms; a low threshold of suspicion is therefore needed for diagnosis.

Granulomatosis with Polyangiitis (GPA)

Granulomatosis with polyangiitis (GPA; formerly Wegener's granulomatosis) classically involves a triad of upper airway, lung and renal disease, but limited or localized forms of the condition occur in up to 30%. It is thought to be an autoimmune disease, associated with cytoplasmic antineutrophil cytoplasmic antibodies (c-ANCAs) which are specific for proteinase-3 (PR3). Any part of the body may be affected and in generalized disease there is often malaise disproportionate to the clinical findings.

GPA has been classified as

- 'Localized' (respiratory tract involvement only with no systemic vasculitis)
- 'Early systemic' or 'generalized' disease

Table 44.1   Granulomatous conditions of the nose and sinuses

Infective	Inflammatory	Neoplastic
Bacteria		
Tuberculosis (*Mycobacterium tuberculosis*)	Sarcoidosis	Extranodal NK/ T-cell lymphoma
Leprosy (*Mycobacterium leprae*)	Granulomatosis with polyangiitis (GPA, Wegener's syndrome)	
Rhinoscleroma (*Klebsiella rhinoscleromatis*)	Eosinophilic granulomatosis with polyangiitis (EGPA; Churg-Strauss)	
Syphilis (*Treponema pallidum*)	Cocaine-induced midline destructive lesion (CIMDL)	
Actinomycosis (*Actinomyces israelii*)	Giant cell granuloma	
Fungal		
Aspergillus (fumigatus/flavus/niger)	Eosinophilic granuloma (Langerhans cell histiocytosis)	
Zygomycosis (*Conidiobolus coronatus, Rhizopus oryzae*)		
Dermateaceae (*Curvularia, Alternaria, Bipolaris*)		
Rhinosporidiosis (*Rhinosporidiosis seeberi*)		
Blastomycosis (*Blastomyces dermatitidis, Cryptococcus neoformans*)		
Histoplasmosis (*Histoplasma capsulatum*)		
Sporotrichosis (*Sporotrichum schenckii*)		
Coccidiomycosis (*Coccidiodes immitis*)		
Protozoa		
Leishmaniasis (*Leishmania* spp.)		

Many cases of early systemic disease progress to generalized disease, approximately 5% remain localized.

The incidence is approximately 10–15 per million per year. The mean age at diagnosis is 40–50 years, although it can occur at any age. Men and women are equally affected. GPA is predominantly a Caucasian disease.

Clinical Presentation

The head and neck is the most common site of involvement at presentation (73–93%). The nose and sinuses are involved in over 80% with symptoms which include the following:

- Nasal obstruction, crusting, discharge, bleeding and facial pain.
- Destruction of the sinonasal architecture with characteristic nasal collapse (25%), septal perforation and ultimately the formation of a single large cavity.
- One-third of patients develop otitis media with effusion.
- Sensorineural hearing loss (35%) and facial nerve paralysis (8–10%).
- Subglottic or upper tracheal stenosis (16%, five times more common in childhood).
- Oral symptoms are rare but 'strawberry' gingival hyperplasia is pathognomonic.
- Ocular manifestations (50%), with visual loss in up to 8%.

Necrotizing vasculitis in the lungs causes cough, haemoptysis and pleuritic pain. Over 75% of patients develop renal involvement. Cutaneous manifestations include ulceration and nodules, and both polymyalgia and polyarthritis have been described. Neurological sequelae include meningitis, mononeuritis multiplex and cranial neuropathies.

Diagnosis

ANCA has two main staining patterns: c-ANCA, 90% of which are PR3-ANCA, and perinuclear (p-ANCA), 90% of which are myeloperoxidase (MPO)-ANCA.

c-ANCA is generally associated with systemic GPA (sensitivity 91%, specificity 99%) and titers correlate with disease activity. However, sensitivity falls to 60% with localized disease. Ten percent of patients with GPA have a positive p-ANCA and up to 30% may be ANCA-negative, particularly in localized disease. A full blood count, erythrocyte sedimentation rate, C-reactive protein, renal function, serum angiotensin-converting enzyme (ACE), urinalysis and chest X-ray or chest computed tomography (CT) should be performed. Tissue biopsy may be helpful in ANCA-negative patents. Systemic nasal biopsy shows specific features for GPA in less than 10%. The probability increases by up to 50% when deep biopsy from major lesions is taken. Paranasal sinus biopsies yield more positive results than nasal specimens.

CT and magnetic resonance imaging (MRI) of the sinuses may show nonspecific mucosal thickening (90%), bony destruction (62%) and new bone formation (78%). The combination of bone destruction and new bone formation on CT is virtually diagnostic, especially when accompanied on MRI by a fat signal from the sclerotic sinus wall, so-called 'tramlining'.

The American College of Rheumatology proposed a clinical classification in 1990 to distinguish GPA from other vasculitides (Table 44.2). The Chapel Hill Consensus, last updated in 2012, added PR3-ANCA to the definition in 1994.

Treatment and Prognosis

Untreated, GPA is a lethal disease with a mean survival of 5 months; a fulminating course with a fatal outcome can occur in as little as 48 hours. The introduction of systemic corticosteroid treatment improved mortality rates to 50%. Treatment aims to induce and maintain remission. Initial treatment typically involves steroids plus cyclophosphamide, methotrexate or rituximab. Methotrexate, azathioprine or mycophenolate mofetil are then used as steroid-sparing agents for maintenance, sometimes with co-trimoxazole.

Table 44.2 1990 American College of Rheumatology criteria for the diagnosis of granulomatosis with polyangiitis (GPA)*

Criteria	Definition
Nasal or oral inflammation	Painful or painless oral ulcers or purulent or bloody nasal discharge
Abnormal chest X-ray	Nodules, fixed infiltrates or cavities
Abnormal urinary sediment	Microscopic haematuria with or without red cell casts
Granulomatous inflammation on biopsy	Granulomatous inflammation within the wall of an artery or in the peri- or extravascular area (artery or arteriole)

* A diagnosis of GPA requires two or more of these four criteria. This rule is associated with a sensitivity of 88.2% and a specificity of 92.0%.

Topical nasal treatment such as douching, intranasal steroids and nasal lubricants may be helpful for symptomatic relief. Surgery is generally reserved for cases that are refractory to medical treatment, or for complications of GPA. Rhinoplasty to correct a saddle nose deformity should be deferred until the disease has been in remission for at least 1 year. Grommets are best avoided because of the risk of chronic otorrhoea.

Eosinophilic Granulomatosis with Polyangiitis (EGPA)

This rare vasculitis of unknown aetiology, formerly known as Churg-Strauss syndrome, is associated with chronic rhinosinusitis with nasal polyps (CRSwNP), allergic rhinitis, asthma and eosinophilia. The mean age at diagnosis is 50 years (range 4–75 years), but there is no gender preponderance. The annual incidence is 0.5–4 per million in Europe, rising to 67 per million in asthmatics.

Clinical Presentation

Asthma occurs in 99% of patients and is characteristically late onset. Sinonasal symptoms are present in up to 93%, with nasal obstruction, rhinorrhoea, anosmia, sneezing, crusting and epistaxis. Neurological symptoms are common, with mononeuritis multiplex in up to 76% and peripheral polyneuropathy in 25%. Central nervous system involvement is less common but is the second most common cause of death. Cutaneous symptoms including papules and nodules occur in up to 50%. Cardiac involvement is less common but is the major cause of mortality, usually from granulomatous myocarditis.

Diagnosis

Diagnosis is based on clinical features illustrated in Table 44.3. The condition should be suspected in anyone with difficult-to-treat CRSwNP, asthma and a systemic eosinophilia as the ANCA is only positive in 40–75% of cases, typically p-ANCA specific for MPO but

Table 44.3 1990 American College of Rheumatology criteria for the diagnosis of eosinophilic granulomatosis with polyangiitis (EGPA)*

Criteria	Definition
Asthma	History of wheezing or diffuse rales on expiration
Eosinophilia	Eosinophilia >10% on white blood cell differential count
Mononeuropathy or polyneuropathy	Development of mononeuropathy, multiple mononeuropathies or polyneuropathy
Pulmonary infiltrates, non-fixed	Migratory or transitory pulmonary infiltrates on radiographs
Paranasal sinus abnormality	History of acute or chronic paranasal sinus pain or radiographic opacification of the paranasal sinuses
Extravascular eosinophils	Biopsy including artery, arteriole or venule, showing accumulations of eosinophils in extravascular areas

* A diagnosis of EGPA requires any four or more of these six criteria. This rule is associated with a sensitivity of 85% and a specificity of 99.7%.

occasionally c-ANCA. Sinonasal imaging shows non-specific widespread opacification, and patients are more likely to develop frontoethmoidal mucocoeles.

Treatment and Prognosis

Treatment is primarily with high-dose systemic steroids, but cyclophosphamide, methotrexate, azathioprine and mycophenolate mofetil may also be helpful. Remission rates are 91% with over 25% relapse. Sinonasal symptoms should be treated with topical nasal steroids, douching and endoscopic sinus surgery as required.

Cocaine-Induced Midline Destructive Lesion (CIMDL)

Cocaine use via intranasal inhalation is known to cause septal perforation but more aggressive midfacial destruction has also been noted. Such cocaine-induced midline destructive lesions (CIMDLs) can mimic localized or systemic GPA as well as neoplasia.

Clinical Presentation

Patients complain of nasal obstruction and bleeding, with change in shape of the nose and nasal regurgitation as the lesion progresses to destroy the nasal framework and palate. Systemic symptoms are rare.

Diagnosis

Nearly 90% of patients have a positive p-ANCA against human neutrophil elastase (HNE); over 50% of patients will also have a positive PR3-ANCA. Histology is often very similar to that of GPA.

Treatment and Prognosis

There is no role for immunosuppression, and patients must stop using cocaine to prevent further progression. Conservative treatment includes nasal douching, debridement of necrotic areas and topical or systemic antibiotic therapy.

Sarcoidosis

Sarcoidosis is a systemic granulomatous condition of unknown aetiology. It is slightly more common in women than men with peak onset between the third and fourth decades. The incidence varies from 6–16 per 100,000 with significant geographical variation. It is 10–20 times more common in African Americans than Caucasians.

Clinical Presentation

Sarcoidosis primarily affects the lower respiratory tract but may involve almost any organ. It involves the upper respiratory tract in up to 18%.

Symptomatology includes the following:

- Nasal obstruction, crusting, bleeding or facial pain (1–4%).
- Characteristic 'strawberry skin' appearance of nasal mucosa with or without ulceration, crusting, septal perforation and adhesions.
- Expansion of the nasal dorsum can be associated with thickening and purplish discoloration of the overlying skin known as lupus pernio, which is a cutaneous manifestation of chronic systemic sarcoid.
- Salivary gland enlargement (5–10%), which is more rarely associated with facial palsy and uveitis (uveoparotid fever, Heerfordt's syndrome).
- Laryngeal involvement (1–5%), especially supraglottitis (85%), with cough, hoarseness, dysphagia and rarely stridor.

Diagnosis

No test is pathognomonic. Diagnosis relies on a combination of clinical features, imaging, histology, biochemical testing and the exclusion of other granulomatous diseases. The classic histological appearance is that of a non-caseating granuloma. Nasal biopsy is only helpful if the mucosa appears clinically abnormal, when over 90% of samples are positive. Serum

ACE is elevated in up to 85% during active disease, but is non-specific. Serum and urinary calcium levels are elevated in 15%. Imaging of the chest allows staging of the disease. CT scanning may show punctate osteolysis of the nasal bones in 25% of patients and will also demonstrate secondary involvement of the sinuses. Bilateral lacrimal gland enlargement may be seen.

Treatment and Prognosis
Sarcoidosis has a variable clinical course; up to two-thirds of patients will spontaneously remit whereas 10–30% follow a chronic course despite systemic therapy.

Some patients require no treatment, but international guidelines suggest systemic or intra-lesional steroid treatment for life-threatening or critical disease. Hydroxychloroquine has been used for cutaneous and sinonasal sarcoidosis. Nasal treatment includes intranasal steroids and douching. Surgery has a limited role, particularly in the presence of active disease. Septal surgery should be avoided as there is an increased rate of septal perforation. Symptomatic laryngeal disease that fails to respond to systemic treatment may be treated with transoral laser and intralesional steroid injection.

KEY POINTS

- Many patients with systemic granulomatous conditions present first to ear, nose and throat (ENT) surgeons. It is important to maintain a low threshold of suspicion to make an early diagnosis and avert more severe systemic disease.
- Any patient with blood-stained discharge and crusting in the nose has a granulomatous condition until proven otherwise.
- No test is completely reliable, and a combination of clinical findings combined with diagnostic investigations is required.
- The sensitivity and specificity of c-ANCA in GPA are 91% and 99%, respectively.
- Secondary or tertiary referral may be required to diagnose and manage the condition.
- Management should be multidisciplinary.
- A range of medications is available, of which steroids combined with cytotoxic drugs are the most frequently used.
- Patients on long-term systemic steroids should be monitored for complications.

---

45. DIAGNOSIS AND MANAGEMENT OF FACIAL PAIN

Introduction
Facial pain is complex. Individuals are often convinced their facial symptoms have an underlying sinus aetiology. There may be a strong psychological component and a significant proportion of patients will have undergone unsuccessful sinus surgery. Recent evidence showed that the majority of migraines with or without aura are diagnosed as 'sinogenic pain'. Of patients referred to ear, nose and throat (ENT) clinic with sinogenic pain, 80% were diagnosed with migraine and additional 8% earned the diagnosis of migrainous headache. Differentiating sinogenic from non-sinogenic symptoms is therefore paramount.

Sinogenic Facial Pain
Pain in sinusitis that is not acute or associated with a complication is rare (Table 45.1). Patients may complain of pressure, fullness or throbbing in the distribution of the

Table 45.1   Definitions of headache caused by rhinosinusitis and the diagnosis of rhinosinusitis

International Headache Society (IHS) definition of headache due to rhinosinusitis
(a) Any headache fulfilling criterion C
(b) Clinical, nasal endoscopic and/or imaging evidence of acute rhinosinusitis

(c) Evidence of causation demonstrated by at least two of the following:
 • Headache has developed in temporal relation to the onset of rhinosinusitis
 • Either or both of the following:
   • Headache has significantly worsened in parallel with worsening of the rhinosinusitis
   • Headache has significantly improved or resolved in parallel with improvement in or resolution of the rhinosinusitis
 • Headache is exacerbated by pressure applied over the paranasal sinuses

(d) In the case of a unilateral rhinosinusitis, headache is localised and ipsilateral to it
(e) Not better accounted for by another IHS diagnosis

Note: See EPOS2020 definition of chronic rhinosinusitis in Chapter 33.

paranasal sinuses or at the vertex of the head. Symptoms may be bilateral or unilateral depending on which sinuses are affected. Exacerbation of these symptoms on bending forward is not diagnostic of rhinosinusitis. Symptoms may be acute, recurrent acute (moderated by repeated short courses of antibiotics) or chronic. There may be associated nasal congestion and/or hyposmia. There should be endoscopic signs of oedema and/or polyposis causing obstruction of outflow drainage pathways, and mucosal disease. Over 80% of patients with endoscopic evidence of purulent secretions have no headache or facial pain. If surgery is performed in cases where facial pain is the dominant symptom without firm clinical evidence of rhinosinusitis, patients largely continue to complain of facial pain postoperatively.

NON-SINOGENIC FACIAL PAIN

The Primary Headaches

Migraine (Paroxysmal)

Migraine is characterised by recurrent, often unilateral, moderate to severe pulsatile or throbbing headaches lasting between 2 and 72 hours. The sufferer may retreat to bed in a dark, quiet room.

In classical migraine (25%) symptoms include:

- Nausea, vomiting, photophobia.
- Prodromal aura: a transient visual, sensory (olfaction or taste), or language or motor disturbance (pins-and-needles or numbness).
- 60% of sufferers exhibit unilateral cranial autonomic symptoms such as nasal discharge and tearing which often leads to confusion in diagnosis and management.

The condition runs in families in two-thirds of cases and is more common in women. Triggers may include stress, hunger, fatigue, hormonal changes, foodstuffs containing tyramine (aged cheeses, smoked fish, cured meats, some types of beer), monosodium glutamate, indoor air quality and lighting. The main aspects of treatment are trigger avoidance, acute symptomatic control and pharmacological prevention.

Acute episodes should be treated with an oral triptan (avoid in cardiovascular disease) and non-steroidal anti-inflammatory drugs (NSAID) or paracetamol ± antiemetic. For migraine prophylaxis, consider topiramate (risk of foetal malformations) or propranolol bearing in mind comorbidities and side effects. If unsuitable, consider amitriptyline or acupuncture. Botulinum toxin type A is useful in those with chronic migraines (15 or more headache days per month of which at least 8 days are with migraines) not responding to other therapies. Review migraine prophylaxis after 6 months.

Tension-Type Headache (Paroxysmal or Continuous)

Usually symmetric and non-pulsatile in nature. The feeling is of tightness, pressure or constriction (vice like) that may be confined to a small area at the glabella or extend across the whole forehead and into the temporoparietal scalp. Consider aspirin, paracetamol or NSAID for acute treatment. For chronic tension-type headaches (continuous or last for more than 15 days per month) consider acupuncture, relaxation training, stress management and/or counselling. Low-dose amitriptyline is also effective.

Cluster Headache (Paroxysmal)

Excruciating unilateral headaches affecting the frontotemporal and retro-orbital regions (Figure 45.1a). Men between the ages of 20 and 50 years are most often affected. Duration ranges from 15 minutes to 3 hours or more, with a rapid onset and without preliminary signs. Clusters often continue for several weeks followed by months or years of remission. Intense pain is caused by dilation of blood vessels creating pressure on the trigeminal nerve. National Institute for Health and Care Excellence (NICE) recommends oxygen therapy and/ or subcutaneous or nasal triptan for acute treatment. Consider verapamil for prophylaxis with electrocardiogram (ECG) monitoring.

Paroxysmal Hemicrania

A severe debilitating unilateral headache affecting the peri-orbital and frontotemporal regions, with an average age of onset of 30 to 40 years. Attacks are short-lasting, ranging from 2 to 45 minutes and frequent, happening more than 5 times a day. Trigeminal autonomic symptoms may occur. Most patients respond to indomethacin within 24 hours. Other treatments include calcium-channel blockers, naproxen, carbamazepine, and sumatriptan.

Trigeminal Neuralgia (Paroxysmal)

Trigeminal neuralgia is characterised by unilateral paroxysms of brief but severe pain followed by asymptomatic periods without pain, although a constant dull ache may persist in some patients. Pain is often described as stabbing or lancinating, burning, pressing, crushing, exploding or shooting, and patients may describe a trigger area on the face so sensitive that touching or even air currents may trigger an episode. Vascular (arterial and venous) compression of the trigeminal nerve roots is the likely cause in most cases. Magnetic resonance imaging (MRI) should be performed to exclude multiple sclerosis or middle fossa pathology. Carbamazepine is the drug of choice for management. Gabapentin, lamotrigine and topiramate are useful as second-line agents. Microvascular decompression produces satisfactory relief in most well-selected cases.

Post-Surgical/Traumatic Neuralgia (Continuous)

Post-traumatic trigeminal neuropathy often misdiagnosed as 'sinus pain' is related to major maxillofacial and minor oral surgery. Third molar surgery and implants are significant contributors. The diagnosis is based on a history of surgery or trauma temporally correlated with the development of the characteristic neuropathic pain which commonly persists 2 months after the injury and can be permanent. Medical therapy is like that used in neuropathic pain conditions depending on the patients' symptoms; drugs to treat neuropathic pain (amitriptyline, gabapentin or pregabalin), infiltration with local anesthetic and corticosteroid and, ultimately, nerve section may offer some symptom relief.

Sluder's Neuralgia and 'Contact Point Pain'

The theory that implicates mucosal contact points within the nose as a cause of headache or facial pain has, unfortunately, become firmly entrenched in otolaryngology folklore. High-quality studies now exist to support the view that the majority of people with contact points experience no facial pain.

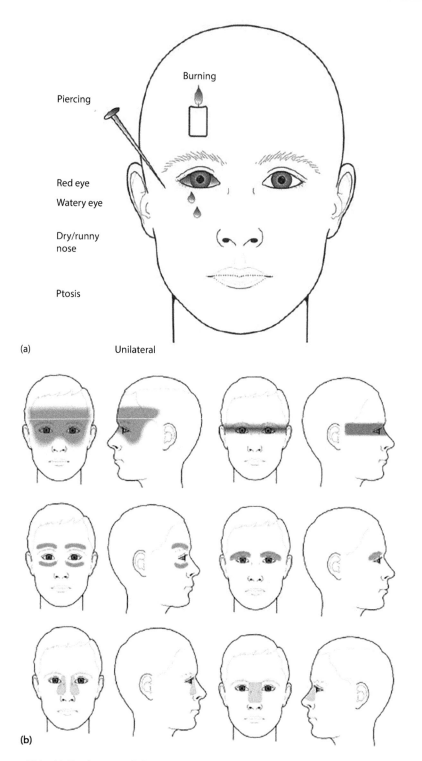

Figure 45.1 (a) The features of cluster headache showing trigeminal autonomic symptoms that may be confused for a sinogenic aetiology. (b) Facial map of the patterns of distribution of mid-facial segment pain.

Mid-Facial Segment Pain (Paroxysmal or Continuous)

Mid-facial segment pain is a type of tension headache that affects the mid-face (Figure 45.1b), and is common. Pain is usually continuous and bilateral. Analgesia overuse is common and nasal surgery relieves pain for several months only. Tension pain and its management have been described above.

Persistent Idiopathic Facial Pain (Atypical Facial Pain)

A diagnosis of exclusion only, persistent idiopathic facial pain is described as a persistent facial pain that does not have the classical characteristics of cranial neuralgias and for which there is no obvious cause. Significant psychological disturbance may exist with the suggestion they are unable to function normally because of their pain. Reassure the patient that you recognise they have genuine pain. Drug treatment revolves around a gradual buildup to the higher analgesic and antidepressant levels of amitriptyline (75–100mg) at night. Second-line treatment includes gabapentin and carbamazepine. Referral to a clinical psychologist or psychiatrist may be helpful.

Other types of facial pain are summarised in Table 45.2.

History Taking in Facial Pain

- **Where is the pain and does it radiate?**
  Bilateral pain is commonly mid-facial segment pain. Migraine, cluster and other trigeminal autonomic headaches, and temporomandibular joint (TMJ) disorders tend to be unilateral.

- **Is it continuous or intermittent?**
  Sinogenic pain and migraine are unlikely to be continuous or present on a daily basis. Pain of this character is more likely to represent tension headache, mid-facial segment pain, analgesia-dependency headache or atypical facial pain. Constant and predominantly unilateral pain, particularly if progressive, may be due to a tumour.

Table 45.2 Other types of facial pain

	Painful teeth	TMJ disorder	Tumour-related pain	Analgesia-dependency headache or medication-overuse headache
Location	Affected tooth	Periauricular areas, deep otalgia, temporoparietal and cervical scalp	Unilateral, dependent on tumour location	Bilateral, symmetrical
Duration	Paroxysmal or continuous	Paroxysmal or continuous	Continuous or progressive	Continuous
Quality	Sharp, well-localised pain	Aching pain worse when chewing with/without clicking, grinding noises when moving jaw	Dull or gnawing pain	Dull, diffuse and band-like headaches
Other	Percussing the offending tooth is often diagnostic	Treatment includes joint rest, NSAIDs, correction of factors (e.g. Custom-made bite guard), physiotherapy, steroid/local anesthetic TMJ injection	Imaging is crucial	On stopping analgesics, headaches disappear or decrease by more than 50% in two-thirds of patients

- **What is the character?**

  Vascular pain tends to be throbbing, with cluster headaches being particularly severe. Mid-facial segment pain, like tension headache, is often described as pressure or bandlike pain. Trigeminal neuralgia may cause intense stabbing pain that is initiated by a trigger.

- **What is associated with it?**

  Sinogenic pain is associated with adverse rhinological symptoms but should be differentiated from trigeminal autonomic symptoms. Migraine may have aura and is often associated with nausea. Cluster headaches are frequently triggered by alcohol and wake the patient. TMJ pain is exacerbated by chewing, and that of trigeminal neuralgia and myofascial pain is provoked by trigger points.

- **What relieves it?**

  Sinogenic pain almost always responds to topical decongestion and antibiotics. Patients with migraine will retreat to a quiet and darkened room. Although mid-facial segment pain may initially respond to simple analgesics, the benefit is usually short-lived.

- **What effect does it have on daily life?**

  Patients with persistent idiopathic facial pain often describe their pain in dramatic detail as severe and unrelenting despite sleeping well and living a relatively normal life. Severe crippling pain that wakes the patient, often a man, is typical of cluster headache.

KEY POINTS

- Comprehensive history is mandatory.
- Normal endoscopy in a symptomatic patient makes sinogenic pain extremely unlikely.
- Psychological illness may exacerbate facial pain.
- Surgery for facial pain is rarely beneficial.
- Rhinosinusitis does not usually cause pain.
- Incidental mucosal thickening on computed tomography (CT) does not automatically equate to a sinogenic cause for facial pain.
- Many headache disorders may have associated trigeminal autonomic symptoms.
- Many patients with chronic facial pain benefit from neuropathic pain management.
- Multidisciplinary management is helpful.

---

46. PRE-ASSESSMENT FOR RHINOPLASTY

Rhinoplasty is one of the most challenging procedures in facial plastic surgery and consideration must be given to both facial aesthetics and nasal function. It is technically difficult to achieve consistently excellent results and, as the surgery is on the most prominent part of the face, the aesthetic outcome is visible to all. Meticulous planning is therefore essential. Assessment should include:

- Consideration of the patient's motivations, anxieties and expectations
- Analysis of the face
- Analysis of the nose
- Examination
- Photography

The Patient

It is essential to obtain a clear history of the patient's complaint and symptoms. Identification of any structural, congenital, traumatic, cosmetic and/or functional issues is crucial. Any past history of nasal surgery, sinonasal disease, diabetes, psychopathology, anticoagulant medication, smoking or cocaine use should be elicited. It is important to understand the patient's motivations, anxieties and expectations.

Identifying High-Risk Patients

High-risk patients are unlikely to be satisfied with surgical results. Examples are patients with body dysmorphic disorder (BDD), those who are unreasonably demanding or overly flattering, patients who insist on secrecy and the so-called surgiholic, as well as obsessive, perfectionist and impolite patients. The simplified acronyms SIMON (single, immature, male, overly expectant/obsessive, narcissistic) and SYLVIA (secure, young, listens, verbal, intelligent, attractive) describe some of characteristics of the high-risk and the ideal patient, respectively.

Body Dysmorphic Disorder

BDD describes an altered perception of one's own appearance that results in distress. It is a subjective feeling of ugliness or physical defect which the patient feels is noticeable to others, although the appearance is within normal limits.

Three questions to ask patients, based on the Diagnostic and Statistical Manual of Mental Disorders (DSM-IV) criteria, have been developed to help surgeons screen for BDD:

1 Are you worried about your appearance in any way?
2 Does this concern or preoccupy you? That is, do you think about it a lot and wish you could worry about it less?
3 What effect has this preoccupation with your appearance had on your life?

Expectations

Determining pre-operative expectations is crucial as poor results are often based on emotional dissatisfaction rather than technical failure. It is therefore important to ask the following:

- What are your outcome expectations?
- How do you anticipate your life will be different following treatment?
- What if your expectations are not met?

Analysis of the Face

Attractive faces are deemed to have ideal measurements and angles, which are reportedly based on the dimensions first described by Leonardo da Vinci.

Facial symmetry is reported to be the basis for a beautiful face, although minor asymmetry may be associated with the perception of beauty. Many patients are unaware of minor facial asymmetries and, if they discover these in the post-operative period, it could lead to dissatisfaction and misunderstanding. It is therefore important to raise these concerns with the patient and document them pre-operatively.

Analysis of facial proportions is performed using the 'rule of thirds' and the 'rule of fifths' to assess the face from a frontal view (Figure 46.1A). The nose ideally occupies one-third of the length of the face and one-fifth of its width. Powell and Humphrey described the ideal angles of the facial aesthetic triangle (Figure 46.1B).

Facial proportions act as a guide and are helpful in planning procedures but should not be taken as absolute. Each rhinoplasty should respect the individual's wishes, gender, ethnicity and character.

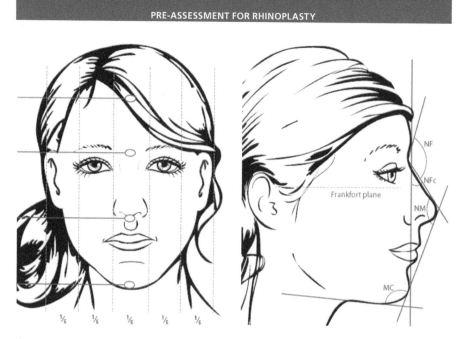

Figure 46.1 (A) The concept of dividing the symmetric face into thirds and fifths. (B) Triangles of Powell and Humphrey. Angles of the aesthetic triangle: nasofrontal (NF) = 115–135, nasofacial (NFc) = 30–40°, nasomental (NM) = 120–132° and mentocervical (MC) = 80–95°.

Analysis of the Nose

Inspection of the External Nose

- *Skin quality*: Thin skin is unforgiving and minor irregularities are easily detectable; refining and narrowing the nasal tip can be challenging where there is thick skin.
- *Deviations*: The nose is divided into thirds. The upper third corresponds to the bony vault, the middle third to the upper lateral cartilages and dorsal septum and the lower third to the lower lateral cartilages, caudal septum and alar base. Deviated noses are described on the basis of direction of the deviation of each third, e.g. classically described C-shaped, one-sided or S-shaped deviations.
- *Length of the nose*: Measured from the nasion to the tip, which is equal to the distance between the stomium and the menton. This can also be calculated mathematically as the distance from the nasal tip to the stomium multiplied by a constant of 1.6. Nasal length: $NT = TS \times 1.6$.
- *Tip projection*: This is a measure of how far the nasal tip lies anterior to the face. Ideal projection is determined using Goode's ratio, where a line drawn from the alar–facial groove to the nasal tip measures 0.55–0.60 of the distance from the nasion to the nasal tip. A ratio less than this equates to an under projected nose and greater than this corresponds to over projection (Figure 46.2A).
- *Lip–chin relationship*: The horizontal distance from the surface of the upper lip to that of lower lip is normally around 2 mm. The anterior surfaces of the upper and lower lips rest on the nasomental line in an aesthetic face (Figure 46.2B). When the chin lies posterior to this line, it is described as retrognathic; when it lies anterior it is prognathic. A retrognathic chin can give the illusion of an over projected nose, and the reverse applies to a prognathic chin. Genioplasty or chin implant procedures are therefore often used in conjunction with rhinoplasty.
- *Dorsum*: The dorsum is inspected from both frontal and lateral views. Tracing the lateral aesthetic lines (also known as the brow-tip line) should reveal a smooth curvilinear line connecting the eyebrow superiorly to the nasal tip inferiorly (Figure 46.3A).

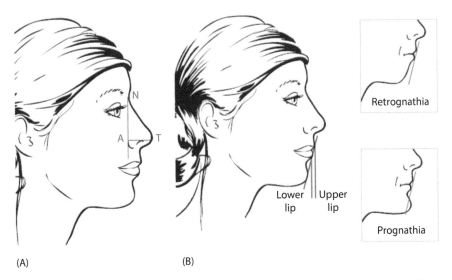

Figure 46.2   (A) Determining tip projection by using Goode's ratio. (B) Lip–chin relationship.

Identification of any irregularities in this smooth curve highlights sources of nasal deformity. In the lateral view, the height of the dorsum is assessed; the dorsum is a straight line in men and in women gently curves with a supratip break delineating the dorsum from the nasal tip.

- *Tip configuration*: There are four tip-defining points identified by light reflection (Figure 46.3A). These represent the domes, the supratip and the infratip. The size and shape of the lower lateral cartilages are assessed, as are asymmetry, bifidity and rotation.
- *Tip rotation*: The ideal dimension of the nasolabial angle in men is 90–95°and in women is 95–105°(Figure 46.3B).
- *Columellar show*: The relationship between the ala and the columella is assessed in the lateral view. The amount of visible caudal septum is ideally limited to 3–5 mm (Figure 46.3B). This is the distance between two parallel lines drawn from the most anterior and the most posterior parts of the nasal vestibule. A degree of columellar show greater than this may be due to either a hanging columella or abnormalities in the alar margins such notching or retraction.
- *Basal view*: The width of the alar base approximates to the intercanthal distance. The ratio of the width of the dorsum of the nose relative to the alar base should be equal to 80%. From the basal view, the nose can also be divided into thirds. The upper third corresponds to the lobule and the lower two-thirds correspond to the columella. A line that transects the columella at the area of medial crural footplate diversion divides the base into two halves. The overall basal view outline conforms to an isosceles triangle with pear-shaped nostrils lying at a 45° angle to the vertical.

Inspection of the Internal Nose
Anterior rhinoscopy and nasal endoscopy should be performed.

- Septum inspection should be made, looking for deviation, spurs, perforation or the presence of a septal button.
- Lateral nasal wall and turbinate inspection can identify congestion, hypertrophy and asymmetry.

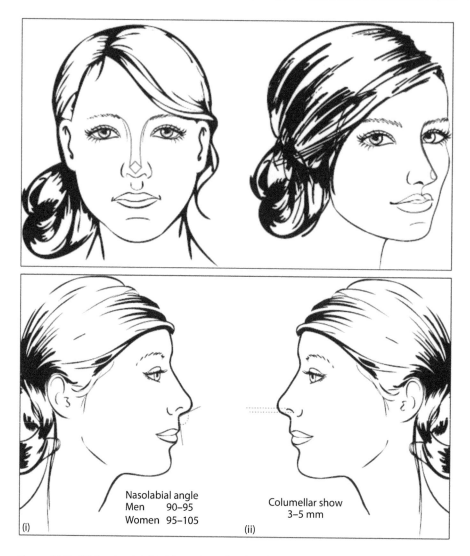

Nasolabial angle
Men   90–95
Women 95–105

Columellar show
3–5 mm

(i)   (ii)

Figure 46.3 (A) Front and right oblique views showing the brow-tip line. Note the four tip-defining points. (B) (i) Nasolabial angle in men and women. (ii) Normal columellar show.

- Internal nasal valve assessment should be carried out during normal quiet respiration at rest, as exaggerated effortful breathing is likely to precipitate transient internal nasal valve collapse in the normal individual.
- Cottle's manoeuvre of opening the internal nasal valve by pulling on the soft tissues of the cheek is non-specific. A better test is to place a Jobson Horne probe in the internal nasal valve to prevent the collapse of the upper lateral cartilage and detect its effect on inspiration.
- Alar collapse is a measure of external nasal valve collapse and must be identified pre-operatively.
- The external nasal valve is not a true valve and is identified by the area bounded by alar cartilages, septum and columella.
- Endoscopy can exclude polyps, purulent discharge or residual adenoidal tissue.

Palpation

- *Skin*: Palpate for an assessment of skin texture and elasticity.
- *Irregularities*: Palpate for underlying irregularities that may be due to skin, soft tissue, cartilage, bone or previous graft material.
- *Nasal bones*: Assess the size, position and presence of palpable steps.
- *Tip recoil*: This is an assessment of the strength of the lower third of the nose and provides a palpable measure of the degree of underlying tip support.
- *Alar cartridges*: Palpate for thickness, strength and shape.
- *Spine and septum*: Assess tip support, and confirm the presence and quantity of septal cartilage.

Photograph Review

Standardised photographs are essential for pre-operative planning. They guide preoperative discussion with the patient, act as an intraoperative reference and are essential for comparison with post-operative results. The standard photographic views obtained for rhinoplasty are frontal, left and right lateral, left and right oblique and basal.

Computer Imaging

Computer morphing of the pre-operative photographs has been found to enhance communication with the patient. However, it is essential to clarify to the patient that image manipulation is only a means of communication and does not imply a specific guaranteed outcome.

Conclusion

Following the systematic assessment and examination of the patient, the proposed surgery can be effectively planned with clear surgical steps. It is good practice to commit the surgical steps to a written plan.

KEY POINTS

- Rhinoplasty is a technically challenging procedure for which both the aesthetics and the function of the nose must be considered.
- Meticulous planning is essential to ensure the best surgical outcomes.

Successful surgery requires realistic patient expectations, careful consideration of facial aesthetics and a detailed examination of the nose.

---

47. RHINOPLASTY FOLLOWING NASAL TRAUMA

Introduction

Forty percent of facial fractures affect the nasal bones, and many of these involve damage to the nasal septum. External forces that are sufficient to cause a bony or cartilaginous deformity can also damage the overlying skin and soft-tissue envelope, commonly leading to a scar or contour abnormality.

A distinction should be made between childhood and adult fractures, as any injury in the growing nose will likely have consequences for future nasal development. Trauma can, of course, be superimposed on preexisting deformities, or in a patient who has had a previous rhinoplasty. In these cases, old photographs indicating pre-injury status are helpful.

Assessment

It should be clearly documented whether the primary issue is functional, aesthetic or both. The assessment and investigation should be carried out in a standardised approach. Firstly, external examination of each third of the nose is done looking for irregularity, asymmetry, deviation and skin injury followed by anterior and posterior rhinoscopy. Attention should be paid to the septum (septal haematoma, and septal displacement) and all levels of the nasal valve. In addition to standard clinical rhinoplasty photographs, a head-down photograph is useful.

Timing of Surgery

Primary Management of Trauma

Management of simple nasal fractures is outlined in Chapter 41.

In cases of an acute saddle nose deformity or complex nasoethmoidal fractures a post-trauma rhinoplasty should be undertaken in the acute or subacute period as septal collapse is difficult to restore later once scarring and fibrosis are established.

Lacerations to the skin over a compound fracture need to be closed primarily but may provide access enabling primary reduction of displaced nasal bones.

'The Missed Opportunity': Subacute

Where the nasal bony pyramid is displaced but the time from injury has passed that of closed manipulation, re-opening the partially healed fractures is necessary to remobilise the bony fragments allowing better realignment.

Post-Trauma Rhinoplasty

General Principles

The key is to create a stable dorsal line connected to the nasal bones, and then correct the position of the anterior and posterior angles, as these two important points determine the support of the tip cartilages, nostril shape and the columella–labial profile.

Wide exposure via the external approach with full septal dissection gives the best control to evaluate the deformity and to reconstruct, mostly with the use of grafts, such as local (septal cartilage), autologous (rib) or allogenic (cadaveric rib).

Rib cartilage can be difficult to use, and choosing the more horizontal sixth or seventh rib via the inframammary or direct approach gives a straighter graft. The goal is to harvest thin, stable and non-calcified cartilage grafts without significant warping.

With these grafts the septal framework (L-frame) can be repaired or a new L-shaped strut must be created. The most important fixation point of this framework is to the nasal spine (via drill hole or into periosteally), which should be midline. The dorsal and posterior cartilage needs to be secured to the residual dorsal septum or affixed to the perpendicular plate and nasal bones.

Upper Third

Deformities commonly involve the cartilage as well as the bone (upper laterals and septum). These deformities can be very difficult to correct by traditional osteotomies and need a different approach with a more controlled re-opening of the old fracture lines, sculpting and re-shaping of the bones by fine rasps or, better, by modern power tools or piezosurgery. The use of securing sutures through the bone and upper septum allows a more satisfactory repositioning than leaving flail segments with little control of how they heal.

Re-sculpting using modern power tools or piezo requires wide undermining via an open septorhinoplasty approach. Collapse or loss of the nasal bone does not occur when the internal periosteal lining is preserved. A significant advantage of using the piezo device is that it will not damage soft tissue. Pre-operative computed tomography (CT) facial bone scanning with three-dimensional (3D) reconstruction allows for more accurate planning.

Final contouring of defects or concavities can be performed with autologous tissue such as diced cartilage either as a paste, with a fascia wrap (diced cartilage wrapped in fascia [DCF]), or molded using a physiological glue (e.g. platelet-rich plasma [PRP]).

Middle Third

The middle-third support is important for the form and function of the nose as this is part of the complex area of the nasal valve.

This area needs to be tensioned between the attachments at the pyriform aperture and the dorsum to prevent dynamic collapse. The principle after adequate septal repair is to support the junctional roof. Spreader grafts are the mainstay of treatment here for the damaged nose and they can be placed according to the aesthetic and functional needs.

For conservation and re-orientation purposes a turn-in flap (spreader flap) can be used as well. Camouflaging techniques to correct the contour may also be considered.

Nasal Tip/Lower Third

Loss of cartilage (mainly septum and lower laterals) can produce multiple deformities in the tip, commonly with associated soft-tissue damage. Loss of tissue volume usually requires reconstruction with grafts, with ear cartilage being a good source.

With an undamaged envelope, tip repair can be achieved by endonasal techniques, but with a more complex problem, the open approach permits wide exposure, release of contractions and accurate repair or grafting.

Commonly used grafts of cartilage are strut or septal extension grafts between the medial crura, shield and cap grafts, rim grafts for nostril sidewall stability and lateral crural grafts, either to augment or to replace a lost framework.

The Skin Envelope

Probably the most frequently traumatised area is at the rhinion where the skin is thinnest. Lacerations should be cleaned, dressed or sutured primarily to prevent tattooing. Adequate sun protection of scars, moisturising, massaging and use of silicone gel daily all contribute to good cosmetic scar result.

In thin, damaged skin and severe subcutaneous tissue loss, fat grafting to the nose can be considered and camouflaging the dorsum skeleton at the time of surgery may be achieved by using autologous temporalis fascia, perichondrium from rib or rectus abdominis fascia and PRP and nanofat injections.

Nasal Trauma and Children

Children's nasal injuries are common and have the potential to disrupt normal growth, particularly with loss of septal cartilage, as happens with a septal abscess.

In general, it is best to defer surgery at least until after puberty and as close to maturity as possible. This deformity increases with age and it can be difficult to resist pressure to operate early before nasal maturity. The timing is variable between sexes and in individuals. Osteotomies do not disturb growth of the nose but damage to the growth centres in the septal cartilage does. The patient's parents need to be warned of a possible second operation when growth has stopped.

Where a saddle occurs, replacement by autologous cartilage is preferred as continued growth may then occur.

KEY POINTS

- Childhood injuries need to be monitored to assess growth.
- Acute saddles require early surgical intervention to restore septal height.
- Cartilage-depleted noses may need rib grafts for reconstruction.
- Secondary procedures are common in the repair of damaged noses.

48. EXTERNAL RHINOPLASTY

Introduction
The external approach is a valuable part of the armamentarium of the rhinoplasty surgeon, offering clear exposure of anatomical deformities, easier bimanual sculpturing, precise graft placement and suturing and excellent teaching opportunities. We present external rhinoplasty principles, anatomy, techniques and extended applications.

Indications
Thorough pre-operative assessment of nasal deformities is key in approach selection. External approach indications include:

- Extensive revision surgery
- Severe trauma
- Elaborate reduction and augmentation
- Tip deformities or rotation
- Extreme over projection correction
- Congenital deformities such as the cleft lip nose

Extended applications include septal perforation repair, nasal dermoid excision and even as a hypophysectomy approach.

Principles of External Rhinoplasty
External or open rhinoplasty, also known as the transcolumellar incision or decortication technique, exposes upper and lower lateral cartilages to the nasofrontal angle, in their undisturbed positions. Correct incision placement and meticulous wound closure is essential. A mid-columella incision is connected to bilateral marginal incisions. Subsequent subperichondrial and subperiosteal dissection, leaving as much soft tissue as possible on the skin flap, preserves its viability.

Division of medial intercrural tissue and the upper lateral cartilage from the quadrilateral cartilage exposes the whole septum and premaxillary spine, allowing treatment of nasal valve problems, dorsal septal deviations and septal perforation repair. The external approach avoids intercartilaginous incisions, thus preserving the valve area. Some minor tip support mechanisms are disrupted, including the lower lateral cartilage soft tissue envelope and medial intercrural ligamentous tissue, which can result in some tip ptosis.

Surgical Technique

Incisions
Common transcolumellar incisions include the step, gullwing and preferably an inverted V, placed above the medial crural footplates, ensuring adequate support and an inconspicuous scar (Figure 48.1a). An initial superficial columellar incision is made to protect the medial crura just beneath. Vertical marginal columellar incisions placed 1.5–2 mm inside the vestibule are joined by careful undermining of the columella skin with scissors, against which the columella incision is completed. The marginal incision is extended until halfway along the lateral crus, by spreading angled Converse/Walter scissors and cutting overlying soft tissue, hugging the caudal edge. (Figure 48.1b–d).

Dissection of the Soft Tissue Envelope
Subperichondrial domal dissection minimises supratip oedema, a pollybeak deformity and bleeding complications. Dissection continues laterally to the hinge area, hugging the lower lateral cartilage, extending cephalically to the scroll area (Figure 48.1e). Midline inter-domal dissection toward the cartilaginous vault avoids a false passage into superficial

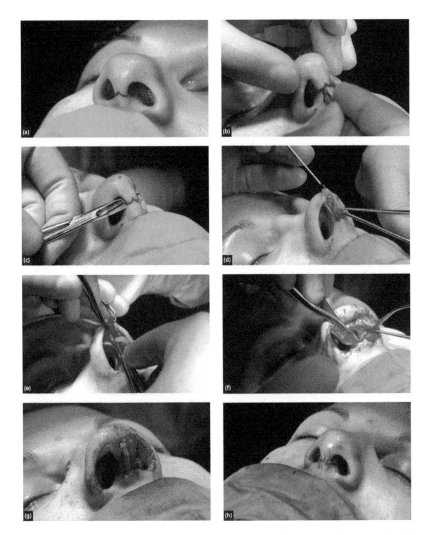

Figure 48.1 External rhinoplasty approach to correct an under projected, asymmetric bulbous tip. (a) Mid-columella inverted-V incision. (b) Superficial incision made through the columella skin. (c) Iris scissors placed behind the incision to protect medial crura. (d) Exposure of the medial crura with development of the columella skin flap. (e) Dissection over the nasal domes with converse scissors. (f) Exposure of the caudal septal cartilage by dissection between medial crura. (g) Columella strut placed between medial crura. (h) Closure of incision after correction of boxy tip deformity.

musculoaponeurotic system (SMAS) tissue. Thick supratip soft tissue can be conservatively thinned, minimising skin vascular compromise.

Dissect the bony pyramid subperiosteally by palpating and incising just above the caudal nasal bones, preventing separation of the upper lateral cartilage from the bony pyramid.

Septal access by medial crura division is preferable (Figure 48.1f). Alternative options include a separate hemitransfixion or Killian's incision. A columella strut in a pocket between medial crura aids tip projection. It extends from 2 mm above the anterior nasal spine to no higher than the angle between the medial and intermediate crura, to preserve the columella-lobular ('double-break') angle. Temporary fixation of medial crura with a needle minimises dome height asymmetry, while fixating with mattress sutures.

Preliminary closure of the columella incision allows final assessment of the supratip area and tip projection, enabling reduction of the cartilage vault or addition of tip onlay or shield grafts (Figure 48.1g). Check overlying soft tissue viability, to prevent skin necrosis.

Incision Closure

Meticulous closure ensures a smooth columella skin line (Figure 48.1h) We prefer a fine absorbable or non-absorbable suture material (6-0 Ethilon, Vicryl Rapide or Prolene), with slight eversion of wound edges. Non-dissolvable sutures are removed 5–7 days postoperatively.

Specific Applications

The Bony Pyramid

Subperiosteal dissection extends halfway along the nasal bones before bony de-humping and lateral, medial and intermediate osteotomies. The open approach allows direct correction of dorsal irregularities.

The Middle Nasal Vault

The internal valve is the smallest area of the nasal airway, bounded by the caudal end of the upper lateral cartilage, inferior turbinate, floor of the nose and septum. In patients with short nasal bones, high bony cartilaginous humps or weak upper lateral cartilages, spreader grafts broaden the valve and prevent a 'pinched' middle third. External rhinoplasty facilitates spreader graft fixation, roof reconstruction and straightening a dorsally deviated septum.

Nasal Tip

Open rhinoplasty exposes the tip in its natural position, facilitating cartilage manipulation and graft fixation. Manipulating the tripod legs (two lateral crura and conjoined medial crura), alters tip projection and rotation. For example, the lateral crural steal enhances tip projection by freeing and medialising the lateral crus from the vestibule skin. Vertical dome division increases the central leg of the tripod, whereas inter-domal sutures can help correct a bifid tip. Other techniques include the columella strut and tongue in groove.

The open approach facilitates tip deprojection, through precise excision of septal cartilage and anterior spine. Techniques include lower lateral cartilage lateral crus volume reduction (complete strip), a complete transfixion incision (separating the paired medial crura from the caudal spine), complete strip procedure and reducing the nasal septum.

Revision Rhinoplasty

External rhinoplasty facilitates precise diagnosis, structural grafting and scar tissue excision. Indications include inadequate or overzealous primary surgery, loss of contour and support.

The Deviated Nose

External rhinoplasty aids bony hump removal in the deviated nose, allowing alteration of the osteotome plane under direct vision. For right-sided deviation, mobilise the left nasal bone, then the bony septum and finally the right nasal bone.

Deviation of the lower two-thirds following septoplasty is often due to dorsal septal deviation and by previously disrupting the septal-upper lateral join. Where mild, shave the convex side, suture to upper laterals and crosshatch the concavity. If severe, a unilateral spreader graft opens the nasal valve, with an onlay graft for residual deviation.

The Tension Nose

Quadrilateral nasal septal overgrowth causes a 'tension nose' with a high nasal dorsum, narrow vault, long anterior nasal spine and stretched overlying skin. Lower lateral cartilages are pushed forward and downward, blunting the nasolabial angle and shortening the upper lip.

Extended Applications

The external approach facilitates large septal perforation repair by exposing the entire septum and excision of nasal dermoids by avoiding poor cosmesis associated with a vertical midline scar.

Conclusions

The external approach is essential for the rhinoplasty surgeon, enabling binocular vision, bimanual manipulation and graft fixation. Precise columella incision, correct dissection and meticulous suturing minimises sequelae, such as prolonged supratip oedema and pronounced transcolumellar scars. Relative disadvantages of increased operating time and difficulty of dorsal assessment are minor and improve with surgical experience.

KEY POINTS

- External rhinoplasty provides unparalleled nasal skeleton exposure, enhanced diagnosis and correction of deformities.
- It is valuable in tip surgery and for precise placement of grafts and sutures
- Reconstitution of tip support with a columellar strut is often required.
- The broken transcolumellar incision gives excellent cosmesis.

49. COSMETIC FACIAL INTERVENTIONS

Blepharoplasty

The term blepharoplasty refers to the modification of the eyelid aesthetics, while maintaining function. Tissues including the skin, orbicularis oculi muscle, septum and fat are variably are excised or repositioned depending on the anatomical defects and desired aesthetic outcome. The indications may be functional, aesthetic or often a combination of both.

In the upper lid skin excess (dermatochalasis), in the early stages it obliterates the natural skin crease, and when advanced results in visual field defects (peripheral in particular) as well as aesthetic changes. In the lower eyelid generally, the aesthetic concerns relate to fat prolapse, resulting in bags under the eyes and elongation of the eyelids, imparting tired a look.

These changes are related to aging with laxity of the periorbital ligaments and skin leading to skin redundancy, changes in the orbicularis muscle (both attenuation and hypertrophy), as well as weakening of the orbital septum that is responsible for holding orbital fat in its anatomical locations. A thorough understanding of the surgical anatomy of the eyebrows, eyelids and mid-face is essential prior to performing a blepharoplasty.

Pre-operative planning should include accurate documentation of patient concerns, medical photographs, a complete ophthalmic assessment and a plan to define and alleviate the anatomical cause of the eyelid abnormality, and an informed discussion. Any additional procedures that may be required such as repositioning of the lacrimal gland, correcting the brow ptosis and lateral canthal procedures should be discussed. Surgery may be carried out under local anaesthetic with sedation or general anaesthetic.

Important surgical references for upper eyelid blepharoplasty include (Figure 49.1):

- Any eyelid ptosis or brow ptosis should be addressed.
- A minimum distance of 7–8 mm should be left between lid margin and the upper eyelid skin crease and approximately 22–25 mm of skin between the inferior aspect of the eyebrow and the eyelid margin.
- The upper eyelid skin crease represents the most superior point of attachment between the skin and the levator aponeurosis. This position is just inferior to the insertion of

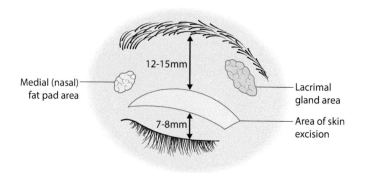

Figure 49.1 Upper lid blepharoplasty surgical markings. A minimum distance of 7–8mm should be left between lid margin and the upper eyelid skin crease; 12–15mm should be left between the inferior aspect of the eyebrow and the upper eyelid skin crease.

the orbital septum onto the levator aponeurosis. The skin crease lies at a higher level in females, approximately 7–8 mm from the lash line, compared with 5–6 mm in males. It is important not to raise the skin crease in males to avoid a 'feminisation' of the eyelid appearance.

In general, the removal of fat from the upper eyelid should be avoided or restricted to the medial fat compartment to prevent 'hollowing' of the eyelid that post-operatively manifests a 'cadaveric' appearance, which is not easily amenable to correction. Other anomalies include a prolapsed lacrimal gland, which can be repositioned by suturing the capsule of the lacrimal gland to the inner aspect of the periosteum of the lacrimal fossa. Rare anomalies such as a prominent supra-orbital rim can be reduced by drilling.

In the lower eyelid the focus is on either excision or re-draping of the prolapsed fat, tightening the orbital septum and, rarely, skin excision in the lateral aspect of the lower eyelid, which is kept to the minimum.

It is important to recognise when a blepharoplasty is inappropriate. This includes risk factors that expose a patient to exposure keratopathy, namely a history of contact lens wear, previous corneal laser refractive surgery, dry eye, facial palsy or thyroid dysfunction (which causes thickening of the subcutaneous region). Postmenopausal women should be specifically warned of the temporary risk of dry eyes immediately post-operatively (which may last weeks). Serious complications include orbital hemorrhage (0.05%) or a retrobulbar hematoma, which may present as severe pain, and result in disrupted cosmesis and/or blindness (which is a surgical emergency).

Non-surgical interventions, such as a chemical brow lift using botulinum toxin in the glabellar area and lateral/superolateral orbital rim, may achieve a 3-mm lift.

Surgical Rejuvenation of the Aging Face

A rhytidectomy (facelift) is an operation that corrects the visible signs of aging primarily in the lower two-thirds of the face and upper neck. This includes redundant facial skin and deep rhytids, jowling or loss of a well-defined mandibular border and improvement of prominent nasolabial folds. Extrinsic aging derives mainly from solar ultraviolet radiation (photoaging), which damages the DNA, and smoking. Skeletal deflation results in poor ligamentous support, resulting in tissue sagging exaggerated by gravity.

Patients should be counselled that rhytidectomy is not effective for superficial rhytids resulting from solar damage or minor depressions secondary to acne scarring. Adjunctive techniques, such as laser resurfacing/dermabrasion/radiofrequency/platelet-rich plasma (PRP) therapy are indicated. A healthy lifestyle should be advocated to maintain the results in the long term.

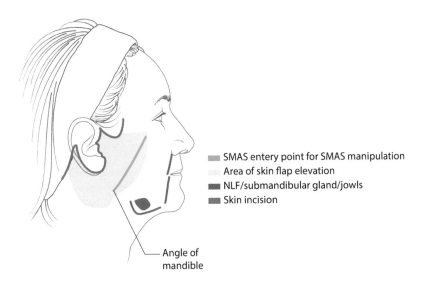

SMAS entery point for SMAS manipulation
Area of skin flap elevation
NLF/submandibular gland/jowls
Skin incision

Angle of
mandible

Figure 49.2 Rhytidectomy surgical principles including the skin incision, area of skin flap elevation and elevation of SMAS flap below the zygomatic arch (ensuring that the frontal, marginal and
greater auricular and buccal nerves are protected), SMAS manipulation (plication, imbrication, or
combination of techniques) and skin re-draping without tension on the suture lines.

The major limitation of facelift surgery is related to the sagging of tissues in the submental
area, and prominence of the submandibular glands.

Good surgical candidates are those who have a strong bony architecture defined by a well-
defined mandible and high hyoid, with good facial soft tissue volume, and skin elasticity.

Pre-operatively, evaluate the patient's skin type (Glogau classification) and note any significant skin pathology. Beware supplements such as vitamin E, Ginkgo biloba and garlic can
also increase bleeding. Patients must stop smoking cigarettes 3–4 weeks before surgery to
avoid vascular compromise, necrosis of skin flaps and skin sloughing post-rhytidectomy.
Pre-operative photographs are essential to aid planning, and medicolegal defence, with standardised full-face frontal, lateral and oblique views.

The surgical principles of rhytidectomy include (Figure 49.2):

- Incision placement is critical to help hide incisions and avoid altering the hairline.
- Post-tragal facelift incision (most female patients).
- Pre-tragal incision (males).

Patient should be marked pre-operatively including incision, area of jowling, submandibular
bulge, nasolabial folds, platysmal banding, surface anatomy of greater auricular and frontal
and marginal mandibular nerves.

Inadequate volume in the face may be addressed by autologous fat transfer intra-operatively,
and with careful planning neck fat may be transferred. Alternatively, fat from of other areas
of the body may be harvested. Other options include injections of appropriate fillers.

The surgical steps include:

- Infiltration with local anaesthetic.
- Elevation of the skin flap.
- Elevation of the superficial musculoaponeurotic system (SMAS) flap, ensuring that
  the frontal, marginal and greater auricular and buccal nerves are protected.
- SMAS manipulation (plication, imbrication or combination of techniques).
- Skin re-draping without tension on the suture lines.

- If there is significant submental laxity, a midline platysmaplasty is performed.
- Liposuction is restricted to the neck and along the lower border of the mandible ensuring any fat in the face is preserved.
- Closure may include surgical drains, use of fibrin glue (under the skin flap) or other techniques to minimise bleeding.
- A full bandage is applied covering the head and the neck.

Complications include:

- Bleeding.
- Haematoma formation (incidence 4%):
  - Small, non-expanding haematomas after 24 hours may be amenable to aspiration or drainage (by opening the existing incision), followed by a pressure dressing.
  - Expanding haematoma constitutes a surgical emergency, requiring immediate wound exploration and clot evaluation.
- Temporary nerve paralysis.
- Permanent nerve paralysis (rare, 0.1%): the most injured nerve is the great auricular nerve, followed by the marginal, buccal and frontal nerves.
- Pixie ear deformity results from improper incision placement around the lobule and/or tension in the suture line because of overzealous skin flap excision, which can be avoided by preventing any excess tension on the lobule.

Patients should be advised of the expected post-operative discourse in which pain becomes more intense after 24 hours but settles within 72 hours. Oedema resolves over several weeks and facial contour stabilises at approximately 4–6 weeks after surgery. Erythema of the incision should fade over several months.

Non-Surgical Rejuvenation of the Aging Face

Non-surgical rejuvenation is gaining popularity because of minimal downtime, less expense and acceptable results. Though the field of anti-aging and facial rejuvenation is advancing rapidly with new information and new therapies, the basic principles remain the same. These include skin care with pharmaceutical and cosmeceuticals used on a daily basis; periodic use of Botulin toxins and fillers; and in some cases more invasive treatments such as chemical peels, heat technology (such as laser, radiofrequency or their variations) and plasma therapy. As new technologies evolve, our goal should be focused on the patient, honesty and achieving a balanced look, which may be part of an overall programme of health and self-improvement. Often this is achieved by a combination of tools.

Prescription topical retinoids form the cornerstone of any topical rejuvenation plan. They act on retinoic acid receptors (RARs) and the retinoid X receptors (RXRs), which are receptors found in all cells, targeting keratinocytes and melanocytes in the epidermis and fibroblasts in the dermis. This leads to epidermal hyperplasia and impaction of the stratum corneum (producing smoother skin with a 'glow'); increased dermal collagen type I, III and VII synthesis; reduced collagen breakdown and normalisation of elastic tissue organisation (improving coarse wrinkling and crepe-like skin texture) and a reduction in melanin synthesis.

Tretinoin and retinaldehyde are the most studied agents. Retinaldehyde is a precursor that is oxidised into the active product retinoic acid (tretinoin commercially). Tretinoin is more irritating, but more effective than retinaldehyde, although large-scale randomised controlled trials (RCTs) are lacking. The rate of this conversion is variable, making it difficult to calibrate the concentration of retinaldehyde required to get the best outcome. Thus, many aesthetic practitioners use tretinoin rather than retinaldehyde in clinical practice. The senior author prescribing regimen starts with 0.025%, building up to 0.1% used at varying intervals. The dose is titrated relative to results versus side effects of the patient. Aesthetic patients generally want results and do tolerate the short-term side effects, learning to find their 'optimal' dose.

Botulinum toxin type A (BTX-A) is a zinc-dependent endopeptidase produced by *Clostridium botulinum*. It acts on cholinergic nerve endings to produce muscle paresis that lasts for around 3 months, and then starts to wear off. When the muscle relaxes, it stops pulling on the skin and the wrinkle caused by the muscle pull fades away. Botulinum toxin has been the most revolutionary anti-aging treatment in recent years. It has an excellent safety profile and has been used extensively for facial rejuvenation with a focus on hyperkinetic wrinkles. It is also used in the dysfunctional paralyzed face to improve facial symmetry or in the scarred face to improve dermal contour with the use of fillers. Generally, an appropriate amount of Botulinum toxin is injected and the patient is reviewed after 2 weeks for further injections if required. This helps to avoid creating an unnatural appearance and a frozen face. Botulinum toxin is contraindicated in patients with underlying neuromuscular junction disorder, allergy to any of its components (human albumin, botulinum toxin), pregnancy and breastfeeding.

Fillers represent products that are inserted into different skin layers to improve angles, lines, folds, scars and flaccidity. The idea is to replace an original volume lost by the aging process or to create volume. Fillers can be temporary or permanent. Although hyaluronic acid is safe, it binds up to one thousand times its weight in water forming a viscous quality similar to 'jelly' that causes an overinflated look. The newer generation biodegradable polycaprolactone-based collagen stimulators restore volume and redefine contours in a more natural way. Severe but rare complications of fillers include undesired aesthetic result, skin necrosis and blindness (which is a surgical emergency). These should be mentioned in the consenting process. Generally, we recommend avoiding the use of permanent fillers, which have additional complications of long-term damage, inflammation, infection and extrusion.

Chemical peeling is the topical application of chemical agents to cause controlled destruction of part or all the epidermis, with or without dermal injury. This leads to desquamation, liquefaction and coagulation of the affected layers, followed by inflammation, and finally regeneration of epidermal and dermal tissues. Indications for chemical peeling include fine lines and wrinkles, pigmentation disorders such as solar lentigines and melasma, superficial acne scars and benign epidermal growths.

KEY POINTS

- Thorough understanding of the surgical anatomy is essential prior to performing a blepharoplasty:
  - Distance between the inferior aspect of eyebrow and the upper lid skin crease on downgaze is two-thirds the distance from the inferior aspect of the eyebrow to eyelid margin.
  - Minimum of 10–12mm should be left between the inferior aspect of the eyebrow and the upper eyelid skin crease in upper lid blepharoplasty.
  - Whitnall's ligament supports the levator muscle complex, hence damage must be prevented.
- Sun damage to the skin, atrophy of tissues and the effects of gravity bring on the changes seen in the aging face patient.
- Facial fat injection is a valuable adjunct to aging face surgery, facial.
- Tretinoin has been shown to be most effective in photographing. Its irritational side effects are reduced by starting a regimen at lower doses and building up to higher doses at varying intervals.
- Newer generation polycaprolactone-based collagen stimulators restore volume and redefine contours in a more natural way.
- Regenerative surgical techniques may enhance graft survival and improve the quality of damaged skin.

HEAD AND NECK

50. SURGICAL ANATOMY OF THE NECK

Embryology

Branchial Arches

The branchial arches emerge at the fourth week of gestation. Each arch has its own nerve, cartilage and artery. The fifth arch obliterates after all the branchial arches become apparent. Between the arches sit internal pouches (lined with endoderm) and external clefts (lined with ectoderm).

Fascia: Anatomy

The neck has superficial and deep fascial planes encasing the structures of the neck. The superficial fascia invests the platysma muscle.

The investing layer of deep fascia forms a cylinder draping most of the structures of the neck. It encloses the sternocleidomastoid, omohyoid, infrahyoid and trapezius muscles, and the parotid gland.

The carotid sheath encloses the common carotid artery, the internal and external carotid arteries, the internal jugular vein and the vagus nerve.

The pretracheal layer has two parts: the muscular encasing the infrahyoid muscles and the visceral containing the trachea, the thyroid gland, the pharynx and upper oesophagus.

The prevertebral fascia encompasses the posterior neck muscles, the scalenes and the vertebrae. The alar fascia is a layer of fascia anterior to the prevertebral fascia, extending from the skull base to level of second thoracic vertebra.

Neck Spaces

Compartments lie between the fascial layers, normally containing loose areolar tissue only. The submandibular, parapharyngeal and retropharyngeal spaces are described further, other spaces include the submental, peritonsillar, prevertebral, carotid, parotid and visceral.

Submandibular Space

The superior limit is the mucosa of the floor of the mouth, the inferior is the investing fascia from the mandible to the hyoid. The anterior and posterior bellies of the digastric muscle form the anteroinferior and posteroinferior boundaries. The mylohyoid muscle divides it into superior and inferior compartments, which communicate around the posterior edge.

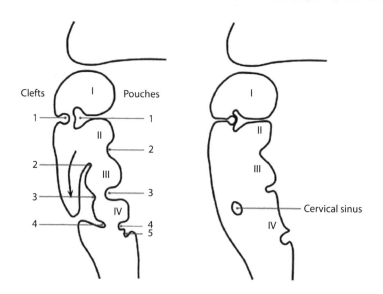

Figure 50.1   Diagram of the branchial apparatus.

Parapharyngeal Space

This inverted pyramid-shaped space extends from the skull base to the hyoid. It is bounded by the superior constrictor muscle medially and pterygoid muscles, the parotid gland and the mandible laterally. The styloid process and its attachments divide it into pre-styloid and post-styloid compartments.

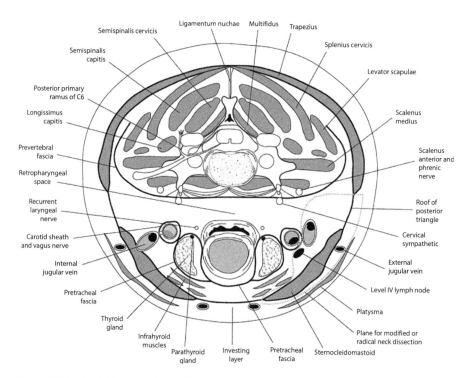

Figure 50.2   Fascial layers of the neck.

Table 50.1 Branchial derivatives

Arch	Nerve	Cartilage	Muscle	Artery	Internal pouch	External cleft
1. Mandibular arch	Trigeminal (mandibular branch V3)	Meckel's cartilage: mandible; malleus head and neck; incus body and short process; hillocks of His 1 (tragus), 2 (helical crus) and 3 (helix)	Mylohyoid, anterior digastric, muscles of mastication, tensor tympani, tensor veli palatini	1st aortic arch: maxillary artery	Eustachian tube, middle ear cleft, medial surface of tympanic membrane	External auditory meatus, lateral surface of tympanic membrane
2. Hyoid arch	Facial	Reichart's: lesser cornu + upper body of hyoid, long process of incus, stapes superstructure, styloid process, hillocks of His 4 (antihelix crus), 5 (antitragus, scapha), 6 (lobule)	Muscles of facial expression, posterior belly of digastric, platysma, stapedius	2nd aortic arch: stapedial artery	Palatine tonsil	Grows over remaining grooves
3.	Glossopharyngeal	Greater cornu + lower body of hyoid	Stylopharyngeus superior and middle constrictor	3rd aortic arch: common carotid artery	Inferior parathyroid glands, thymic duct	Obliterated
4.	Vagus–superior laryngeal nerve	Thyroid lamina	Cricothyroid	4th aortic arch: aorta on left, subclavian artery on right	Superior parathyroid glands	Obliterated
6.	Vagus–recurrent laryngeal nerve	Cricoid, arytenoid cartilages	Inferior constrictor, intrinsic muscles of larynx	6th aortic arch: ductus arteriosus and pulmonary artery	Ultimobrachial body (forms parafollicular C cells of thyroid)	Obliterated

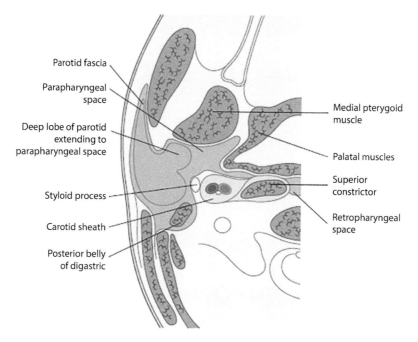

Figure 50.3   Parapharyngeal space.

Retropharyngeal Space

Connecting the two parapharyngeal spaces is the retropharyngeal space. It extends from the skull base to the level of the carina. The anterior boundary is the buccopharyngeal fascia, the posterior boundary is the alar fascia.

The 'danger space' lies posterior to the retropharyngeal space, between the alar and the prevertebral fascia, extending to the level of the diaphragm.

Cervical Lymphatics

Level I: Level Ia is the single midline zone between the two anterior bellies of digastric and the hyoid. Ib lies between the anterior and posterior bellies of the digastric muscle and the mandible.

Level II: Extends from the skull base to the level of the inferior border of the hyoid bone. The accessory nerve subdivides into IIa and IIb.

Level III: Extends from the level of the inferior border of the hyoid to the inferior aspect of the cricoid cartilage.

Level IV: This zone extends from the level of the inferior border of the cricoid to the clavicle.

Level V: Extends from a superior apex formed by the junction of the trapezius and sternocleidomastoid muscles to the clavicle inferiorly. The anterior limit is the posterior border of the sternocleidomastoid and the posterior limit is the anterior border of trapezius. Subdivided into Va and Vb at the level of the inferior border of the cricoid.

Level VI: Another single midline zone between the common carotid arteries laterally, from the inferior aspect of the hyoid down to the innominate artery.

Important Nerves

The Facial Nerve

The facial nerve's main function is motor innervation to the muscles of facial expression. It also provides motor supply to the posterior belly of digastric and the stylohyoid. The trunk of the nerve exits the temporal bone via the stylomastoid foramen. It traverses the parotid

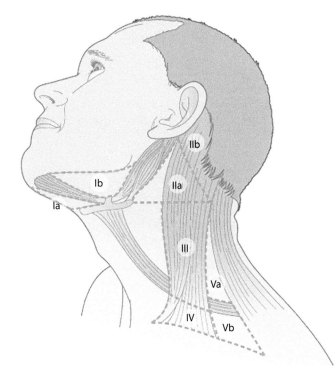

Figure 50.4   Lymph node zones and subzones.

gland, dividing into five main branches. Known as the 'pes anserinus', these branches are the temporal, zygomatic, buccal, marginal mandibular and cervical.

Glossopharyngeal Nerve
The glossopharyngeal nerve exits the skull via the anterior jugular foramen, passing between the internal jugular vein and the internal carotid artery. It curves around the stylopharyngeus muscle, deep to hyoglossus and enters the constrictor muscles. Fibres are distributed to the tonsil, pharynx, posterior tongue and minor salivary glands of the oral mucosa and oropharynx.

Vagus Nerve
The vagus nerve leaves the skull via the middle compartment of the jugular foramen. The nerve runs posteriorly in the carotid sheath, between the internal jugular vein and common carotid artery. The vagus nerve gives off the following branches in the neck: auricular branch (Arnold's nerve), carotid body branches, pharyngeal branch, superior laryngeal nerve, cardiac branches, and the recurrent laryngeal nerve.

The left recurrent laryngeal nerve leaves the vagus and loops around the ligamentum arteriosum and arch of the aorta before ascending in the tracheo-oesophageal groove. The right recurrent laryngeal has a more variable path but usually hooks around the subclavian artery before passing medially toward the tracheo-oesophageal groove. The right nerve is non-recurrent in 1% of people.

Spinal Accessory Nerve
The nerve exits the skull via the middle compartment of the jugular foramen. It passes deep to the posterior belly of the digastric, then crosses level II, penetrating the sternocleidomastoid muscle, which it supplies. It usually leaves the posterior aspect of the muscle one centimetre above Erb's point, where the cervical plexus branches emerge, before running across

level V. This is variable and the nerve may not pass through the muscle. The nerve enters the deep surface of the trapezius at the junction of its lower and middle third.

Hypoglossal Nerve

The hypoglossal nerve provides motor innervation to the intrinsic muscles of the tongue and all extrinsic muscles except the palatoglossus. It exits the skull via the hypoglossal canal, and runs deep to the internal jugular vein. It curves around the carotid bifurcation as it heads anteriorly, passing inferior to the greater horn of the hyoid before coursing superiorly.

Salivary Glands

Parotid Glands

The parotid glands are the largest salivary glands. They extend from the zygomatic arch superiorly to the upper part of the neck inferiorly. Medially, they fill the gap between the mandible and the mastoid. They extend close to the lateral wall of the oropharynx. The anatomy of the facial nerve is described above. The nerve divides the gland into superficial (80%) and deep (20%) lobes. The nerve lies superficial to the retromandibular vein. The parotid duct (of Stensen) originates within the gland; it emerges from the anterior border of the parotid gland, turning medially at the anterior border of the masseter, before entering the oral cavity opposite the second upper molar.

Submandibular Glands

These are the second largest salivary glands. They lie in the submandibular triangle formed by the anterior and posterior bellies of the digastric and the margin of the mandible, and wrap around the posterior border of mylohyoid. The facial artery enters or grooves the gland posteriorly.

The gland's fibrous capsule is crossed by the facial vein, and the marginal mandibular branch of the facial nerve.

The submandibular duct emerges from the medial surface of the superficial part of the gland; the lingual nerve begins anteromedial to the duct but crosses underneath to continue posterolaterally.

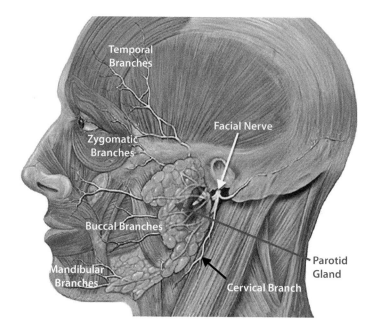

Figure 50.5   Anatomy of the parotid gland.

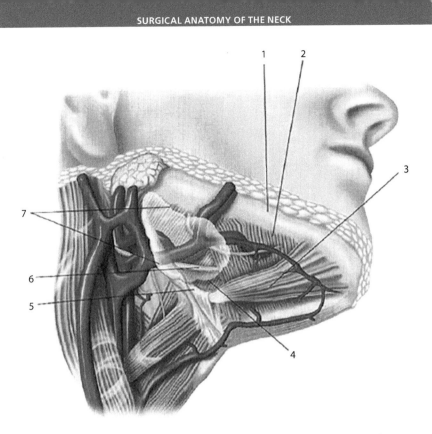

Figure 50.6 Submandibular glands. 1. Mandible. 2. Mylohyoid. 3. Anterior belly of digastric. 4. Submandibular gland. 5. Hyoid. 6. Hypoglossal nerve. 7. Facial artery.

Sublingual Glands

The sublingual glands are the smallest of the named salivary glands and have no true capsule. They lie beneath the mucosa of the floor of the mouth. There is no dominant duct drainage; most of the small excretory ducts open directly on the summit of the sublingual fold, but some may open into the submandibular duct.

The Pharynx

Anatomically, the pharynx is divided into distinctive subdivisions: the nasopharynx, the oropharynx and the hypopharynx.

The boundaries of the nasopharynx are the two posterior nasal apertures (anteriorly), the sloping inferior body of the sphenoid bone and the occipital bone (posterosuperiorly), the soft palate (inferiorly) and the superior constrictor muscle (posterolaterally).

The clinical boundaries of the oropharynx are a horizontal line drawn at the level of the hard palate (superiorly), a horizontal line drawn through the floor of the valleculae (inferiorly) and a vertical plane defined by anterior boundary of the palatoglossal folds (anteriorly).

The boundaries of the hypopharynx are the level of the hyoid bone (superiorly) and the lower margin of the cricoid cartilage (inferiorly). The missing anterior segment corresponds to the laryngeal inlet.

Pharyngeal Muscles

The pharyngeal muscular wall is relatively thin and comprises three circular constrictor muscles. They are assisted by three longitudinal muscles, which act as elevators and dilators. The constrictors sit within each other like three stacked cups and overlap on their posterior aspect.

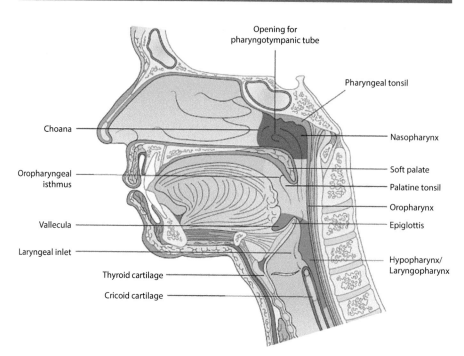

Figure 50.7   Sagittal section of the head and neck.

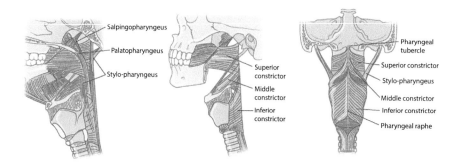

Figure 50.8   Muscles of the pharynx. Left, sagittal section. Middle, lateral view. Right, posterior view.

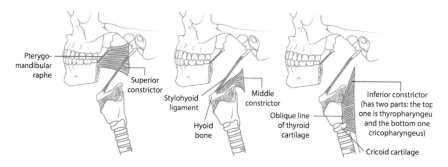

Figure 50.9   Attachments of the constrictor muscles of the pharynx. Left, superior constrictor. Middle, middle constrictor. Right, inferior constrictor.

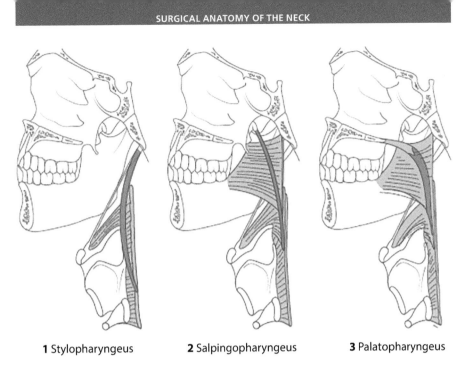

1 Stylopharyngeus   **2** Salpingopharyngeus   **3** Palatopharyngeus

Figure 50.10   Attachments of the longitudinal muscles of the pharynx. 1, Stylopharyngeus. 2, Salpingopharyngeus. 3, Palatopharyngeus.

The Larynx

The supraglottis commences at the epiglottis and aryepiglottic folds. Its lower border is a horizontal line drawn through the apex of the laryngeal ventricle. The glottis extends caudally from this line and includes the vocal cords. The line of demarcation between the glottis and the subglottis is a line drawn 1cm below the free edge of the vocal fold. The subglottis becomes the trachea at the lower border of the cricoid.

The framework of the larynx consists of the hyoid bone, and the thyroid, cricoid, epiglottic, arytenoid, corniculate and cuneiform cartilages.

The intrinsic ligaments of the larynx connect the cartilages together and form an internal framework. The conus elasticus attaches to the upper border of the cricoid and is stretched between the inner surface of the thyroid cartilage anteriorly and the vocal process of the arytenoid behind. The free upper border of this membrane is the vocal ligament.

Muscles of the Larynx

The extrinsic muscles attach the larynx to neighboring structures and maintain the position of the larynx.

The intrinsic muscles are paired and the majority act to move the arytenoid at the cricoarytenoid joint. The posterior cricoarytenoid is the only abductor of the larynx.

The cricothyroid muscle does not insert into the arytenoid cartilages; it brings the thyroid and cricoid cartilages closer together in a visor-like motion and therefore stretches the vocal folds.

All the intrinsic muscles of the larynx are supplied by the recurrent laryngeal nerve, except the cricothyroid, which is supplied by the external branch of the superior laryngeal nerve.

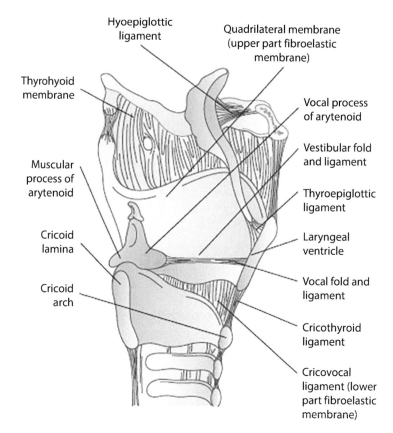

Hyoepiglottic ligament

Quadrilateral membrane (upper part fibroelastic membrane)

Thyrohyoid membrane

Vocal process of arytenoid

Muscular process of arytenoid

Vestibular fold and ligament

Cricoid lamina

Thyroepiglottic ligament

Cricoid arch

Laryngeal ventricle

Vocal fold and ligament

Cricothyroid ligament

Cricovocal ligament (lower part fibroelastic membrane)

Figure 50.11 Sagittal section across the larynx looking laterally.

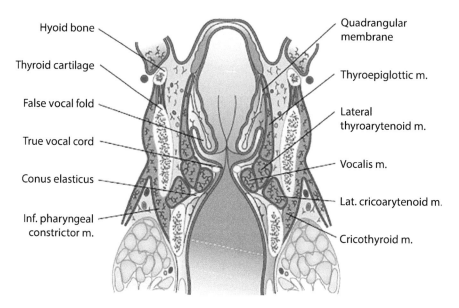

Hyoid bone

Quadrangular membrane

Thyroid cartilage

Thyroepiglottic m.

False vocal fold

Lateral thyroarytenoid m.

True vocal cord

Vocalis m.

Conus elasticus

Lat. cricoarytenoid m.

Inf. pharyngeal constrictor m.

Cricothyroid m.

Figure 50.12 Coronal section through the larynx looking anteriorly.

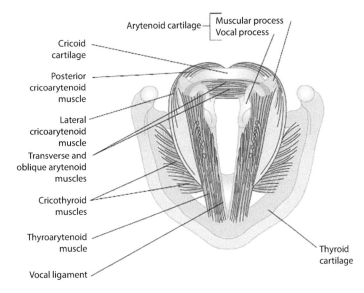

Figure 50.13 Dissected view of the larynx from above.

The vocal folds have a superficial squamous epithelium, beneath which is the lamina propria. This has three distinct layers. The superficial layer is Reinke's space. The intermediate and deep layers make up the vocal ligament. The vocalis muscle lies lateral and deep to the vocal ligament.

51. AETIOLOGY OF HEAD AND NECK CANCER

Introduction
Squamous cell cancer constitutes the most common head and neck malignancy and is related to tobacco and/or alcohol usage, or infection with human papillomavirus (HPV). Non-squamous malignancy includes thyroid cancer, salivary gland cancer and sarcomas. These malignancies are not associated with tobacco and/or alcohol usage.

Squamous Malignant Tumours
Squamous cell carcinoma of the head and neck encompasses cancer of the oral cavity, oropharynx, larynx and hypopharynx, nasopharynx, nasal cavity and paranasal sinuses.

Tobacco and Smoking
The main aetiological factors for oral cavity cancer are smoking and alcohol. Tobacco contains over 30 known carcinogens such as polycyclic aromatic hydrocarbons and nitrosamines. There is a synergistic interaction with alcohol due to the increased mucosal absorption of these carcinogens due to increased solubility of the carcinogens in alcohol compared with aqueous saliva. The use of filtered cigarettes reduces this exposure and stopping smoking reduces the risk of head and neck cancer. The risk of oral cancer is reduced by 50% for those who have discontinued for more than 9 years, but it is unlikely that it ever returns to the baseline. Pipe and cigar smokers have an increased risk of oral cancer.

Oral cancer is strongly associated with different forms of smokeless tobacco consumed by chewing. These include bidi, chutta, paan, khaini and toombak. This is particularly common in the Indian subcontinent and accounts for the high incidence of oral cancer in these countries. When marijuana is smoked, a wide range of potential carcinogens are released and absorbed, with an overall risk of 2.6 compared to non-users.

Alcohol

Alcohol is believed to act in a synergistic fashion with tobacco; however, some case control and cohort studies have shown an increased risk of cancer even in non-smokers. Alcohol itself is not a carcinogen, so possible carcinogenic mechanisms include alcohol acting as a solvent, non-alcohol constituents of alcoholic drinks, the alcohol metabolite acetaldehyde, activation of the cytochrome p450 system, decreased activity of DNA repair enzymes or T cells or the associated nutritional deficiencies associated with heavy alcohol intake.

Dental Factors

Poor oral hygiene is associated with oral cancer. This may be due to chronic inflammation of the gingiva or an alteration in the oral microbiome. There is some evidence suggesting mouthwashes containing alcohol may also be important.

Infections

In oral cancer, several viruses have been implicated in carcinogenesis including HPV, human immunodeficiency virus (HIV) and herpes simplex virus (HSV).

Human Papillomavirus

Some authors have dismissed a link between oral cavity cancer and HPV infection due to low prevalence. In contrast, other authors have reported that the infection of oral cavity cells by HPV is not rare, and the relationship is not resolved.

Human Immunodeficiency Virus

A study from New York showed HIV infection in 5% of head and neck cancer patients. Due to the depressed immunity in HIV patients, the head and neck cancers observed were more advanced in the HIV group.

Herpes Simplex Virus

Several studies have shown that patients with oral cancer have higher antibodies to HSV. However, there is little evidence that HSV gene sequences are present in oral cancer cells or any evidence of gene integration.

Nutritional Factors

Several studies suggest high fruit and vegetable intake is associated with a decreased risk of head and neck cancer. This may be due to increased intake of the antioxidants or free radical scavenging vitamins A, C and E.

Genetic and Immunologic Predisposition

Although smoking is the main risk factor, not all people who smoke develop head and neck cancer. There are several genetic conditions that are associated with increased risk of head and neck cancer including Li-Fraumeni syndrome (*p53* gene mutation), Fanconi's anaemia, Bloom syndrome and ataxia-telangiectasia.

Patients treated with bone marrow transplants and organ transplants have an increased incidence of skin cancer and oral cavity cancer, possibly due to the long-term use of immunosuppressive drugs.

Cancer of the Oropharynx

Recent studies have shown a dramatic change in the aetiology of oropharyngeal cancer from a cancer caused by smoking and alcohol to a cancer now predominantly caused by HPV. The increase in tonsil and base of tongue cancer over the last decade is largely due to HPV infection of the palatine and lingual tonsils, and it has been called an epidemic of HPV-associated oropharyngeal cancer.

HPV exists in many different serotypes and HPV 16, 18, 31, 33, 35 and 39 are associated with head and neck cancer and HPV 16 and 18 are the most common types associated with squamous cell carcinoma. The E6 and E7 open reading frames (ORFs) of the high-risk HPVs are important. They bind to and inactivate tumour suppressor genes *p53* and *pRb,* respectively, allowing uncontrolled cell proliferation, resulting in genomic instability and cellular transformation.

Patients with HPV-positive tonsil cancer tend to be young, non-smokers and non-drinkers. The molecular characteristics are completely different from HPV-negative tonsil cancers. HPV-positive tonsil cancers have shown a better prognosis.

Cancer of the Larynx and Hypopharynx
The numbers of new cases of laryngeal cancer are falling by around 2% to 3% a year, mainly because fewer people are smoking.

Tobacco and Alcohol
There is a strong association between laryngeal cancer and cigarette smoking. Environmental tobacco smoke also increases the risk of laryngeal cancer. The combined use of tobacco and alcohol increases the risk of laryngeal cancer by 50% over the estimated risk if these factors were considered additive. The risk is greater for hypopharyngeal cancer than laryngeal cancer.

Other Factors
Laryngeal cancer is also associated with nickel and mustard gas exposure and there may be association with asbestos exposure. Postcricoid carcinoma is associated with previous radiation and sideropenic dysphagia - between 4% and 6% of patients have a history of Plummer-Vinson syndrome.

Cancer of the Nasopharynx
Nasopharyngeal cancer (NPC) is endemic in southern China and Hong Kong with an incidence rate of 50 per 100 000.

There are three subtypes: World Health Organisation (WHO) type 1, keratinising squamous cell carcinoma; WHO type 2, non-keratinising (differentiated) carcinoma and WHO type 3, undifferentiated carcinoma. In North America, type 1 accounts for 68% of cases whereas in the Far East, types 2 and 3 account for 95% of cases. There is a genetic association, with different types of HLA types, and a familial association. The most important environmental factor is infection by Epstein-Barr virus (EBV).

Dietary factors are also important. People who live in affected areas where NPC is common typically eat diets very high in salt-cured fish and meat. Studies indicate that foods preserved in this way that are cooked at high temperatures may produce chemicals that can damage DNA.

Cancer of the Nasal Cavity and Paranasal Sinuses
Cancers of the nasal cavity and paranasal sinuses are rare. As in all head and neck cancer, smoking tobacco is a risk factor for nasal cavity cancer. Occupational factors are also important including exposure to dust from wood, textiles and leather and possibly flour.

Non-Squamous Malignant Tumours
Carcinoma of the Thyroid
Differentiated thyroid cancer (DTC) accounts for 80% of thyroid cancers, split into papillary and follicular cancer. Other thyroid tumours include poorly differentiated cancer (10%), anaplastic (5%) and medullary thyroid cancer (MTC; 5%). The incidence of papillary thyroid cancer is increasing, which is partly the result of the incidental detection of early thyroid cancer because of increasing use of imaging.

Thyroid cancer is more common in areas of the world where diets are low in iodine, but there is not a strong epidemiological relationship between iodine intake and cancer. A history of radiation treatment in childhood is a known risk factor. Inherited medical conditions such as Gardner syndrome, familial polyposis and Cowden disease have an increased incidence of thyroid cancer. Certain families also have an increased incidence of papillary thyroid cancer.

MTC originates from the parafollicular C cells, secretes calcitonin and occurs in both sporadic and hereditary forms. Seventy-five percent of MTC occurs as a sporadic form and 25% as a hereditary form. The hereditary forms can occur in the hereditary syndrome multiple endocrine neoplasia syndrome type A (MEN-2A), in MEN-2B or as a single component in a hereditary disease (familial MTC). Both MEN-2 syndromes are autosomal dominant genetic disorders characterised by mutations in the *RET* proto-oncogene.

Salivary Gland Carcinomas

Exposure to radiation to the head and neck area increases the risk of salivary gland cancer. Some studies have also suggested that working with certain metals (nickel alloy dust) and minerals (silica dust) may increase the risk for salivary gland cancer. In men, smoking and heavy alcohol consumption was also associated with higher risk, but not in women. Hormonal dependence may also be important; early menarche and nulliparity are associated with increased risk, whereas older age at full-term pregnancy and long duration of oral contraceptive use are associated with reduced risk.

Sarcomas of the Head and Neck

Sarcomas of the head and neck constitute less than 1% of head and neck malignancies. They are divided into those arising from soft tissue (STS) and those arising from bone (osteosarcoma).

Genetic Predisposition

Studies have shown that some groups of individuals are at an increased risk of developing STS. Among them are genetically predisposed individuals, such as those suffering from neurofibromatosis (who are at risk of malignant peripheral neuroectodermal tumour [MPNT]), Li-Fraumeni syndrome and children with retinoblastoma (who are predisposed to osteosarcoma, rhabdomyosarcoma and fibrosarcoma). Other heritable syndromes associated with an increased risk of STS include Gardner syndrome and nevoid basal cell carcinoma syndrome.

Radiation, Viruses and Other Factors

Previous exposure to irradiation is another well-documented risk for both STS and osteogenic sarcoma in other sites, but the head and neck is less commonly affected. Patients with chronic lymphoedema have an increased incidence of STS formation. Patients with Paget's disease of bone, particularly the skull, are predisposed to osteogenic sarcoma. The role of viruses in the pathogenesis of STS has been investigated, but apart from the association of HIV with Kaposi's sarcoma there is no conclusive proof available for a viral aetiology.

KEY POINTS

- Squamous cell cancer is the most common head and neck malignancy, and it is related mainly to alcohol and tobacco use.
- HPV is now the leading cause of cancer of the oropharynx.
- Other malignancies of the head and neck such as thyroid cancer, salivary gland cancer and sarcomas are not related to alcohol or tobacco usage. The main causes of these cancers are less clear. Prior exposure to radiation in the head and neck area is one of the few identified risk factors.
- Genetic predisposition to head and neck cancer is rare and is present in a few inherited conditions such as Fanconi's anaemia and Li-Fraumeni syndrome. MTC is a well-known example of a hereditary thyroid cancer secondary to a specific mutation in RET oncogene.

There is an important role of head and neck cancer prevention through alcohol and tobacco cessation, HPV vaccination and close follow-up of risk groups such as genetic conditions carriers.

52. MOLECULAR BIOLOGY AND GENE THERAPY

Molecular Genetics: DNA Structure and Function

Hereditary information in eukaryotes is stored in the form of double-stranded deoxyribonucleic acid (DNA) and is referred to as the genome. DNA forms a double helix structure bonding complementary pairs of nucleotides, such as adenine (A) with thymine (T) and cytosine (C) with guanine (G). Within the coding part of DNA nucleotides on each strand are grouped in triplets, known as codons. Each codon sequence determines a single specific amino acid. Some codons are 'stop' codons, constituting a signal for arrest of translation. The overwhelming majority of DNA (99.9%) exists in the cell nucleus as the nuclear genome and the remaining DNA forms the mitochondrial genome, encoding 37 genes.

Each DNA molecule is packaged into a chromosome by complex folding of the DNA around proteins. Diploid human cells contain 22 pairs and a pair of sex chromosomes (XX or XY) that determines the sex of the organism. One of each pair of chromosomes is maternally inherited and the other is paternally inherited. The ends of the chromosomes are capped by telomeres, which are specialised structures that are involved in cell mortality. During normal cell division, DNA replication is achieved by the separation of the two strands by DNA helicase. Each separated single strand then acts as a template for forming a new complementary strand.

A gene is a region of the chromosomal DNA that produces a functional ribonucleic acid molecule (RNA). It comprises regulatory DNA sequences that determine when and in which cell types that gene is expressed; exons are coding sequences and interspersed introns are non-coding DNA sequences.

Transcription is the intra-nuclear process driven by the RNA polymerase whereby one DNA strand acts as a template for the synthesis of an RNA strand (uracil replaces thymine in RNA). This primary RNA transcript then undergoes post-transcriptional processing, or splicing. The mature mRNA migrates into the cytoplasm where it acts as a template for the synthesis of a polypeptide during translation, via ribosomes. Successive amino acids are added creating a polypeptide chain from to the triplet code on the mRNA, resulting in protein synthesis.

Other Regulators of Gene Expression

Small interfering RNAs (siRNAs; double stranded) and microRNAs (miRs; single stranded) are biologically significant post-transcriptional regulators of gene expression. siRNAs and miRs are non-coding RNA molecules that base pair with mRNA via the RISC complex, preventing their translation into proteins. In addition, long non-coding RNAs (ncRNAs) have been identified that are thought to regulate various aspects of gene expression and they have been implicated in a number of diseases, including aging and cancer.

Molecular Aberrations of Cellular Biology

DNA mutation may occur as a result of base substitutions, as well as nucleotide insertions and deletions. Insertions and deletions of nucleotides are very rare in coding DNA. Base substitution is a more common form of mutation in coding DNA, which may have a range of consequences on the function of the gene: a loss of function; a gain in function, often due to stabilisation of the active protein or no net functional effect. An example of a silent substitution yielding no functional effect is seen when an amino acid may be encoded by different codons (e.g. GUA, GAC, GUG and GUU all encode valine), so a substitution of the third base results in no change to the amino acid. At the other extreme is the nonsense mutation, whereby a base substitution results in an early stop codon, which leads to truncation of the polypeptide and a dramatic reduction in function.

A proto-oncogene may be converted into an oncogene by a point mutation or by a simple increase in the copy number of the gene (gene amplification) resulting in an overproduction of protein. Loss of function of a tumour suppressor gene is also oncogenic, which can occur a number of ways, including a missense mutation causing loss of protein function, an early stop codon and transcriptional silencing. The methylation status of CpG islands surrounding the promoter regions of genes determines whether a particular gene is expressed within a cell, such that methylation of a CpG island 'switches off' the gene that it is regulating. Many tumour suppressor genes are now recognised to be inactivated by hypermethylation of the promoter region in malignant tumours. With inactivation of a tumour suppressor gene, it must be considered there are two alleles, with the theory that both alleles must be non-functioning and known as Knudson's 'two-hit' hypothesis. This is well explained by hereditary tumours, where an inherited mutation eliminates the function of one allele, the so-called loss of heterozygosity (LOH), with a second somatic mutation ('hit') required to facilitate the oncogenic potential of the mutations. It is now known that tumour suppressors do not all fit this model, and they can be haploinsufficient (gene only functions in the presence of two wild-type alleles), dominant negative (where one mutated allele has an effect that dominates over the effect of the wild-type allele) or gain of function.

Gene Sequencing

Recently a variety of next-generation sequencing (NGS) methods have been applied to the field. Methods involved include constructing a library of DNA fragments, which are amplified using polymerase chain reaction (PCR). The sequence of the DNA is determined by synthesis, with different NGS platforms using different sequencing chemistry to determine which complementary bases have been added to the original DNA strands. Using massive parallel sequencing, this method is performed much more quickly and efficiently than traditional Sanger sequencing.

Proteomics and Metabolomics

Proteomics is the profiling of proteins in cells and serum by two-dimensional gel analysis separating proteins by charge and mass, by X-ray crystallography and by mass spectrometry. Proteomics has the ability to identify post-translational modifications, some of which are cancer cell specific, which would not be detected by genetic or expression profiling. The power of this approach is particularly evident in cancer studies as it has the ability to compare the entire protein pattern of tumour tissue and normal tissue in a manner analogous to comparative genomic hybridisation.

Metabolomics is the global analysis of metabolites but is a relatively new discipline and no single technique is suitable for the analysis of all different types of molecule. Therefore, a mixture of techniques such as gas chromatography, high-pressure liquid chromatography and capillary electrophoresis are used to separate metabolites and the molecules are then identified using methods such as mass spectrometry. Metabolomics has already been applied to the detection of oral cancer in saliva and serum.

Gene Therapy

Gene therapy offers a novel paradigm that leads to the destruction of tumour cells in cancer patients. To date, the approaches to target specific cancer cells fall into four basic categories: (1) chemosensitisation, (2) cytokine gene transfer, (3) inactivation of protooncogene production and (4) selective oncolytic viruses.

Selective sensitisation of cancer cells using gene therapy would be an ideal way to kill cancer cells. Using this approach, the expected gene is delivered only to cancer cells and then a second therapy (e.g. radiotherapy or chemotherapy) is used to induce killing in the cells that express the transgene. Efficiency and targeting have been shown to be difficult *in vivo* largely due to the bystander effect, where an infected cell spreads the expressed genes to the cells surrounding it via cell–cell contacts, reducing the method efficiency in the targeted cells.

The host immune response has been shown to play a role in cancer eradication. In addition to generalised suppression increasing the risk of carcinogenesis, it has been shown that individuals with head and neck cancer lack an effective local immune response even early in the disease. This dysfunction occurs as a result of the normal immune system not recognising the tumour cells. Causes of this include immunological ignorance, downregulation of major histocompatibility complexes and loss of costimulatory receptor and pathways. In some tumours, the cytokine stimulatory pathways (interleukin [IL]-2, interferon-gamma and IL-12) that normally upregulate the normal tumour immune response are suppressed. One method to break this immune dysregulation is to overexpress the downregulated cytokines.

Restoring the function of a key cellular gene whose dysfunction has resulted in cancer progression is a major goal of gene therapy. The most common mutations of key genes in squamous cell cancer of the head and neck are *p53* and *p16*. *p53* plays a role in triggering cell death in many different pathways involving apoptosis. Gendicine®, a drug with modified adenovirus harbouring *p53* gene, was approved in China in 2004, becoming the first gene therapy approved for clinical use in humans. However, the western version of Ad-p53 (Advexin®) for the treatment of head and neck cancer was refused approval by the U. S. Food and Drug Administration in 2008.

The future of restoring function via correction of genetic defects found in cancer may lie with clustered regularly interspaced short palindromic repeats (CRISPR)/CRISPR-associated nuclease 9 (Cas9) gene editing. CRISPR-Cas9 utilises the DNA cutting action of the Cas9 protein to create double-stranded DNA breaks, has relative high efficiency and accuracy for disruption gene transcription and can be adapted for editing gene transcription. Safety trials for the delivery of CRISPR-edited T cells into patients have started.

With increased knowledge of the genetic defects in cancer, delivery vectors aimed selectively at tumour cells provide another research challenge. The translation of molecular biology research into clinical practice, 'from laboratory to bedside,' is without a doubt the greatest challenge facing the clinician scientist. Progress so far has been largely at the level of disease classification, premorbid diagnosis and patient counselling. However, several discrete arms to translational research have hinted at the future role of genetic analysis determining the likely effectiveness of existing anti-cancer treatments.

KEY POINTS AND FUTURE RESEARCH

- Genetic sequencing data potentially provides more accurate diagnosis and prognosis than conventional histopathological techniques.
- There is the potential for therapeutic restoration of DNA or protein function, as well as exploitation of a genetic abnormality for targeting therapy.
- Although genomics and other omics has generated a large body of data, cancers are complicated tissues. Future research may shift toward understanding the cancer environment and how perhaps to target this in future therapeutic strategies.
- Our increased understanding of cellular oncogenesis will lead to the development of novel cancer therapies in the years to come.
- Gene therapy is likely to be a part of these therapies.

A head and neck oncologist will need to understand both the viral vectors and their strategies of implementation to offer a full range of treatment to the cancer patient.

53. IMAGING OF THE NECK

Introduction
Current imaging options for the head and neck include:

- *Plain X-rays*: They are limited to detecting ingested radiopaque foreign bodies, assessing the dentition in oncological patients and those presenting with floor of mouth abscesses.
- *Ultrasound (US)*: It is quick, non-invasive, readily available, inexpensive and does not use ionising radiation. It is heavily operator dependent. Widely used for evaluating neck lumps, lymph nodes, thyroid and salivary glands, and guiding fine-needle aspiration (FNA) or core biopsies.
- *Computed tomography (CT)*: This is used extensively in staging cancer patients and detecting neck masses or abscesses. The entire neck can be scanned in a few seconds, and images reconstructed in any plane. Intravenous iodinated contrast agent necessary due to its low soft-tissue resolution. Radiation dose and dental artifact are an important consideration.
- *Magnetic resonance imaging (MRI)*: This produces images with excellent soft-tissue contrast. It does not use ionising radiation. Contraindicated in certain patients with metallic foreign bodies, prosthesis and implanted devices. Long acquisition times result in motion artifact.
- *Positron emission tomography (PET)*: This is a functional imaging technique where hypermetabolic cells accumulate tracer, usually fluorine-18-labellfed 2-fluoro-2-deoxy-D-glucose (FDG). The combination of CT and PET allows accurate anatomical localisation, which is especially useful in assessing patients with an unknown primary, and in post-treatment patients.
- *Contrast swallow*: This is useful for assessing the presence of leaks following laryngeal/pharyngeal surgery. Videofluoroscopy is important in assessing head and neck cancer patients with dysphagia before or after treatment.
- *Sialography*: This provides excellent luminal depiction of glandular anatomy; however, it is invasive and can cause trauma or be unsuccessful.
- *Scintigraphy*: This provides good quantification of gland function but poor anatomical correlation and radiation burden.

Head and Neck Cancer
Cross-sectional imaging helps to assess the size, location and deep extension of tumour, involvement of surrounding structures, presence of distant metastases and allows post-therapy surveillance and assessment of treatment.

Nasopharyngeal Cancer (NPC)

- Locally aggressive, early metastases despite early primary.
- CT allows assessment of the primary tumour and metastases (Figure 53.1).
- MRI better at demonstrating soft-tissue extent, intracranial extension and skull base bone marrow changes (Figure 53.2).
- PET-CT for staging, assessment of recurrence and evaluating the nasopharynx in patients presenting with unknown primary.

Oral Cavity Tumours

- Challenging radiologically due to surrounding anatomy.
- Small tumours often not visualised by imaging.

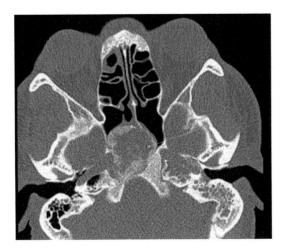

Figure 53.1   Axial CT showing nasopharyngeal carcinoma (white arrow) and retained secretions left mastoid air cells (black arrow) due to Eustachian tube obstruction.

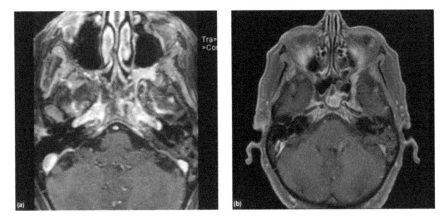

Figure 53.2   MRI showing left nasopharyngeal cancer extending into the pterygopalatine fossa (black arrow) and vidian canal (white arrow) (a) and into the foramen rotundum (black arrow) (b).

- CT shows better evaluation of cortical bone (Figure 53.3), but dental amalgam is a frequent diagnostic issue.
- MRI is better at characterising local tumour extent, perineural spread and bone marrow involvement.

Oropharyngeal Tumours

- Oropharyngeal tumours include tonsil, base of tongue, soft palate and posterior pharyngeal wall cancers.
- Often present with a nodal mass and no obvious primary tumour.
- CT/MRI both useful imaging modalities.
- PET has a higher sensitivity for detection of primary tumour and cervical metastases.
- PET-CT is slightly complicated by the normal physiological uptake in the oropharynx (Figure 53.4).
- Post-treatment PET-CT to assess therapy response.

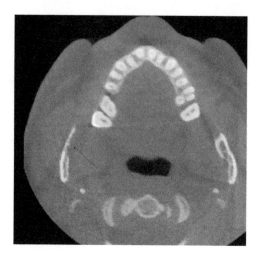

Figure 53.3   Axial CT showing destruction of the inner cortex of the right mandible (arrow) in a histologically proven intraosseous squamous cell carcinoma.

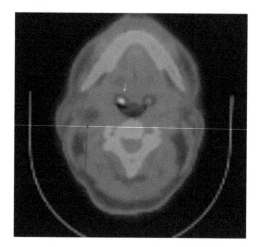

Figure 53.4   PET-CT showing increased activity in the right tongue base (white arrow) in a patient presenting with a right-sided neck mass (black arrow) and no apparent primary on clinical examination or conventional CT. Note the normal physiological activity in the left tongue base.

Hypopharyngeal Tumours

- Hypopharynx consists of the pyriform sinus/fossa, post-cricoid region and posterior hypopharyngeal wall.
- Imaging importantly evaluates the larynx, thyroid cartilage, and nodal status, and usually results in tumour upstaging.
- CT generally preferred modality (Figure 53.5).
- PET-CT for detection of residual/recurrent tumour following treatment.

Laryngeal Tumours

- Most common head and neck malignancy; the majority are squamous cell carcinoma (SCC).
- Imaging allows evaluation of submucosal disease, laryngeal cartilage and extra-laryngeal structure involvement, state of the airway and nodal status.

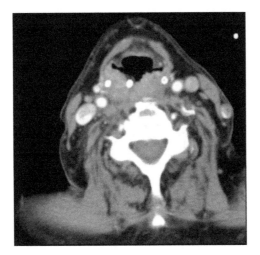

Figure 53.5   Axial contrast CT showing a large hypopharyngeal posterior wall tumour extending into the prevertebral muscles.

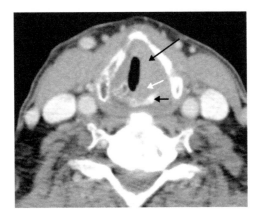

Figure 53.6   Axial contrast CT showing a large left transglottic tumour (long black arrow) with completely destroyed left arytenoid (white arrow) and sclerotic left cricoid cartilage (short black arrow).

- CT is the preferred modality (Figure 53.6).
- US can be used to identify extra-laryngeal spread (Figure 53.7).
- PET-CT, CT or MRI is used for detection of residual/recurrent tumour following treatment.

Neck Lumps

The imaging of patients presenting with a neck lump depends on the age of the patient, clinical history and location of the mass.

Thyroglossal Duct Cyst

- Intimately related to the hyoid bone, most below (65%) or at level of hyoid bone (15%).
- 75% occur in the midline, remainder up to 2 cm off the midline.
- Imaging helps identify relationship to hyoid, presence or absence of normal thyroid tissue, and any solid material within the cyst (Figure 53.8).

Head and Neck   267

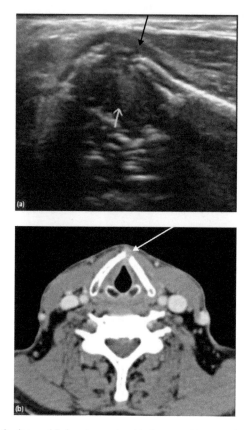

Figure 53.7 US of the larynx (a) showing a sizeable laryngeal tumour (green arrow) extending through a defect in the thyroid cartilage (black arrow) with the corresponding axial CT (b) confirming extra-laryngeal spread of tumour (white arrow).

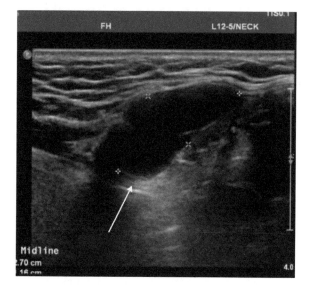

Figure 53.8 US showing a midline infrahyoid homogenous anechoic cystic mass with posterior wall enhancement (white arrow) in keeping with a thyroglossal duct cyst.

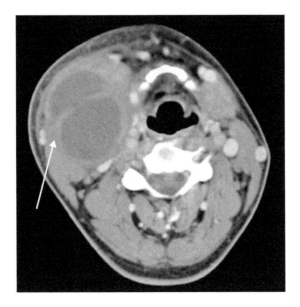

Figure 53.9 Axial contrast CT showing a septated thick-walled right level 2 mass (white arrow) displacing the submandibular gland anteriorly and deep to sternomastoid in keeping with an infected second branchial cleft cyst.

Second Branchial Cleft Cyst

- Classically present as a level II neck mass, superficial to the carotid sheath, posterior to the submandibular gland (SMG) and along the anteromedial border of sternomastoid (Figure 53.9).
- If a beak is identified pointing medially on US, then cross-sectional is warranted to exclude a sinus/fistula.
- Metastatic SCC should be considered until proven otherwise in patients over 40 years.

Ranula

- This is a retention cyst. May be confined to the floor of mouth or extends into submandibular space through a defect in the mylohyoid muscle (plunging ranula).
- US shows unilocular, well-defined cystic submental mass related to the sublingual gland.
- CT shows solitary, low-attenuation, non-enhancing thin-walled mass.
- MRI shows mass of low T1 and high T2 signal.

Lipoma

- US shows a characteristically striped or feathery mass.
- CT shows similar low attenuation as surrounding fat.
- MRI shows high T1/T2 signal, low on fat suppression sequences.

Vascular Malformations

- This is common in the head and neck. They are venous and lymphatic malformations, or a combination.
- Venous malformations are commonly found in the masticator space especially within the masseter.

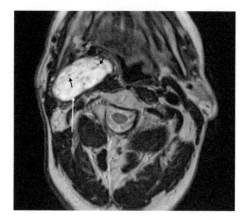

Figure 53.10   Axial T2-weighted MRI showing a high signal right carotid space mass (white arrow) containing several signal voids (small black arrows) consistent with a paraganglioma.

- US shows heterogenous echo pattern with multiple sinusoidal spaces.
- MRI shows striking high signal on T2-weighted sequences.
- Most common lymphatic malformation is a cystic hygroma, usually posterior triangle.
- Imaging shows multiloculated mass, invaginates between vessels/other structures to occupy multiple contiguous spaces.

Paraganglioma

- They occur anywhere along the carotid sheath. Most common is a carotid body tumour (CBT).
- CBTs occur at the bifurcation of the common carotid artery with characteristic splaying of the internal and external carotid arteries.
- MRI shows characteristic 'salt and pepper' appearance (Figure 53.10) with the 'pepper' or low-signal representing flow voids of feeding vessels.

The Hot Neck

- Patients with pyrexia, pain, neck swelling, trismus, restricted neck movements or odynophagia should be considered to have neck sepsis.
- The most common sources are tonsillar or odontogenic infection.
- Imaging to assess whether surgical intervention is required (Table 53.1).
- Odontogenic infections require an orthopantomogram (OPG) to assess dentition.
- US is the first-line investigation in children and any superficial infection.
- Contrast CT of the neck and mediastinum are done to assess deep neck spaces, extent of infection and any complications such as vascular thrombosis, neural dysfunction and mediastinitis.

Table 53.1   Imaging in the hot neck: What the surgeon needs to know

Is there an abscess or just inflammatory change?
If an abscess is present, in which space/spaces?
How large is the abscess?
Extent of abscess
Is the mediastinum involved?
Is the airway compromised?
Is there jugular vein thrombosis?

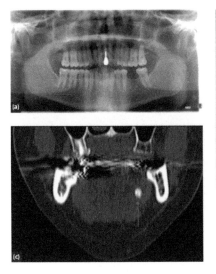
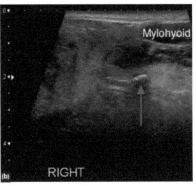

Figure 53.11 Sialolithiasis (a) OPG demonstrates a right-sided SMG calculus. (b) US demonstrates an echogenic calculus with acoustic shadow. (c) CT demonstrates a distal left submandibular ductal calculus.

SALIVARY GLAND OBSTRUCTION AND SIALADENITIS

Sialolithiasis

- SMG is more commonly affected than the parotid.
- 15% of calculi are radiolucent.
- US/CT are most sensitive (Figure 53.11).
- Sialography is useful to plan therapeutic stone retrieval, lithotripsy or balloon sialoplasty. Up to 15% failure rate, can cause ductal trauma or provoke acute sialadenitis.
- MR sialography using non-interventional, T2 weighted technique relies on inherent salivary flow and high sensitivity/specificity (Figure 53.12).

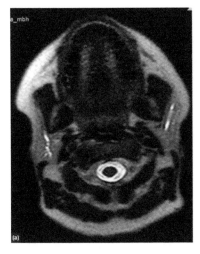
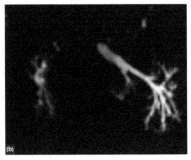

Figure 53.12 MR sialography. (a) T2-weighted axial image to illustrate ductal fluid. (b) Highlighted ductal pattern.

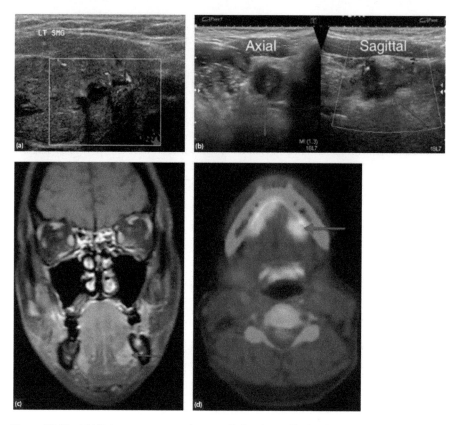

Figure 53.13 (a) US demonstrates an obstructed left submandibular duct. (b) US reveals a sublingual space mass lesion, which was subsequently confirmed histologically as an adenocarcinoma in the sublingual gland. (c) Coronal MRI shows a bulky enhancing mass in the left sublingual space. (d) PET-CT illustrates avid salivary gland lesion.

Salivary Strictures

- Preferentially affect parotid ducts.
- Two-thirds focal stricture, one-third multiple/diffuse strictures.
- US/sialography/MR sialography are able to depict stricture. CT us less useful.
- Type of obstruction important to guide onward treatment decisions.

Sialadenitis

- This affects often elderly, immunosuppressed, malnourished patients with poor oral hygiene.
- US used in acute setting to exclude abscess, obstructive stone/stricture or underlying neoplasm (Figure 53.13).
- Chronic sialadenitis causes gland atrophy. US/sialography/scintigraphy used to determine useful gland function.

Dry Mouth and Glandular Hypofunction

The presentation of a non-obstructive, non-suppurative multisite glandular swelling or even a unilateral asymmetric, atypical finding may be secondary to a diffuse inflammatory or systemic condition.

Sjögren's Syndrome

- OPG may show accelerated dental decay.
- Diagnosis, labial mucosal biopsy, antibody screening, abnormal US/sialography/scintigraphy.
- US may show atrophic hypoechoic pseudocystic regions and eventual fatty replacement.

Sarcoidosis

- Multisystem disorder.
- Bilateral parotid gland enlargement.
- US shows fatty infiltration, facilitates FNA cytology (FNAC)/core biopsy.

IGG4-Related Systemic Disease

- This is a relatively newly recognised multisystem disorder; raised serum IgG4 concentrations.
- US shows geographic textural abnormality and hypervascularity, facilitates FNAC/core biopsy.
- CT/MRI shows enhancement of salivary tissue.

Radiotherapy

- Can induce debilitating xerostomia; usually subjective patient reporting.
- US/CT/MRI shows reduced gland volume and ductal ectasia/fibrosis.
- Salivary flow studies/sialography/scintigraphy identify impaired glandular function/stricture formation.
- New intensity-modulated radiation therapy (IMRT) techniques use reduced dose delivery to salivary glands.

Salivary Masses and Suspected Neoplasms

Benign Neoplasms
Pleomorphic Adenomas

- 90% occur in the superficial lobe of the parotid.
- On US is lobulated, clearly defined, echo-poor, homogenous.
- MRI if malignancy is suspected to evaluate deep lobe lesions and facial nerve weakness; surveillance if managed non-operatively. Low signal T1, T2 bright appearance. (Figure 53.14).

Warthin's Tumour

- On US is well-defined, heterogenous, hypoechoic septated/cystic lesion and often bilateral.
- MRI, T1 bright appearance (Figure 53.15).

Oncocytomas

- These are rare, commonly present as solitary parotid lesions and 10% bilateral.
- Difficult to distinguish from benign/low-grade tumours on imaging.
- MRI shows cystic degeneration, T1 hypointense/isointense and T2 fat-saturated.

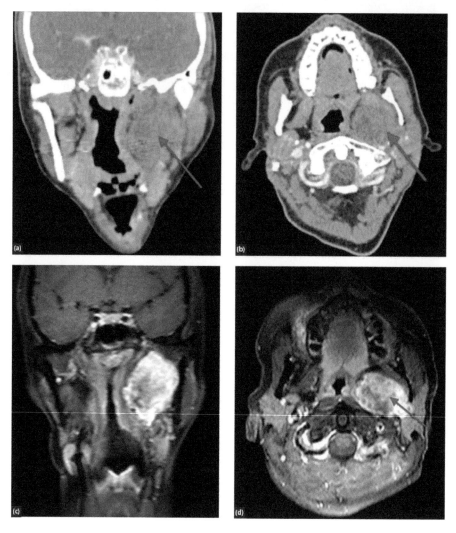

Figure 53.14 Deep lobe Pleomorphic Adenoma (PA) (a and b) on contrast-enhanced CT. (c and d) Post-gadolinium, fat-saturated MR images.

Malignant Neoplasms

Approximately 20% of all parotid, 50% of submandibular and 90% of sublingual gland tumours are malignant. Imaging may appear deceptively benign. US suggestive of malignancy may show inhomogeneity, posterior acoustic shadow, raised inherent vascular flow and ill-defined/infiltrative margins.

Mucoepidermoid Tumours

- Most common parotid malignancy; they make up 12–29% of all salivary malignancies.
- MRI shows cystic change, abundant hypointense fibrous tissue.

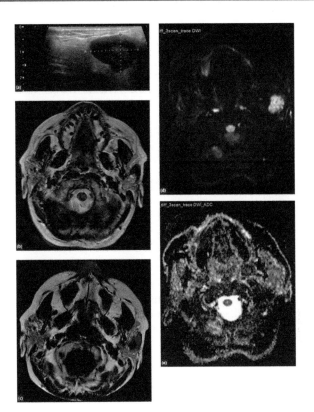

Figure 53.15 (a) US of well-circumscribed, heterogenous Warthin's lesion. (b) Axial T2W MR of left parotid Warthin's. (c and d) DWI of a Warthin's. (e) Matched ADC (apparent diffusion coefficient) image demonstrating hypercellularity.

Adenoid Cystic Carcinomas

- Second most common salivary gland lesion. They are the most common malignant tumousr within SMGs.
- MRI shows T2 hypointense signal, T1 bright intralesional bleeds. May identify local perineural spread.

54. MANAGEMENT OF LARYNGOTRACHEAL TRAUMA

Introduction
The laryngotracheal region provides the important functions of airway maintenance, airway protection, phonation and swallow. Injury to structures in this region are diverse and rare but can result in severe morbidity and mortality.

Anatomy
The laryngotracheal complex is relatively well protected and can deflect significant traumatic force before being injured. The larynx is divided into three subsites: supraglottis, glottis and subglottis. The subglottis is continuous with the trachea inferiorly and contains a complete cartilaginous ring structure (cricoid) which is the most sensitive and vulnerable region to even trivial trauma.

Epidemiology and Aetiology of Laryngotracheal Injury

The majority of traumatic laryngotracheal injuries occur in males, with an incidence of up to 1 in 5000 emergency presentations and up to 2000 deaths annually reported in the United Kingdom. The mechanism of injury to the larynx can be classified as either external trauma (blunt or penetrating) or internal injury (inhalation or iatrogenic). Central to all laryngotracheal injuries, irrespective of mechanism, is the potential for a compromised airway.

Blunt Injuries

Blunt injuries can be further subclassified into the following:

- *Crush injury*: This is sustained especially in motor vehicle accidents where a hyperextended neck is thrust forward exposing the larynx to anterior crushing forces.
- *Clothesline injury*: This is a high-velocity impact of the larynx with a stationary object. This can lead to instant exsanguination from cricotracheal separation or a crushed larynx.
- *Strangulation injury (e.g. hanging) injury*: This may initially be minor but may lead to subsequent laryngeal oedema and compromised airway.

Penetrating Injuries

Penetrating laryngotracheal injuries can cause varying degrees of damage depending on the location and the nature of the weapon used. Injury to neurovascular and soft-tissue structures can result in oedema, inflammation, haemorrhage, scarring and anatomical disruption. Gunshot wounds tend to cause a broad spectrum of damage, whereas stab wounds follow a more predictable course of injury.

Inhalational Injuries

Inhalational injuries to the larynx and trachea occur following inhalation of toxic gases, exposure to fires or ingestion of toxic substances. This may involve the transfer of high levels of thermal energy, causing significant airway oedema. Early securement of the airway is essential as delayed oedema can occur.

Iatrogenic Injuries

Iatrogenic injuries to the laryngotracheal complex can occur following instrumentation of the airway (e.g. endotracheal intubation or elective laryngeal surgery such as microlaryngoscopy). Factors such as high cuff pressure, prolonged duration of intubation, use of large diametre endotracheal tubes and patient-specific factors such as diabetes have all been identified as contributing to post-intubation injury.

Pathophysiology of Laryngeal Trauma

The complexities and complications associated with chronic laryngeal injury are variable, unpredictable and often not discernible at the outset. The potential problems include

- Scarring, subluxation and ankylosis of the arytenoids and cricoarytenoid joints
- Fibrosis of the laryngeal muscles disrupting the mucosal wave
- Anterior and posterior glottic webbing, and supraglottic and subglottic scarring
- Neural injury can lead to muscle palsy
- Unstable cartilage fractures, malunion or non-union

Functionally these may lead to progressive shortness of breath, airway obstruction, glottic incompetence, dysphonia, aspiration and dysphagia.

Classification of Laryngeal Trauma

Classification systems help to provide a unified approach to the assessment and management of laryngeal injuries. Several classification systems for traumatic laryngeal injury exist. Fuhrman et al. classify laryngotracheal injuries into five groups (Box 54.1). Classification of posterior glottic stenoses, described by Bogdasarian and Olson, is based on the structures involved (Figure 54.1).

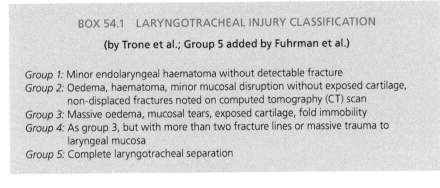

BOX 54.1   LARYNGOTRACHEAL INJURY CLASSIFICATION

(by Trone et al.; Group 5 added by Fuhrman et al.)

Group 1: Minor endolaryngeal haematoma without detectable fracture
Group 2: Oedema, haematoma, minor mucosal disruption without exposed cartilage, non-displaced fractures noted on computed tomography (CT) scan
Group 3: Massive oedema, mucosal tears, exposed cartilage, fold immobility
Group 4: As group 3, but with more than two fracture lines or massive trauma to laryngeal mucosa
Group 5: Complete laryngotracheal separation

Evaluation of Laryngotracheal Trauma

Assessment and management of laryngotracheal injury following the principles of advanced trauma and life support (ATLS) and a multidisciplinary team approach is essential (Figure 54.2). Like any other traumatic event, the primary goal is to assess and where necessary to protect the airway. Urgent review of patients is vital as those initially exhibiting only subtle symptoms can progress to complete airway obstruction from progressive oedema.

The most common presenting symptoms include dysphonia, dyspnoea, dysphagia, neck pain and haemoptysis. Patients with penetrating neck injuries may present with haemodymic

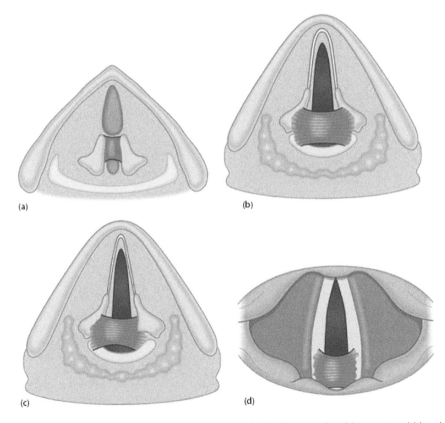

Figure 54.1   Classification of posterior glottic stenosis. (a) Type I, isolated inter-arytenoid band. (b) Type II, posterior glottic mucosal tunnel, but no arytenoid cartilage ankylosis. (c) Type III, ankylosis and immobility of one arytenoid joint. (d) Type IV, ankylosis and immobility of both arytenoid joints.

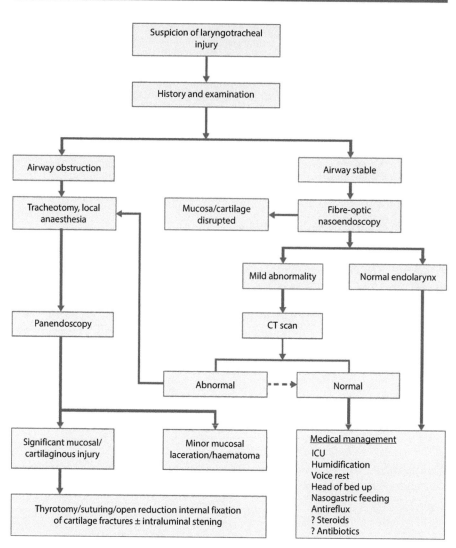

Figure 54.2   Management algorithm for patients presenting with laryngotracheal trauma.

instability, externally visible neck wounds, bleeding, bruising or an expanding haematoma. Clinical signs suggestive of airway obstruction include stridor, tachypnoea and accessory muscle use.

Airway Management

A thorough history and examination including fibreoptic nasoendoscopy can be obtained. Fibreoptic nasoendoscopy can aid in assessing patency of the airway, vocal fold movement, presence of lacerations, haematomas and exposed cartilage.

Options for acute management of the threatened airway include

- Endotracheal intubation
- Fibreoptic awake intubation
- Tracheostomy under local anaesthetic
- Cricothyroidotomy (in an emergency situation)

An emergency tracheostomy should be performed in a controlled environment such as the theater setting, under local anaesthetic with the patient breathing spontaneously. In the struggling patient inhalational anaesthesia with inspired oxygen may be administered. Muscle relaxants should be avoided as positive pressure ventilation may aggravate an air leak and surgical emphysema. To avoid the area of laryngotracheal injury, the tracheostomy incision is ideally placed slightly lower than usual.

In paediatric laryngeal trauma, airway control consists of inhalational anaesthesia allowing for spontaneous ventilation and securing the airway with rigid bronchoscopy and tracheostomy.

Once the airway is secured, further evaluation and exploration of the laryngotracheal injury can occur by means of a laryngotracheobronchoscopy and pharyngo-oesophagoscopy.

Imaging
Imaging is used in conjunction with rather than as a replacement for operative exploration. The gold standard imaging modalities are computed tomography (CT) with three-dimensional (3D) reconstruction and magnetic resonance imaging (MRI). Radiological findings may demonstrate cartilage fractures, haematoma, oedema, cricoarytenoid joint dislocation or subluxation, subcutaneous air and airway stenosis. CT angiography is helpful in assessing the integrity of vascular structures, especially in penetrating trauma involving zones 1 and 3 of the neck.

Management of Laryngotracheal Injuries
Non-Operative Approach
Airway stability is integral to non-operative management and assumes protection by the patient's own reflexes or by an endotracheal tube. This generally includes patients with group 1 and 2 laryngeal injuries. These injuries include minor mucosal lacerations without exposed cartilage or bone, small haematomas or undisplaced single fractures of the laryngeal cartilaginous framework.

Non-operative management of these patients involves admission to a level 2/3 environment for airway monitoring for at least 24 hours and treatment with constant humidification, head elevation, nil by mouth and voice rest. Systemic corticosteroids, nebulised adrenaline, inhibition of gastro-oesophageal reflux and antibiotics may also be considered.

Operative Approach
Surgery is aimed at airway preservation, prevention of secondary sequelae of healing and restoration of function via repair of endolaryngeal and other concomitant injuries.

Endoscopic
Endoscopic evaluation of the laryngotracheal complex can be performed in the acute and chronic setting. Imaging can be taken for documentation and therapeutic interventions can be performed. These potentially include, in the acute setting, aspiration of vocal fold haematomas, suturing and re-approximation of vocal folds and stent insertion to support the laryngeal framework and prevent adhesions, especially at the anterior commissure. In the chronic setting division of webs and adhesions, cordotomy, cordectomy, arytenoidectomy or injection thyroplasty can be undertaken under endoscopic vision. Endoscopic balloon or bougie dilatation can also be used for cricopharyngeal stenosis, and balloon dilatation with laser can be used for the endoscopic management of laryngotracheal stenosis.

Open

An open approach to traumatic laryngotracheal injury is recommended for patients with group 3 and 4 injuries or laryngeal fractures that are deemed unsuitable for endoscopic repair. Laryngeal fractures are repaired by raising the perichondrial layer and stabilising the fracture with wires, adaption alloy miniplates or alternatively non-metallic biodegradable plates which will absorb over 1.5 to 3 years. Group 5 injuries (complete cricotracheal separation) require emergency tracheostomy and immediate repair.

An open approach is used less often in the chronic setting, and it usually addresses functional deficits relating to airway, voice and swallow. Cricotracheal resection may be performed for chronic subglottic stenosis, type I Isshiki open thyroplasty to medialise a paralyzed vocal fold, and cricopharyngeal myotomy for cricopharyngeal stenosis. Reconstruction where there is cartilage loss may involve local muscle flaps, such as strap muscle or sternocleidomastoid, or the use of free grafts, such as rib cartilage. Longer term stents may be used where there has been significant damage to the laryngotracheal complex.

Future Directions

Laryngeal Tissue Engineering

Growth factors, such as basic fibroblast growth factor (bFGF), transforming growth factor (TGF)-β3 and granulocyte-macrophage colony-stimulating factor (GM-CSF), have been used experimentally and have shown some promising results in vocal fold regeneration and reduction of scar formation. The potential use of stem cells in a suitable scaffold as a therapy for future reconstruction is also promising based on *in vivo* and *in vitro* animal studies. However this area of research is currently limited to the laboratory stage.

Laryngotracheal Transplantation

The concept of laryngotracheal transplantation has been present for decades but still remains in its infancy. It is only suitable for a subset of patients who have endured severe trauma, requiring laryngectomy, and carries with it the challenges of a prolonged recovery and life-long immunosuppression. There have been isolated reports of successful laryngeal transplant with long-term survivorship despite issues with chronic rejection.

Conclusion

- The aetiology of trauma to the larynx and trachea is wide-ranging, resulting in complex and potentially life-threatening injuries.
- A multidisciplinary approach will enable airway protection and assessment of the extent of injury to determine the best management and timing of any potential operative intervention.
- Depending on the degree of injury, patient comorbidities and treatment-specific factors, treatment may involve operative or non-operative techniques.
- Chronic upper aerodigestive tract dysfunction is a likely sequela and requires prolonged rehabilitation.

Further Reading

Bell RM, Krantz BE, Weigelt JA. ATLS: a foundation for trauma training. *Ann Emergency Med* 1999; **34**: 233–237.

Lee WT, Eliashar R, Eliachar I. Acute external laryngotracheal trauma: diagnosis and management. *Ear Nose Throat J* 2006; **85**: 179–184.

Rossbach MM, Johnson SB, Gomez MA, et al. Management of major tracheobronchial injuries: a 28-year experience. *Ann Thoracic Surg* 1998; **65**: 182–186.

55. PHARYNGITIS

Introduction
Pharyngitis is defined as inflammation of the pharynx. It can be generalised or localised to a specific area (tonsillitis). The presenting symptom is usually a sore throat, and this is the most common presentation for primary care consultation. Most cases of pharyngitis are due to infection: viral in 40–60% and bacterial in 5–30% of cases. Non-infectious causes include dry air, allergy/post-nasal drip, chemical injury, gastro-oesophageal reflux disease (GERD), smoking, neoplasia and endotracheal intubation.

Gabhs Bacterial Pharyngitis
Group A beta-haemolytic streptococci (GABHS) are the most common cause of bacterial pharyngitis and are spread via respiratory secretions through close contact. The incubation period is 1–5 days and individuals are most infectious in the early stages of the disease.

The classical history is a sore throat, fever, chills, malaise, headaches, anorexia and abdominal pain. Although indistinguishable from viral aetiologies, several features are suggestive of GABHS, such as pharyngeal erythaema, enlarged tonsils, tonsillar exudate, fever, cervical lymphadenopathy, soft palate petechiae and a scarlet fever rash.

Scottish Intercollegiate Guidelines Network (SIGN) guidelines recommend that the Centor clinical prediction score should be used to differentiate between GABHS and viral pharyngitis, therefore, assisting the decision on antibiotic prescription.

The Centor score gives 1 point each for

- Tonsillar exudate
- Tender anterior cervical lymph nodes
- History of fever
- Absence of cough

The likelihood of GABHS infection increases with increasing score and is 25–86% with a score of 4 and 2–23% with a score of 1.

A full blood count may show leukocytosis, which is highly suggestive of bacterial infection. Rapid antigen detection tests (RADTs) or throat swabs for culture are not currently advocated in the United Kingdom.

Streptococcal pharyngitis usually has a 5–7-day self-limiting course. Non-steroidal anti-inflammatory drugs (NSAIDs) and paracetamol are effective for symptom relief. Chlorhexidine gluconate and benzydamine hydrochloride mouthwashes can alleviate the intensity of pharyngeal discomfort and a single dose of oral or intramuscular corticosteroids (in conjunction with antibiotic therapy) can reduce pain and hasten symptom resolution.

The use of antibiotics is discretionary, and most guidelines recommend that antibiotics should not be prescribed for symptomatic management, especially with less severe presentations (e.g. 0–2 Centor criteria). Penicillin is the antimicrobial agent of choice for GABHS. For adults, oral penicillin V 500 mg, four times daily for 10 days is prescribed. Alternatives include narrow-spectrum cephalosporins (cephalexin) or macrolides (azithromycin, clarithromycin). Avoid ampicillin-based antibiotics, including co-amoxiclav, due to the risk of rash in infectious mononucleosis (IM).

Complications of Gabhs Pharyngitis
Complications can be regarded as suppurative (peritonsillar, parapharyngeal and retropharyngeal abscesses) and non-suppurative (rheumatic fever, post-streptococcal reactive arthritis/glomerulonephritis, scarlet fever and paediatric autoimmune neuropsychiatric disorders associated with streptococcal infections [PANDAS]).

Peritonsillar Abscess

A peritonsillar abscess (PTA) is a collection of pus between the fibrous capsule of the tonsil and the superior constrictor muscles, usually at the upper pole. There has been an increase in the incidence of PTA, with GABHS and anaerobes such as *Fusobacterium necrophorum* and *Streptococcus milleri* clearly identified as causative organisms. The history is progressive, unilateral sore throat over 3–4 days with odynophagia, trismus, ipsilateral otalgia, headache, fever and lymphadenopathy. The patient often develops a 'hot potato' voice and, on examination, trismus is virtually pathognomonic. The tonsil is displaced medially by the hyperaemic, bulging mucosa over the peritonsillar space and the jugulodigastric nodes are tender and enlarged.

Drainage of pus is often curative and bacteriological specimens do not need to be sent to the laboratory routinely. This can be performed by either needle aspiration or an incision and drainage (with scalpel and forceps). Although drainage is the primary treatment, antibiotics are recommended for resolution of infection. A combination of benzylpenicillin and metronidazole is the preferred choice. In patients with penicillin allergy, erythromycin/clarithromycin should be used. The use of a single dose of intravenous steroid in addition to antibiotic therapy significantly reduces throat pain, time in hospital, fever and trismus. Interval elective tonsillectomy after recurrent PTA is recommended.

Non-Gabhs Bacterial Pharyngitis

Pathogens in non-GABHS include *Haemophilus influenza, Moraxella catarrhalis, Corynebacterium haemolyticum, Mycoplasma pneumonia* and *Borrelia* species. Sexually transmitted bacterial infections such as *Neisseria gonorrhoeae, Chlamydia trachomatis* and *Treponema pallidum* can also lead to tonsillopharyngeal infections. Anaerobic bacteria can also be co-pathogens in GABHS infections, with a synergistic effect leading to suppurative complications.

Although diphtheria (*Corynebacterium diphtheria*) has almost been eradicated due to vaccination, this condition can rapidly lead to significant airway obstruction or delayed exotoxin-induced myocarditis and neuritis, therefore, a high diagnostic suspicion needs to be maintained.

Viral Pharyngitis

Viral pharyngitis is common. Rhinovirus, parainfluenza and corona are the most common etiological agents, but adenovirus, coxsackie, herpes simplex, Epstein-Barr virus (EBV), cytomegalovirus (CMV) and human immunodeficiency virus (HIV) may also be causal. Symptoms are similar to those of GABHS pharyngitis, although milder and features coryza, exanthema and cough and treatment is usually symptomatic.

Infectious Mononucleosis (Glandular Fever)

Glandular fever is a common, acute, systemic viral infection caused by EBV. IM is primarily a disease of young adults and the incubation period is 5–7 weeks. The most common symptom is tender cervical adenopathy, accompanied by sore throat. Pharyngeal signs range from acute follicular tonsillitis, profuse exudate, petechiae on the soft palate and sometimes a PTA. Airway obstruction can be seen, as well as periorbital oedema (Hoagland sign) and cranial nerve neuropathies.

The diagnosis is made from the clinical picture, together with mononucleosis on the peripheral blood film. CMV infection and toxoplasmosis can give a similar clinical picture. Traditionally, the Hoagland criteria was used to confirm the diagnosis of IM: >50% lymphocytes and >10% atypical lymphocytes with fever, pharyngitis, adenopathy and a positive serological test. The serological Paul Bunnell and monospot tests are similar in terms of sensitivity (63–95%) and specificity (84–100%). The gold standard is serological evidence of EBV-specific immunoglobulin M (IgM) antibody.

The systemic manifestations of EBV infection include generalised lymphadenopathy, hepatosplenomegaly, rubelliform skin rash and, rarely, gastrointestinal, cardiovascular, respiratory, neurological and haematological manifestations. The oncological risks following EBV-related IM include Hodgkin's disease, Burkitt's lymphoma, lymphoproliferative disorders in immunocompromised patients and the development of nasopharyngeal carcinoma. A history of IM significantly increases the risk of future multiple sclerosis.

Treatment is symptomatic for mild to moderate cases. Antivirals are generally not recommended, apart from severe manifestations when used as an adjunct to corticosteroids. Steroids are indicated for acute upper airway oedema rather than symptom control. Contact sports should be avoided for 4–6 weeks even in the absence of splenic enlargement because of the risks of splenic rupture.

Non-EBV Viral Pharyngitis
CMV infection in the immunocompetent host rarely results in clinically apparent disease. Infrequently, a mononucleosis-like syndrome with mild pharyngitis can be seen, particularly in older adults. Symptoms are similar to IM, but lymphadenopathy is less common.

Type 1 herpes simplex infection primarily involves the oral cavity/oropharynx, affecting younger children, causing severe vesicular and ulcerative stomatitis of the lips, tongue, gums, buccal mucosa and oropharynx. The treatment is supportive with analgesics and fluids. Acyclovir is active against herpes virus but is effective only if started at the onset of infection.

Herpes zoster pharyngitis arises from reactivation of the virus after previous chickenpox (i.e. shingles/cold sores). The pharyngeal features include odynophagia, vesicles and shallow ulcers in the distribution of cranial nerves V, IX and X. Treatment with antivirals should be started within 72 hours of onset of the lesions. Acyclovir has previously been the drug of choice, but valacyclovir/famciclovir are equally effective and have more convenient dosing regimens with decreased incidence of post-herpetic neuralgia.

Hand, foot and mouth is caused by coxsackieviruses and is characterised by a vesicular eruption in the oral cavity/oropharynx causing dysphagia and dehydration, with vesicles on the hands and feet. It is normally accompanied by pyrexia, malaise and vomiting. The illness is short-lived and mainly affects young children. Currently, it is not susceptible to antiviral agents or vaccination, therefore, prevention requires public health interventions and surveillance.

Non-Specific Chronic Pharyngitis
Non-specific chronic pharyngitis is common and relies on a history of long-standing variable throat discomfort without any specific aetiological factors, with often little to find on clinical examination. Aetiological factors include heavy smoking, industrial/occupational irritants, chronic sinusitis with post-nasal drip, acid reflux, poor dental hygiene, psychological stress or *Chlamydia pneumoniae* infection. Exclusion of malignancy is imperative and treatment is supportive by removing causative factors.

Specific Chronic Pharyngitis
Syphilis is a spirochaete infection (*T. pallidum*) acquired through sexual intercourse. The most frequent extragenital sites for the primary lesion (chancre) are the lips, tongue, buccal mucosa and tonsil. Secondary syphilis occurs 4–6 weeks after the primary lesion and features fever, headache, malaise, generalised lymphadenopathy, mucocutaneous rash and sore throat. The pharynx displays hyperaemia and inflammation and there may be mucus patches or 'snail track' ulcers. Serological tests for syphilis include Venereal Disease Research Laboratory (VDRL), rapid plasma reagin (RPR) and tests to detect specific treponemal antibodies. Penicillin is the treatment of choice, with 2.4 mega units intramuscularly in a single dose.

Pharyngeal tuberculosis (TB) is uncommon, but occasionally, can be seen in patients with widespread miliary TB. Lupus vulgaris is a low-grade cutaneous form of TB and has been described in the nasal cavities and pharynx. The diagnosis is usually made by association with pulmonary disease, and systemic treatment with triple therapy (isoniazid, rifampicin and pyrazinamide) is first line.

Toxoplasmosis is caused by the protozoan *Toxoplasma gondii*. Infection is usually asymptomatic, but some patients may have a sore throat with malaise, fever and cervical adenopathy. Serological diagnosis is often restricted due to cost. The disease is usually self-limiting and therefore treatment is unnecessary.

Scleroma is a chronic infective condition caused by *Klebsiella rhinoscleromatis*. The disease begins in the nose and only secondarily spreads to the pharynx where it produces granulomatous lesions and scarring.

Candidiasis

Oropharyngeal candidiasis (OPC), or thrush, is a common infection typically caused by the yeast *Candida albicans*. For symptomatic infection to occur, there must be local mucosal disease, a history of radiotherapy or immunocompromise (diabetes/immunosuppressive drugs). When symptomatic, it presents with pain and dysphagia and examination reveals small white/creamy-white plaque-like lesions on the tongue, palate, buccal mucosa or oropharynx (pseudomembranous lesions). Mild disease responds well to local therapy such as nystatin drops or lozenges and for moderate to severe disease, oral fluconazole is recommended.

HIV and AIDS

Pharyngeal presentation of HIV disease includes acute seroconversion illness (pyrexia, pharyngitis, malaise, mucous membrane ulceration, cervical lymphadenopathy), opportunistic infections (*Candida*, TB, syphilis, CMV, *Cryptococcus*), oral hairy leukoplakia (OHL), oral aphthous ulceration, lymphoid tissue hyperplasia and neoplastic lesions (non-Hodgkin's lymphoma [NHL], Kaposi's sarcoma [KS], squamous cell carcinoma [SCC] of the head and neck, Hodgkin's disease, myeloma and leiomyosarcoma in children).

Role of Tonsillectomy

The referral criteria for tonsillectomy in the presence of recurrent sore throats that are used currently in the United Kingdom are based on the following SIGN guidelines:

- Sore throats are due to acute tonsillitis.
- The episodes of sore throat are disabling and prevent normal functioning.
- Seven or more well-documented, clinically significant, adequately treated sore throats in the preceding year
  or
- five or more such episodes in each of the preceding years
  or
- three or more such episodes in each of the preceding 3 years.

Further Reading

Scottish Intercollegiate Guidelines Network (SIGN). The management of sore throat and indications for tonsillectomy. *National Clinical Guideline*. Edinburgh: SIGN; April 2010.

Centor R, Witherspoon J, Dalton H, et al. The diagnosis of strep throat in adults in the emergency room. *Med Decis Making* 1981; 1(3): 239–246.

National Institute for Health and Clinical Excellence (NICE). Respiratory tract infections: antibiotic prescribing. Prescribing of antibiotics for self-limiting respiratory tract infections in adults and children in primary care. *NICE Clinical Guidelines, CG69*. Issued: July 2008.

56. UPPER AIRWAY OBSTRUCTION AND TRACHEOSTOMY

Introduction
The upper aerodigestive tract, larynx, trachea and bronchi form the conduit between the external environment and the lungs to facilitate gas exchange. The larynx acts to protect the airway from aspiration during swallowing and is the primary organ for phonation. The narrowest site of the adult airway is the glottis and abnormal narrowing of the laryngotracheal complex causes breathlessness, particularly on exertion.

Pathophysiology of the Airway
In laminar airflow, airway resistance is dictated by the diametre of the airway and by the density of inspired gas (Poiseuille's law):

$$R = \frac{8nl}{\pi r^4}$$

where R = resistance, n = viscosity, l = length and r = radius.

Laryngotracheal Stenosis
In adults, approximately 50% of airway stenosis is seen post-intubation. Major risk factors include duration of ventilation, sizing of ventilation tubes, excessive cuff pressures and the patient's response to injury. Other aetiologies include bilateral vocal cord palsy, granulomatosis with polyangiitis (GPA), idiopathic subglottic stenosis (ISS), supraglottic stenosis, previous papilloma treatment, glottic web, tracheomalacia, vascular lesion, amyloidosis and congenital subglottic stenosis.

Diagnosis and Management
A history must establish previous prolonged ventilation, the duration of shortness of breath and coexisting medical problems. Voice changes and chronic cough are common but exertional dyspnoea is the main symptom. Chronic airway obstruction is sometimes misdiagnosed as asthma or chronic obstructive pulmonary disease.

Examine the severity of stridor, chest recession, body morphology (body mass index) and neck scars. Perform fibreoptic nasal endoscopy to assess vocal cord mobility, evidence of laryngopharyngeal reflux (LPR), pooling of secretions in the hypopharynx and the degree of stenosis if visible. If a tracheostomy is in place, the lower airway can also be assessed if the patient will tolerate temporary removal of the tracheostomy tube.

Investigate with a high-resolution computed tomography (CT) scan and request respiratory function testing to determine the severity of airway compromise but also to monitor the response to treatment. If there is any evidence of disordered swallowing, fibreoptic endoscopic evaluation of swallowing (FEES) or videofluoroscopy are helpful. Treat LPR with a twice daily proton pump inhibitor and an alginate suspension after the evening meal. Always manage patients within a multidisciplinary team including an ENT and thoracic surgeon, respiratory physician and speech and language therapist.

Intra-Operative Assessment
The definitive airway assessment is airway endoscopy. Flexible bronchoscopy allows assessment of the dynamic airway and rigid bronchoscopy is essential in tracheal stenosis. Suspension microlaryngoscopy, with jet ventilation, allows binocular vision with two hands free for surgery and use of the carbon dioxide laser where required. Prior to suspension, map the stenotic segment (by measuring the distance from the lips/teeth at the proximal and distal extremities of the stenosis) then grade the severity of the stenosis using the Myer–Cotton grading system (Table 56.1).

Table 56.1   Myer-Cotton grading system

Grade I	No obstruction to 50% obstruction
Grade II	51–70% obstruction
Grade III	71–99% obstruction
Grade IV	No detectable lumen

Surgery for Laryngotracheal Stenosis

Traditionally, endoscopic surgery for stenosis is employed in the first instance. Inflammatory stenoses may respond to steroid injection, radial cuts (laser or cold steel) or dilatation. Such procedures often need to be repeated periodically. More mature stenoses may require topical mitomycin-C application or tracheobronchial stents. Failure of endoscopic treatment may require open tracheal or cricotracheal resection.

Idiopathic Subglottic Stenosis

ISS is a rare, slowly progressive, fibro-inflammatory process of unknown aetiology, leading to narrowing of the airway in the subglottis. The diagnosis is one of exclusion and must follow the anatomical description above with no history of intubation or tracheostomy in the last 2 years, no neck trauma or surgery, no neck radiotherapy and be antineutrophil cytoplasmic antibody (ANCA) and angiotensin-converting enzyme (ACE) negative. Tissue for histology must be sent to exclude other inflammatory conditions or a low-grade neoplasm.

The majority of patients can be managed with endoscopic airway surgery once or twice a year. Aggressive laser ablation of the stenosis is not advised as this will risk more severe stenosis recurrence. Cricotracheal resection has been used to treat this condition but there are concerns over the post-operative voice due to the resection being in close proximity to the vocal cords. A laryngofissure and posterior cricoid split can instead be performed.

Granulomatosis with Polyangitis

GPA is an immune disorder characterised by inflammation of small- and medium-sized vessels. Most patients have other manifestations such as nasal crusting, subglottic stenosis and lungs or kidneys involvement. The presence of a positive cytoplasmic antinuclear cytoplasmic antibody (cANCA) test may aid diagnosis, but a definitive diagnosis will be made by tissue histology.

Approximately 25% of GPA patients have involvement of the larynx, trachea and bronchi; however, subglottic involvement is most commonly seen. Intra-lesional corticosteroid injections, radial cuts and dilatation will treat the majority of new stenoses, but tracheostomies and long-term stents may be required.

Sarcoidosis

A diagnosis of sarcoidosis depends on the presence of typical clinical features and non-caseating granulomatous inflammation on histology with the exclusion of other known causes of granulomas (tuberculosis, leprosy, syphilis and fungal disease).

Anatomically, laryngeal sarcoid has a predilection for the supraglottic region, particularly the epiglottis, aryepiglottic folds and arytenoids. Vocal cord paralysis is also reported as a result of perineural invasion. Laryngeal disease tends to progress slowly with a relapsing and remitting course.

High-dose systemic steroids have been recommended as the first-line treatment, but endoscopic steroid infiltration and laser reduction surgery have been used.

Bilateral Vocal Cord Mobility Impairment

Bilateral vocal cord mobility impairment (BVCMI) produces a reasonable voice but with a degree of dyspnoea as the vocal cords tend to lie in the median or paramedian position. There are three principal causes: bilateral laryngeal denervation (neck and chest malignancy or thyroid surgery), bilateral cricoarytenoid joint fixation (trauma or rheumatoid arthritis) and inter-arytenoid scarring (following endotracheal intubation).

Surgery is directed at improving the aperture of the posterior glottis. Endoscopic partial posterior cordectomy and partial arytenoidectomy can be performed using the CO_2 laser or where there is potential for recovery in time, a tracheostomy or vocal cord suture lateralisation procedure may be performed temporarily. Various reinnervation operations have been described; however, these are infrequently performed. Inter-arytenoid scarring can be treated with posterior laryngeal mucosal advancement flaps or posterior cricoid split with cartilage grafting; however, aspiration is almost universal post-operatively.

Acute Upper Airway Obstruction

The causes of upper airway obstruction are varied with some being immediately apparent whereas others are subtle. Aetiologies of rapidly progressive airway obstruction include penetrating or blunt trauma to the head and neck region, infections or oedema of the upper airway, vocal cord paralysis and foreign body inhalation. Primary malignancy of the head and neck may also present with acute airway obstruction.

Symptoms and Signs

In the absence of acute trauma to the upper airway, presenting symptoms include dyspnoea, cough, voice change, dysphagia, pain on swallowing or referred otalgia. Stridor denotes turbulent airflow and heralds complete airway obstruction. Inspiratory stridor is usually from obstruction at and above the glottic larynx, whereas expiratory stridor is from the intrathoracic airway and biphasic from the subglottis and trachea.

On examination, there may be increased work of breathing and accessory muscles of respiration use. Dysphonia indicates a laryngeal injury, and the greater the degree of hoarseness, the greater the severity. Drooling implies either pharyngeal or oesophageal obstruction or the avoidance of swallowing due to pain and bleeding denotes mucosal trauma or exposure of a vascular structure by an invasive lesion. Significant pharyngeal trauma and fractures of the laryngeal skeleton or trachea may give rise to surgical emphysema, which may independently worsen the upper airway obstruction.

Management

In resuscitation scenarios, the principle of an ABCDE approach is adopted. Examine to exclude or address any immediately reversible causes of airway obstruction as it should be secured by the least invasive technique that the attending clinician is capable of without delay. Where the airway is sufficiently stable but no cause for the airway compromise has been identified, the examination should include a transnasal fibreoptic endoscopy.

Medical Interventions

Administer high-flow oxygen via a face mask with a reservoir bag and use of humidification if practically possible. Heliox (80% helium:20% oxygen) results in less turbulent flow and allows the patient to experience reduced resistance during breathing. Steroids reduce mucosal oedema. Broad-spectrum antibiotics should be given in any case where acute infection is suspected. Adrenaline nebulisers also can help to reduce airway oedema.

Airway Interventions and Cricothyroidotomy

Simple airway adjuncts such as an oral Guedel airway or nasopharyngeal airway may assist with situations of supraglottic airway compromise. Endotracheal intubation is the intervention of choice where there has been a loss of respiratory drive necessitating assisted ventilation, or in cases of progressive upper airway obstruction. The usual route of intubation is via the mouth. An alternative route is transnasal intubation using endoscopic guidance.

In the emergency setting of 'can't intubate, can't oxygenate' (CICO), a surgical cricothyroidotomy using the 'scalpel–bougie' technique is supported by the Difficult Airway Society in the United Kingdom for front of neck airway (FONA) as the safest and quickest way to secure the airway. Extend the patient's neck, palpate the cricothyroid membrane in the midline and incise the skin vertically and the underlying membrane horizontally using a size 10 scalpel. Insert an airway bougie and railroad a size 6 endotracheal tube over the bougie into the airway.

Tracheostomy

Indications of tracheostomy:

- Upper airway obstruction
- Prolonged ventilation
- Removal of secretions
- Part of another procedure (major head and neck surgery/laryngectomy/pharyngolaryngectomy)

Effects of tracheostomy:

- Laryngeal bypass – loss of cough and phonation
- Reduction in respiratory dead space
- Loss of nasal mucosa filtration and humidification
- Increased risk of infection
- Tube acts as foreign body leading to local inflammation

Complications:

- Immediate (haemorrhage, air embolism, local damage)
- Intermediate (extubation, obstruction, subcutaneous emphysema, infection, fistulae)
- Late (tracheocutaneous fistula, tracheal stenosis)

The procedure should be carried out in an operating theatre under sterile conditions, under general or local anaesthesia. The patient should be supine, with the neck extended. A horizontal incision is sited halfway between the sternal notch and the lower border of the cricoid cartilage. Incise the skin and dissect through the subcutaneous tissues to the strap muscles, which are retracted laterally, following blunt dissection in the midline to separate them. The thyroid isthmus should be clamped, divided and transfixed. The anterior tracheal wall is identified and the tracheotomy should be made between the second and fourth tracheal rings. Before entering the trachea, select an appropriately sized tracheostomy tube and check that the cuff and all connecting equipment works properly. Having informed the anaesthetist that the trachea is about to be opened, the tracheotomy can be performed (vertical slit, horizontal slit or tracheal window). The anaesthetist should withdraw the endotracheal tube and, when the tip is immediately above the tracheotomy, withdrawal can stop and the tracheostomy tube should be inserted. The cuff should be inflated and the tube connected to the ventilator. The incision should be closed loosely and the tracheostomy tube secured in position with tapes and sutures.

KEY POINTS

- Assessment of the airway should be part of an overall systematic approach to managing the critically ill patient.
- The assessment should determine the level(s) of airway obstruction.
- Action should be decisive.
- The least invasive intervention that will bypass the level of the lowest obstruction should be used.
- Any intervention should be carried out by someone who is experienced in the use of that technique.

Further Reading

1. The National Tracheostomy Safety Project. http://www.tracheostomy.org.uk

2. Frerk C, Mitchell VS, McNarry AF, et al. Difficult Airway Society 2015 guidelines for management of unanticipated difficult intubation in adults. *Br J Anaesth* 2015; **115**(6): 827–848.

3. Pracy JP, Brennan L, Cook TM, et al. Surgical intervention during a can't intubate can't oxygenate (CICO) event: emergency front of neck airway (FONA). *Clin Otolaryngol* 2016; **41**(6): 624–626.

57. VOICE DISORDERS AND LARYNGITIS

The assessment and evaluation of a patient with a voice disorder should be done in a multidisciplinary clinic by a laryngologist and a speech therapist. Persistent or progressive dysphonia may suggest an organic lesion in the larynx, while intermittent dysphonia may suggest a functional disorder.

History

History should differentiate:

- Dysphonia/hoarseness: any impairment of voice or difficulty speaking
- Dysarthria: difficulty in articulating words
- Dysarthrophonia: dysphonia in conjunction with dysarthria (e.g. cerebrovascular accident)
- Dysphasia: impairment of the comprehension of spoken or written language
- Odynophonia: pain when talking

It is important to know the patient's occupation and professional and recreational voice usage. It is valuable to use self-administered questionnaires and the perceptual rating of voice questionnaire to assess the voice (Figure 57.1). These tools help with understanding the severity of the voice problem and help in measuring outcomes after treatment.

Examination

Examination should include:

- Neck for stigmata of previous surgery or masses
- Nasal cavity
- Findings implying cranial nerve or neurological disease

Laryngoscopy can be supplemented with stroboscopy, laryngography, or digital acoustic voice analysis. Videolaryngostroboscopy is the standard of care for a voice clinic.

Management

There are four broad categories of voice disorders:

- Inflammatory
- Structural or neoplastic
- Neuromuscular
- Muscle tension

Similarly, treatment for voice pathology can be split into the five modalities shown in Figure 57.2.

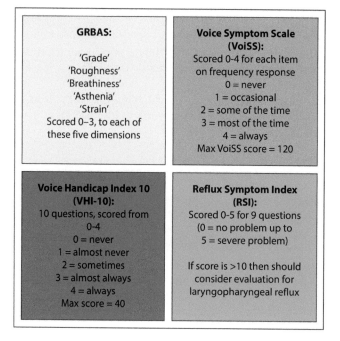

GRBAS:	Voice Symptom Scale (VoiSS):
'Grade' 'Roughness' 'Breathiness' 'Asthenia' 'Strain' Scored 0–3, to each of these five dimensions	Scored 0-4 for each item on frequency response 0 = never 1 = occasional 2 = some of the time 3 = most of the time 4 = always Max VoiSS score = 120
Voice Handicap Index 10 (VHI-10):	**Reflux Symptom Index (RSI):**
10 questions, scored from 0-4 0 = never 1 = almost never 2 = sometimes 3 = almost always 4 = always Max score = 40	Scored 0-5 for 9 questions (0 = no problem up to 5 = severe problem) If score is >10 then should consider evaluation for laryngopharyngeal reflux

Figure 57.1 Commonly used objective assessment measures.

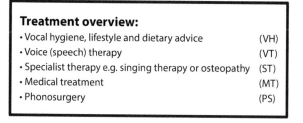

Treatment overview:
- Vocal hygiene, lifestyle and dietary advice (VH)
- Voice (speech) therapy (VT)
- Specialist therapy e.g. singing therapy or osteopathy (ST)
- Medical treatment (MT)
- Phonosurgery (PS)

Figure 57.2 Treatment overview.

Specific Voice Disorders and Their Management

Laryngitis

Laryngitis is a descriptive term indicating a degree of erythema, oedema, epithelial change that may include ulceration, leukoplakia, and/or stiffness of the mucosa of the vocal fold. Often there is an increased amount of thick mucus present. Most acute laryngitis is associated with upper respiratory tract infections. Chronic laryngitis has close links with smoking, alcohol, reflux, occupational exposures, social activities, allergies, and vocal/throat hygiene. The voice is usually hoarse (rough, strained, breathy, or whispery), which may be due to vocal fold stiffness from the inflammatory process and/or secondary to muscle tension imbalance. The majority of acute infections are self-limiting. Treatment of chronic laryngitis consists of voice hygiene (VH) with reduced use/abuse and rest.

Arytenoid Granuloma

Arytenoid granulomas are benign inflammatory lesions that arise from the perichondrium of the vocal processes (Figure 57.3). They result from trauma-related injury, predominately secondary to intubation or repeated impact from throat clearing/coughing. Reflux is accepted as an important aetiological factor, and it also slows down the healing process.

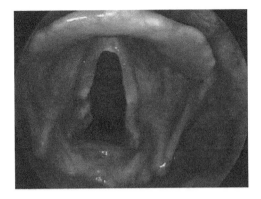

Figure 57.3   Arytenoid granuloma.

Symptoms:

- Dysphonia and/or vocal fatigue
- Tickling sensation
- Discomfort

Management:

- Reducing laryngeal irritants, i.e. stopping smoking, improving VH, treating any reflux. voice therapy (VT), which includes raising awareness of, and reducing, hyperfunctional vocally abusive behaviour.

Phonosurgery (PS) does not usually cure arytenoid granulomas when used in isolation as there is a high rate of recurrence.

- Botulinum toxin injections into the thyroarytenoid muscle can be helpful in difficult cases to stop impact, allowing healing.

Vocal Fold Polyps

Vocal fold polyps are benign swellings of greater than 3 mm that arise from lamina propria of the vocal folds (Figure 57.4).

- Most common cause of structural dysphonia.
- Often solitary, but occasionally bilateral.

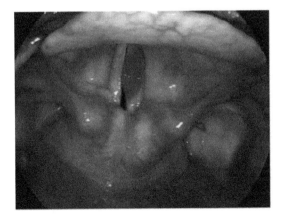

Figure 57.4   Right-side haemorrhagic vocal fold polyp.

- More common in men than in women.
- Smoking association.
- Predominately presents at age 30–50 years.
- Occasionally, a sulcus, mucosal bridge, or intracordal cyst is found immediately opposite on the contralateral vocal fold. These are thought to cause polyp formation; therefore, contralateral examination is crucial.

Symptoms:

- Dysphonia: voice is lowered in pitch and cuts out in speech.
- Lost vocal dynamic range partially.
- Straining to speak.
- Very seldom, large polyps can cause dyspnoea and episodes of choking.

Management:

- VT, but unlikely to result in polyp resolution.
- Treatment of concomitant inflammatory conditions.
- Most polyps need surgery
  - PS options include laser or cold steel.
  - The goal of surgery is to restore the smooth edge of the vocal cord to allow full closure and normal vibration.

Vocal Fold Nodules

Vocal fold nodules are small bilateral swellings (less than 3 mm in diameter) that develop on the free edge of the vocal fold at the maximal contact area (Figure 57.5).

- Associated with certain occupations (e.g. teaching, singing).
- In children, found more often in boys than in girls.
- In adults, strikingly more frequent in women, predominately less than 30 years old.

Aetiology of vocal nodules is thought to be voice abuse rather than overuse.

Symptoms:

- Voice often husky and breathy.
- Worsening symptoms with voice use.
- Often associated with discomfort on phonation.
- Phonation may become a little deeper in pitch and associated with breaks.

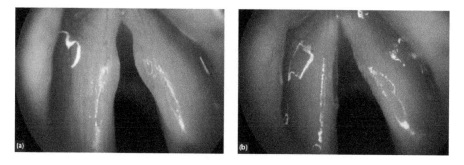

Figure 57.5 Vocal fold nodules. Bilateral, symmetric phonatory lesions along the anterior one third of the membranous vocal folds (a). After VT, the nodules remained, and the lesions were resected with CO_2 laser PS (b).

Management:

- If nodules are not causing significant problems, they should be left alone.
- Aggravating factors, such as inadequate lubrication, infections, and reflux, should be treated to reduce their irritant effects.
- Mainstay for persistent vocal nodules is VT with VH. Not infrequently, the voice and function improve, but the nodules persist.
- Surgery should be reserved for those who fail voice therapy and remain symptomatic. Surgical aim is precise excision of the nodule alone, with no exposure of the underlying ligament.

Pseudocysts

Pseudocysts are so named because the lesion has no cyst wall but is filled with serous fluid, having an appearance similar to that of a blister.

- Likely due to phonotrauma.
- Initial management is VH.
- PS might be necessary if symptoms are recalcitrant to therapy.

Reinke's Oedema

Reinke's oedema is a result of oedema of the subepithelial space (Reinke's space), as shown in Figure 57.6.

- Almost exclusively found in smokers.
- Hypothyroidism may be found as a concomitant feature.
- Reinke's space contains lakes of oedema.
- The sex distribution is equal, but the pitch-lowering effects on the voice are more conspicuous in women.
- Age at presentation is 40–60 years.

Symptoms:

- Deepening of the pitch of the voice in women
- Gruffness
- Inability to raise the pitch of the voice
- Choking episodes
- Reflux symptoms

Management:

Conservative measures like VH and smoking cessation manage symptoms well in most cases. Treat underlying hypothyroidism, infections, or reflux. VT may help in a well-motivated patient.

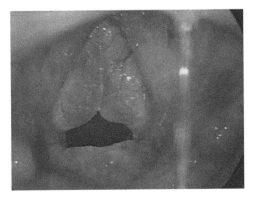

Figure 57.6   Reinke's oedema.

Surgical treatment should be considered if:

- Leukoplakia is present and a histological diagnosis is necessary.
- Gross oedema causes choking episodes or airway embarrassment.
- The inability to accomplish pitch elevation of the voice is problematic.

There is significant potential for worsening the patient's condition by causing scarring after PS. Reduction glottoplasties are performed using cold steel or laser. Care should be taken minimise epithelial excision due to the risk of causing a permanent scar and hoarseness. The myxematous material is aspirated/removed/vaporised, and then the epithelial edges are apposed, after excision of redundant mucosa as necessary. Often, good results are obtained by simply treating one side.

Cysts

Cysts are found less frequently than polyps and nodules, and sulci and mucosal bridges even less so. There are two primary types of cyst: mucous retention cyst and epidermoid cyst. A mucous retention cyst (Figure 57.7) is a blocked minor salivary gland.

Epidermoid cysts (Figure 57.8) are lined by squamous epithelium and are filled with keratin and cholesterol debris. They are thought to arise as a result of voice abuse/misuse. For both types of cysts, a definitive diagnosis is only possible by microlaryngoscopy and cordotomy (Figure 57.9).

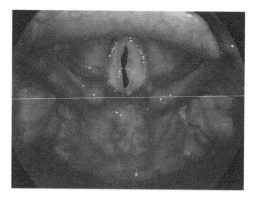

Figure 57.7   Mucous retention cyst.

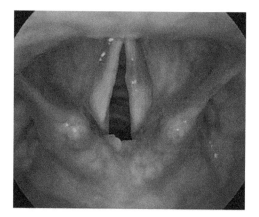

Figure 57.8   Epidermoid cyst.

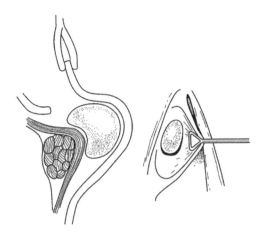

Figure 57.9   Epidermoid cyst approached via cordotomy and mucosal flap.

Adult Laryngeal Papilloma

- Associated with human papillomavirus (HPV) genotypes 6 and 11
- Bimodal incidence
- Juvenile: 2–4 years
- Adult: 20–40 years
- Small risk of malignant transformation in adult papilloma

Presentation:

- Progressive dysphonia
- Dyspnoea
- Stridor

Treatment:

- Endoscopic excision. Options include:
  - Cold steel
  - Microdebrider
  - Laser
- Adjuvant treatments:
  - Cidofovir—falling out of favour due to carcinogenic potential
  - Interferon-α—rarely used due to significant risk of side effects and morbidity, including neurological sequelae, leukopenia, cardiac dysfunction, and hepatorenal failure
  - Bevacizumab—antiangiogenic monoclonal antibody that appears to work and is in the process of undergoing randomised controlled trials (RCTs)
  - Photodynamic therapy—starting to emerge, but more evidence is needed before it becomes widely used
- HPV vaccine—quadrivalent vaccine for HPV 6/11/16/18 is now offered to males and females at ages 11–12 years in the United Kingdom
- Tracheostomy—should be avoided if possible due to risk of seeding the stoma or distal airways

Vocal Cord Palsy/Paresis

Vocal cord palsy/paresis often presents with breathy voice and symptoms of aspiration. An obvious laryngeal paresis will show asymmetry of movement on abduction and adduction, where the affected side 'lags behind' the normal side. Asymmetry maybe subtle and may only be apparent on prolonged endoscopic observation while asking the patient to phonate and then sniff repeatedly. Bilateral palsies/paresis present with upper airway symptoms, dyspnoea, stridor, and respiratory compromise.

Causes include:

- Iatrogenic injury (surgery)
- Malignant disease
- Trauma
- Idiopathic
- Neurological disease

It is fundamental to rule out malignancy with computed tomography (CT) of the skull base to thorax. Some centres use electromyography (EMG) to evaluate the laryngeal musculature.

Management:

- VT—strategies to allow compensation and decrease aspiration.
- Surgery
  - Injection medialisation procedure—endoscopic administration of absorbable semi-permanent materials (e.g. hydroxyapatite, collagen)
  - Laryngeal framework surgery—which may include insertion of an implant
  - Laryngeal reinnervation
- Bilateral palsies/paresis may need a tracheostomy acutely, but a range of other procedures may be used to improve the airway, such as a cordectomy.

Muscle Tension Dysphonia (MTD)

Muscle tension imbalance causing MTD is one of the biggest causes or contributors to voice disorders. Although it is often a diagnosis of exclusion (i.e. the vocal folds look normal and move normally), it is often present with inflammatory, structural, and neurological conditions as the laryngeal muscles try to overcome a deficiency in voice production. MTD can lead to trauma and structural changes in the vocal fold mucosa. MTD therefore ecompasses a group of conditions characterised by an imbalance of the synergist and antagonist muscles affecting vocal fold position and tensioning. Muscles are hyperfunctional or hypofunctional, giving recognizable patterns of clinical presentation and laryngeal appearance.

The degree of dysphonia is variable, ranging from an intermittent problem related to a particular voice task (e.g. teaching) to severe and constant hoarseness. Other symptoms include:

- Pitch: too high or low
- Reduced range
- Sensation of tightness, constriction, or lump in the throat
- Effortful voice production
- Discomfort on speaking or singing
- Vocal fatigue

Treatment consists of identifying precipitating causes and treating as appropriate, such as:

- Vocal hygiene and lifestyle advice
- Voice therapy targeted at specific muscle groups
- Laryngeal manipulation
- Behavioural therapy
- Medical treatment (e.g. reflux management)

Spasmodic Dysphonia (SD)

SD is a voice disorder arising from a focal dystonia involving certain laryngeal muscles but reflecting central motor processing issues/abnormalities. It is a task-specific dystonia: the spasm occurs only on phonation, and it can be overridden by vegetative phenomena, such as laughing, chanting, or singing. There is a background of normal speech overlaid with vocal spasms that are not under voluntary control. This leads to the typical strained and strangled speech pattern of adductor dysphonia (more common) and the breathy pattern of abductor dysphonia. SD is readily controlled with injections of botulinum toxin to the affected muscle groups, combined with VT to eliminate hyperfunction.

> **KEY POINTS**
>
> When assessing a patient, it is important to consider the following questions:
>
> - What are the patient's expectations? (Always ask this in voice consultations.)
> - Is there any suspicion of a malignant or premalignant condition?
> - Could the potential complications of an intervention, particularly surgical treatment, create more problems than the intervention can help?

Further Reading

Costello D, Sandhu G. Practical Laryngology, 2015.

Mohan S, Young K, Judd O. A Practical Guide to Laryngeal Framework Surgery, 2018.

58. DYSPHAGIA AND ASPIRATION

Dysphagia

Dysphagia is the term used to describe difficulty with swallowing solids, liquids, or both. It implies impairment of one or more of the phases of swallowing. Dysphagia usually arises as a complication of another health condition (see Table 58.1). It can be divided into oropharyngeal (high) dysphagia and oesophageal (low) dysphagia.

Aspiration

Aspiration is the entry of food or liquid into the airway below the true vocal folds. It may be due to incompetent or inadequate airway protection and ill-timed, uncoordinated events before, during, or after the swallow has triggered. Silent aspiration is defined as foreign material entering the trachea or lungs without an outward sign of coughing or attempts at expulsion.

Clinical Assessment

The history should include the onset, duration, progression, and severity of the symptoms, as well as the types of food that give problems. Typically, malignant dysphagia presents with a short and progressive history, including a need to change to foods with softer textures and more liquid consistency, and associated weight loss. Conversely, in neuromyogenic dysphagia it can be more difficult to swallow fluids.

A fibreoptic endoscopic examination of the upper aerodigestive tract should be performed in all cases of dysphagia. The assessment of swallow (fibreoptic endoscopic evaluation of swallowing— FEES) is very useful in identifying aspiration, in evaluating secretion management, and for visual feedback to the patient during compensatory procedures to aid swallowing and reduce aspiration. The examination can be performed at the bedside, and ideally a digital recording is made. Foodstuffs of different textures that have been dyed with food colouring to enhance their visibility can be given. Bolus flow during swallow, laryngeal penetration and aspiration, and post-swallow residue should be documented. Endolaryngeal sensation can also be assessed.

Table 58.1 Causes of dysphagia and aspiration

Congenital	Oesophageal motility disorder
Cleft lip and palate	Achalasia
Cerebral palsy	Oesophageal spasm
Vascular rings	Presbydysphagia
Oesophageal atresia	
Laryngeal cleft	
Tracheo-oesophageal fistula	
Infection	**Neoplastic**
Pharyngitis	Benign tumours
Deep neck space infection	Malignant tumours
Inflammatory	**Neurological**
Laryngopharyngeal reflux	Cerebrovascular accident
Gastro-oesophageal reflux	Parkinson's disease
Eosinophilic oesophagitis	Multiple sclerosis
Patterson-Brown-Kelly syndrome	Myasthenia gravis
Scleroderma	Vocal cord palsy
Systemic lupus erythematosus	
Sjögren's syndrome	
Traumatic	**Miscellaneous**
Foreign body	Chemotherapy-radiotherapy
Food bolus	Pharyngeal pouch
Caustic burns	Globus pharyngeus
Head and neck trauma	
Spinal trauma	

Barium swallow or water-soluble contrast swallow testing provides a useful outline of the pharyngeal and oesophageal anatomy and is particularly useful for assessment of pharyngeal pouches and dysmotility.

Where concern about a malignant cause exists, cross-sectional imaging and examination of the upper aerodigestive tract under general anaesthesia are indicated.

Swallowing Rehabilitation
Successful rehabilitation of patients with dysphagia depends upon accurate diagnosis. In recent years, dysphagia rehabilitation has broadened from an almost exclusive use of peripheral muscle strengthening to incorporate techniques designed to maximize central control.

Oral Motor Exercises
Originally, oral motor exercises were developed for improving articulatory precision related to speech. Subsequently, these exercises were logically expanded and transferred to swallowing rehabilitation, with the goal of improving oral-phase movements and facilitating tongue-driving forces involved in the pharyngeal phase of swallowing.

Effortful Swallow
The instructions for the effortful swallow technique are simply to 'swallow hard.' Because increased effort resulted in increased pressure on the bolus, this technique was routinely applied to reduce pharyngeal residue in patients with pharyngeal motility disorders. However, a potential complication of the effortful swallow is decreased anterior hyoid movement during swallowing.

Mendelsohn Manoeuvre
Following initiation of swallowing, peak hyolaryngeal excursion is maintained for several seconds before relaxing and completing the swallow. The presumed benefit of the Mendelsohn manoeuvre is prolonged suprahyoid contraction, which results in prolonged upper oesophageal sphincter (UOS) opening for improved bolus flow into the oesophagus.

Masako Manoeuvre

In the Masako manoeuvre, the patient is instructed to protrude their tongue and gently hold it between their incisors. This can be used specifically to overcome the significantly increased anterior bulge of the posterior pharyngeal wall seen in patients who have undergone base of tongue resection.

Head-Lift (Shaker) Exercise

The head-lift exercise strengthens the floor of the mouth. The individual lies on their back and raises their head until they can see their feet. Strengthening the muscles of the floor of the mouth that are involved in both the oral and pharyngeal phases of swallowing increases laryngeal excursion, increases the width and duration of UOS opening, and consequently decreases UOS intrabolus pressure in healthy elderly individuals.

Expiratory Muscle Strengthening

Expiratory muscle strength training (EMST) is quickly emerging into more widespread clinical practice and is a promising approach for managing pharyngeal swallowing impairment and airway protection. EMST is designed to strengthen the contraction of the expiratory musculature by directing expiratory airflow through a one-way, spring-loaded valve that remains open in the presence of positive airflow.

Maximising Central Control

Increased understanding of the neural control of swallowing—particularly the role of the cerebrum in swallowing neural networks—has brought about a significant paradigm expansion in the collective approach to swallowing impairment.

Skill Training

Relearning or modifying the complex sequence of swallowing events at the level of central control is gaining increasing recognition as a type of skill-based training for use after neurological impairment. To further strengthen this approach, the use of biofeedback from electromyography and manometry is being explored.

Stimulation

The development of brain imaging and stimulation techniques has significantly expanded our understanding of the neurophysiological mechanisms of swallowing. Approaches like transcranial magnetic stimulation and direct current stimulation, designed to improve swallowing function through extrinsic modulation of central neuronal circuits involved in swallowing motor control, are being explored.

Chronic Aspiration

Prevention of aspiration occurs primarily through reflex laryngeal closure, laryngeal elevation, and cessation of breathing during swallowing, and any aspirated contents are expelled through coughing. A certain amount of aspiration is normal in humans, especially during sleep, and it is tolerated without complications in healthy subjects with normal tracheobronchial ciliary function and normal immunology.

The response to even small quantities of aspiration will depend on the pH of the aspirate, the microorganisms present, and the person's pulmonary and immunological status. Aspiration may lead to cough or, in some cases, life-threatening pulmonary complications. In cases where the cough reflex is reduced or absent, silent aspiration may occur. Acute, severe aspiration of a large bolus may cause airway obstruction and may prove fatal, whereas chronic, small-volume aspiration may risk pneumonia or respiratory failure through chronic pulmonary emphysematous disease or bronchiectasis.

Principles of Management

The management aims are to protect the airway, to avoid life-threatening respiratory complications, and to achieve adequate nutrition, while also considering the psychological and social aspects of food and feeding.

Surgery for Aspiration

Cricopharyngeal Myotomy

If pooling of secretions in the hypopharynx due to a hypertonic or uncoordinated cricopharyngeal sphincter, myotomy may help. Trial of medical myotomy using botulinum toxin can be utilized before considering either transoral laser myotomy or an external approach.

Laryngeal Incompetence

Vocal fold medialisation can help to reduce chronic aspiration if vocal fold immobility and positioning are contributory. Injection thyroplasty can be used as a trial before considering a permanent thyroplasty technique.

Glottic closure techniques for aspiration have been described but are not commonly used. They are prone to breakdown and render patients dependent upon tracheostomies. Many surgeons would advise narrow field laryngectomy over these techniques.

Pharyngeal Pouch

A pharyngeal pouch (Zenker's diverticulum) is a posterior pulsion diverticulum occurring in a natural weakness (Killian's dehiscence) between the fibres of the thyropharyngeus and cricopharyngeus. It is associated with an oesophageal motility disorder in the majority of cases.

The symptomatic patient complains of dysphagia, regurgitation of food, coughing, aspiration or repeated chest infections. Treatment is indicated when symptoms affect quality of life or pose a risk to the patient's health.

Endoscopic techniques transect the diverticulo-oesophageal wall so that material does not collect in the pouch. This transection also divides the cricopharyngeus and some upper oesophageal muscle fibres, and it quite neatly performs a synchronous myotomy. Division of this dividing wall has evolved from using electrocoagulation, the CO_2 laser, and, more recently, endoscopic stapling devices. Unfortunately, the endoscopic approach is not always feasible if there is poor access, and it is not always suitable for very small or very large pouches; furthermore, there is still a small incidence of post-operative leaks with the risk of mediastinitis. In some cases, it is necessary to perform an external approach diverticulectomy combined with a cricopharyngeal myotomy. This does, however, mean a longer hospital stay and increased morbidity.

Laryngeal Suspension

In severe cases of aspiration where there is reduced laryngeal elevation, excessive pooling of hypopharyngeal secretions, and reduced laryngeal sensation, or severely discoordinated swallowing, the aspiration poses a significant risk to life. If there is also limited likelihood of recovery of swallow function, yet life expectancy is still reasonable, then the safest option is to consider a narrow-field laryngectomy.

There are, however, some intermediate measures to consider before taking such a drastic step. Laryngeal suspension techniques aim to elevate the larynx away from hypopharyngeal secretions and also to pull open the upper oesophageal inlet.

Laryngectomy

A narrow-field laryngectomy removes the laryngeal skeleton but spares the hyoid, the strap muscles, and the hypopharyngeal mucosa, allowing for a multilayer closure with reduced incidence of a fistula. Preservation of pharyngeal mucosa also means that pharyngeal closure can be achieved using a linear stapling device and feeding can commence within 5–7 days.

Discussion

The ideal surgical procedure for chronic aspiration would be simple, associated with few complications, allow speech and swallowing, and be easily reversible without long-term sequelae.

The majority of patients with a reversible neurological deficit tend to show recovery within a few months, and it is the practice in most units to manage these patients with tracheostomies and feeding tubes, although this may be far from ideal. There are therefore very few indications for reversible procedures. Dysphagia with mild aspiration due to dysfunction of the cricopharyngeus muscle, weakness of the hemilarynx, or reduced pharyngeal constrictor activity can usually be managed with a cricopharyngeal myotomy or vocal cord medialisation with or without excision of the redundant pharyngeal mucosa. Laryngeal or laryngohyoid suspension may be considered in more severe cases.

The difficult decision is with patients who are not going to recover a safe swallow or who are experiencing either a neurological condition that is progressive or severe scarring and contracture related to radiotherapy treatment. Supportive procedures described above may be helpful for a while, but there will come a time when a laryngectomy may become the procedure of choice. It provides a definitive separation of the respiratory and digestive tracts. Feeding tubes and tracheostomies are avoided and depending on residual dexterity and neurological function surgical voice restoration may be possible.

Further Reading

1. Ludlow CL. Central nervous system control of the laryngeal muscles in humans. *Respir Physiol Neurobiol* 2005; 147(2–3): 205–222.

2. O'Keeffe ST. Use of modified diets to prevent aspiration in oropharyngeal dysphagia: is current practice justified? *BMC Geriatr* 2018; 18: 167.

3. Katoh M, Ueha R, Sato T, Sugasawa S, Goto T, Yamauchi A, Yamasoba T. Choice of aspiration prevention surgery for patients with neuromuscular disorders: report of three cases. *Front Surg* 2019; 6: 66.

59. SALIVARY GLAND TUMOURS

Incidence

- The incidence of salivary gland cancer (SGC) is 7–12 per 1,000,000. Benign salivary neoplasms are more common, occurring in up to 6 per 100,000.
- Most tumours (80%) arise in the parotid glands, of which 30% are malignant, and 10% arise in the submandibular glands, 40% being malignant. Less than 1% occur in the sublingual and minor salivary glands (MiSG), where the majority (70–90%) are malignant.
- Benign tumours affect all age groups, with a peak incidence in the sixth decade.
- Malignancy is relatively more likely in younger patients.

Risk Factors

- Salivary malignancy increases with exposure to environmental factors, low-dose ionizing radiation, and aflatoxins.
- Smoking is related to development of Warthin's tumours.

Clinical Presentation

Most parotid and submandibular gland tumours are slow-growing and asymptomatic. The patient eventually becomes aware of a firm mass. A small number of tumours cause discomfort by obstructing salivary flow. Deep lobe parotid tumours may be impalpable clinically, but they may displace the tonsil and palate medially, causing stertor, sleep disordered breathing, altered voice, and Eustachian tube dysfunction.

MiSG are found throughout the entire upper aerodigestive tract and the signs and symptoms of MiSG tumours depend upon the anatomical site involved. The most common sites are the oral cavity/oropharynx, and the tumours often present as firm submucosal swellings.

The following symptoms and signs suggest the tumour may be malignant:

- Pain
- Paraesthesia
- Rapid growth
- Facial/other nerve palsy
- Skin involvement
- Fixity
- Irregularity
- Ulceration
- Associated lymphadenopathy

Investigation

Imaging

- Image guidance facilitates fine-needle aspiration cytology (FNAC) or core biopsy, and it increases the 'hit rate'.
- Imaging provides complimentary diagnostic information.
- Imaging assists with diagnosis and in evaluating the urgency of resection.
- Imaging aids staging of tumour.
- Ultrasound is usually adequate for most lesions.
- Consider cross-sectional imaging for large tumours (>3 cm), deep lobe/parapharyngeal space involvement, or suspicion of malignancy.
- MRI is generally preferred due to better definition of tumour–normal salivary gland interface, and it is not affected by dental artefact.
- Imaging features that suggest malignancy include an irregular capsule, extracapsular invasion, hypervascularity, and features consistent with necrosis.

FNAC and Core Biopsy

- Malignant tumours must be detected and accurately characterized pre-operatively wherever possible, as the staging, workup, and surgery may differ.
- FNAC has an accuracy for the diagnosis of benign lesions of around 95%, and an accuracy of 80% for malignancy.
- Core biopsy can improve diagnostic accuracy further or may be used as a second-line method if FNAC suggests possible malignancy. Theoretical risk of tumour seeding has been suggested.
- Even if FNAC suggests benign disease, removal of the tumour for further histopathology analysis remains mandatory.

Common Benign Tumours

Pleomorphic Adenomas (PAs)

PAs are derived from intercalated duct/myoepithelial cells. Most parotid PAs are within the superficial lobe, but a small proportion arise in or involve the deep lobe. Most patients with a PA should be advised to have surgery on the basis of definitive histology, the tumour's continued growth if left untreated, and the small chance of malignant transformation (1–5% per decade). The mucoid nature and exceptionally thin/absent capsule make PAs extremely fragile, and they can rupture during surgery, inevitably seeding the operative field and increasing the risk of recurrence.

Choice of Operation

- Controversy exists about the extent of parotidectomy—total superficial parotidectomy, partial superficial parotidectomy (the tumour and a cuff of normal tissue), or extracapsular dissection.
- Despite a total or partial superficial parotidectomy, there is often one margin adjacent to the facial nerve (FN) that would be exposed anyway. On this basis, a careful extracapsular dissection may be justified.
- Deep lobe tumours generally require total conservative parotidectomy.
- Parapharyngeal space PAs can be excised via a cervicoparotid or transmandibulotomy/transpharyngeal approach. Transoral robotic surgery offers an alternative.
- PAs of the submandibular gland are treated with extracapsular excision of the gland (higher rate of marginal mandibular injury).
- PAs of the MiSG are treated with wide local excision.

Recurrence of PAs

- Most recurrences are multicentric (overall recurrence rate up to 2%).
- Recurrences typically occur a decade after the original surgery.
- It is important to repeat imaging and FNAC, because there is a higher rate of malignant change within recurrent tumours (3%).
- In general, all remaining parotid tissue should be resected. If there is significant risk to FN, limited surgery may be considered.
- Recurrent PA of submandibular gland should be treated with selective neck dissection (Levels I–III), which will remove the tissue that harbours recurrent disease.
- Radiotherapy is effective in reducing further recurrence of PA, and it should be considered following revision surgery.

Warthin's Tumour (Adenolymphoma)

Warthin's tumours are thought to arise from salivary duct inclusions within intraparotid lymph nodes. They account for 20% of benign parotid tumours and are frequently bilateral. Malignant change is exceedingly rare. FNAC and imaging can provide a diagnosis. The tumour can be managed either conservatively with observation, or with surgery.

Surgery: Parotid Gland

Management of Complications

- *Facial weakness*: Facial nerve injury is a significant morbidity. Risk of facial nerve damage is related to the extent of the disease, type of resection, and surgical experience. Neuropraxia usually recovers within 4–6 weeks, and more severe injuries, in 6–12 months. Risk of permanent facial palsy is 1–2%.
- *Sensory loss*: Sensory loss in the distribution of the greater auricular nerve (GAN) is unavoidable. Some improvement is seen 12 months post-operatively.
- *Cosmetic defects*: The incision rarely causes huge concern. Loss of bulk behind the mandibular ramus may be visible and can be mitigated with fat transfer if necessary.
- *Frey's syndrome*: Gustatory sweating/flushing may be socially embarrassing, but it affects only a minority of patients. Conservative surgery may decrease the risk. Application of an antiperspirant or subdermal botulinum toxin injection may be necessary.
- *Salivary fistula or collection (sialocele)*: Sialocele occurs a few days after surgery and can be tense and painful. Collections are aspirated, and aspiration may need repeating.

Antibiotics may be considered to prevent/treat secondary infection. Hyoscine patches or botulinum toxin injection can reduce saliva production. Both leaks and collections almost always settle.

- *Stump neuroma of GAN*: When the GAN is cut, the stump can form a painful neuroma, often some time after surgery. It can be managed by simple local excision and burying of the fresh nerve end in the muscle.
- *First bite syndrome*: Rarely, intense pain occurs in the parotid gland when the patient is just about to eat, but the pain quickly passes. This syndrome is generally self-limiting. Treatment with botulinum toxin or antineuropathic agents can be effective.

Operative Procedure

The fundamental principle of a parotidectomy is exposure of the FN and then removal of the gland and diseased tissue from around it. The branching pattern of the FN can vary, and the nerve may be displaced from its normal position by tumour. The FN monitor can aid identification of the nerve and manipulation of the tissues around it. The FN trunk can be identified by several anatomical landmarks:

- *Tragal pointer*: inferior portion of cartilaginous external auditory canal. FN lies 1 cm deep and inferior to its tip.
- *Tympanomastoid suture*: FN lies immediately deep and inferior to this at its point of exit from the skull.
- *Posterior belly of the digastric muscle*: FN leaves the skull immediately anterior to the attachment of this muscle.
- *Styloid process*: lies deep to the exit of the FN from the skull, so care must be taken using this landmark.
- *Retrograde dissection*: of terminal FN branches.

Surgery: Submandibular Gland

Unlike the parotid, where only a part of the gland is removed, total resection of the submandibular gland is always indicated for tumours of the submandibular gland.

Informed Consent

- *Marginal mandibular nerve weakness*: weakness of the angle of the mouth, most noticeable on smiling/puckering the lips. Permanent weakness 2–3%.
- *Lingual and hypoglossal nerve damage*: is unusual but possible (<1%). Tongue motor dysfunction impairs articulation and mastication, but rapidly compensates.

Malignant Tumours

Introduction

SGC is rare, and it is complex owing to its heterogeneity, both in histological appearance and in clinical behaviour. The vast majority of salivary gland malignancies are epithelial tumours (> 80%), the remainder being mesenchymal or haematolymphoid tumours. Patients are staged using the TNM system (See Staging of Head and Neck Cancer). MiSG cancers are staged as per the anatomic site they originate in.

Common Malignant Tumours

- *Acinic cell carcinoma (AcCC)*: 3% of all SGC, up to 17% in parotid gland. Considered low grade, with good survival. Long natural history, long-term follow-up required.
- *Mucoepidermoid carcinoma (MEC)*: high incidence in MiSG. Prognosis mainly influenced by clinical stage, histological grade, and surgical margins. Low-grade tumours have excellent prognosis.
- *Adenoid cystic carcinoma (AdCC)*: mainly occurs in MiSG, lesser incidence in major salivary glands. Often diagnosed at an advanced stage, and complete excision may not be possible due to complex anatomical location. Propensity for perineural

extension and neuronal skip lesions. Tendency for local recurrence and distant metastases (often pulmonary) despite aggressive treatment.

- *Polymorphous adenocarcinoma (PAC):* 75% arise from MiSG, frequently in palate. Local recurrence may occur even with negative margins and can occur very late in follow-up.
- *Carcinoma ex pleomorphic adenoma:* 25% of salivary gland cancers. Tend to arise in major glands. Carry a poor prognosis.

Treatment
Parotid, Submandibular, and Sublingual Glands

- Surgery is the preferred treatment of parotid and submandibular gland cancers.
- The extent of surgery depends on the size of the lesion, its relationship to FN, and extraparotid tissue invasion.
- The majority of parotid cancers (80%) are located in the superficial parotid lobe, with a normal functioning FN. A standard superficial partial parotidectomy would be adequate for the majority of small cancers.
- Total parotidectomy may be advocated in locally advanced, high-grade tumours, because intraparotid lymph nodes that may harbour metastatic disease may be overlooked.
- FN-preserving parotidectomy, allowing for microscopic remnant disease if unavoidable, followed by radiotherapy in a patient with a pre-operatively functioning FN, is considered the standard of care.
- Gross tumour involvement of the FN requires nerve resection followed by immediate cable grafting. GAN is usually adequate for this purpose.
- For submandibular gland malignancy, the minimally required surgery is a gland resection within a Level I–III neck dissection.
- The N+ neck requires surgery (Levels I–V). N0 neck should be treated electively surgically or by radiotherapy, depending on the risk factors (tumour >4 cm, histological high-grade).
- Post-operative radiotherapy in advanced disease or in the presence of poor prognostic features improves locoregional control and survival.
- Radiotherapy can be used in unresectable disease or in patients who are not surgical candidates. Chemotherapy remains of palliative use in salivary gland cancer.

MiSG Cancer

- Treatment of MiSG cancer is wide local resection with clear margins. Radiotherapy to the primary site is generally recommended for most patients, unless tumour is a low-grade variant.
- Treatment of the neck is considered in patients with N+ or high-grade cancers, but risk of occult metastasis is otherwise low.

Histiotyping, Grading, and Prognosis
Histological diagnosis can be difficult in SGC. A reclassification rate of up to 29% has been observed. Different histological subtypes are divided into low, intermediate, and high grades as a surrogate marker for biological behaviour (Box 10.1). However, a clear relationship between histological subtype, grading, and biological aggressiveness is often lacking. Furthermore, grading often has little therapeutic relevance, as most salivary gland cancers are treated similarly with surgery and post-operative radiotherapy. Treatment results for both major and minor salivary gland cancers are comparable, with 60–70% 5-year survival and 50–60% 10-year survival. Prognosis varies widely depending on patient, tumour, and treatment related factors.

Further Reading

World Health Organization Classification of Head and Neck Tumours (4th edition) 2017: Salivary gland tumours.

60.   PARAPHARYNGEAL SPACE

Parapharyngeal Tumours

Lesions of the parapharyngeal space are rare, accounting for only 0.5% of head and neck masses. However, they may involve a wide spectrum of primary pathologies.

Anatomy

The parapharyngeal space is an inverted, pyramidal-shaped neck space filled with fat and areolar tissue (Figure 60.1). Its superior base comprises the sphenoid and temporal bones and includes the jugular and hypoglossal canal and the foramen lacerum. Its inferior apex is at the greater cornu of the hyoid bone. It has three sides, medial, lateral, and posterior, and an anterior leading edge that is the pterygomandibular raphe.

The medial surface is distensible and comprises the superior pharyngeal constrictor muscle, the buccopharyngeal membrane, and the pharynx. The lateral surface, which is relatively immobile, comprises the medial pterygoid muscle, the ramus of the mandible, the deep lobe of the parotid gland, and the posterior belly of the digastric muscle. The posterior surface is part of the prevertebral fascia, bordered by the carotid sheath posterolaterally and the retropharyngeal space posteromedially.

Two fascial condensations in the parapharyngeal space are of surgical importance. The aponeurosis of Zuckerkandl and Testut (Figure 60.2) is fascia that joins the styloid process to the tensor veli palatini. It divides the parapharyngeal space into the pre-styloid and post-styloid compartments. The pre-styloid compartment contains adipose tissue, lymphatics, ectopic salivary gland tissue, small nerves and vessels, a small branch of the trigeminal nerve to the tensor veli palatini muscle, and branches of the ascending pharyngeal artery and pharyngeal venous plexus.

The post-styloid compartment is posteromedial and contains the internal carotid artery, internal jugular vein, cranial nerves IX to XII, the cervical sympathetic chain, lymph nodes, and glomus bodies.

The stylomandibular ligament is formed by a band of the cervical fascia that extends from near the apex of the styloid process to the angle and posterior border of the mandible (Figure 60.3). It and the posterior border of the mandible form the stylomandibular tunnel. The tunnel is a deep relation of the deep lobe of the parotid gland. Tumours of the deep lobe can extend into the parapharyngeal space through this tunnel, giving rise to a dumbbell-shaped tumour.

Primary Pathology

A comprehensive review of the literature identified 70 different histological subtypes of lesions, of which 82% were benign and 18% were malignant. The most common tumours were of salivary gland origin (45%). These arose in the pre-styloid compartment. The vast majority (75%) were benign and most (64%) were pleomorphic adenomas. Adenoid cystic carcinoma and mucoepidermoid carcinoma were the most common primary malignancies. The second most common tumours were neurogenic in origin, accounting for 41%. The majority of these lesions were benign, and of these 52% were paragangliomas, 27% were schwannomas, and 9% were neurofibromas.[1]

Secondary Pathology

The parapharyngeal space may be directly invaded by malignancy from the nasopharynx, tonsil, retromolar trigone, palate, and tongue base.

The most common metastases to the parapharyngeal space are from nasopharyngeal cancer. Parapharyngeal nodes may also be involved in oropharyngeal and maxillary sinus cancers. Rarely, these nodes may be involved with metastases from distant sites, such as breast, colon, and prostate cancer.

Clinical Presentation and Evaluation

Parapharyngeal tumours are usually asymptomatic oropharyngeal masses, found on incidental examination. They may present with nasal obstruction, snoring, or hearing loss due to Eustachian tube occlusion. Rarely, they may present with cranial nerve dysfunction causing hoarseness, dysphagia, or cough, due to pressure on, or involvement of, the hypoglossal, vagus, or glossopharyngeal nerve.

Bimanual palpation helps assess tumour mobility and size, and appreciation of the displacement of the tonsil or the posterior pharyngeal wall provides clues to whether the lesion has its origins from the pre-styloid or post-styloid compartment.

Imaging and Other Investigations

Imaging of the parapharyngeal space is essential to planning surgical resection. Multiplanar imaging with fine-slice computed tomography (CT) and magnetic resonance imaging (MRI) provides the detail required. Further information regarding vascularity and relationship to the neurovascular structures can be gained from angiography. Therapeutic interventions, such as pre-operative embolization, or balloon occlusion studies can be performed at the same time.

Knowledge of the displacement patterns of fat and the internal carotid artery within the parapharyngeal space will aid in the localization of lesions.

Some lesions will have characteristic appearances on cross-sectional imaging that can provide diagnostic information.

Treatment

Lesions of the parapharyngeal space are predominantly treated by surgery. The aim of surgery is to remove the lesion with minimal morbidity. Adjuvant radiotherapy is reserved for malignant lesions or recurrent benign lesions with a high risk of recidivism. Chemotherapy is administered when indicated by specific histology, such as rhabdomyosarcoma, positive margin status, tumour histology, and perineural and lympho-vascular spread. Radiotherapy has also been used in patients who are considered a high surgical risk or for unresectable lesions.

The choice of surgical technique is dependent on the tumour size, its relationship to the parotid gland and skull base, and whether the tumour is malignant.

Transcervical Approach

The transcervical approach is ideal for small benign lesions independent from the deep lobe of parotid.

The procedure is performed under a general anaesthetic with a nasotracheal tube, which allows an extra centimetre of anterior distraction of the mandible. A skin crease incision 5 cm below the mandible protects the marginal mandibular branch of the facial nerve. The platysma is divided and the fascia of the submandibular gland is raised with the superior flap to protect the facial nerve. The submandibular gland can be mobilized or excised. The stylomandibular ligament is divided, allowing the mandible to be distracted. The parapharyngeal space is located between the digastric muscle, the mandible, and the medial pterygoid muscle insertion on the mandible.

Transcervical–Transparotid Approach

The transcervical–transparotid approach is well suited for lesions arising from the deep lobe of the parotid gland, for vascular tumours (as it allows access to vessels in the neck), and for the resection of malignant lesions. The transcervical incision is extended into a modified Blair's incision. Parotidectomy increases access to the parapharyngeal space. Management of the facial nerve is determined by the pre-operative functional status and the histology of the lesion being excised.

Mandibulotomy

A mandibular osteotomy further improves access and may be necessary for infiltrative malignant lesions and those high in the space and/or involving the skull base. A tracheostomy or overnight intubation may be required to protect the airway. Mandibulotomy can lead to a longer hospital stay, delay in return to normal nutrition, and additional complications, such as temporomandibular joint dysfunction and malunion.

Transoral Robotic Surgery (TORS)

The advent of robotics and modern endoscopic systems has made the transoral approach more viable for tumours of the parapharyngeal space.

Technical advantages of TORS include a three-dimensional high-resolution image with magnification, as well as the tremor filtration and motion scaling that allow delicate dissection.

The improved angled visual access enables the superior and inferior extents of tumours to be visualised via a transoral approach.

The ideal indications for TORS parapharyngeal space resection are benign salivary gland tumours occurring in the pre-styloid compartment, displacing the carotid artery posteriorly and laterally. These are the majority of parapharyngeal space tumours. Schwannomas and other benign neural tumours that are not deforming the carotid artery and not displacing the carotid artery medially are suitable for resection.

Complications of Surgery

Complications relate to vascular injury, lower cranial nerve injury, tumour spillage, tumour recurrence and first bite syndrome. First bite syndrome is thought to be due to loss of sympathetic innervation to the parotid gland, which leads to increased sensitivity of the myoepithelial cells to parasympathetic stimulation.

Further Reading

1. Riffat F, Dwivedi RC, Palme C, et al. A systematic review of 1143 parapharyngeal space tumors reported over 20 years. *Oral Oncol* 2014; **50**(5): 421–430.

2. López F, Suárez C, Vander Poorten V, et al. Contemporary management of primary parapharyngeal space tumors. *Head & Neck* 2019; 41: 522–535.

61. STAGING OF HEAD AND NECK CANCER

Introduction
Many factors affect the outcome of patients with a malignant head and neck tumour. The factors relate to the tumour, the host, and management. Staging of head and neck cancer is a system designed to express the relative severity, or extent, of the disease. It is meant to facilitate an estimation of prognosis and to provide useful information for treatment decisions.

General Rules for Staging
The TNM system is based on three components:

- *T*: extent of the primary tumour
- *N*: absence or presence and extent of regional lymph node metastases
- *M*: absence or presence of distant metastases

The five major sites of the head and neck (oral cavity, oropharynx, larynx, hypopharynx, and paranasal sinuses) share the same TNM system. Different systems are used for the nasopharynx and thyroid (see Head and Neck Endocrine section), because they are sufficiently different with respect to risk factors, behaviour, and treatment.

Histopathological Grading
The histological grading of squamous cell carcinoma represents estimation by the pathologist of the expected biological behaviour of the neoplasm. The grades are:

- *GX*: Grade of differentiation cannot be assessed
- *G1*: Well-differentiated
- *G2*: Moderately differentiated
- *G3*: Poorly differentiated
- *G4*: Undifferentiated

The pathological TNM classification is represented by pT, pN, and pM. The extent of the tumour in terms of the location and level of the lymph nodes should be documented. In addition, the number of nodes that contain tumour and the presence or absence of extranodal extension of the tumour should be recorded.

Stage Grouping
A tumour with four degrees of T, three degrees of N, and two degrees of M will have 24 potential TNM categories. Therefore, it has been felt necessary to condense the categories into a convenient number of TNM stage groups (Table 61.1). The grouping adopted is designed to

Table 61.1   TNM stage grouping

Stage 0	Tis	N0	M0
Stage I	T1	N0	M0
Stage II	T2	N0	M0
Stage III	T1, T2	N1	M0
	T3	N0, N1	M0
Stage IVA	T1, T2, T3	N2	M0
	T4a	N0, N1, N2	M0
Stage IVB	Any T	N3	M0
	T4b	Any N	M0
Stage IVC	Any T	Any N	M1

Table 61.2   Stage grouping of human papillomavirus (HPV)-related (p16-positive) oropharyngeal cancer

Stage I	T1, T2	N0, N1	M0
Stage II	T1, T2	N2	M0
	T3	N0, N1, N2	M0
Stage III	T1-T3	N3	M0
	T4	Any N	M0
Stage IV	Any T	Any N	M1

Table 61.3   Stage grouping for nasopharyngeal cancer

Stage I	T1	N0	M0
Stage II	T1	N1	M0
	T2	N0-1	M0
Stage III	T1-2	N2	M0
	T3	N0-2	M0
Stage IVA	T4	N0-2	M0
Stage IVB	Any T	N3	M0
Stage IVC	Any T	Any N	M1

ensure, as far as possible, that each group is more or less homogeneous with respect to survival. Carcinoma in situ is categorized as stage 0, cases with distant metastases as stage IV. The exception to this grouping system is p16-positive oropharyngeal and nasopharyngeal cancers (Tables 61.2 and 61.3).

Method of Staging

Computed tomography (CT) and magnetic resonance imaging (MRI) are now established as the mainstay investigations in the pre-operative workup of patients with head and neck cancer. Scans to evaluate the primary site should be performed prior to biopsy to avoid the effect of upstaging from the oedema caused by biopsy trauma.

Endoscopy and biopsy should be performed by a senior surgeon and should include a description and photographic documentation or diagrammatic representation. Panendoscopy is recommended only for symptomatic patients or patients with primary tumours known to have a significant risk of a second (synchronous) primary tumour.

The cTNM classification, based on examination, imaging, endoscopy, and biopsy, should be clearly documented in the case file only when all the staging information (including imaging) is collated.

Tumour Staging

Lip and Oral Cavity

The oral cavity extends from the skin-vermilion junction of the lips to the junction of the hard and soft palate above and to the line of the circumvallate papillae below. The anatomic sites and subsites are as follows:

- Lip:
  - External upper lip (vermilion border)
  - External lower lip (vermilion border)
  - Commissures

- Oral cavity:
  - Buccal mucosa
  - Mucosa of the upper and lower lips

Table 61.4 TNM clinical classification for lip and oral cavity tumours

T – Primary tumour	
T1	Tumour 2 cm or less in greatest dimension and 5 mm or less depth of invasion
T2	Tumour 2 cm or less in greatest dimension and more than 5 mm but no more than 10 mm depth of invasion or tumour more than 2 cm but not more than 4 cm in greatest dimension and depth of invasion no more than 10 mm
T3	Tumour more than 4 cm in greatest dimension or more than 10 mm depth of invasion
T4a	Lip: tumour invades through cortical bone, inferior alveolar nerve, floor of mouth, or skin (chin or nose)
T4a	Oral cavity: tumour invades through cortical bone, into deep/extrinsic muscle of tongue, maxillary sinus, or skin of face
T4b	Lip or oral cavity: tumour invades masticator space, pterygoid plates, or skull base, or encases internal carotid artery

- Cheek mucosa
- Retromolar areas
- Buck-alveolar sulci, upper and lower (vestibule of mouth)
- Upper alveolus and gingiva (upper gum)
- Lower alveolus and gingiva (lower gum)
- Hard palate
- Tongue—dorsal surface, lateral borders anterior to vallate papillae (anterior two thirds), and inferior (ventral) surface
- Floor of mouth

The eighth edition of the staging system recognises the importance of depth of invasion and this is shown in Table 61.4.

Pharynx

The pharynx is divided into three regions: nasopharynx, oropharynx, and hypopharynx. The eighth edition staging manual has been divided into three separate entities—nasopharyngeal cancer, HPV-associated (p16-positive) oropharyngeal cancer, and hypopharyngeal and non-HPV-associated (p16-negative) oropharyngeal cancer—to better reflect the variety of diseases arising in the pharynx.[1, 2]

Each region is subdivided into specific sites as summarized below.

Oropharynx

The oropharynx is the portion of the pharynx extending from the plane of the superior surface of the soft palate to the superior surface of the hyoid bone (or floor of the vallecula). It includes:

- Anterior subsites (glosso-epiglottic area)
- Base of tongue (posterior to the vallate papillae or posterior third)
- Vallecula
- Lateral subsites
- Lateral wall
- Tonsil
- Tonsillar fossa
- Tonsillar pillar
- Posterior wall
- Superior subsites
- Inferior surface of soft palate
- Uvula

Table 61.5a   Oropharyngeal cancer: p16-negative cancers or p16 immunohistochemistry not performed

T – Primary tumour	
T1	Tumour 2 cm or less in greatest dimension
T2	Tumour more than 2 cm but not more than 4 cm in greatest diameter
T3	Tumour more than 4 cm in greatest dimension or extension to lingual surface of the epiglottis
T4a	Tumour invades any of the following: larynx, deep extrinsic muscles of tongue (genioglossus, hyoglossus, palatoglossus, and styloglossus), medial pterygoid, or mandible and hard palate.
T4b	Tumour invades any of the following: lateral pterygoid muscle, pterygoid plates, lateral nasopharynx, or skull base, or it encases the carotid artery.

Table 61.5b   Oropharyngeal cancer: p16-positive cancers

T – Primary tumour	
T1	Tumour 2 cm or less in greatest dimension
T2	Tumour more than 2 cm but not more than 4 cm in greatest diameter
T3	Tumour more than 4 cm in greatest dimension or extension to lingual surface of the epiglottis
T4	Tumour invades any of the following: larynx, deep extrinsic muscles of tongue (genioglossus, hyoglossus, palatoglossus, and styloglossus), medial pterygoid, mandible and hard palate, lateral pterygoid muscle, pterygoid plates, lateral nasopharynx, or skull base, or it encases the carotid artery

The classification of p16-positive and p-16 negative oropharyngeal tumours is shown in Tables 61.5a and 61.5b.

Nasopharynx

The nasopharynx begins anteriorly at the posterior choana and extends along the plane of the airway to the level of the free border of the soft palate. It includes:

- Superior wall
- *Posterior wall*: from the level of the junction of the hard and soft palates to the superior wall
- *Lateral wall*: including the fossa of Rosenmüller
- *Floor*: superior surface of the soft palate

The classification of nasopharyngeal tumours is shown in Table 61.6.

Hypopharynx

The hypopharynx extends from the superior border of the hyoid bone to the lower border of the cricoid cartilage. It includes the piriform sinuses, the postcricoid area, and the lateral and posterior pharyngeal walls.

- The postcricoid area (pharyngo-oesophageal junction) extends from the level of the arytenoid cartilages and connecting folds to the inferior border of the cricoid cartilage, thus forming the anterior wall of the hypopharynx.
- Piriform sinus extends from the pharyngo-epiglottic fold to the upper end of the oesophagus. It is bounded laterally by the thyroid cartilage and medially by the hypopharyngeal surface of the aryepiglottic fold and the arytenoid and cricoid cartilages.

Table 61.6 Nasopharyngeal tumours

	T – Primary tumour
T1	Tumour is confined to nasopharynx or extends to oropharynx and/or nasal cavity without parapharyngeal involvement
T2	Tumour extends to parapharyngeal space and/or has infiltration of the medial pterygoid, lateral pterygoid, and/or prevertebral muscles
T3	Tumour invades bony structures of skull base, cervical vertebra, pterygoid structures, and/or paranasal sinuses
T4	Tumour has intracranial extension and/or involvement of cranial nerves, hypopharynx, orbit, or parotid gland, and/or infiltration beyond the lateral surface of the lateral pterygoid muscle

Note: Parapharyngeal extension denotes posterolateral infiltration of tumour beyond the pharyngo-basilar fascia.

- Posterior pharyngeal wall extends from the superior level of the hyoid bone (or floor of the vallecula) to the level of the inferior border of the cricoid cartilage and from the apex of one piriform sinus to the other.

The current staging for hypopharyngeal tumours is summarised in Table 61.7.

Larynx

The anatomical sites and subsites of the larynx are:

- *Supraglottis:*
  - Suprahyoid epiglottis (including tip and lingual [anterior] and laryngeal surfaces)
  - Aryepiglottic fold, laryngeal aspect
  - Arytenoid
  - Infrahyoid epiglottis
  - Ventricular bands (false cords)
- *Glottis:*
  - Vocal cords
  - Anterior commissure
  - Posterior commissure
- *Subglottis*

Tables 61.8, 61.9, and 61.10 detail the T stages for the various laryngeal cancer sites.

Table 61.7 Hypopharyngeal tumours

	T – Primary tumour
T1	Tumour is limited to one subsite of hypopharynx and is 2 cm or less in greatest dimension
T2	Tumour invades more than one subsite of hypopharynx or an adjacent site, or measures 2–4 cm in greatest dimension, without fixation of hemilarynx
T3	Tumour measures >4 cm in greatest dimension, or involves fixation of hemilarynx or extension to oesophagus
T4a	Tumour invades any of the following: thyroid/cricoid cartilage, hyoid bone, thyroid gland, oesophagus, or central compartment soft tissue
T4b	Tumour invades prevertebral fascia, encases carotid artery, or invades mediastinal structures

Note: Central compartment soft tissue includes prelaryngeal strap muscles and subcutaneous fat.

Table 61.8   Supraglottic tumour stages

	T – Primary tumour
T1	Tumour is limited to one subsite of supraglottis with normal vocal cord mobility
T2	Tumour invades mucosa of more than one adjacent subsite of supraglottis or glottis or region outside the supraglottis (e.g. mucosa of base of tongue, vallecula, medial wall of piriform sinus) without fixation of the larynx
T3	Tumour is limited to larynx with vocal cord fixation and/or invades any of the following: postcricoid area, pre-epiglottic tissues, or paraglottic space and/or with minor thyroid cartilage erosion (e.g. inner cortex)
T4a	Tumour invades through thyroid cartilage and/or invades tissues beyond the larynx, e.g. trachea, soft tissues of the neck, including deep/extrinsic muscles of the tongue (genioglossus, hyoglossus, palatoglossus, and styloglossus), strap muscles, thyroid, and oesophagus
T4b	Tumour invades prevertebral space or mediastinal structures or encases carotid artery

Table 61.9   Glottic tumour stages

	T – Primary tumour
T1	Tumour is limited to vocal cord(s) (may involve anterior or posterior commissure) with normal mobility
	T1a—tumour is limited to one vocal cord
	T1b—tumour involves both vocal cords
T2	Tumour extends to supraglottis and/or subglottis, and/or with impaired vocal cord mobility
T3	Tumour is limited to larynx with vocal cordu fixation and/or invades paraglottic space, and/or with minor thyroid cartilage erosion (inner cortex)
T4a	Tumour invades through thyroid cartilage or invades tissues beyond the larynx, e.g. trachea, soft tissues of neck including deep/extrinsic muscle of tongue (genioglossus, hyoglossus, palatoglossus and styloglossus), strap muscles, thyroid, and oesophagus
T4b	Tumour invades prevertebral space or mediastinal structures or encases carotid artery

Table 61.10   Subglottic tumour stages

	T – Primary tumour
T1	Tumour is limited to subglottis
T2	Tumour extends to vocal cord(s) with normal or impaired mobility
T3	Tumour is limited to larynx with vocal cord fixation
T4a	Tumour invades through cricoid or thyroid cartilage and/or invades tissues beyond the larynx, e.g. trachea, soft tissues of neck including deep/extrinsic muscle of tongue (genioglossus, hyoglossus, palatoglossus, and styloglossus), strap muscles, thyroid, and oesophagus
T4b	Tumour invades prevertebral space or mediastinal structures or encases carotid artery

Nasal Cavity and Paranasal Sinuses

The anatomical sites and subsites are:

- *Nasal cavity*:
  - Septum
  - Floor
  - Lateral wall
  - Vestibule
- *Maxillary sinus*
- *Ethmoid sinus*

Tumour `staging is documented in Tables 61.11 and 61.12.

Table 61.11   Maxillary sinus tumours

	T – Primary tumour
T1	Tumour is limited to the antral mucosa with no erosion or destruction of bone
T2	Tumour causes bone erosion or destruction, including extension into hard palate and/or middle nasal meatus, except extension to the posterior wall of maxillary sinus and pterygoid plates
T3	Tumour invades any of the following: bone of posterior wall of maxillary sinus, subcutaneous tissues, floor or medial wall of orbit, pterygoid fossa, or ethmoid sinuses
T4a	Tumour invades any of the following: anterior orbital contents, skin of cheek, pterygoid plates, infratemporal fossa, cribriform plate, and sphenoid or frontal sinus.
T4b	Tumour invades any of the following: orbital apex, dura, brain, middle cranial fossa, cranial nerves other than maxillary division of trigeminal nerve, nasopharynx, and clivus

Table 61.12   Nasal cavity and ethmoid sinus tumours

	T – Primary tumour
T1	Tumour is restricted to one subsite of nasal cavity or ethmoid sinus without bone erosion
T2	Tumour involves two subsites or extends to involve an adjacent site within the nasoethmoidal complex, with or without bony invasion
T3	Tumour extends to invade the medial wall or floor of the orbit, maxillary sinus, palate, or cribriform plate
T4	Tumour invades any of the following: anterior orbital contents, skin of nose or cheek, minimal extension to anterior cranial fossa, pterygoid plates, and sphenoid or frontal sinuses
T4b	Tumour invades any of the following: orbital apex, dura, brain, middle cranial fossa, cranial nerves other than maxillary division of trigeminal nerve, nasopharynx, and clivus

Salivary Glands

The staging classification (Table 61.13) applies only to carcinomas of the major salivary glands. Tumours arising in minor salivary glands (mucus-secreting glands in the lining membrane of the upper aerodigestive tract) should be staged according to their anatomical site of origin (e.g. lip). There should be histological confirmation of the disease. The anatomical sites and subsites are:

- Parotid gland
- Submandibular gland
- Sublingual gland

Unknown Primary

There should be histological confirmation of squamous cell carcinoma with lymph node metastases but without an identified primary carcinoma. Current recommended diagnostic

Table 61.13   Salivary gland tumours

	T – Primary tumour
T1	Tumour is 2 cm or less in greatest dimension without extraparenchymal extension*
T2	Tumour is more than 2 cm but no more than 4 cm in greatest dimension without extraparenchymal extension*
T3	Tumour is more than 4 cm and/or with extraparenchymal extension
T4a	Tumour invades skin, mandible, ear canal, or facial nerve
T4b	Tumour invades base of skull or pterygoid plates or encases carotid artery

*Extraparenchymal extension is clinical or macroscopic evidence of invasion of skin, soft tissues, or nerve, except those listed under T4a and T4b. Microscopic evidence alone does not constitute extraparenchymal extension for classification purposes.

methods include an early PET CT scan with targeted biopsies based on the findings. Transoral laser or robotic excision of the tonsil and tongue base mucosectomy are also recommended in cases that remain unknown. Histological methods should be used to identify Epstein-Barr virus (EBV) and HPV/p16-related tumours. If there is evidence of EBV, the nasopharyngeal classification is applied. If there is evidence of HPV and positive immunohistochemistry p16 overexpression, the p16-positive oropharyngeal classification is applied. One key change from previous versions of the TNM system is the elimination of the T0 category in sites other than the nasopharynx, high risk HPB (HR-HPV)–associated oropharyngeal carcinoma (OPC), and salivary gland cancers (which can be identified by their unique histology). If no primary lesion can be identified, then the lymph node may have emanated from any mucosal site, so there is no rationale to support retaining the T0 designation outside of the virally associated cancers of the oropharynx and nasopharynx.

Skin Carcinoma of the Head and Neck

Head and neck skin cancer is now presented in a separate chapter in the eighth edition of the American Joint Committee on Cancer (AJCC)/Union for International Cancer Control (UICC) staging manual. The classification applies to cutaneous carcinomas of the head and neck region excluding the eyelid (as an anatomical site), Merkel cell carcinoma, and malignant melanoma. The T stage is presented in Table 61.14, and the N stages are the same as nodal metastases from other sites of the head and neck. The following sites are recognised:

- Lip
- External ear
- Other and unspecified parts of the face
- Scalp and neck

Malignant Melanoma of the Upper Aerodigestive Tract

The classification in Table 61.15 applies only to mucosal malignant melanomas of the head and neck region. The regional lymph nodes are staged according to the site in the upper aerodigestive tract of the tumour. Because malignant melanoma are aggressive tumours, T1 and T2, are omitted as are stages I and II.

Table 61.14   Head and neck skin cancer

T1	Tumour is 2 cm or less in greatest dimension
T2	Tumour is >2 cm and <4 cm in greatest dimension
T3	Tumour is >4 cm in greatest dimension or has minor bone erosion or perineural invasion or deep invasion*
T4a	Tumour has gross cortical bone/marrow extension
T4b	Tumour has skull base or axial skeleton invasion including foraminal involvement and/or vertebral foramen involvement to the epidural space

*Deep invasion is defined as invasion beyond the subcutaneous fat or >6 mm (as measured from the granular layer of adjacent normal epidermis to the base of the tumour). Perineural invasion for T3 classification is defined as clinical or radiographic involvement of named nerves without foramen or skull base invasion or transgression.

Table 61.15   Malignant melanoma of the upper aerodigestive tract

TX	Primary tumour cannot be assessed
T0	No evidence of primary tumour
T3	Tumour is limited to the epithelium and/or submucosa (mucosal disease)
T4a	Tumour invades deep soft tissue, cartilage, bone, or overlying skin
T4b	Tumour invades any of the following: brain, dura, skull base, lower cranial nerves (IX, X, XI, XII), masticator space, carotid artery, prevertebral space, or mediastinal structures

Regional Lymph Nodes

Lymph nodes are described as ipsilateral, bilateral, contralateral, or midline; they may be single or multiple and are measured by size, number, and anatomical location. Midline nodes are considered ipsilateral nodes, except with thyroid cancers. Direct extension of the primary tumour into lymph nodes is classified as lymph node metastasis.

Lymph nodes are subdivided into specific anatomical sites and are grouped into seven levels for ease of description (Table 61.16).

The definitions of the N categories (Table 61.17) are the same for most head and neck sites (oral cavity, p16-negative pharyngeal carcinoma, laryngeal carcinoma, sinus carcinoma, salivary gland carcinoma). The AJCC/UICC manual's eighth edition recognises the importance of extranodal extension (previously called extracapsular spread).

The latest edition of the AJCC/UICC manual has also introduced two separate staging systems (cTNM and pTNM) for neck metastases of HPV-related (p16-positive) oropharyngeal cancer (Tables 61.18a and 61.18b). Studies have shown a significant difference in outcome based on the number of pathologically positive lymph nodes, defining two categories: those with 1 to 4 (N1) versus 5 or more (N2) positive nodes. As the number of nodes can only be counted in the neck dissection specimen, a separate N system based on histological assessment of the neck dissection specimen has been created (pTNM). Recognizing that lymph node size >6 cm does not have a prognostic role in surgically treated necks, no pN3 category exists.

Table 61.16   Nomenclature for anatomical sites of lymph nodes

Level I	Contains the submental and submandibular triangles, bounded by the posterior belly of the digastric muscle, the hyoid bone inferiorly, and the body of the mandible superiorly
Level II	Contains the upper jugular lymph nodes and extends from the level of the hyoid bone inferiorly to the skull base superiorly
Level III	Contains the middle jugular lymph nodes from the hyoid bone superiorly to the cricothyroid membrane inferiorly
Level IV	Contains the lower jugular lymph nodes from the cricothyroid membrane superiorly to the clavicle inferiorly
Level V	Contains the posterior triangle lymph nodes, bounded by the anterior border of the trapezius posteriorly, the posterior border of the sternocleidomastoid muscle anteriorly, and the clavicle inferiorly
Level VI	Contains the anterior compartment lymph nodes from the hyoid bone superiorly to the suprasternal notch inferiorly. On each side, the medial border of the carotid sheath forms the lateral border
Level VII	Contains the lymph nodes inferior to the suprasternal notch in the upper mediastinum

Table 61.17   Clinical N stage

NX	Regional lymph nodes cannot be assessed.
N0	No regional lymph node metastasis
N1	Metastasis in a single ipsilateral lymph node, 3 cm or less in greatest dimension without extranodal extension
N2	N2a—Metastasis in a single ipsilateral lymph node, more than 3 cm but not more than 6 cm in greatest dimension without extranodal extension
	N2b—Metastasis in multiple ipsilateral lymph nodes, none more than 6 cm in greatest dimension, without extranodal extension
	N2c—Metastasis in bilateral or contralateral lymph nodes, none more than 6 cm in greatest dimension, without extranodal extension
N3a	Metastasis in a lymph node more than 6 cm in greatest dimension without extranodal extension
N3b	Metastases in a single or multiple lymph nodes with clinical extranodal extension

Table 61.18a   Clinical nodal (N) stage for HPV-related (p16-positive) oropharyngeal cancer

Nx	Regional lymph nodes cannot be assessed
N0	No regional lymph node metastases
N1	One or more ipsilateral lymph nodes, none larger than 6 cm
N2	Contralateral or bilateral lymph nodes, none larger than 6 cm
N3	Lymph node(s) larger than 6 cm

Table 61.18b   Pathologic N stage for HPV-related (p16-positive) oropharyngeal cancer

Nx	Regional lymph nodes cannot be assessed
pN0	No regional lymph node metastases
pN1	Metastasis in 4 or fewer lymph nodes
pN2	Metastasis in more than 4 lymph nodes

The natural history and response to treatment of cervical nodal metastases from the nasopharynx are different in terms of their impact on prognosis; thus, they justify a different N classification (Table 61.19).

Table 61.19   N staging for nasopharyngeal cancer

N – Regional lymph nodes	
NX	Regional lymph nodes cannot be assessed
N0	No regional lymph node metastasis
N1	Unilateral metastasis, in cervical lymph node(s), and/or unilateral or bilateral metastasis in retropharyngeal lymph nodes, 6 cm or less in greatest dimension, above the caudal border of cricoid cartilage
N2	Bilateral metastasis in cervical lymph node(s), 6 cm or less in greatest dimension, above the caudal border of cricoid cartilage
N3	Metastasis in cervical lymph node(s) greater than 6 cm in dimension and/or extension below the caudal border of cricoid cartilage

Note: Midline nodes are considered ipsilateral nodes, and the supraclavicular triangle is defined by the lines joining the following three points: the superior margin of the clavicle at its sternal and acromial ends, and the point where the line of the neck meets the shoulder.

KEY POINTS

- Staging of head and neck cancer is a system designed to express the relative severity, or extent, of the disease. It is meant to facilitate an estimation of prognosis and to provide useful information for treatment decisions.
- Classification of the anatomical extent of head and neck cancer as determined clinically and histopathologically is called the TNM system.
- Radiological investigations to evaluate the primary site should be performed prior to biopsy to avoid the effect of upstaging from the oedema caused by biopsy trauma.
- The clinical (pretreatment) classification (cTNM) based on examination, imaging, endoscopy, and biopsy should be clearly documented in the case file only when all the information is collated.
- Individual TNM classifications should be assembled into four stage groups (stages I–IV), each with similar survival outcomes.
- The AJCC/UICC staging manual should be available in every theatre, multidisciplinary team meeting, and clinic to assist in applying the correct stage.

62. LARYNGEAL MALIGNANCY

The most common type of laryngeal cancer is squamous cell carcinoma. The incidence is higher in men, and the cancer is most common after the age of 60 and less common before age 40. Smoking remains the most common aetiological factor, with alcohol an independent risk factor, but in combination the two have a multiplicative risk. After smoking cessation, the risk reduces and reaches the level of never smokers after 20 years.

Clinical Presentation

Glottic cancer alters the voice early by affecting wave patterns along the vocal cord. Supraglottic lesions may be asymptomatic until they are quite large, and their initial presentation with a neck lump due to nodal metastasis is common. Voice alteration is different in quality from that seen with glottic and subglottic cancer, with altered phonation progressing to a 'hot potato' voice. Early symptoms from subglottic disease can be vague, with a feeling of globus or foreign body sensation in the throat.

With increasing lesion size, maximum phonation time decreases, the voice becomes breathy (cord fixation), aspiration may be seen, and eventually the patient develops airway obstruction with dyspnea and stridor. Dysphagia, odynophagia, haemoptysis, and referred otalgia signify advanced disease.

Assessment

An initial assessment is made using the flexible nasoendoscope; the information gathered is often complementary to what is gained during rigid endoscopy and includes cord mobility and a panoramic view of the larynx.

Imaging for laryngeal mass lesions should include cross-sectional imaging and chest imaging. Magnetic resonance imaging (MRI) has higher sensitivity than computed tomography (CT) in assessing cartilage invasion.

Rigid endoscopic assessment under general anaesthesia not only should assess the extent of the tumour and take a biopsy, but also should be done by a surgeon who can make the decision whether the tumour can be resected transorally. Anatomical constraints may make even small tumours unresectable.

Laryngeal Dysplasia

The clinical significance of laryngeal dysplasia lies in its propensity for malignant transformation (between 11% and 25%). The British Association of Otolaryngologists Head and Neck Surgeons have generated consensus on the management of this condition and follow-up (Figures 62.1 and 62.2).

Early-Stage Laryngeal Cancers

It is currently believed that in early cancers, surgery and radiotherapy as single modalities offer equivalent survival outcomes. Both treatment options should be considered and discussed in the multidisciplinary team and with the patient.

Voice outcomes are comparable for T1 glottic cancers treated by either modality. Even in patients who undergo a type III cordectomy, vocal function often returns to pre-operative levels. Transoral laser microsurgery (TLM) is a same-day procedure, whilst radiotherapy involves several weeks of daily treatment. For these reasons, lesions that are limited to one vocal cord (T1a) and accessible for resection with adequate margins are commonly treated by TLM. When the tumour involves the anterior commissure or extends across two subsites (T1b or T2), voice outcome is more variable with TLM, and the choice between radiotherapy and TLM is made depending on patient factors (e.g. occupation, distance away from hospital) and tumour factors (e.g. access for resection).

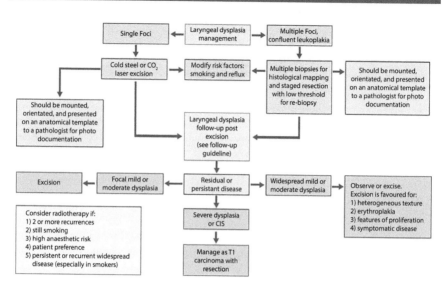

Figure 62.1 Management of laryngeal dysplasia based on a multiprofessional consensus.

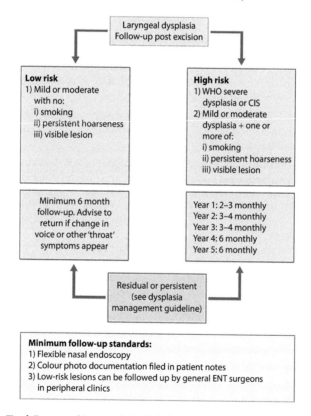

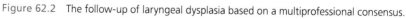

Figure 62.2 The follow-up of laryngeal dysplasia based on a multiprofessional consensus.

T3 Laryngeal Cancer

Non-Surgical Treatment

Radiation therapy alone or in combination with systemic therapy (concurrent chemo-therapy or cetuximab) offers organ preservation in appropriately selected patients without compromising survival. The landmark VA study (see further reading) showed that in patients responding to induction chemotherapy, the laryngeal preservation rate was 64% at 2 years, with similar survival rates at 2 years (68%) as surgery followed by radiotherapy. Salvage laryngectomy rates were significantly lower for T3 disease than for T4 disease (29% versus 56%). A higher proportion of patients with a fixed cord underwent salvage laryngectomy.

A subsequent trial by the Intergroup RTOG 91–11 demonstrated that laryngeal preservation rates with concurrent chemoradiotherapy was superior to sequential induction chemotherapy followed by radiotherapy and to radiotherapy alone (88% versus 75% versus 70%) with similar survival rates. This benefit decreases with age and is non-significant over 70 years of age and therefore less appropriate in patients above this age.

Partial Laryngectomy
The current evidence suggests both open partial laryngectomy and TLM can be useful organ-preserving methods for the treatment of T3 squamous cell laryngeal cancer.

Total Laryngectomy
Total laryngectomy is a bona fide treatment for T3 laryngeal disease, especially in patients who have a fixed cord. For endolaryngeal tumours with no pathological evidence of neck disease, a total laryngectomy with adequate margins is all that will be needed. These patients will not need reconstructive interventions because adequate pharynx will be available to create an adequately wide neopharynx.

T4 Laryngeal Cancer
There is general agreement that laryngeal cancer that extends outside the framework of the larynx should be treated by primary surgery—most commonly, a total laryngectomy. The reasons for this consensus are that tumours invading the cartilage do not respond well to radiation, and even if tumour control is achieved, there is a high risk of a nonfunctional larynx, chondronecrosis, and gastrostomy dependence.

Neck Management
For glottic cancer, estimates for the incidence of microscopic lymph node metastasis by disease stage are: <5% (T1), 7% (T2), 14% (T3), and 33% (T4). For T1 tumours, treatment of the primary site alone will suffice. T2 tumours are less prone to metastatic spread, but, given the ~7% risk of occult spread, there is no consensus on whether the neck should be treated in this setting.

For all supraglottic cancers and advanced glottic tumours, the neck needs to be addressed even if there is no clinical or radiological evidence of disease. For midline supraglottic cancers, both sides of the neck should be treated.

Adjuvant Treatment
Post-operative radiotherapy in patients at risk of locoregional recurrence can improve locoregional control and survival. Indications are: pT4 tumours, close or involved resection margins, involved node larger than 3 cm, multiple positive nodes, extracapsular spread, perineural invasion, and vascular invasion. Adjuvant chemoradiotherapy should be considered with a positive resection margin and/or extracapsular spread.

Recurrent Disease
Residual or recurrent laryngeal cancer following radiotherapy is aggressive and carries a poor prognosis. Options for those with recurrent cancer are based on the initial treatment received and the stage of the recurrent disease. Salvage total laryngectomy is often recommended, even for early cancers.

Open partial laryngectomy has been demonstrated to have very good outcomes with recurrent cancer. TLM's role is limited in recurrent cases, due to the difficulty of identifying the extent of the tumour and interpreting resection margins. It is suggested that, where suitable, patients should be offered open partial laryngectomy in preference to TLM for recurrent tumours, unless the cancer is limited to the mid cord. In cases not suitable for open partial laryngectomy, total laryngectomy should be offered.

Transoral Laser Microsurgery (TLM)

TLM is a minimally invasive surgical approach to functional laryngeal preservation. Patient selection is key to the success of the technique, as inadequate endoscopic access to facilitate satisfactory oncologic resection is the main contraindication to TLM.

For glottic cancer, the specimens resected by TLM will have much smaller margins than the margins obtained in open surgery, with margins of 1 mm being acceptable. Working closely with the pathologist is vital for correct interpretation of specimens. For supraglottic cancer, surgical margins of at least 5 mm are required. Glottic and supraglottic transoral resections should be classified using the European Laryngological Society system (Table 62.1). There is usually no need to reconstruct the surgical defect; the tumour bed is left exposed and readily accessible for additional resections to achieve negative margins.

Small superficial T1a glottic tumours may be excised en bloc with the CO_2 laser (see Figure 62.3). More complex tumours benefit from an initial cut through tumour to assess depth of invasion. The way that the laser cuts through normal tissue is very different from

Table 62.1   European Laryngological Society classification of cordectomies

Definition	Type		Description
Subepithelial cordectomy	I		Resection passing through the superficial lamina propria
Subligamental cordectomy	II		Resection including vocal ligament
Transmuscular cordectomy	III		Resection through vocalis muscle

Table 62.1 (Continued)

Definition	Type	Description
Total cordectomy	IV	Resection from the vocal process to the anterior commissure— depth reaches or includes the internal perichondrium of the thyroid cartilage
Extended total cordectomy	Va	Resection includes the contralateral vocal fold and anterior commissure
	Vb	Resection includes the arytenoids
	Vc	Resection includes the subglottis

Table 62.1 (Continued)

Definition	Type	Description
	Vd 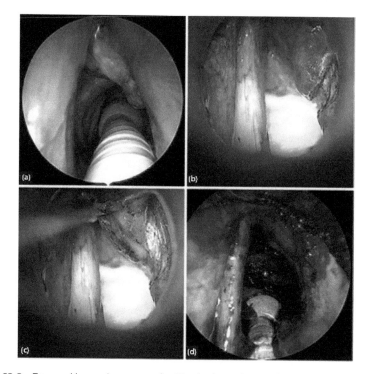	Resection includes the ventricle and false cords
Anterior commissurectomy	VI	Resection of the anterior commissure

Figure 62.3 Transoral laser microsurgery for T1a glottic carcinoma. (a) Pre-operative. (b) Tumour divided to assess depth. (c) The deep margin followed with the laser. (d) Post-resection.

its cut through tumour, and the difference can be appreciated under the operating microscope. Once the deep margin of the tumour is identified, it can be followed and the tumour removed.

Open Partial Laryngectomy

The goal of open partial laryngectomy is complete tumour removal, while preserving the functional integrity and separation of larynx and pharynx. Preservation of at least one functional cricoarytenoid unit is essential. The cricoarytenoid unit consists of an arytenoid cartilage, the cricoid cartilage, the associated musculature, and the nerve supply from the superior and recurrent laryngeal nerves for that unit. It is the cricoarytenoid unit, not the vocal folds, that allows for physiologic speech and swallowing without the need for a tracheostoma.

Procedures that can be applied to glottic disease include several vertical hemilaryngectomy modifications and horizontal supracricoid laryngectomy with cricohyoidoepiglottopexy (CHEP). For supraglottic disease, supraglottic laryngectomy and supracricoid laryngectomy with cricohyoidopexy (CHP) may be considered.

Further Reading

Department of Veterans Affairs Laryngeal Cancer Study Group, Wolf GT, Fisher SG, Hong WK, Hillman R, Spaulding M, Laramore GE, Endicott JW, McClatchey K, Henderson WG. Induction chemotherapy plus radiation compared with surgery plus radiation in patients with advanced laryngeal cancer. *N Engl J Med* 1991; 324(24): 1685–1690.

Mehanna H, Paleri V, Robson A, Wight R, Helliwell T. Consensus statement by otorhinolaryngologists and pathologists on the diagnosis and management of laryngeal dysplasia. *Clin Otolaryngol* 2010; 35(3): 170–176.

Steiner W. Results of curative laser microsurgery of laryngeal carcinomas. *Am J Otolaryngol* 1993; 14: 116–121.

63. HYPOPHARYNX

Introduction

The hypopharynx is the caudal part of the pharynx, also called laryngopharynx, extending from the hyoid bone to the lower margin of the cricoid cartilage. Hypopharyngeal cancers are distinctly different from laryngeal cancers in terms of presentation, management, and prognosis. Hypopharyngeal cancers make up 5–10% of head and neck cancers, and the presentation is often vague, with up to 80% presenting as stage III or IV disease. These factors lead to overall poorer outcomes than are experienced with other head and neck cancers.

Epidemiology

Hypopharyngeal cancers are rare, making up less than 0.5% of all cancers and tend to occur in individuals over 50 years old.

Subsites of cancer (in order of most frequent to least) are:

- Piriform sinus (PS)
- Posterior pharyngeal wall (PPW)
- Postcricoid area (PC)

PS and PPW lesions are more common in males, whereas PC lesions are predominant in females.

Table 63.1 Common sites of hypopharyngeal tumour local extension

Primary site	Local affected area
Lateral wall PS	Thyroid cartilage
Medial wall PS	Paraglottic space, impeding vocal cord movement
Pyriform apex	Via cricothyroid membrane to involve thyroid gland or recurrent laryngeal nerve
PC	Cricoid and/or tracheal cartilages Via cricothyroid membrane to involve thyroid gland High risk of extension to cervical oesophagus with submucosal spread or skip lesions due to rich oesophageal submucosal lymphatic plexus
PPW	Prevertebral fascia, and tending to be exophytic into the lumen

Etiology

Hypopharyngeal cancer has multifactorial etiology, including:

- Tobacco.
- Alcohol.
- Age (mean age of presentation is 65 years).
- Human papillomavirus (HPV) is present in 10.9% of hypopharyngeal cancers (although HPV-associated cancer is more common in the oropharynx).
- Iron-deficiency dysphagia (associated with Plummer-Vinson syndrome) for PC tumours.

Local Spread

Tumours at different subsites of the hypopharynx tend to locally extend in individual ways (Table 63.1). The local effects have significant impact on therapeutic options. It is obvious from the table that PC tumours vary substantially in symptoms and subsequent treatment. It is important to note that lateral PS and PC tumours are the tumours most likely to affect laryngeal cartilage in the table.

Regional Spread

Hypopharyngeal tumours have the highest propensity for early nodal metastases: up to 70% of patients may have lymph node metastases at presentation. There is also a high incidence of occult nodal metastases, up to 40% in early disease. Therefore, it is essential to treat the neck.

Distant Spread

Among all head and neck cancers, hypopharyngeal primaries have the highest incidence of distant metastases at presentation (17–24%) and during follow-up, with more than 50% of failures due to distant metastases.

Symptomatology

Hypopharyngeal tumours are detected late, because the patients are often asymptomatic in the early stages. The earliest symptom may be mild non-specific throat discomfort. In fact, globus sensation may be the only presenting complaint, with normal clinical findings. Half of patients present with a neck mass.

Investigations

- Endoscopy via flexible transnasal oesophagoscopy or rigid endoscopy.
- Fine-needle aspiration cytology (FNAC) for palpable neck node.
- Cross-sectional imaging by computed tomography (CT) or magnetic resonance imaging (MRI), depending on local protocols. Chest CT is indicated in all patients to examine for synchronous tumours.
- PET CT is a useful imaging modality in the assessment for distant metastasis.

For staging of hypopharyngeal cancer, see Chapter 61.

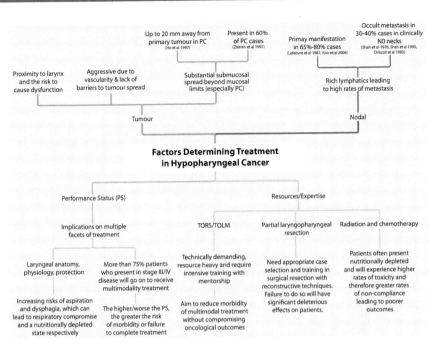

Figure 63.1 Factors determining treatment in hypopharyngeal cancer.

Factors Determining Treatment in Hypopharyngeal Cancer

Treatment decisions in cancer are guided by the biology of the disease and the peculiarities of the organ affected. Tumour and nodal factors, performance status of the patient, resources, and technical expertise dictate the management (Figure 63.1).

Treatment of Early Hypopharyngeal Cancers

Early cancers are potentially curable, and the goals of treatment should be to maximise chances of cure with function preservation. Stage I/II (T1 and T2) hypopharyngeal cancers should be treated with a single modality, either radiation therapy or larynx conservation surgery. Figure 63.2 gives an overall view of options for management of early disease.

There are some advantages of transoral over open approaches: transoral approaches avoid disruption of laryngeal skeleton and soft tissues; allow preservation of innervation, which aids with swallowing outcomes; and prevent orocervical fistula formation. However, contraindications include: oral submucous fibrosis, full-thickness involvement of the pharyngeal muscles, or involvement of thyroid cartilage, base of tongue, arytenoids, or cervical oesophagus.

Treatment of Advanced Hypopharyngeal Cancer

In advanced hypopharyngeal cancers with cord fixity and/or cartilage erosion (T3/T4a), the main issue is treating the disease whilst preserving the laryngeal form and function. In patients with good performance status, no comorbidities, and intact laryngeal framework and function (T1–3,N0–2c), the standard of care is concurrent chemotherapy with radiation. In patients with compromised laryngeal framework (T4a) or dysfunction, the standard of treatment is surgery *with* adjuvant radiation therapy. Lastly, patients with intact laryngeal function but extralaryngeal spread through the membranes without cartilage involvement undergoing neoajuvant chemotherapy with response assessment may be considered for organ preservation.

Non-Surgical Organ Preservation Strategies for Advanced Disease

Non-surgical organ preservation aims for good locoregional control with function preservation (i.e. no aspiration or need for tracheostomy and feeding tubes after completion of treatment). However, careful patient selection is essential to ensure optimal results.

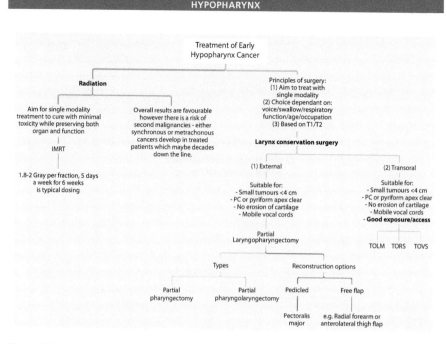

Figure 63.2   Treatment options for early hypopharyngeal cancer (TOLM = transoral laser micro-surgery, TORS = transoral robotic surgery, TOVS = transoral video-assisted endoscopic surgery).

Chemoradiotherapy for Advanced Hypopharyngeal Cancer

Concomitant chemoradiation in hypopharyngeal cancers was found to be better than induction chemotherapy. Single-agent cisplatin is the standard of care, but there is a decreasing effect of chemotherapy in patients over 70 years old. Chemoradiation is generally accepted as the gold standard of treatment in advanced laryngeal cancers without frank cartilage erosion.

Salvage Surgery After Organ Preservation

The premise for offering organ preservation is the ability to salvage if the treatment does not succeed. Communicating this is critical in counselling the patient whilst planning treatment.

Residual Local Disease

The hypopharynx is at the highest risk for locoregional and distant spread. Control rates after primary radiotherapy/chemoradiation are low, with around 30–50% of patients having residual/local recurrences. Most of these patients tend to have unresectable lesions. When the case is salvageable, most often the surgery is laryngopharyngectomy with pharyngeal reconstruction, but the outcomes are bleak, with a successful salvage rate of only 17.1%.

Salvage laryngopharyngectomies have an increased rate of complications, especially pharyngocutaneous fistulae, which may occur in up to 50%. Pharyngocutaneous fistulae in turn increase the incidence of carotid artery blowouts. Mortality in surgically treated hypopharyngeal cancers is a reality, with average hospital mortality rate for laryngopharyngectomy around 6%, with the gastric pull-up group having the highest incidence, 11%. Because of the low salvage potential and the high rate of complications, it is imperative to carefully choose patients for organ preservation, and the surgical team should have a low threshold for using vascularised tissue from non-radiated areas to reconstruct.

Surgery for Advanced Hypopharyngeal Cancers

Surgery for hypopharyngeal cancer involves the larynx as well as the hypopharynx. The larynx is usually entirely removed unless the lesion is lateralised. The pharynx is usually

Surgery is advocated for:	Surgery is contraindicated for:
Good general condition/PS	Poor general condition/PS
Involved laryngeal framework	Metastatic disease
Compromised laryngeal function then it should be removed to allow airway protection	Disease extension to areas of unresectability or poor feasibility: root of neck, prevertebral involvement, superior extension into the oropharynx, lateral extension involving carotid artery (T4b)
Salvage surgery following radiation or concurrent chemoradiation	

Figure 63.3   Arguments for and against surgery in advanced disease.

resected either partially or circumferentially, and most patients will need appropriate reconstruction to restore pharyngeal continuity and minimise the risk of pharyngocutaneous fistulae. Adjuvant radiation/chemoradiation is an *essential* part of the multimodal therapy for stage III/IV hypopharyngeal cancers treated surgically. Pros and cons of surgery in advanced hypopharyngeal cancer are shown in Figure 63.3.

Surgical Procedures for Advanced Hypopharyngeal Cancer

Figure 63.4 shows the surgical options for advanced hypopharyngeal cancer as well as reconstruction options.

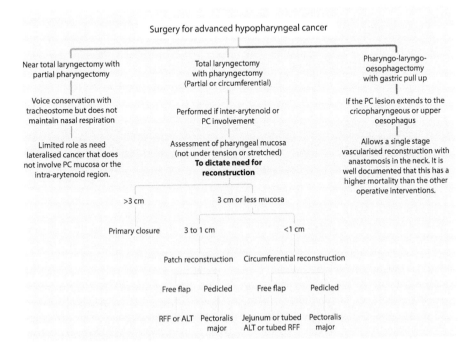

Figure 63.4   Surgical options for hypopharyngeal cancer (RFF = radial forearm flap, ALT = anterolateral thigh).

Management of Neck Disease in Advanced Hypopharyngeal Cancer

In stage III and IV cancers, the patient either has manifest neck nodes (N1–N3) or has advanced primary (T3/T4) tumour. With neck nodes, the surgical plan is usually bilateral neck dissection at Levels II–V. In patients with advanced primaries and no neck nodes, the surgical plan will entail bilateral neck dissection at Levels II–IV. The neck dissection needs to be tailored to individual disease, with consideration of retropharyngeal nodes.

Adjuvant Therapy

Following surgery in advanced stage III and IV hypopharyngeal cancers, adjuvant therapy with either radiation therapy or concurrent chemoradiotherapy is an essential part of the treatment protocols.

Disease Surveillance

The patients should be monitored for second primary cancers in the upper aerodigestive tract; second primaries are seen in up to 50% of patients.

KEY POINTS

- Accurate staging is essential. Workup should include evaluation for synchronous primaries and distant metastasis.
- Laryngeal function should be accurately evaluated prior to treatment, especially while considering organ preservation.
- Unimodality treatment is recommended for stage I and II disease.
- Multimodality treatment is recommended for stage III and IV disease.
- The overall 5-year, tumour-specific survival is less than 30%, although the survival of treated patients rises to 50%.

Further Reading

Garneau JC, Baskt RL, Miles BA. Hypopharyngeal cancer: A state of the art review. *Oral Oncology* 2018; 86: 244–250.

Paleri C, Rollands NJ. (Eds.) Head and Neck Cancer: United Kingdom National Multidisciplinary Guidelines, 5th edition, 2016.

---

64. OROPHARYNX

Introduction

There has been a rapid increase in the incidence of human papillomavirus (HPV)-associated oropharyngeal squamous cell carcinoma (HPV+ OPSCC) over several decades. This disease entity presents in younger, fitter, more affluent patients who drink less alcohol and smoke less tobacco than patients who present with HPV-negative disease (HPV– OPSCC). HPV+ tumours typically present with multiple cervical lymph nodes (with a high prevalence of extracapsular spread), but they respond more favourably to treatment. OPSCC treatment results in high levels of early and long-term toxicity; consequently, greater numbers of younger patients are cured of their disease but are left with poor swallowing outcomes. Although most patients with HPV+ OPSCC do well, a subgroup of patients still do poorly. There is an urgent need to find novel de-intensified treatments that maintain the advantageous survival outcomes but confer better swallowing outcomes for patients with HPV+ OPSCC, as well as defining treatments that will improve survival for patients with HPV– OPSCC.

Surgical Anatomy of the Oropharynx

The pharynx is divided into three parts: the nasopharynx, oropharynx, and hypopharynx. The oropharynx is bounded superiorly by the soft palate, inferiorly by the lingual surface of the epiglottis, anteriorly by the palatoglossal arches and vallate papillae of the tongue, and laterally by the pharyngoepiglottic folds. The section of posterior pharyngeal wall included in the oropharynx lies anterior to the vertebral bodies of C2/C3 and extends from a horizontal line drawn through the hard palate cranially to a horizontal line drawn through the hyoid bone caudally.

Surgical access to the structures of the oropharynx may be achieved transorally, anteriorly via mandibulotomy, or inferiorly and laterally from the neck.

Tumours of the Oropharynx

Apart from mucous retention cysts of the vallecula/tonsil and papillomas, benign oropharyngeal tumours are rare. Deep lobe parotid tumours, commonly pleomorphic salivary adenomas, while not strictly tumours of the oropharynx, may present as an asymmetric mass protruding into the pharynx and/or soft palate. Thus, peritonsillar bulging in the absence of infective symptoms should not be confused with quinsy, and instead should be suspected to be a deep lobe parotid tumour.

Lymphomas in the oropharynx are rare and are almost exclusively non-Hodgkin lymphomas arising in the lymphoid tissue of the palatine tonsil or base of tongue (BOT).

Salivary gland cancers account for up to 6% of all head and neck malignancies. Approximately 20% of all salivary gland tumours arise in the minor salivary glands (MiSG), and they are malignant 80% of the time. The most common sites of such tumours are the hard and soft palate, and the four most common malignant subtypes are mucoepidermoid carcinoma, adenoid cystic carcinoma, adenocarcinoma, and salivary duct carcinoma. Surgical resection with adequate surgical margins is the primary treatment of choice. Post-operative radiotherapy (RT) is used, particularly in patients with high-risk factors (T3/4, close/involved margins, high-grade tumour, perineural/perivascular invasion, and N+ disease), although the radiosensitivity of MiSG cancers is highly variable.

Oropharyngeal Squamous Cell Carcinoma (OPSCC)

Squamous cell carcinoma is the most common malignancy presenting in the oropharynx. While alcohol and tobacco use are well documented individual and synergistic risk factors for the development of head and neck SCC, evidence confirms that HPV, specifically genotype 16, is an additional independent risk factor for OPSCC.

Two diagnostic strategies are commonly used to detect HPV DNA within tumour cells—in situ hybridization (ISH) and polymerase chain reaction (PCR). Contamination or previous infection could render tests positive without confirming downstream biological activity of HPV; therefore, quantitative reverse transcription PCR (qRT-PCR) and RNA-based chromogenic ISH (RNA-ISH) can be used. More often, however, immunohistochemistry of p16 overexpression is used as a surrogate marker, although up to 30% of p16-positive tumours are HPV negative. Immunohistochemistry is inexpensive and widely available and is well established in treatment protocols. The overexpression of p16 correlates well with clinical outcome.

Clinical Presentation

It is recognized that the presentation of HPV+ OPSCC differs significantly from that of HPV– OPSCC. HPV+ OPSCC typically presents with a small primary tumour and multiple, enlarged, cystic cervical lymph nodes as well as a high prevalence of extracapsular spread (ECS). In contrast, HPV– OPSCC presents as a more typical head and neck cancer, with larger primary tumours and relatively lower tumour burden in cervical lymph nodes. In OPSCC, 60% of tumours arise in the tonsil and 30% in the BOT.

Local extension of OPSCC can give rise to a range of symptoms, including odynophagia, persistent throat pain, referred otalgia, dysphagia, altered speech, impaired tongue movement, and bleeding. Incidental discovery of painless enlarged cervical lymph node(s) is a very common presentation, especially for HPV+ OPSCC. If the presenting lymph node is solitary, it is commonly in Level II, while multiple involved lymph nodes will present as a chain extending from Level II to Level IV.

Clinical Examination

Patients require a thorough examination of the upper aerodigestive tract (UADT), with inspection of the oral cavity and oropharynx and transnasal flexible fibreoptic endoscopy. High-quality clinical photographs are important for recording pertinent clinical findings. Examine the neck thoroughly to determine the presence of lymph node involvement as well as the nodes' size, consistency, and mobility.

Investigations

- Cross-sectional imaging—computed tomography(CT) or magnetic resonance imaging (MRI)—of the head and neck.
- CT scan (or PET CT) of the thorax and upper abdomen.
- Examination under anaesthesia (EUA) of the UADT and biopsy of the presenting primary tumour.
- Ultrasound (US) of the neck if enlarged nodes are identified and US fine-needle aspiration cytology (FNAC) of any suspicious neck nodes.

Management

The management of oropharyngeal carcinoma is challenging. HPV status is highly prognostic in OPSCC patients treated with chemoradiotherapy (CRT): 3-year overall survival is 82.4% in HPV+ cancer, compared to 57.1% in HPV− cancer. Currently, HPV+ and HPV− OPSCC are managed using the same treatment protocols, but the improved prognosis associated with HPV positivity highlights the need for de-intensified treatment strategies that maintaining the patients' survival outcomes. Treatment intensification is also needed to enhance survival in patients with HPV− OPSCC and the subgroup of patients with HPV+ OPSCC who do badly. At present, there are no high-quality data comparing surgical and non-surgical approaches, and RT and CRT are the accepted standards of care in many centres throughout the world for early and late-stage OPSCC, respectively.

In general, the treatment options are:

- For T1–T2 N0: Radical RT or transoral surgery and neck dissection (with post-operative CRT if there are adverse pathological features on histology)
- For other stages: primary CRT or surgery and adjuvant (chemo)radiotherapy

Radiotherapy (RT)/Chemoradiotherapy (CRT)

The rationale for the use of RT or CRT in treating OPSCC is functional organ preservation while achieving high cure rates. Early-stage T1–T2 N0–N1 OPSCC can be effectively treated with RT alone (70 Gy in 35 fractions). For more advanced T and/or N stage OPSCC, CRT is the standard of care, with a RT dose equivalent of 70 Gy delivered in 35 fractions together with concurrent cisplatin at a dose of 100 mg/m^2 given on days 1, 22, and 43 of the schedule. Radical RT may be given alone to patients with advanced disease who are not fit for concurrent treatment, particularly if they are more than 70 years old, when the benefits of concurrent chemotherapy are reduced.

The dose of adjuvant RT after surgery in head and neck cancers is 57.6 Gy to the primary site with up to 63 Gy to areas of ECS. RT should begin ideally within 5 weeks and no later than 6 weeks post-operatively. The indications for post-operative RT and CRT for OPSCC depend on pathological risk factors for recurrence and include primary tumour factors, such as close (1–5 mm) or positive (<1 mm) margins, T3–4 stage, and perineural and/or lymphovascular invasion, and nodal factors, such as ECS of nodal disease and/or N2–N3 nodal stage. Patients with ECS and/or microscopically involved (<1 mm) surgical resection margins experience significant benefit in terms of overall and disease-free survival from post-operative CRT compared to RT alone.

Transoral Surgery (TOS)

Transoral laser microsurgery (TLM) and transoral robotic surgery are minimally invasive surgical techniques for T1–T3 tumours with considerably less long-term functional deficit than open surgery. TOS is usually performed with neck dissection, either simultaneously or as a staged procedure. Adjuvant treatment is required in most patients, usually due to advanced nodal disease.

TOS is generally well tolerated, with a median length of hospital stay of approximately 4.4 days. Acute complications include haemorrhage (2.4%) and fistula (2.5%). Temporary tracheostomy tubes are needed in 12% of patients at the time of surgery but most are decannulated prior to discharge. Temporary nasogastric tubes are required in up to 47% of patients post-operatively but most patients can manage an oral diet by 4 weeks after surgery. Long-term functional outcomes after TOS appear favourable in small studies.

Transoral Robotic Surgery (TORS)

Currently, the daVinci® Surgical System is the most popular platform for robotic surgery. It consists of three parts: a 'patient-side' that cart deploys surgical instruments within the patient's body; a 'surgeon's console', which is remotely placed where three-dimensional display, foot pedals to control cautery, and hand controls for the instruments are found; and the 'vision cart', which houses the video processor and screens to project the procedure to the operating assistant and other observers.

Despite evidence supporting the safety and feasibility of TORS, there are no randomised studies comparing oncological outcomes of surgery versus CRT for OPSCC to date.

Free flap inset with the robot transorally after oropharyngectomy can now also be performed.

Management of the Neck

In the clinically/radiologically N0 neck, the prevalence of micrometastatic nodal disease is between 10% and 30%; therefore, elective treatment of the neck is recommended by either a selective neck dissection or RT. With surgery, dissection of Levels II, III, and possibly Level IV should be performed. In N0 necks, lateralised tumours require an ipsilateral neck dissection, with non-lateralised tumours needing a contralateral neck dissection for pathological staging purposes only. In N+ necks undergoing surgery, it is usual to dissect Level IIb.

Treatment Failure

Significantly more locoregional relapse is found in the HPV– OPSCC group than in the HPV+ OPSCC group, although the rate of distant metastasis does not differ significantly between the groups. The most common pattern of distant spread is to the lung, bone, and liver.

KEY POINTS

- The incidence of oropharyngeal cancer is increasing, and most of the increase is attributable to a rise in HPV-related disease (HPV+).
- HPV+ oropharyngeal squamous cell carcinoma (HPV+ OPSCC) constitutes a discrete disease entity, presenting in patents who are younger than patients presenting with HPV– disease.
- Despite presenting with clinicopathological features usually associated with poor disease outcome (N+ with ECS), HPV+ tumours respond better to treatment.
- Attention has turned to potential de-intensified treatment strategies for HPV+ OPSCC, in order to maintain advantageous survival outcomes whilst reducing treatment-related early and long-term toxicity.
- Significant expertise exists in transoral robotic surgery (TORS) for oropharyngeal surgery, and several ongoing randomised trials will clarify the role of this modality in head and neck cancer treatment.

Further Reading

1. De Almeida JR, Byrd JK, Wu R, et al. A systematic review of transoral robotic surgery and radiotherapy for early oropharynx cancer: a systematic review. *Laryngoscope* 2014; 124: 2096–3002.

2. Howard J, Masterson L, Dwivedi RC, et al. Minimally invasive surgery versus radiotherapy/chemoradiotherapy for small-volume primary oropharyngeal carcinoma. *Cochrane Database Syst Rev* 2016; 12 CD010963.

3. Holsinger FC, McWhorter AJ, Menard M, et al. Transoral lateral oropharyngectomy for squamous cell carcinoma of the tonsillar region: I. Technique, complications, and functional results. *Arch Otolaryngol Head Neck Surg* 2005; 131: 583–591.

65. NASOPHARYNGEAL CARCINOMA

The nasopharynx is situated deep inside the head, and carcinoma arising in the epithelium of the nasopharynx has a different aetiology, epidemiology, and biology than other cancers of the upper aerodigestive tract.

Epidemiology

The incidence of nasopharyngeal carcinoma demonstrates one of the largest geographical variations among all head and neck cancers, and the incidence in endemic areas can be 50 times higher than in low-prevalence areas. The highest incidence is found in Southern China, including Taiwan, Hong Kong, and Macau. Migrants originating from high-incidence areas also have a high incidence of nasopharyngeal carcinoma, although the risk decreases in second- or third-generation offspring of migrants. Populations from Malaysia, Indonesia, Arabia, North Africa, Thailand, and the Philippines, as well as Inuits, have intermediate incidence of nasopharyngeal carcinoma. Caucasians and populations from Northern China and East Asia have a low incidence.

Aetiology

Consumption of salted fish and eating preserved foods, especially at a young age, are aetiological factors. Smokers have a moderate increase in risk. The aetiology of nasopharyngeal carcinoma is the result of a complex interplay of genetic factors, early latent infection by Epstein–Barr virus (EBV) as well as subsequent EBV reactivation, and exposure to environmental carcinogens.

EBV is found only in the poorly differentiated and undifferentiated forms of nasopharyngeal carcinoma, which are the prevalent subtypes in high-incidence areas. The exact role of EBV in the development of nasopharyngeal carcinoma is still unknown. It is postulated that the combination of genetic susceptibility, environmental factors, and EBV infection all contribute.

Pathology

The most common histological form of nasopharyngeal cancer in endemic areas is the non-keratinising type. The histology of keratinising squamous cell carcinoma (SCC) is similar to that of other SCC in the upper aerodigestive tract. However, the non-keratinising type has some distinctive histological features. The malignant cells are infiltrated with lymphocytes and plasma cells; the term lymphoepithelial carcinoma is used to describe this. Lymphoepithelial carcinoma can also be found in salivary glands, paranasal sinuses, and lungs. When lymphoepithelial carcinoma is found outside the nasopharynx, it is important to distinguish between primary cancer and metastatic nasopharyngeal carcinoma.

EBV is ubiquitous in all the cancer cells in non-keratinising nasopharyngeal carcinoma. Immunostaining for EBV in cancer cells can help to differentiate between nasopharyngeal carcinoma and different types of head and neck cancer, especially in tissue obtained from metastatic lymph nodes. Immunostaining for EBV-encoded small ribonucleic acid (EBER) is commonly used to detect EBV inside the cancer cells.

Other cancers that occur in the nasopharynx include salivary gland carcinomas, sarcomas, lymphomas, and malignant melanomas.

Clinical Features
Early cancers of the nasopharynx produce minimal and trivial symptoms. Local features can be divided into nasal, otological, cervical, and neurological findings. Common nasal symptoms are blood-stained nasal discharge, post-nasal drip, obstruction, cacosmia, or a smell of blood.

Otological symptoms are usually caused by Eustachian tube dysfunction (i.e. ipsilateral hearing loss, tinnitus, and sensation of blockage). Otoscopic examination reveals a middle ear effusion. The nasopharynx should always be examined in adults with unexplained persistent middle ear effusion.

An enlarging upper neck mass is the most common reason for patients to be referred. Up to 70% of patients have enlarged neck lymph nodes on presentation (most frequently Level II and upper Level V). Lymphatic spread occurs in an orderly fashion from superior to inferior, with skip metastases rare.

Nasopharyngeal carcinoma patients can present with metastatic neck lymph nodes from an unknown primary. Imaging modalities like magnetic resonance imaging (MRI) and positron emission tomography (PET) may reveal the presence of a small cancer in the nasopharynx. Testing for EBV can also point to a nasopharyngeal primary.

Neurological symptoms include headache (usually vertex or occiput), facial pain, midface numbness, cranial nerve palsies (most commonly V2, V3, and VI). Rarely, patients present with ophthalmoplegia, decreased vision, and proptosis.

Diagnosis
A full head and neck examination is essential in all patients. Care should be taken to look for otitis media with effusion, cranial nerve palsies, and cervical lymphadenopathy.

Antegrade nasopharyngoscopy should be performed with either a rigid or a flexible endoscope. Most of the cancers are readily apparent under endoscopy, presenting as a mass with abnormal capillaries on the surface and with areas of ulceration (Figure 65.1).

Once a tumour is identified, biopsy of the lesion can usually be performed concurrently or under general anaesthesia (Figure 65.2).

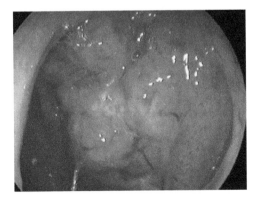

Figure 65.1   View of a tumour in the left nasopharynx through a 0° rigid nasoendoscope.

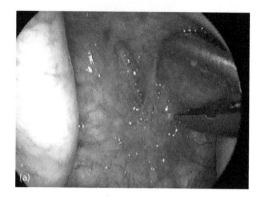

Figure 65.2 Biopsy of the left nasopharynx.

Laboratory Tests

Serum EBV IgA antibiodies against viral capsin antigen, early antigen, and EBV nuclear antigens are elevated in patients with nasopharyngeal carcinoma and can be used as tumour markers in screening for the cancer. These serological markers are not useful for monitoring of treatment efficacy and screening for recurrence. Plasma EBV DNA is a more sensitive and specific tumour marker for nasopharyngeal carcinoma that is useful for prognostication, monitoring of treatment response, and screening for tumour recurrence.

Imaging

MRI is the imaging modality of choice for delineating the extent of disease in the skull base. CT is useful in detecting cortical bone erosion in the skull base but cannot often differentiate between normal structures and tumour invasion in the skull base. PET CT is a useful adjunct to delineate the extent of disease, nodal metastasis, and distant metastasis.

Staging

Nasopharyngeal carcinoma has biological behaviour and prognosis vastly different from SCC of the head and neck region, and the staging system for it is also different (see Staging of Head and Neck Cancer).

Primary Treatment

Non-Surgical Treatment

Radiotherapy is the cornerstone of locoregional treatment for all stages of nasopharyngeal carcinoma without distant metastases. Early-stage disease, including stage I and low-risk stage II nasopharyngeal carcinoma, can be treated with radical radiotherapy alone. Stage II disease with higher tumour load and stage III or IV disease require combination chemotherapy and radiotherapy. The current standard of care for advanced nasopharyngeal carcinoma is concurrent cisplatin during radiotherapy followed by adjuvant cisplatin and fluorouracil. Epidermal growth factor receptor tyrosine kinase inhibitors like cetuximab have not been shown to be beneficial.

Intensity-modulated radiotherapy (IMRT) is the standard of care for radiation treatment of nasopharyngeal carcinoma. With IMRT, local control rates of over 90% have been reported. The complications of conventional two-dimensional radiotherapy, such as hearing loss, xerostomia, temporal lobe neuropathy, trismus, and neck fibrosis, are reduced.

Salvage Treatment

Salvage treatment for nasopharyngeal carcinoma is moderately successful but with significant morbidities. Because patients with recurrences have already been exposed to the toxicities of previous treatment, the choice of the salvage treatment needs to take into account the tolerance of the normal tissue.

Radiotherapy for Local Failures

Radiotherapy for local failures can be delivered by external beam or by local brachytherapy. The main limiting factor in re-irradiation is the radiation tolerance of vital organs like brainstem, optic chiasma, and temporal lobe.

Brachytherapy delivers a high dose of radiation with limited penetration inside the nasopharynx to treat local failures without deep invasion.

Surgery for Local Failure

The nasopharynx is notoriously difficult to access surgically. Most routes of access require facial incisions and multiple osteotomies and transgress a significant amount of normal tissue to expose the nasopharynx. Therefore, surgical resection of the nasopharynx, namely nasopharyngectomy, is reserved for salvaging radiation failures. The decision to offer nasopharyngectomy for salvaging local failures depends on the location of the tumour and the general condition of the patient. Tumours that show internal carotid artery encasement, extensive skull base infiltration, or intracranial extension are not suitable for salvage surgery.

Surgical approaches to the nasopharynx include the transpalatal (inferior) approach, the transcervico-mandibulo-palatal approach, the midfacial degloving (anterior) approach, the maxillary swing (anterolateral) approach (Figure 65.3), the facial translocation (anterolateral) approach, the lateral skull base approach, the endoscopic-endonasal approach, and robot-assisted approaches.

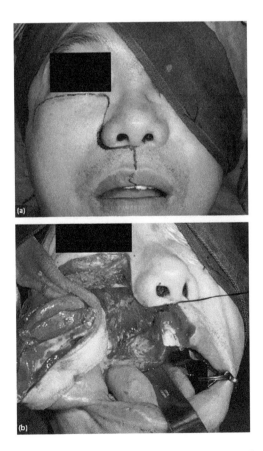

Figure 65.3 (a) Weber-Ferguson-Longmire incision and (b) view after swinging the maxilla laterally.

Nodal Failures

Radical neck dissection is considered the standard of care for management of nodal failures. The rationale for performing radical neck dissection instead of a lesser operation is that there are usually multiple involved nodes, the incidence of extracapsular involvement is high (< 70%), and further radiation may not be possible.

Further Reading

Hildesheim A, Wang C-P. Genetic predisposition factors and nasopharyngeal carcinoma risk: a review of epidemiological association studies, 2000–2011: Rosetta Stone for NPC: genetics, viral infection, and other environmental factors. *Semin Cancer Biol* 2012; 22(2): 107–116.

Lee A, Sze W, Au J, et al. Treatment results for nasopharyngeal carcinoma in the modern era: the Hong Kong experience. *Int J Radiat Oncol Biol Phys* 2005; 61(4): 1107–1116.

Tsang RK, Wei WI. Salvage surgery for nasopharyngeal cancer. *World J Otorhinolaryngol Head Neck Surg* 2015; 1(1): 34–43. (open access)

66. NASAL AND SINUS MALIGNANCY

Sinonasal malignancies are an uncommon heterogeneous group of tumours. They are often misdiagnosed as benign conditions. Extension of these tumours into the orbit, brain, and infratemporal fossa causes profound symptoms, with significant implications for morbidity and prognosis. Surgery and radiotherapy remain the mainstays of treatment. The prognosis is relatively poor compared with that for tumours at other head and neck subsites.

Epidemiology

- Rare, with incidence of 0.5–1 per 100,000 per year.
- 0.2–0.8% of all malignancies.
- <3% of upper aerodigestive tract neoplasms.
- Predominately develop in the fifth and sixth decades of life.
- Incidence in men is twice the incidence in women.
- The misconception that certain races are more susceptible than others to sinus malignancies is explicable by occupational exposure to carcinogens.

Incidence of Sinonasal Malignancy by Subsite

- Maxillary sinus—the most common (55%)
- Nasal cavities (35%)
- Ethmoid sinuses (9%)
- Frontal sinuses (1%)
- Sphenoid sinuses (1%)

Aetiology

Multiple occupational exposures to carcinogenic compounds have been identified, including (but not limited to):

- Hard wood—adenocarcinoma
- Soft wood—squamous cell carcinoma (SCC)
- African mahogany
- Nickel—SCC
- Smoking
- Chemicals (e.g. chromium, polycyclic hydrocarbons, aflatoxin)

Primary	Anterior	Posterior	Medial	Lateral	Superior	Inferior
Frontal sinus	Skin	Ant. Cranial fossa, frontal lobes				Ethmoid sinus, nasal cavity
Ethmoid sinus	Skin	Sphenoid nasopharynx, clivus, pituitary	Nasal cavities, cribriform plate	Orbit	Ant. Cranial fossa, frontal lobes	Nasal cavity
Maxillary sinus	Cheek, skin	Ptergopalatine, infratemporal fossae, mid. Cranial fossa	Nasal cavity	Cheek, skin	Orbit	Palate
Sphenoid sinus	Ethmoid sinuses	Clivus, pituitary gland, posterior cranial fossa		Middle cranial fossa, cavernous sinus	Pituitary gland, hypothalamus	Nasopharynx
Nasal cavities	Skin	Sphenoid sinus, nasopharynx		Maxillary sinus	Ant. Cranial fossa, frontal lobes	Palate

Figure 66.1   Patterns of local spread.

Local Extension

Sinonasal malignancies commonly spread by local invasion. Extension is possible into the orbit due to proximity and the thin barrier of bone and intracranially due to olfactory nerve fibres extending into the nasal cavity. Periosteum, perichondrium, and dura appear to act as temporary barriers and to resist tumour expansion to some extent. The anterior maxilla and orbital floor are very thin and readily destroyed by tumour.

Patterns of local spread are summarised in Figure 66.1.

Ohngren's line runs from the medial canthus of the eye to the angle of the mandible. Tumour position in relation to this line historically had implications for prognosis. Superiorly based tumours tend to be more aggressive and poorly differentiated, whereas tumours arising inferior to the line are more amenable to treatment and, consequently, have a better prognosis. The advent of craniofacial resection and radiation treatments has rendered this classification less relevant.

Lymphatic Drainage

The lymphatic drainage of the nose and paranasal sinuses predominantly splits into anterior and posterior drainage.

- The anteroinferior part of the nasal cavity and the skin of the nasal vestibule drain via the anterior pathway to the first-echelon facial, parotid, and submandibular lymph nodes.
- The remainder drains via the posterior pathway into retropharyngeal nodes.

Both routes subsequently drain to the upper deep cervical chain. Lymphatic spread to regional nodes becomes apparent in 25–35% of patients at some time during the course of their disease. Nodal involvement at presentation is found in 10% of patients.

Distant metastases at the time of presentation are unusual; sites for metastases are bone, brain, liver, lung, and skin.

Staging

For staging of nasal and paranasal sinus malignancy, please refer to Chapter 61.

Histopathological Subtypes

Squamous cell carcinoma (SCC)
- Most common sinonasal malignancy.
- Transformation of schneiderian membrane papillomas is a recognised risk.

- Adenocarcinoma
- Adenoid cystic carcinoma
- Olfactory neuroblastoma
  - Arises from olfactory neuroepithelium, hence it is a neuroendocrine tumour with paraneoplastic capabilities
  - Bimodal distribution, with peaks at 20 and 50 years of age
  - Classified by Kadish system
- Sinonasal undifferentiated carcinoma (SNUC)
- Mucosal melanoma
  - Nasal cavity and the septum are usually the sites of origin
- Haemangiopericytomas/glomangiopericytoma
  - Rare neoplasms of pericytes within the outer capillary wall
- Biphenotypic sinonasal sarcoma
  - New addition to the WHO classification for head and neck tumours
  - A low-grade sarcoma with neural and myogenic phenotype

Clinical Features

- Unilateral stuffiness/blockage
- Bleeding or spotty nasal secretions
- Nasal distortion (late sign)
- Facial pain with or without progressive infraorbital nerve sensory change
- Epiphora
- Progressive trismus, mainly due to invasion of the pterygopalatine and infratemporal fossae
- Oral masses and teeth mobility
- Proptosis and diplopia
- A visible swelling of the cheek

Imaging

- Dual modality with computed tomography (CT) and magnetic resonance imaging (MRI)
  - Allows accurate assessment/staging of bony and soft tissue architecture, respectively (Figure 66.2)

Biopsy

Ideally, biopsies are performed under general anaesthesia, to reduce the rate of non-diagnostic samples and complications and to allow sampling from within the sinus itself.

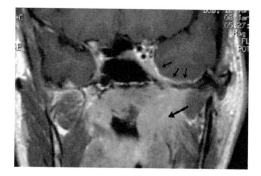

Figure 66.2 MRI and CT scans are complementary and help distinguish between tumour, retained secretions, and dural infiltration. This patient had an extensive tumour that had spread into the cavernous sinus and that had infiltrated the dura of the temporal lobe (small arrows) and the infratemporal fossa (large arrow). The spread was not apparent on the CT scan, which had shown a relatively small tumour affecting the sphenoid.

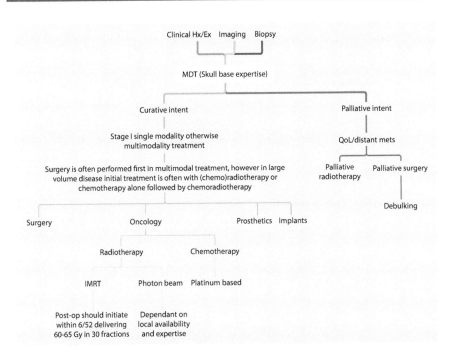

Figure 66.3   General principles of management of sinonasal tumours.

Treatment—General Principles

In general, cases should be carefully discussed in a multidisciplinary forum with skull base expertise to determine treatment approach and also to facilitate smooth and timely transfer between specialties, thereby avoiding unnecessary delays in adjuvant therapy. Figure 66.3 outlines general principles of management, with the proviso that certain tumours require more specific management strategies. Multimodality therapy (surgery, radiotherapy, and chemotherapy) has generally been demonstrated to be the most effective approach in the treatment of SCC and SNUC, whereas olfactory neuroblastoma is treated with surgery and post-operative radiotherapy.

Other than the stage of disease, the patient's wishes, and concurrent comorbidity, there are relatively few contraindications to treatment. Local invasion of the anterior cranial fossa and skull base are not necessarily contraindications given the development of modern surgical techniques. Distant metastases confer a poor prognosis and by definition render the patient incurable. Involvement of the facial skin is also not a contraindication to treatment. The involved area is best excised and repaired with flap, which can be a rotational or a free flap.

Surgery for Maxillary Tumours

A variety of operations for maxillary tumours have been described, the choice of which is determined by the extent of the tumour and amount of bone that needs to be removed. Figure 66.4 gives an overview of surgical options for maxillary tumours.

Midface Approaches

In the midface, an appropriate soft-tissue approach is required to facilitate bony resection, and three are commonly described (Figure 66.5). The selection of the specific approach depends on the pre-operative assessment of tumour location and anatomical considerations for resection to allow for surgery with curative intent. The principles of surgery are soft-tissue approach, osteotomies, resection, and reconstruction.

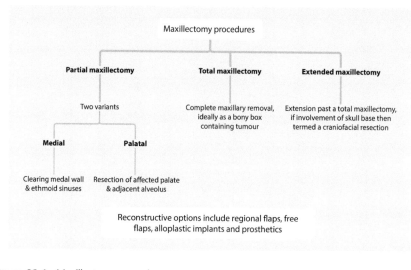

Figure 66.4   Maxillectomy procedures.

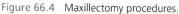

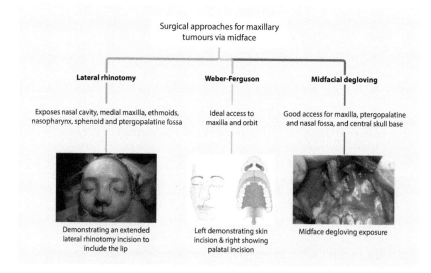

Figure 66.5   Approaches to the midface.

Neck Dissection

The rate of occult metastasis is less than 10%, with no suggestion in retrospective reviews that elective selective neck dissection contributes to an improved rate of neck control or overall survival.

Reconstruction and Rehabilitation of the Midface

Patients requiring extensive ablative surgery will predominately need post-operative radiotherapy. Meticulous rehabilitation, be it biological or prosthetic, aims to ensure a good cosmetic and functional outcome with separation of the nasal and oral cavities. Low defects not compromising the orbit adnexa can often be treated effectively with obturators. Where a dental obturator is used, healing of the bony cavity can be rapid, but it is beneficial to apply a split-thickness skin graft to the under surface of the facial skin flap. After the facial incision is closed, the cavity should be immediately fitted with a temporary prosthesis to cover

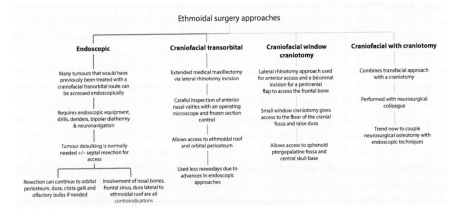

Ethmoidal surgery approaches

Endoscopic	Craniofacial transorbital	Craniofacial window craniotomy	Craniofacial with craniotomy
Many tumours that would have previously been treated with a craniofacial tranorbital route can be accessed endoscopically	Extended medical maxillectomy via lateral rhinotomy incision	Lateral rhinotomy approach used for anterior access and a bicoronal incision for a pericranial flap to access the frontal bone	Combines transfacial approach with a craniotomy
Requires endoscopic equipment, drills, deriders, bipolar diathermy & neuronavigation	Careful inspection of anterior nasal vaities with an operating microscope and frozen section control	Small window craniotomy gives access to the floor of the cranial fossa and raise dura	Performed with neurosurgical colleague
Tumour debulking is normally needed +/– septal resection for access	Allows access to ethmoidal roof and orbital periosteum	Allows access to sphenoid ptergopalatine fossa and central skull base	Trend now to couple neurosurgical osteotomy with endoscopic techniques
Resection can continue to orbital periosteum, dura, crista galli and olfactory bulbs if needed	Involvement of nasal bones, frontal sinus, dura lateral to ethmoidal roof are all contraindications	Used less nowadays due to advances in endoscopic approaches	

Figure 66.6   Approaches to access and manage the ethmoid complex surgically.

the palate and restore normal facial contours. The temporary prosthesis is changed at 14-day intervals until there is appropriate healing to allow fitting the final prosthesis. Larger defects necessitate flap reconstruction, often in the form of a free flap. Options for composite (bone and muscle) flaps include (but are not limited to):

- Deep circumflex iliac artery (DCIA) bone flap
- Scapula tip flap

Surgery for Ethmoid Tumours
Figure 66.6 describes surgical approaches to the ethmoids. Surgical technique selection depends on patient, tumour (location, extent), and surgical experience.

Management of the Orbit
Attempts to preserve the orbital contents and diminish mutilation often result in orbital recurrence. If the orbital muscles, globe, or orbital apex are involved, a lid-sparing exenteration is required. The lids provide good skin cover of the defect and can also be used to cover osseointegrated implants, which can be placed at the time of the surgery. Orbital involvement despite exenteration significantly affects survival.

Prognosis
The overall prognosis for sinonasal malignancy is directly related to the degree of local control. Prognosis varies very significantly between different pathologies.

- For olfactory neuroblastoma and adenoid cystic carcinoma, 5-year survival rates are high, but patients may continue to develop relapses for several decades after treatment.
- SNUC and malignant melanoma have very poor 5-year survival rates.

KEY POINTS

- Sinonasal malignancies can be difficult to differentiate from non-neoplastic lesions.
- Sinonasal malignancies are uncommon, representing <1% of all malignancies and <3% of all upper aerodigestive tract cancers.
- Sinonasal malignancies tend to present late.
- The main treatment modalities are surgery and radiotherapy.
- Olfactory neuroblastoma and adenoid cystic carcinoma may relapse after a decade; therefore, patients should be followed up for at least 15 years.

Further Reading

Kak I, Perez-Ordoñex B. Sinonasal tract pathology: an updated review of select entities. *Diagnostic Histopatholgy* 2019; 25(7): 2650273.

Paleri C, Rollands NJ. (Eds.) Head and Neck Cancer: United Kingdom National Multidisciplinary Guidelines, 5th edition, 2016.

Sethi N, Pearson A, Bajaj Y. Key Clinical Topics in Otolaryngology, 2016.

67. BENIGN AND MALIGNANT DISEASE OF THE ORAL CAVITY

Common Disorders of Teeth and Periodontium

Dental Caries

- Dynamic imbalance occurs between demineralisation and remineralisation of enamel.
- Bacteria in dental plaque generate acid environment.
- Progression leads to cavitation and invasion of dentinal tubules.
- Treatment is with restoration of integrity.

Tooth Wear

- Non-plaque-mediated chemical dissolution of tooth tissue (erosion)
- Non-masticatory tooth-to-tooth contact (attrition)
- Friction of exogenous material against tooth surface (abrasion)

Dental Infections

- *Pulpitis:* dental pulp inflammation, usually secondary to caries. Treatment is root canal or extraction rather than antibiotics.
- *Acute dentoalveolar abscess:* pain, swelling, erythema, and suppuration usually adjacent to causative tooth. Treatment is root canal surgery or extraction with or without systemic antibiotics.
- *Pericoronitis:* acute localised infection around a partially erupted tooth.
- *Periodontal disease:* plaque-related inflammation of the gingival or periodontal tissues.

Gingival Abnormalities

- *Pigmentation:* localised or generalised, with many causes, including melanoma, Kaposi's sarcoma, smoking, and Addison's disease.
- *Redness:* local or general, and can be attributed to lichen planus, allergies, or herpetic stomatitis.
- *Swellings:* can be local (epulides) or general, related to systemic causes.
- *Ulceration:* most common causes neoplasm, aphthous ulcers, or bacterial infections.

Dental Trauma

- Common especially in childhood. Avulsed permanent teeth need immediate reimplantation, avulsed deciduous teeth should be left out. Other dental trauma requires dental practitioner follow-up. Be vigilant for non-accidental injury.

Infections of the Jaw

- *Alveolar osteitis (dry socket):* localized inflammation after dental extraction. Management is curettage of the socket to promote blood clot formation.

- *Osteomyelitis:* acute or chronic. Treatment is with surgical debridement and systemic antibiotics.
- *Osteonecrosis:* secondary to medication related osteoradionecrosis of the jaw (MRONJ) or radiotherapy.

Cysts of the Jaw

Inflammatory

- *Radicular cyst:* most common inflammatory cyst. Occurs around apex of non-vital tooth. Diagnosis is with vitality testing. Treatment is with surgical enucleation.

Developmental

- *Dentigerous cyst:* Develops around crown of unerupted tooth. Mostly unilocular. Treatment is either enucleation or marsupialisation.

Non-Odontogenic Developmental Cysts

- *Nasopalatine duct cyst:* embryological remnant of nasopalatine duct. Often incidental radiological finding.

Non-Epithelial Bone Cyst

- *Aneurysmal bone cyst:* controversial because there is no cyst lining. Scalloped appearance on radiography. Biopsy confirms no lining and healing then occurs.
- *Ameloblastoma:* locally invasive odontogenic bone tumour. Appears uni- or multicystic on x-ray. Histopathological diagnosis is mandatory.

Disorders affecting the Oral Mucosa

Benign Oral Mucosal Changes

- *Frictional keratosis:* adaptation of oral mucosa to increased trauma.
- *Leukoedema and nicotinic stomatitis:* generalised white change of the oral mucosa. Most commonly seen in smokers. Sometimes red spots on white background when openings of minor salivary glands are visible.
- *Fordyce spots:* small yellow/white sebaceous spots commonly on the buccal mucosa from developmental substitution of minor salivary for sebaceous glands.
- *Tongue coating:* true coating of the tongue is rare. Occasional overgrowth and staining, 'brown hairy tongue', is rarely pathological.
- *Geographic tongue:* synchronous turnover with thinning of the mucosa of the tongue leads to red patches. Appearance moves across tongue. No curative treatment available.
- *Median rhomboid glossitis:* red, depapillated, smooth, rhomboidal area on dorsum of tongue. Mostly asymptomatic but occasionally associated with immunosuppression. No treatment required.
- *Mucosal swellings:* Fibroepithelial polyps, viral warts, and lipomas are common reasons for referral.

Changes in Mucosa Colour

- *White:* commonly with mucosal thickening by acanthosis or hyperkeratosis. Established squamous cell carcinoma (SCC) can present as a white patch, but dysplasia presents this way less frequently.
- *Red:* reflects thinning of the mucosa or increased vascularity (e.g. dysplasia or malignancy).
- *Pigmentation:* localised or generalised. Intraoral melanomas are rare.
- *Grey/blue:* often related to foreign bodies, such as dental amalgam or heavy metal poisoning. Dark blue lesions are mostly venous malformations.

Table 67.1 Clinical features of aphthous ulcers by type

Type of aphthous ulceration	Clinical features
Minor	Most common Usually <10 mm in diameter Last 2–3 weeks Non-keratinised mucosa Heal without scarring Can be multiple, but fewer than 10
Major	Diameter >10 mm Can last up to 3 months Non-keratinised or keratinised mucosa Heals with or without scarring Usually single, but maximum of 3
Herpetiform	Least common Diameter <5 mm Last for up to 2 weeks Heal without scarring Large numbers—up to 100 Can coalesce into large groups

Oral Ulceration

- *Aphthous ulceration*: immunological ulcers that are multifactorial in origin (Table 67.1).
- *Erythema multiforme*: immunological hypersensitivity reaction that can affect an individual system or multiple systems (Stevens-Johnson syndrome). Intraorally, it presents as widespread oral ulceration leading to tissue damage and swollen, crusted lips. Multiple drug triggers. Treated with high-dose systemic steroids.

Systemic Diseases and the Mouth

Skin Diseases

- *Pemphigus and pemphigoid*: autoimmune disorders driven by immunoglobulins, resulting in separation of epithelial cells (pemphigus) or of basement membrane (pemphigoid). Significant variability in skin lesion presentation. All patients should have ophthalmological assessment due to conjunctival scarring.
- *Lichen planus*: very common T-cell-mediated attack on basement membrane. Can be white (acanthosis), red (atrophy/ulceration), or mixed. Lesions tend to be intermittent and recurring. Diagnosis is via incisional biopsy. Treatment is usually symptomatic, with topical steroids.
- *Scleroderma*: either in isolation or as part of CREST. May significantly affect mouth opening.

Gastrointestinal Disorders

- *Ulcerative colitis*: aphthous ulceration during periods of disease activity.
- *Crohn's disease*: can present early in disease process with swelling, angular cheilitis, mucosal tagging, cobblestone appearance of mucosa, linear ulceration, or gingival inflammation.
- *Orofacial granulomatosis*: features of Crohn's disease but no GI disorder. Likely immunological. Exclusion diet initially (e.g. benzoate, sorbate, cinnamon, and chocolate). Systemic immunotherapy occasionally required.

Viral Diseases

- *Herpes simplex virus (HSV)*: HSV 1 or 2 can cause primary herpetic stomatitis. Recurrent lesion can present as persistent ulceration on palate.
- *Herpes zoster virus (HZV)*: multiple oral vesicles, which may be neuropathic.
- *Epstein–Barr virus (EBV)*: neck swellings, hairy leukoplakia, and nasopharyngeal cancer.
- *Human herpesvirus 8 (HHV8)*: Kaposi's sarcoma.
- *Human immunodeficiency virus (HIV)*: rarely associated with oral lesions following to highly active antiretroviral therapy (HAART).

Fungal Infections

Types of candidiasis	Predisposing factors
Acute pseudomembranous candidiasis (thrush)	Local or systemic immunosuppression
Acute atrophic candidiasis	Broad-spectrum antibiotics
Erythematous candidiasis	None, ageing
Chronic atrophic candidiasis	Denture wearing, esp. at night
Chronic hyperplastic candidiasis	Tobacco smoking
Median rhomboid glossitis	Tobacco smoking, local immunosuppression
Angular cheilitis	Denture wearing, diabetes
Chronic mucocutaneous candidiasis	Immune deficiency

Orofacial Pain

- *Trigeminal neuralgia*: Unknown origin; classically, electric shooting pain with a trigger zone on face. Single branch of trigeminal nerve often affected. Carbamazepine is first-line management.
- *Cluster headaches*: unilateral pain with ptosis, facial erythema/swelling, lacrimation, and nasal discharge. Inhaled oxygen or triptan beneficial.
- *Atypical odontalgia*: intense toothache with no dental pathology.
- *Oral dysesthesia*: Altered sensation, such as feeling of dryness, burning, numbness, or change in taste. No underlying pathology. Occasional haematinic deficiency. Reassurance often helpful.
- *Temporomandibular disorder*: common.

Malignant Tumours of the Oral Cavity

Introduction

The oral cavity is lined by stratified squamous epithelium of varying degrees of keratinisation. Primary tumours can be derived from mucosa, salivary glands, neurovascular tissues, bone, or dental tissues. Over 90% of tumours are squamous cell carcinoma (SCC). There has been an increase of over 20% of oral cancer in patients under the age of 65, with HPV-associated oropharyngeal carcinoma playing an increasing role. Globally, tobacco and alcohol remain the main aetiological factors. Five-year survival rates are 80% if the cancer is confined to the mucosa, 40% for those with regional spread, and 20% with distant disease.

History

- Thorough symptom history, including for metastatic disease
- Medical history
- Social history
- Possible site-specific history (e.g. claudication)

Examination

- Palpation for cervical lymphadenopathy
- Systematic oral examination with two dental mirrors
- Flexible nasoendoscopy
- Dental examination

Initial Investigations

- Photographs
- Incisional biopsy of all suspicious lesions
- Fine-needle aspiration cytology of suspicious lymphadenopathy
- Orthopantogram
- Routine blood values

Staging Investigations

- Computed tomography (CT) +/− chest CT
- Magnetic resonance imaging (MRI)
- Ultrasound (USS) +/− fine needle aspiration cytology (FNA) of lymphadenopathy
- Positron emission tomography (PET)/PET-CT

Surgical Margins

- To ensure >5 mm pathological margin post-shrinkage, 1-cm soft-tissue and bony margins are standard.
- Royal College of Pathologists classify >5 mm as clear, 1–5 mm as close, <1 mm as positive.
- Post-operative adjuvant therapy depends on margin status and lymph node involvement.

Surgical Access

- *Mandibulotomy*: Extend neck dissection incision anteriorly and include lip-split procedure. Osteotomy performed anterior to mental foramen to reserve mental nerve function.
- *Visor approach with lingual release*: Intraoral mucosal incision is made in lingual gingival sulcus bilaterally, allowing 'drop down' of oral tissues.
- *Upper cheek flap*: Can be a combination of conventional Weber-Ferguson (lip split extending into lateral rhinotomy incision) with subciliary extension (Diffenbach extension) or medial canthal extension (Lynch extension).

Key Points Regarding Tumour Location

Buccal Carcinoma

- Commonest site for oral cancer in Southeast Asia.
- Associated with betel/paan consumption.
- Good surgical reconstruction to prevent post-operative trismus.
- Up to 26% of patients have occult nodal metastasis at presentation.
- Consider selective neck dissection (Levels I–III) if tumour is >4 mm thick.

Floor of Mouth Carcinoma

- One of the most common sites of oral cancer.
- Leukoplakia of the floor of mouth has a 1–2.9% annual transformation rate.
- Anterior lesions may require treatment of both sides of neck.
- Tendency for cervical metastasis to occur with thinner tumours.

Tongue Carcinoma

- One of the most common sites of oral cancer.
- Usually presents at stage I/II disease.
- Neck dissection should include Levels I–IV because of skip lesions.
- Reconstruction should maximise function of residual tongue and may involve local or distal pedicled and free flaps.

Retromolar Carcinoma

- 6–7% of oral carcinomas.
- Frequently presents as stage III/IV disease with extension into adjacent sites.

Maxillary Alveolus and Hard Palate

- Carcinoma of the maxillary alveolus is three times less common than cancer of the mandibular alveolus.
- Carcinoma of the hard palate represents only 1–3% of oral cancers.
- Palatal carcinoma is associated with reverse smoking.
- All patients should have dental impressions as part of their workup.
- Some degree of bone removal is nearly always required.
- Selective neck dissection is often required.

Mandibular Alveolus

- Represents approximately 10% of oral cancers, although the rate is up to 30% in the Japanese population.
- 94% of tumours invade bone.
- Alveolar carcinoma is a surgical disease requiring a rim or segmental resection of the mandible.

Management of the Mandible

- Bone involvement may be erosion or invasion.
- MRI, CT, SPECT, and periosteal stripping are complementary in assessing bone involvement.
- Bone margins should be dictated by overlying soft-tissue margins.
- Rim resection should be conducted when oncologically acceptable.

Lip Reconstruction

Principles of Lip Reconstruction

- Nerve supply of reconstructed lip should be preserved if possible, to maintain oral continence.
- Preservation of muscle-carrying vermilion tissue.
- Lip tissue should preferentially be used to reconstruct defects.
- Muscles should be normally oriented if possible.
- Adjacent tissue, such as cheek, should be considered if the defect is too large.
- Free-tissue reconstruction is used only if local tissue is insufficient.

Reconstruction of the Vermilion

- *Vermilion flap*: defects close to the white roll and include advancement or 'switch' flaps from opposite lip.
- *Mucosal advancement flaps*: useful for total vermilionectomy defects.

Reconstruction of the Upper Lip

- *Wedge excision*: defects up to one third of lip.
- Cheek flap (e.g. nasolabial) can used for defects up to one half of lip.
- Abbe-Sabattini flap can be used if commissure is not involved (see Figure 12.17).
- Total lip reconstruction is rare, but a folded radial forearm flap can be used.

Reconstruction of the Lower Lip

- *Defect up to one third of lip*: simple wedge excision
- *Defect between one third and one half of lip*:
  - Wedge excision
  - *Karapandzic technique*: unilateral or bilateral full-thickness mucomusculocutaneous flaps supplied by branches of facial artery (see Figure 12.14)
  - *Johanson's step technique*: square or rectangular segments removed lateral to defect in stepwise fashion (see Diagram 12.16)
  - *Lip switch*: Abbe-Sabattini flap or Estlander for commissure reconstruction (see Figure 12.18)
- Defect greater than one half of lip
  - Freeman modification of Bernard von Burow technique (Figure 12.20)
  - Free tissue transfer

Further Reading

1. D'Cruz AK, Vaish R, Kapre N, et al. Elective versus therapeutic neck dissection in node-negative oral cancer. *N Engl J Med* 2015; 373(6): 521–529. doi:10.1056/NEJMoa1506007
2. Field EA, Longman L, Tyldesley WR. (2003). *Tyldesley's Oral Medicine*. Oxford: Oxford University Press.
3. Stell PM, Maran AGD, Watkinson JC, Gilbert RW. (2012). *Stell and Maran's Textbook of Head and Neck Surgery and Oncology*. London: Hodder Arnold.

68. MANAGEMENT OF THE UNKNOWN PRIMARY IN HEAD AND NECK CANCER

Introduction

Head and neck squamous cell carcinoma (HNSCC) that presents as carcinoma of unknown primary (CUP) represents a challenge. Improvements in diagnostic techniques have enabled the identification of a higher proportion of primary sites in patients presenting with CUP. The most common presentation of CUP in the head and neck is human papillomavirus (HPV)-associated oropharyngeal carcinoma (HPV + OPSCC). With the continued increased incidence of HPV+ OPSCC, it is likely that the incidence of CUP will also increase.

Definition

In the head and neck, the definition of a true unknown or occult primary carcinoma is the presentation of metastatic neck lymphadenopathy without the development or manifestation of an index primary tumour within a preceding 5-year period. CUP is diagnosed in a patient when there is proven squamous cell carcinoma (SCC) in one or more cervical lymph nodes, with an absence of an obvious primary tumour despite rigorous clinical examination, appropriate imaging, and examination under anaesthesia +/− biopsy.

In patients with a true CUP, the primary tumour may never become evident or may remain undetected on initial presentation, only to later become clinically evident. However, the most likely primary sites are often treated by inclusion in radiation fields, such that the primary never becomes clinically evident. An alternate hypothesis suggests that the primary tumour has been destroyed by the patient's immune system after early metastasis to the cervical lymph nodes.

Incidence

The universal availability of cross-sectional imaging and standardized diagnostic protocols has reduced the incidence of CUP in HNSCC significantly. The incidence reported in the current literature is around 5% of HNSCC. It is increasingly recognized that high-risk (HR) HPV-related HNSCC tends to present with regional disease and a clinically unrecognised primary focus, and most patients presenting with CUP will likely have a primary site in the oropharynx.

Nomenclature

Recent changes to the TNM staging system published in the 8th edition of the American Joint Committee on Cancer (AJCC) *Cancer Staging Manual* included changes to CUP staging. A T0 category is no longer assigned to p16– OPSCC and other non-HR HPV cancers (e.g. larynx, oral cavity, and hypopharynx). This is because, in these tumours, an exact primary site is by definition unable to be established. In contrast, cytology specimens from an enlarged lymph node in which the presence of metastatic carcinoma is confirmed can be tested for HPV and Epstein-Barr virus (EBV) status, which safely allows the primary site to be determined as either oropharynx or nasopharynx, respectively. Therefore, classification systems for p16+ OPSCC and nasopharyngeal cancer maintain T0 categories.

Evaluation and Diagnosis

Clinical Assessment

Patients presenting with metastatic lymphadenopathy with an occult primary should undergo a structured diagnostic workup, as recommended by evidence-based guidelines.

- *History*: A thorough history is essential. Social history, such as smoking and alcohol consumption, or a history of multiple sexual partners and orogenital contact, may supply clues to the location of the primary tumour.
- *Clinical Examination*: The site of the node is an indicator of the primary site. Nomograms based on epidemiological data and lymph node distribution have been created to help predict the primary site. Fibreoptic nasopharyngolaryngoscopy should be performed, with special attention to sites where a small primary focus may be missed (e.g. nasopharynx, base of tongue (BOT), infrahyoid epiglottis, and piriform sinus). Novel endoscopic techniques, such as narrow-band imaging (NBI), have shown some utility in the clinic setting, being able to identify neoplastic tissue at an earlier stage than conventional endoscopy.
- *Imaging*: Cross-sectional imaging, such as multiplanar computed tomography (CT) and/or magnetic resonance imaging (MRI) and fluorodeoxyglucose (FDG) positron emission tomography (FDG-PET) CT should be performed prior to an assessment under general anaesthesia.
- *Examination under anaesthesia*: If the primary site is not identified with imaging, then the patient should undergo panendoscopy under a general anaesthetic, with biopsies of the nasopharynx and BOT as well as tonsillectomy. Using this protocol, most CUP cases turn out to be oropharyngeal primaries (either tonsillar or BOT).

Endoscopic Biopsy of the Nasopharynx

Blind biopsies of the nasopharynx often provide a poor yield of primary site diagnosis. It is therefore recommended that biopsies from this site should be guided using rigid endoscopes, especially where abnormalities have been noted on imaging.

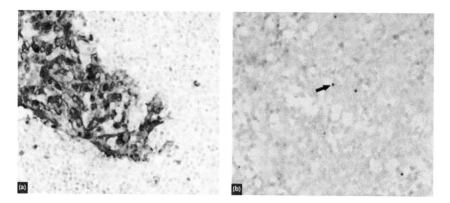

Figure 68.1 Photomicrograph showing immunohistochemistry of a lymph node from a patient with metastatic HNSCC of unknown primary suggesting a tonsil origin. (a) Positivity to p16 in the tonsil (b) identified malignant cells in the tonsil.

Bilateral Tonsillectomy

In the HR HPV era, there is greater recognition that tumours can be multifocal at presentation and that the primary may reside in the contralateral tonsil in up to 10% of cases, providing a basis for bilateral tonsillectomy (Figure 68.1). Furthermore, bilateral tonsillectomy could reduce the need for bilateral irradiation to the neck, thus leading to reduced morbidity. Where patients have undergone previous tonsillectomy but have tonsillar remnants, the excised remnants should be sent for analysis because primary tumours may be found in them.

Tongue Base Biopsies

Blind biopsies of the BOT are often unsatisfactory because occult carcinomas rarely arise from the mucosal surface and are often deeper. BOT mucosectomy, a procedure that has developed with the advent of robotic techniques (which offer superior manoeuvrability and access), allows sampling of the entire BOT mucosa and is able to identify a primary site in over 50% of patients who are PET negative and have no tonsil primary (Figures 68.2 and 68.3). Interestingly, around 10% can have contralateral foci. However, the morbidity of this procedure cannot be underestimated, with the risk of bleeding, need for tube feeding, and the potential for pharyngeal stenosis.

Pet Scanning

FDG-PET CT scanning is now a key modality in the evaluation of the unknown primary. It provides anatomical localisation of the avid lesion. A negative PET CT result does not eliminate the requirement for panendoscopy and multiple-site biopsies. FDG-PET CT is only

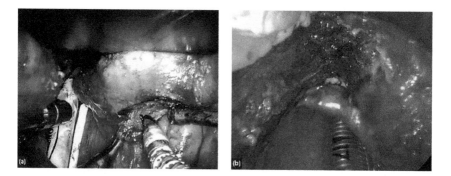

Figure 68.2 (a) Robotic tongue base mucosectomy in progress and (b) completed procedure.

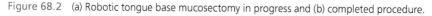

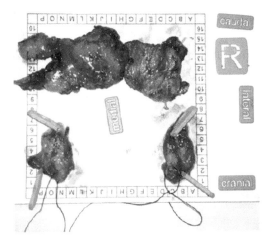

Figure 68.3 Bilateral tonsillectomy and robotic tongue base mucosectomy specimen oriented and mounted for pathological examination.

useful if it is performed before anaesthesia and biopsy, because the post-biopsy inflammatory response may increase the uptake of FDG, causing a false-positive result (Figure 68.4). Studies have determined the sensitivity and specificity of PET scanning in identifying the primary site in CUP to be as high as 92%.

Nice Recommendations

The National Institute for Health and Clinical Excellence (NICE) made the following recommendations for patients with a neck lump thought to arise from a head and neck cancer. The recommendations are summarised in an algorithm in Figure 68.5. Ultrasound-guided fine-needle aspiration cytology (FNAC) or core biopsy, with a cytopathologist or a biomedical scientist present to assess the adequacy of the cytology sample, may help streamline the diagnostic process. Similarly, an FDG-PET scan can be carried out as the first investigation to detect the primary site.

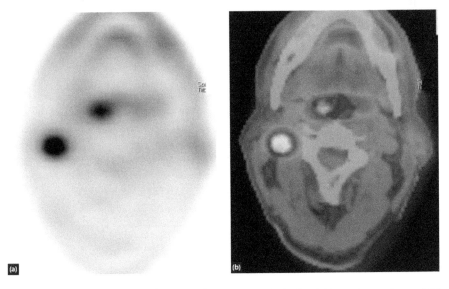

Figure 68.4 FDG-PET CT scan demonstrating tracer uptake in the right oropharynx in a patient presenting with metastatic SCC of the right neck.

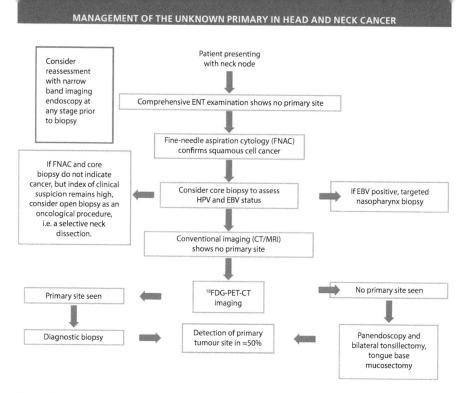

Figure 68.5 Suggested algorithm for the management of the unknown primary.

Clinical Management

In the absence of high-level evidence, the optimal management of CUP continues to generate debate. CUP management can be organized into the treatment of early disease (N1 with no extracapsular spread) and advanced disease (extracapsular spread, N2 and N3; Table 68.1). In early disease, single-modality therapy can be considered, either in the form of neck dissection (ND) alone without adjuvant treatment and a 'watch and wait' approach to the primary, or radiotherapy (RT) alone in patients who pose a high surgical risk. Advanced cases require combined modality therapy.

Surgical Management of the Neck

Traditionally, most units favour ND up front, followed by either RT or chemoradiotherapy (CRT) as indicated. Selective neck dissection (SND) is a valid option for patients with N2a and N2b disease, because the risk of metastases in Levels I and V is low in patients with CUP unless they present with N3 disease. Surgery allows adequate pathological staging of the neck

Table 68.1 Treatment recommendations from ENT-UK Multidisciplinary Treatment Guidelines (2016)

Stage	Surgery	Radiotherapy	Chemotherapy
T0N1M0 (No ECS)	SND or MRND (modified radical ND)	No, unless for mucosal sites	No
T0N1M0 (ECS)	SND or MRND	Yes, to neck	Should be considered
T0N2M0	SND or MRND	Yes: ipsilateral, but contralateral should be considered	Should be considered
T0N3M0	MRND or RND	Yes: ipsilateral, but contralateral should be considered	Should be considered

and therefore tailoring of onward treatment. Performing surgery in a non-irradiated neck is also advantageous in minimising morbidity. However, this approach could potentially cause a treatment delay if any unexpected surgical complications occur. Primary RT or CRT will reduce the need for surgery but may render surgery difficult and with an increased risk of complications.

However, recent randomized trials have reported that PET-CT-guided active surveillance following radical CRT showed similar survival outcomes to up-front ND followed by CRT and led to considerably fewer NDs, fewer complications, and lower costs. Although this was in the setting of the known primary, the data are robust enough to warrant a re-examination of the current approach using primary surgery in CUP.

Branchial Cyst Carcinoma
The evidence for the existence of branchial cyst or branchiogenic carcinoma is tenuous. Many patients with CUP may present with a cystic lateral neck mass. There is enough evidence to recommend that all patients over 35 years old with lateral cystic masses must be presumed to have cancer until proven otherwise, and therefore they should be entered into a CUP investigation protocol even if the initial FNAC is not suggestive of metastatic SCC.

RT to the Neck and the Putative Primary Site
The recommended RT fields remain controversial, with some centres offering unilateral radiation to the neck and ipsilateral likely primary sites, while others propose bilateral neck treatment and 'total mucosal irradiation'.

Bilateral neck irradiation tends to give better local control and disease-free survival than unilateral treatment, but the improvement in overall survival is not always seen. Unfortunately, bilateral irradiation is associated with increased morbidity in terms of pain, xerostomia, and long-term dysphagia with increased feeding tube dependence.

Intensity-modulated radiotherapy (IMRT) with bilateral neck radiation has the potential for reduced acute and late toxicity and a significant reduction in morbidity. IMRT is currently the standard of care for head and neck cancers in several countries.

Recommended Treatments

- cT0N1M0 without ENE (extranodal extension): single-modality treatment either with SND or involved field RT alone
- pT1N0M0 with ENE: post-operative RT if ENE is identified
- T0N2M0 and T0N3M0: primary CRT followed by PET-CT guided surveillance or combined modality treatment, ND followed by RT or CRT

Treatment Outcomes
Most series show improved overall and disease-free survival with combined modality treatment. Survival results are dependent upon the N category at presentation, with an expected 5-year survival of 70–100% for N1 cancers, 30–60% for N3, and 52–75% for all stages of HNSCC with unknown primary site.

Patterns of Failure
The pattern of failure largely depends on the initial treatment protocol. If RT is used, disease recurrence is usually in the neck and distant metastases. FDG-PET CT scan is probably the best method for detection and diagnosis of recurrences. Distant metastases often occur within a year of treatment completion and are most often in the lung. The incidence of recurrence in the potential primary site is extremely variable, and mainly occurs in patients treated with surgery alone.

> **KEY POINTS**
>
> - CUP in HNSCC is an increasingly rare entity and accounts for fewer than 5% of cases.
> - The diagnostic workup should include history, examination, cross-sectional imaging, and examination under anaesthesia as well as biopsies.
> - Treatment of CUP should be based on the stage of the disease process, with a single modality used for early-stage disease and a combined modality used for patients with advanced disease.
> - The survival outcomes are generally good for early and late-stage disease.

Further Reading

Mackenzie K, Watson M, Jankowska P, et al. Investigation and management of the unknown primary with metastatic neck disease: United Kingdom National Multidisciplinary Guidelines. *J Laryngol Otol* 2016; **130**: S170–S175.

Mehanna H, McConkey CC, Rahman JK, et al. PET-NECK: a multicentre randomised Phase III non-inferiority trial comparing a positron emission tomography-computerised tomography-guided watch-and-wait policy with planned neck dissection in the management of locally advanced (N2/N3) nodal metastases in patients with squamous cell head and neck cancer. *Health Technol Assess* 2017; **21**: 1–122.

Paleri V, Roland NJ. Head and neck cancer: United Kingdom national multidisciplinary guidelines. *J Laryngol Otol* 2016; **130**: S1–S224.

69. METASTATIC NECK DISEASE

The most important prognostic factor in head and neck squamous cell cancer (HNSCC) is the presence or absence, level, and size of metastatic neck disease. Patients with lymph node involvement in HNSCC have a significantly reduced chance of survival compared to those who have no lymph node metastases.

Elective removal of regional lymph nodes serves as a staging procedure to ascertain whether metastatic disease is present and to identify high-risk patients who might benefit from systemic adjuvant therapy; it is not expected to diminish the metastatic potential.

Neck Levels
Currently, six neck levels representing the sites of first-echelon nodes within the head and neck are recognised (Figure 69.1).

Neck Dissection Terminology
The terminology of the Committee for Neck Dissection Classification of the American Head and Neck Society is used (Table 69.1 and Figure 69.2).

However, division of SND into named subtypes has been superseded by recommendations that the levels or sublevels removed during SND be precisely stated in the operative notes.

Region-Specific Lymphatic Drainage
In a landmark study of 1,155 patients with previously untreated HNSCC published by Lindberg in 1972,[1] the topographical distribution of clinically evident cervical metastases was set out. This identified distinct patterns of spread to the neck based on the primary site

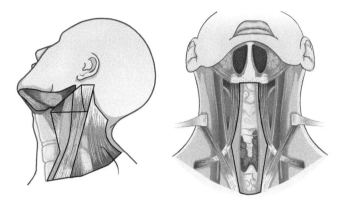

Figure 69.1   The lymph node levels of the neck.

Table 69.1   Classification of neck dissection techniques

Radical neck dissection (RND)	Removal of Levels I–V, accessory nerve, internal jugular vein, and sternocleidomastoid (SCM)
Modified radical neck dissection (MRND)	Removal of Levels I–V dissected; preservation of one or more of the accessory nerve, internal jugular vein, or SCM (types I, II, III, respectively)
Selective neck dissection (SND)	Preservation of one or more levels of lymph nodes
Extended radical neck dissection (ERND)	Removal of one or more additional lymphatic and/or non-lymphatic structures(s) relative to a radical neck dissection, e.g. Level VII, retropharyngeal lymph nodes, hypoglossal nerve

(Table 69.2). Histological proof of this concept was produced in 1990 by Shah in a series of 1,119 neck dissections.

Metastatic Behaviour in the Previously Treated Neck
Surgery and radiotherapy significantly disrupt the natural lymphatic drainage of the head and neck. Thus, the patterns of drainage described above will not be applicable to disease recurrence following treatment.

Occult Nodal Disease
The term occult disease is used to describe the presence of metastases in the neck nodes that cannot be clinically or radiologically identified. These are most commonly from a primary in the oropharynx.

Cystic Neck Metastases
Cystic neck metastases are usually of oropharyngeal origin, with the most common sites being the tonsil or tongue base. Human papillomavirus (HPV)-related tumours are more often associated with cystic metastases than HPV-negative tumours.

Prognostic Nodal Features
Prognostic nodal features are summarised in Box 69.1. In a study of 1,330 patients, Lefebvre et al. demonstrated that irrespective of T category, extra-nodal extension (ENE), three or more positive nodes and positive Level IV nodes doubled the risk of regional recurrence and trebled the risk of distant metastases.[3]

Clinical Staging
The joint UICC and AJCC classifications for regional cervical lymphadenopathy have had substantial changes made to them in the 8th edition (see Chapter 61).

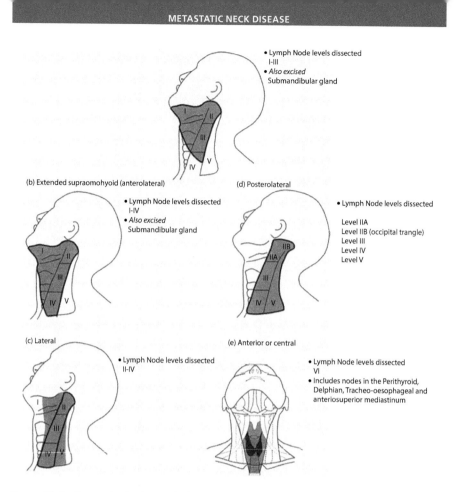

Figure 69.2 Types of selective neck dissection (a) Levels I–III (supraomohyoid); (b) Levels I–IV (extended supraomohyoid); (c) Levels III–IV (lateral); (d) Levels III–IV (posterolateral); (e) Levels VI–VII (anterior/paratracheal).

Table 69.2 Patterns of lymphatic drainage

Primary site	Echelon nodes
Oral cavity	Levels I, II, and III
Oropharynx	Levels II, III, and IV
Larynx	Levels II, III, and IV
Hypopharynx	Levels II, III, and IV
Thyroid	Levels IV, VI, and VII

BOX 69.1 PROGNOSTIC NODAL FEATURES

- Site
- Size
- Number
- Extra-nodal extension (ENE)
- Matting

Assessment of Cervical Lymphadenopathy

Fine-Needle Aspiration Cytology (FNAC)

FNAC is easy to perform, can be reported immediately, and has overall accuracy rates exceeding 90%. The technique is particularly useful in the assessment of a palpable node when searching for an unknown primary, because the cytological aspirate can be subjected to tests that may help in the search for the primary tumour. HPV or Epstein–Barr virus (EBV) transcripts (or their surrogate markers) will point to a primary site in the oropharynx or nasopharynx, respectively. Trucut biopsy of the lymph node, particularly under ultrasound guidance, is increasingly being used.

Ultrasound

Ultrasound can detect the presence of malignant cervical lymph nodes with sensitivity rates between 70% and 90%. When ultrasound is combined with FNAC, the rate increases to 90%.

Computed Tomography (CT)

The diagnostic accuracy of CT scanning in detecting malignant cervical lymphadenopathy is higher than clinical examination. The criteria used for categorising metastatic deposits include lymph nodes with a short-axis diameter larger than 1 cm, a cluster of three or more borderline enlarged nodes larger than 0.8 cm, and nodal necrosis or patchy enhancement within the nodes.

Magnetic Resonance Imaging (MRI)

MRI can detect cervical lymphadenopathy with overall similar accuracy rates to CT, although meta-analyses have found CT to perform better than MRI. However, MRI may be better in evaluating the N0 neck and in the presence of deep invasion.

PET CT

Currently, the widespread role of PET-CT is confined to detecting the occult primary, detecting unknown distant metastases in certain clinical settings, and assessing residual and recurrent disease after irradiation. The PET-CT detection rate for nodes less than 1 cm is reported at 71%. Thus, this modality has a poor detection rate (0–30%) in the setting of the N0 neck.

Treatment of Metastatic Neck Disease

The N0 Neck

General consensus in the literature is that it is prudent to treat the neck when the risk of occult spread is more than 15–20%. In fact, many surgeons and oncologists would perform elective neck treatment for smaller probability (5–15%) of occult metastases. At least in oral cavity cancer, this approach has been proven to have a significant impact upon both overall and disease-free survival.

Although there are no prospective trials, retrospective data from studies with large numbers suggest that elective neck dissection (END) and irradiation are equally effective in controlling subclinical disease. Generally, when the primary tumour is being treated with radiotherapy, then elective treatment should be with radiotherapy. When the primary tumour is treated with surgery, then elective neck surgery should be carried out (Figure 69.3).

In the presence of advanced primaries at high risk of occult spread or midline cancers, contralateral neck treatment is often warranted.

The N+ Neck

The treatment offered to the neck often depends on the modality used to treat the primary site, as seen in the suggested algorithms for patients undergoing primary chemoradiation (Figure 69.4) and primary surgery (Figure 69.5).

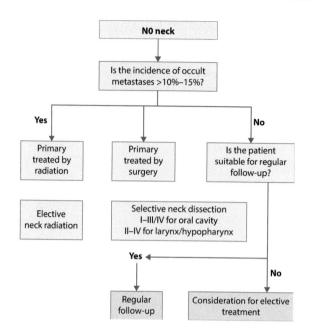

Figure 69.3   Algorithm for the management of the N0 neck.

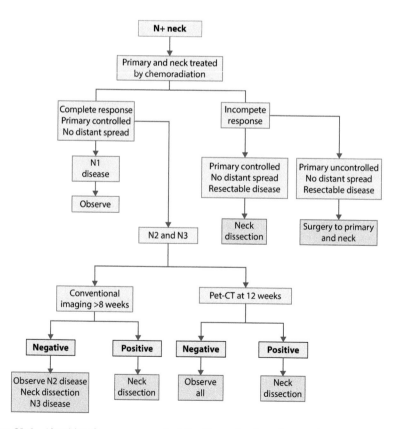

Figure 69.4   Algorithm for management of the N+ neck when chemoradiation is the primary modality.

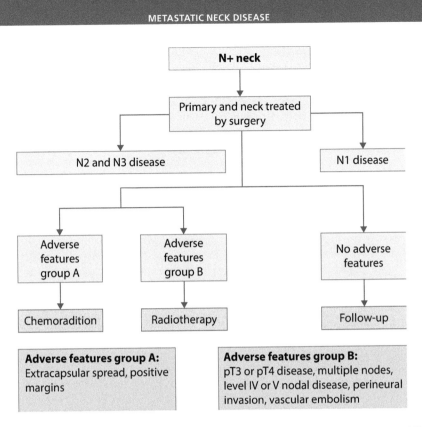

Figure 69.5 Algorithm for the management of the N+ neck when surgery is the primary modality.

Adjuvant radiotherapy or chemoradiotherapy is indicated for surgically managed N2 and N3 disease and for N1 disease with poor prognostic features.

If the N+ neck is treated with primary radiotherapy or chemoradiotherapy, response to treatment should be determined with a 12-week PET CT scan. Complete responders can be safely observed. Incomplete responders should be offered neck dissection. Surgical procedures after chemoradiotherapy are associated with more complications.

Treatment Outcomes

Regional control rates in the N0 neck are good regardless of modality, with failure rates of 3–7%. Recurrence rates in the N+ neck vary depending upon stage and presence of ENE. Where the primary tumour has been controlled, overall recurrence rates range from 10% in the N1 neck without ENE, 20–30% for N2 disease, and up to 85% for N3 disease.

Future Research

The following areas need to be addressed:

- Imaging of low-volume disease
- Significance of occult cancer in the neck
- Molecular detection of occult neck disease and its significance
- Sentinel node biopsy for occult neck cancer, in non-oral-cavity cancer
- Selective neck dissection for palpable disease
- Super-selective neck dissection for residual disease after chemoradiation
- Management of the contralateral neck
- Quality of life after various treatment modalities

Further Reading

1. Lindberg R. Distribution of cervical lymph node metastases from squamous cell carcinoma of the upper respiratory and digestive tracts. *Cancer* 1972; **29**: 1446–1449.

2. Shah JP. Patterns of cervical lymph node metastasis from squamous carcinomas of the upper aerodigestive tract. *Am J Surg* 1990; **160**: 405–409.

3. D'Cruz AK, Vaish R, Kapre N, et al. Elective versus therapeutic neck dissection in node-negative oral cancer. *N Engl J Med* 2015; **373**: 521–529.

70. PROSTHETIC MANAGEMENT OF ORAL AND FACIAL DEFECTS

Introduction
Successful complex oral and facial rehabilitation with prosthesis requires detailed planning by a specialist multidisciplinary team. Members of the team include maxillofacial prosthodontists and extended team members, including hygienists, technicians, and the primary care dental professionals. Osseointegrated implants are an essential tool in the reconstruction of oral and facial defects, and their use (primary or secondary) should form part of treatment planning.

Pre-Operative Assessment
Where prosthetic rehabilitation is likely, early assessment by the maxillofacial prosthodontist is important. All dentate patients should be screened with detailed examination and radiographs to decide on retention or extraction of teeth and potential support available to for the prosthesis. Modification of risk factors (e.g. smoking or excess alcohol consumption) should be attempted at this time to reduce risks related to implant/prosthesis failure.

Management of the Maxillary Defect
The use of obturators in the reconstruction of maxillary defects has gradually been reduced, with increased use of predictable free vascularised tissue transfer. The management decision should take into account the size and location of tumour, tumour subtype, prognosis, and the patient's fitness for surgery. Ideally, very large defects are managed with free tissue transfer, but defects up to Brown 2 can be successfully managed with an obturator.[1]

Preparation must begin before surgery with careful planning of resection margins, in particular alveolar margin bony cuts because they are integral to the accuracy and fit of the prosthesis. Depending on the size and location of the defect, components to aid the retention of the prosthesis can be incorporated. These include clasps on remaining teeth, circumzygomatic wires, and concomitant insertion of osseointegrated implants.

Table 70.1   Advantages and disadvantages of prosthetic use

Advantages	Disadvantages
Early rehabilitation	Unknown prognosis for patient
Implants placed before radiotherapy	Unknown oral function post-surgery
Psychological patient benefit	Anatomical difficulties for placement
Reduced number of surgeries	Cost implications if implants not used

Surgical Modifications to Facilitate Obturator Provision

- Where possible, bony cuts through the maxillary alveolus should be made through edentulous bone or tooth extraction socket.
- Incisions through hard palate mucosa should be made lateral to bone cuts, to create keratinised mucosal flap to cover cut edge of bone.
- Grafting of cheek defects is done with split-thickness skin graft to produce a scar band and aid retention.
- Consider excision of the inferior turbinate to provide more vertical space and to prevent future trauma.
- Relining of the obturator with addition of cured silicone to provide rigid support to the cheek and engage undercuts in the resection and aid retention in the immediate post-operative period.
- Modify and further reline 1–3 weeks after surgery (general anaesthetic (GA) may be required) to maintain oronasal/oroantral seal.
- Further relines may be required until definitive impressions for the prosthesis can be performed.

Multipart Maxillary Obturators and the Use of Osseointegrated Implants

Trismus is a common complication of combined surgery and radiotherapy, and it can lead to difficulties in taking impressions as well as insertion of the final prosthesis. Separately constructed components that can be held together with magnets may help circumvent this problem. The use of implants (e.g. zygomatic implants) can help minimise the size of the prosthesis required and aid retention.

Prosthetic Management of Facial Defects

Facial defects can either be surgical or congenital. Traditional methods of reconstruction utilised a combination of skin adhesive, undercuts, and spectacle frames, which have all largely been superseded by implant retention.

Preparation of the defect edges can help maximise the aesthetic result. Smoothing of sharp corners, removal of unsupported soft tissue, and the possibility of lining of the defect wall with split-thickness skin grafts should all be considered as part of the planning process. Preservation of nasal bones is advantageous if possible, to provide vertical support for the prosthesis and spectacles. Reduction of the projection of the nasal septum helps create space within the defect for implant frameworks and reduces secretions in the area of the prosthesis.

Restoration of the Dentition after Ablative Surgery

Head and neck cancer patients often have extensive dental needs. Neglected dentition is common, and when it is paired with either segmental or bony rim resection, it results in dental rehabilitation challenges. Soft and hard free-tissue reconstructive techniques can often lead to bulky flaps obstructing the dental envelope; however, they may also provide a foundation for osseointegrated implant rehabilitation.

A decision about the patient's dentition needs to be made prior to surgery, and the patient should be given realistic expectations. Reduced tongue movement after surgery can lead to functional problems that are challenging to address with conventional dental prostheses. Osseointegrated implants help to overcome these difficulties.

Primary Dental Implant Placement

Installation of osseointegrated implants at the time of primary surgery helps provide effective prosthetic rehabilitation within a reasonable time. The majority of patients complete their dental rehabilitation and demonstrate improvements in quality-of-life scores.

Primary dental implant placement is usually in conjunction with soft-tissue reconstruction. Advances in 3D planning software are beginning to allow primary planned implants in composite flaps, but this approach is usually limited to benign rather than malignant reconstructions.

Secondary Dental Implant Placement

For many patients, decisions about dental rehabilitation are best left until they are fully recovered from the effects of cancer treatment. Functional deficits, patient motivation, and disease control all form part of the planning process. CT-based computerised techniques are used to assist planning for bony healing and osteosynthesis plates and screws. Computer software can also be used to fabricate stereo lithic drilling guides for exact placement.

Management of the peri-implant soft tissues is another important aspect of optimal oral rehabilitation. Reduction of excess tissue, refashioning of sulcal depth, and keratinised soft-tissue grafting can all be considered.

Implant Placement in Irradiated Jaws

Radiotherapy is a significant risk factor for failure of dental implants. To improve implant survival, changes in implant design, 3D planning, and improved surgical techniques have been employed.

Further Reading

1. Brown JS, Shaw RJ. Reconstruction of the maxilla and midface: introducing a new classification. *Lancet Oncol* 2010; 11(10): 1001–1008. doi:10.1016/S1470-2045(10)70113-3

2. Butterworth CJ, Rogers SN. The zygomatic implant perforated (ZIP) flap: a new technique for combined surgical reconstruction and rapid fixed dental rehabilitation following low-level maxillectomy. *Int J Implant Dent* 2017; 3(1): 37. doi:10.1186/s40729-017-0100-8

3. Freudlsperger C, Bodem JP, Engel E, Hoffmann J. Mandibular reconstruction with a prefabricated free vascularized fibula and implant-supported prosthesis based on fully three-dimensional virtual planning. *J Craniofac Surg* 2014; 25(3): 980–982. doi:10.1097/SCS.0000000000000551

71. GRAFTS AND FLAPS IN HEAD AND NECK RECONSTRUCTION

Large defects with no tissue laxity for closure require graft or flap reconstruction.

A graft is tissue with no blood supply, and its survival depends on gaining a blood supply from the recipient bed. A flap is a piece of tissue with its own blood supply.

Principles

In planning, consider three key aspects of defects: What is missing? What is required? What is available?

The reconstructive 'toolbox' concept means picking the ideal reconstruction for a defect. Reconstructions consider 'cosmetic subunits' and 'relaxed skin tension lines' (RSTLs) for incisions.

Skin Grafts

Introduction

Grafts are classified by composition (e.g. skin, fat, mucosa, cartilage, bone, or composite, such as a septal-mucosal graft). Skin grafts are of two types: split-thickness skin grafts (STSGs) or

Table 71.1 Comparison of split-thickness skin grafts (STSGs) and full-thickness skin grafts (FTSGs)

Factor	STSGs	FTSGs
Amount of dermis	Epidermis and variable dermis	Epidermis and all dermis
Primary graft contraction	Less contraction	More contraction
Secondary graft contraction	More contraction	Less contraction
Common harvest areas	Thighs, buttocks	Periauricular/supraclavicular (for colour) Upper arm/groin (for size)
Harvest technique	Dermatome or Watson knife	Blade
Size of graft	Large	Limited
Donor-site healing	Secondary intention	Primary intention
Chance of take	More likely	Less likely
Robustness	Less robust	More robust
Colour match	Abnormal pigmentation	Better colour match
Sensory recovery	Limited	Better

full-thickness skin grafts (FTSGs), and they differ in dermal content. They are compared in Table 71.1.

Skin Graft Healing

Graft survival depends on gaining a blood supply from the recipient bed. This process is 'take'. Take is affected by graft, recipient, and systemic factors. Graft factors include tissue thickness. Local factors include recipient bed vascularity (exposed bone and tendon and radiotherapy prevent take), bleeding, infection, and shearing. Potential systemic problems include smoking, poor nutrition, and diabetes.

Flaps

Principles

Flaps are indicated for extensive defects, exposed vital structures, poor vascularity, radiotherapy, and cosmesis.

Types

Flaps are named according to anatomy (e.g. blood supply or muscle for flap) or by the classification shown in Table 71.2. Common flaps discussed in this chapter are shown in bold type in the table..

Local Flaps

Consider defect, location, cosmetic units, and RSTLs when choosing flap.

Advancement Flaps

For single-pedicle flap, parallel incisions are advanced on one side of defect (e.g. Rintala flap on nose). For bipedicle flap, parallel incisions are pedicled at either end and are raised in the centre and 'bucket-handled' (e.g. tripier flap for eyelid). V-Y flaps are raised as 'V', are advanced with a deep or lateral pedicle, and are closed as 'Y' (e.g. nasolabial flap for alar defect).

Pivot Flaps—Transposition Flaps
Rhomboid Flap

Rhomboid flap is random pattern. To create rhomboid shape around defect: note RSTLs, note LMEs (lines of maximal extensibility) parallel to this—these make two sides of the rhomboid—then draw two further parallel lines meeting the LME lines to make a rhomboid shape with all sides equal length, and two angles of 60° and two angles of 120°. From the 120° angles, drop a line equal in length to one side of the rhomboid. From this, draw a line parallel to the flap. Two options are available from each line, thereby giving a choice of four flaps.

Table 71.2 '5 Cs' classification of flaps

Classification	Flap	Explanation
1. Circulation	Random pattern	No defined pedicle (e.g. some local flaps on face) Length:Breadth ratio is up to 4:1 on face (i.e. smaller than axial flaps)
	Axial	Direct—named artery in subcutaneous tissue, such as nasolabial fold flap (NLF) with facial artery
		Fasciocutaneous—vessel runs in fascia, usually from septocutaneous vessel that passes between muscles to fascia Classified by Cormack and Lamberty (1984)
		Musculocutaneous—vessel in muscle with perforators to skin Importantly, muscle has axial supply but skin has random pattern. Classified by Mathes and Nahai (1981): dominant pedicles supply whole muscle, minor pedicle only part
		Perforator flap • Direct (cutaneous) perforator • Indirect muscle/musculocutaneous perforator (e.g. deep inferior epigastric perforator (DIEP) flap) • Indirect septal/septocutaneous, such as **anterolateral thigh (ALT)** flap
2. Composition	Various	Cutaneous, fasciocutaneous, fascial, musculocutaneous, muscle, osseocutaneous, osseous
3. Contiguity	Local	Tissue transferred is adjacent to defect (e.g. NLF flap for cheek)
	Regional	Tissue transferred in same region (e.g. cervicofacial, **nasolabial**, facial artery myomucosal, submental, **forehead**, temporoparietal fascial, temporalis)
	Distant	Tissue transferred from distance (e.g. supraclavicular artery island, deltopectoral, **pectoralis major**, latissimus dorsi, trapezius)
	Free flap	Tissue transferred as transplant • Upper limb: **radial forearm**, lateral arm • Torso: subscapular (latissimus dorsi, scapular), abdomen (rectus, DIEP), deep circumflex iliac artery (DCIA) • Lower limb: ALT, **gracilis**, free fibular • Enteric: jejunum
4. Contour	Advancement	Move forward without any rotation or lateral movement (e.g. **single-pedicle or bipedicle or V-Y flap)**
	Pivot	Move at a fixed pivot point that is line of maximal tension of flap Transposition flap 'pivots' around point (e.g. **rhomboid / bilobed**) **Rotation flap** 'rotates' around pivot point
5. Conditioning	'Delay'	Flap undergoes prior 'delay' procedure to improve vascularity

Bilobed Flap

A bilobed flap is a random pattern flap that consists of two transposition flaps. Pivot point is 1 radius away, with axis via horizontal line through the defect. First flap is slightly smaller and adjacent to the defect, with axis 45° from pivot point of first axis. Next flap is half the size of the first and adjacent to it, with axis 90° from first axis. The first flap transposes to the primary defect, the second flap to the secondary defect, and the tertiary defect is closed directly.

Pivot Flaps—Rotation Flaps
The primary defect is 'triangulated', and the flap is designed as a semicircle with the radius 3 times the arc length of the triangulated defect and the circumference 8 times the arc length of the defect. The pivot point is the distal part of the flap. Upon movement, a 'back-cut' may be needed for closure, which moves the pivot point toward the defect to reduce tension but decreases flap vascularity.

Locoregional Flaps
Nasolabial Flaps (NLF)
Background: First documented by Indian Sushruta in 600 BC. Transposition flap.

Anatomy: Axial flap based on facial and angular artery; therefore, can be proximally or distally based. Width is 1–2 cm.

Use: Proximally/superiorly based for nasal side wall and alar defects. Distally/inferiorly based for alar/perialar defect, upper lip and commissure, and anterior oral cavity.

Advantages: Good colour match, inconspicuous donor scars in aesthetic junctions.

Disadvantages: Blunt alar groove unless planned correctly, can be bulky, and, if short, pulls up alar.

Technique:

- Plan: Base is determined by defect location. Plan length in reverse from pivot point. Template defect on distal flap to check width and check that donor closes.
- Place incisions along aesthetic junction (i.e. nose/cheek junction, alar groove, nasolabial fold).
- Procedure: Raise subcutaneous flap from tip to base. Transpose and inset and close donor. For intraoral defects, a tunnel is placed traversing the facial muscles and buccinators.

Forehead Flaps (Paramedian)
Background: Original description by Indian Sushruta in 600 BC. Workhorse for nasal defect.

Anatomy: Forehead is divided into 3 zones—paramedian, median, and lateral. Paramedian is based on supratrochlear +/- supraorbital vessels.

Use: For external/internal nasal defects, eyelids/medial canthus, and midface reconstruction.

Advantages: Good colour match, moderate size and thickness, potentially hairless, and donor has good aesthetic result even with secondary intention healing.

Disadvantages: Requires a minimum of two stages. Need correct design or nose contracts. Arc of rotation and short forehead limit reach or are a problem if large flaps are needed. One-stage solution includes dropping pivot point, accepting alopecia/hairy reconstruction, or use of specific design (e.g. Millard flap). Two-stage options are first-stage 'delaying' flap or tissue expansion.

Technique

- Plan: Assess height of forehead. Find origin of supratrochlear artery (1 cm medial to supraorbital foramen above midpoint of pupil). Line drawn vertically up is axis of flap. Plan pedicle length in reverse from pivot point and template defect on distal flap. Keep 'extra' 15% in pedicle length from pivot.
- Procedure: Incise around the flap and pedicle, raise flap distal to proximal in plane under frontalis, and 1 cm superior to the supraorbital ridge, go subperiosteal to protect the vessel. Rotate and inset flap into defect. Graft underside of pedicle for haemostasis. If unable to close donor, then dress. Flap is thinned +/− pedicle division at 3 weeks.

Distant Flaps
Pectoralis Major Flaps
Background: Previously workhorse, now used for salvage cases. Muscle or musculocutaneous (rarely osteomyocutaneous).

Anatomy: Main supply from pectoral branch (to sternocostal head) and deltoid branch (to clavicular head) of the thoraco-acromial artery. Pectoral branch emerges near junction of middle and outer thirds of clavicle. Also supply from internal mammary perforators and lateral thoracic artery.

Use: Pedicled proximally for salvage neck cases (e.g. resurfacing), pharynx patches, oral reconstruction (e.g. mandible +/− bone), and cutaneous defects up to the level of the zygomatic arch.

Advantages: Large area of muscle with good donor closure, reliable blood supply with straightforward harvest, potentially two-team.

Disadvantages: Muscle is bulky. Large skin paddles require split skin graft (SSG) violating breast in females. Osteomyocutaneous flap using fifth rib has unreliable bone.

Technique for myocutaneous flap

- Patient position: Supine with arm abducted on arm table
- Plan:
  - Pre-operatively check for pectoralis major (absence of sternocostal head indicates Poland's syndrome).
  - Pedicle: Extend a line from acromium to xiphoid and a line from the sternal notch, meeting first perpendicularly; the point where the lines meet is where the vascular pedicle runs towards the xiphisternum. Next, mark two thirds along the clavicle from the sternal notch to the coracoid; the pedicle runs curved from here to the bisection point.
  - Skin: Plan length in reverse from pivot point. Template defect as paddle on distal pedicle. Skin paddle is vertical (lateral sternal edge, medially nipple, sixth rib) or oblique or horizontal in fold in women. Skin paddle distal to pectoralis is random pattern and needs rectus sheath (not reliable).
  - Muscle: Access incision from proximal paddle to axilla or along fold (latter gives less access).
  - 'Defensive approach': Mark deltopectoral flap. The boundaries are clavicle, deltopectoral groove, fourth rib, sternum, and intercostal spaces for perforators. Area not harvested is 'lifeboat'.

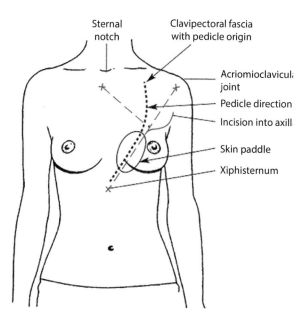

Figure 71.1 Myocutaneous pectoralis major flap markings.

Table 71.3 Free flap aims and options for various defects

Defect	Aims	Options
Cutaneous	Cover with correct thickness and colour	Small/Moderate: Radial forearm flap (RFF) Moderate/Large: ALT, latissimus dorsi, scapula, DIEP
Oral cavity	Volume, mobility, palatal closure	Small/Moderate: RFF Moderate/Large: ALT, scapula, DIEP
Pharynx (tubed)	Mucosalised conduit, motility for swallowing, speech with tracheoesophageal puncture (TEP)	F/C: ALT (adequate speech but risk of stricture) Enteric: Jejunum (good swallow but poor speech)
Mandible	Length, height (osseointegration), composite tissue	Workhorse: Fibula, DCIA Uncommon: Scapula/radius
Other	Functional transfer (e.g. for facial palsy)	Gracilis, ALT

- Procedure: Incise skin paddle to muscle, raise adjacent anterior fasciocutaneous flaps to expose anterior muscle, release inferior border of muscle, raise posterior flap in subpectoral plane, leaving pectoralis minor behind, ligate lateral thoracic artery branch laterally and internal mammary perforators medially, visualise pedicle under clavicular head, create window, and pass flap into neck.

Free Flaps
General Considerations

a. Flap choice (for options, see Table 71.3)
Recipient factors include defect size, location, tissue composition, bed (e.g. radiation), and available vessels. Donor factors include best size and composition match, pedicle length and diameter, donor morbidity, and ability to two-team. Patient factors include age and comorbidity.

b. Recipient vessels
Radical neck dissections sacrifice the jugular vein, but selective dissection gives more venous options. External carotid branches are used (e.g. superior thyroid for pharyngeal reconstruction, facial for variety in skin and oral reconstruction, and superficial temporal vessels for scalp defects). Transverse cervical vessels are a secondary option if they were preserved in dissection.

c. Postoperative care
First 72 hours to 1 week are critical. Monitor for flap (artery and vein), theatre (anesthetic, neuropraxia) and systemic (clot, chest, cardiac) complications. Suboptimal systemic factors (e.g. blood pressure) or local factors (e.g. compression, haematoma) affect perfusion. Flap monitoring is done clinically (e.g. colour, capillary refill, turgor, temperature), by hand-held or implantable Doppler.

Radial Forearm Flap (RFF)
Background: Fasciocutaneous workhorse flap (rarely osseocutaneous).

Anatomy: Based on radial artery (RA), with venous drainage by venae comitantes (VCs) or cephalic vein. Skin perforators extend vertically from RA through septum to skin. Lateral antebrachial cutaneous nerve provides sensation. Palmaris longus (PL) tendon (and bone) can be ~10 cm.

Use: Cutaneous defects. Mucosal defects (e.g. floor of mouth/tongue, buccal mucosa, palate, and oropharynx/tongue base). Composite defects (e.g. lip with PL sling).

Advantages: Consistent anatomy and easy raise. Long pedicle up to 15 cm. Large vessels 3–5 mm. Moderate skin island. Thin and pliable. Option for a sensate flap (e.g. for oral cavity). Good colour match in darker skin. Allows two-team approach.

Disadvantages: Sacrifice of major vessel (RA). Minimal volume if large dead space. May be hairy. Donor requires unsightly graft (ipsilateral forearm graft or hatchett flap improves this).

Technique

- Patient position: Supine, tourniquet, hand table.
- Plan: Allen's test, outline superficial veins (e.g. cephalic), plan flap centering on RA.
- Procedure: Start ulnar, go subfascial and over PL and flexor carpi radialis (FCR) to artery. Radial incision is next, protecting superficial radial nerve and move over brachioradialis to artery, keeping cephalic vein within flap if needed and keep paratenon on tendons. Distal incision controlling the distal end of the artery/vein. Raise pedicle, keeping it with septum and skin to antecubital fossa.

Anterolateral Thigh Flap (ALT)

Background: Fasciocutaneous workhorse flap.

Anatomy: Profunda femoris gives lateral circumflex femoral artery, which has two branches. Descending branch gives ALT perforators, ascending branch to tensa fascia lata (TFL) is used as flap 'lifeboat'. Descending branch in mid-lateral thigh gives skin perforators, which are either septocutaneous (20%) or musculocutaneous (in vastus lateralis; 80%). Nerve supply is lateral femoral cutaneous nerve.

Use: Cutaneous defects anywhere, oral cavity, skull base, and tubed for total pharynx reconstruction.

Advantages: Large skin island (38 cm × 15 cm) with the donor closed primarily. Thin and pliable but can incorporate the vastus lateralis for bulk. Long pedicle (15 cm) with good diameter (1–3 mm). Allows two-team approach.

Disadvantages: Perforator anatomy is variable, so dissection is challenging. Perforator susceptible to compression. In thicker thigh, flap is bulky and donor needs SSG. Colour match poor. Hair-bearing skin transferred.

Technique

- Patient position: Supine with sandbag under ipsilateral hip.
- Plan: Draw line between iliac spine and superolateral patella. At midpoint, draw circle of radius 3 cm. Doppler perforators (one is sufficient, but two are ideal for big flaps).
- Procedure: Longitudinal incision 2 cm medial to line. Take 1 cm cuff of fascia medially. Move subfascially laterally until perforators are identified. Release perforators down to pedicle. Follow descending branch proximal. Template defect over perforator. Cut posterior skin incision subfascially and isolate perforator.

Gracilis Flap

Background: Muscle flap usually for facial reanimation.

Anatomy: Profunda femoris gives the medial circumflex femoral artery, which enters deep aspect of gracilis 8–10 cm below the pubic tubercle. Flap can be innervated by the obturator nerve.

Use: Good for functional transfer (i.e. facial reanimation).

Advantage: Constant anatomy.

Disadvantages: Skin paddle not reliable, muscle is a little bulky, and pedicle is moderate length (6 cm) and diameter (1–2 mm).

Technique

- Patient position: Supine with hip abducted and externally rotated.
- Plan: Line from insertion of adductor longus on pubic ramus to medial femoral condyle.
- Procedure: Longitudinal incision 3 cm behind line. Incise to fascia. Raise fascia posteriorly and find pedicle on deep aspect of gracilis. Divide other distal perforators. Raise anterior fascia, protecting the pedicle. Chase pedicle between adductor longus and brevis. Cut nerve. Divide tendinous insertions.

Conclusions

Grafts and local flaps are beneficial for small defects. Locoregional or distant flaps are important in salvage cases (e.g. free flap failed or vessel depleted neck) but disadvantages include lack of size or reach and being bulky. Free tissue transfer improves functional outcomes and can transfer large volumes of composite tissue in a single stage procedure. The disadvantages include complex and lengthy operations with chance of failure and systemic post-operative complications.

KEY POINTS

- Reconstructive principles include the 'toolbox', 'subunits', and RSTLs.
- There are key differences between and within grafts and flaps.
- Specific areas and defects require specific flaps.

Further Reading

1. Gabrysz-Forget F, Tabet P, Rahal A, Bissada E, Christopoulos A, Ayad T. Free versus pedicled flaps for reconstruction of head and neck cancer defects: a systematic review. *J Otolaryngol Head Neck Surg* 2019; 48(1): 13.

2. Huang TC, Cheng HT. ALT vs. jejunum: have we found the ideal flap for circumferential pharyngoesophageal reconstruction? A meta-analysis of comparative studies. *J Plast Reconstr Aesthet Surg* 2019; 72(2): 335–354.

3. Largo RD, Garvey PB. Updates in head and neck reconstruction. *Plast Reconstr Surg* 2018; 141(2): 271e–285e.

72. RADIOTHERAPY AND CHEMOTHERAPY

RADIOTHERAPY

Introduction

Radiotherapy, either as a single modality or combined with synchronous chemotherapy, is capable of high rates of tumour control. Head and neck radiotherapy uses photons produced in a linear accelerator. The photon beam produced can be shaped using collimators that are able to move, enabling delivery of intensity-modulated radiotherapy (IMRT), and the gantry of the linear accelerator can move around the patient's head to deliver different beam angles (dynamic IMRT). Photons cause tissue ionization and free-radical formation, which causes cell death through single- or double-strand breaks in DNA. The differential response between tumour and normal tissues in their ability to repair DNA breaks is utilised by oncologists to maximise the therapeutic ratio.

Radiotherapy Process

Preparation

- Multidisciplinary meeting (MDT)
- Patient information, education, discussion
- Consent
- Consideration of prophylactic versus reactive feeding tube placement
- Dental assessment

Immobilisation

Use a patient-specific mask to immobilise the head and shoulders. This is subject to regular departmental audit, and the data are used to inform the planning target volume (PTV) margins.

Imaging

Computed tomography (CT) with IV contrast: 2-mm slice, in mask. Fused with prior diagnostic images.

Target Volume

The oncologist will define the gross tumour volume (GTV) based on MRI and CT. A small margin is added (5–10 mm) to allow for microscopic spread/limitations of fusion/imaging employed; this forms the high-dose clinical target volume (CTV) that will receive treatment. Adjacent areas and nodal regions felt to be at high risk of harbouring microscopic disease may be included in a prophylactic CTV to receive a smaller dose. PTV margins (normally 3–5 mm) are added to both CTVs.

Organs at Risk

Organs at risk are anatomical structures with critical functional properties located in the vicinity of the target volume (i.e. spinal cord, brainstem, contralateral parotid, brain, and mandible). Other regions which need contouring in an attempt to reduce toxicity include oral mucosal volume, laryngeal framework, and swallowing muscles.

Peer Review of Contours

The CTV defined by the oncologist should be peer reviewed, particularly in complex cases.

Treatment Planning

The departmental dosimetrists produce an IMRT plan, which is reviewed by the oncologist and subjected to quality assurance.

Delivery

The treatment planned is delivered over the defined number of weeks. At each treatment session, a cone-beam CT or megavoltage image is taken to check positioning and to assess any changes in contour due to weight loss or tumour shrinkage, which may affect dosimetry.

Supportive Care

Supportive care is reviewed weekly during treatment by various members of the MDT.

Altered Fractionation

Although 70 Gy in 35 fractions (overall treatment time, 46 days/7 weeks) is one of the most common radiotherapy dosing schedules, prior to chemoradiation's being accepted as standard treatment, several different fractionation schemes had been studied. Acceleration is a reduction in the overall treatment time below the standard 46 days. Hyperfractionation is use of <2 Gy per fraction, and hypofractionation is use of >2 Gy per fraction. Altered fractionation may be required if radiotherapy appointments are missed, for example. Dose escalation is an increase in the total physical dose above 70 Gy.

A meta-analysis of altered fractionation grouped trials found an overall survival benefit only in the hyperfractionated dose-escalated group. This survival benefit is approximately the same as that seen with the addition of synchronous chemotherapy to standard radiotherapy.

Dose-Escalated Radiotherapy or Synchronous Chemoradiotherapy

The addition of synchronous chemotherapy to standard radiotherapy has been associated with an 8% survival advantage, which is the same benefit that can be achieved with dose-escalated radiotherapy. Studies show, however, that synchronous chemotherapy, rather than dose-escalated hyperfractionated radiotherapy, is more beneficial when local control and the risk of grade 3 mucositis are considered.

CHEMOTHERAPY

Introduction

Chemotherapy alone cannot cure head and neck cancer. It is used in conjunction with surgery and radiotherapy to improve outcomes, such as better local control, organ preservation with continued organ function, and decreased incidence of subclinical micro-metastatic spread. Chemotherapy is given for its direct tumouricidal effect at both the local primary and distant metastatic sites. If given with radiotherapy, it can have a radiosensitising effect, making cancer cells more susceptible to radiotherapy and increasing the cancer cell kill.

Induction (Neoadjuvant) Chemotherapy

Chemotherapy can be used as induction or neoadjuvant treatment before the primary treatment (more often surgery than radiotherapy) in order to shrink an advanced primary tumour or to reduce and render fixed cervical nodes mobile, potentially enabling technically easier surgery. If induction chemotherapy can improve local control, then there is a greater chance of functional organ preservation, and the initial response to chemotherapy can give prognostic information.

However, because most patients who have induction chemotherapy go on to have concurrent chemotherapy as well, there is a risk that the subsequent definitive radiotherapy will not be completed or will require breaks in delivery because of the morbidity caused by induction chemotherapy, and this could result in poorer outcomes.

Overall, evidence has failed to show a survival benefit with induction chemotherapy compared to primary surgery or radiotherapy alone, and there is debate about the benefit of induction chemotherapy followed by concurrent chemoradiotherapy over concurrent chemoradiotherapy alone.

Concurrent or Concomitant Chemotherapy

Concomitant chemotherapy is chemotherapy given at the same time as radiotherapy. It can be administered after neoadjuvant treatment, as a stand-alone treatment, or as an adjuvant after primary treatment. It is given for its direct cell-killing effect and for sensitising cancer cells to the effects of radiotherapy. The most commonly use concurrent chemotherapy regimens use cisplatin (100 mg/m^2 at days 1, 22, and 43 of radiotherapy), either alone or with 5-FU (1 g per day on days 1 to 4).

Increased toxicity produced by adding platinum chemotherapy to radiotherapy can be considerable, with more marked mucositis, dysphagia, nephrotoxicity, ototoxicity, myelodysplasia, and neutropenia. Chemotherapy toxicity can also interfere detrimentally with radiotherapy delivery, causing breaks in treatment, which are associated with poorer outcomes.

Evidence shows there is a survival benefit of chemotherapy when it is added to radiotherapy alone, giving a 6.5% decrease in mortality at 5 years. In absolute terms, however, this benefit was not seen in patients over 70 years old, but patients over age 70 formed a very small number of the total patients reviewed.

If cisplatin is contraindicated because of renal function status/neuropathy/tinnitus/deafness, carboplatin can be considered, because it causes less nephrotoxicity, ototoxicity, and peripheral neuropathy, but it is more myelosuppressive. Also, carboplatin is not thought to be as tumouricidal as cisplatin; for this reason, the epidermal growth factor receptor (EGFR) inhibitor cetuximab can be used instead when cisplatin is contraindicated.

Adjuvant Chemotherapy

Adjuvant chemotherapy is given after the principal treatment. When primary surgery has been the definitive treatment, and when adjuvant chemotherapy is given with adjuvant radiation, it has been shown to improve local control and to increase survival. This benefit is seen in patients who have a higher risk of recurrence, as indicated by positive surgical margins, nodal involvement (especially in multiple nodes), or extracapsular spread.

Targeted Biological Agents

Targeted therapies in head and neck cancer, such as the monoclonal antibody cetuximab, were developed with the recognition that EGFR overexpression occurs in most head and neck cancers (in up to 90% in some studies) and is associated with a poorer prognosis.

Initial hopes were that cetuximab would have less toxicity than standard chemotherapy and therefore could be given to older patients and those with poorer performance status. Although cetuximab has been shown to cause less nephrotoxicity, ototoxicity, and peripheral neuropathy, it causes more intense grade 3 and grade 4 radiation dermatitis.

In patients with HPV-positive oropharyngeal tumours, the De-ESCALaTE HPV trial compared the standard regimen of concurrent radiotherapy with cisplatin to the regimen of cetuximab and radiotherapy. The cetuximab group showed no benefit in terms of reduced toxicity, but instead showed significant detriment in terms of tumour control (higher 2-year recurrence and lower 2-year overall survival); therefore, cisplatin is recommended as the standard of care.

Chemotherapy for Recurrent or Metastatic Head and Neck Cancer

Chemotherapy or targeted biological agents may be indicated for patients with recurrent and/or metastatic disease, although patients with metastatic disease have a median survival of approximately 6–12 months. Often, the most important considerations are the fitness and performance status of the patient and whether they could tolerate the proposed chemotherapy, as well as how much it would reduce their pre-treatment quality of life, for whatever limited survival time they have.

Locoregional Failure

Locoregional failure has been reported in up to 50% of patients with head and neck cancer. In these patients, if salvage surgery or retreatment with radiotherapy/chemoradiotherapy is being considered, it is important to assess for the presence of distant metastatic disease and to exclude second primary tumours. Metastatic disease is not an absolute contraindication to salvage treatments, as locoregional failure and metastatic disease can receive two separate management plans. If locoregional control can be achieved relatively easily by a salvage procedure, the presence of metastatic disease (especially small-volume metastatic disease) should not necessarily stop treatment to the locoregional site.

Distant Metastases

Chemotherapy is often indicated as part of a best supportive care package for distant metastases, but it has not been shown to significantly extend survival. The presence or absence of symptoms will influence when patients receive chemotherapy, and chemotherapy may be appropriate when the patient still has a suitable performance status to receive and benefit from it, with the trade-off being an improved symptom profile for the inevitable morbidity caused by the chemotherapy. A shared decision-making approach is required to allow a fully informed decision.

The most common regimens use cisplatin or carboplatin with 5-FU, and they give an expected response rate of approximately 40%. Carboplatin is used more often, because although it is deemed slightly less effective than cisplatin, it is less toxic and is considered to be more appropriate in the palliative setting. Elderly patients appear to respond to platinum-based chemotherapy in the metastatic setting, but they experience more toxicity. Cetuximab with cisplatin and 5-FU can increase both response rate and improve short-term survival slightly. Cetuximab as a single agent has a low response rate of approximately 10–15%.

KEY POINTS

- Concurrent chemoradiotherapy is the standard of care for treatment of locally advanced head and neck cancer, with a confirmed absolute survival benefit of 6.5% at 5 years.
- Targeted biological agents, such as cetuximab, have roles to play in both advanced head and neck cancer and recurrent or metastatic disease, but those roles are still being established.
- Elderly patients benefit least in terms of survival with the use of concurrent chemotherapy.

Further Reading

1. Nutting CM, Morden JP, Harrington KJ, et al. PARSPORT trial management group. Parotid-sparing intensity modulated versus conventional radiotherapy in head and neck cancer (PARSPORT): a phase 3 multicentre randomised controlled trial. *Lancet Oncol* 2011; 12(2): 127–136.

2. Pignon JP, le Maître A, Maillard E. MACH-NC Collaborative Group. Meta-analysis of chemotherapy in head and neck cancer (MACH-NC): an update on 93 randomised trials and 17,346 patients. *Radiother Oncol* 2009; 92(1): 4–14.

3. Mehanna H, Robinson M, Hartley A, Kong A, Foran B, Fulton-Lieuw T, et al. Radiotherapy plus cisplatin or cetuximab in low-risk human papillomavirus-positive oropharyngeal cancer (De-ESCALaTE HPV): an open-label randomised controlled phase 3 trial. *Lancet Oncol* 2019; 393(10611): 51–60.

73. IMMUNOTHERAPY IN HEAD AND NECK CANCERS

Introduction

Cancer is a genetic disease that develops when DNA is damaged or wrongly decoded. This alters gene expression and impairs normal protein function.

Genetic changes leading to cancer have two general effects:

- Overactivity of genes that stimulate cell growth, survival, and spread
- Underactivity of genes that repress these processes

Thus, the fundamentals of cancer are derangements of the interplay between growth and repression.

Oncogenes and Tumour Suppressor Genes (TSG)

Two classes of genes, oncogenes and TSG, are fundamental to understanding cancer biology.

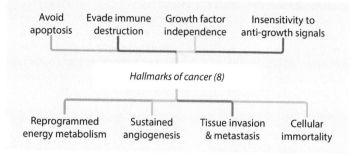

Figure 73.1   Hallmarks of cancer.

Oncogenes are mutated versions of normal cellular genes (called proto-oncogenes) encoding proteins that control cell proliferation, survival, and spread. Abnormalities in proto-oncogenes cause uncontrolled cell division, enhanced cell survival, and dissemination. A single mutated copy can promote cancer. Oncogenes are activated in three ways to cause cancer: mutation, amplification, and translocation.

TSGs are genes whose normal function inhibits cell proliferation and survival. The function of both copies of a TSG must be lost in order to promote cancer (so-called phenotypic recessiveness). Mutated TSGs are responsible for the majority of inherited cancer syndromes, although such syndromes are not a significant cause of head and neck cancers.

Hallmarks of Cancer
Eight key transformations that drive malignant processes, termed the 'hallmarks of cancer', are summarised in Figure 73.1. These properties underpin immunotherapy, which exploits fundamental biological differences between normal and malignant cells.

Biological Targeting
Improvements in our knowledge of cancer biology have enabled development of novel targeted therapies against cancers. This chapter focuses on three specific themes that appear most promising:

- Targeting growth factor independence
- Radiosensitisers
- Enhancing antitumor immune responses

Targeting Growth Factor Independence
Squamous cell carcinoma of the head and neck (HNSCC) frequently displays upregulated epidermal growth factor receptor (EGFR) signalling. EGFR (a.k.a. HER1) is a member of the c-erb family of transmembrane type I receptor tyrosine kinases, which has four members (HER1–4). Binding to EGFR leads to a cascade of intracellular second messengers that subsequently alter gene expression, which means that a protein binding on the cell surface influences cell behaviour.

Growth factor independence can lead to sustained signalling in pathways that control essential functions: growth, apoptosis, angiogenesis, invasion, and DNA damage repair. Monoclonal antibodies (MAbs) and tyrosine kinase inhibitors (TKI) block these pathways by acting on different aspects of the receptor signalling pathway.

Curative Anti-EGFR MAbs
Several EGFR-targeted MAbs have been tested in clinical practice. Clinical trials confirmed the efficacy of cetuximab in combination with chemotherapy or radiotherapy. Subsequently,

Table 73.1   Clinical trials of anti-EGFR MAbs

Trial	Study info	Summary
RTOG-0522 (Ang 2014)	Locally advanced disease; radiation plus cisplatin ± concurrent cetuximab	No difference in LRC or OS
CONCERT-1 (Mesia 2015)	Untreated stage III–IVb disease; chemoradiotherapy (CRT) ± concurrent panitumumab	No benefit for LRC or OS Panitumumab had greater toxicity
CONCERT-2 (Giralt 2015)	Unresected stage III–IVb disease; platinum-based CRT vs. radiation plus panitumumab only	No benefit for LRC or OS Panitumumab had greater toxicity
De-ESCALaTE HPV (Mehanna 2019)	HPV+ oropharyngeal cancers; patients randomised to radiotherapy with either cisplatin or Cetuximab	Cetuximab was deleterious for both OS and recurrence rate

research in locally/regionally advanced HNSCC demonstrated that patients receiving radiotherapy and cetuximab have prolonged locoregional control (LRC) and overall survival (OS) when compared to patients receiving radiotherapy alone (Bonner 2006). Cetuximab was associated with a higher incidence of rash and infusion reactions, but supplementary analysis demonstrated that skin reactions represented a biomarker of favourable outcome. Further trials (Table 73.1) have not shown improved outcomes. The data indicate that, in the curative setting, anti-EGFR MAb therapy should be restricted to the use of cetuximab plus radiotherapy.

Palliative Anti-EGFR MAbs

The EXTREME study treated patients with untreated recurrent/metastatic HNSCC with cisplatin or carboplatin plus 5-fluorouracil. Patients were then randomised to receive cetuximab; the cetuximab arm had prolonged median OS and median progression-free survival, as well as improved response.

Therefore, it appears that triple-agent therapy with platin/5-fluorouracil and cetuximab may be beneficial for patients as first-line therapy for relapsed/metastatic disease. In practice, this regimen is often not used due to concerns about additional toxicity from adding cetuximab to standard treatment.

Curative TKI

Currently, there is no clear indication for the use of TKI in the treatment of newly diagnosed HNSCC. Trials that substantiate this are shown in Table 73.2.

Table 73.2   Clinical trials of tyrosine kinase inhibitors (TKI)

Treatment/ Trial	Study info	Summary
Gefitinib (Saarilahti 2010) (Cohen 2010)	CRT ± concurrent gefitinib Chemotherapy ± concurrent gefitinib	Can be safely combined with CRT (either standard cisplatin-based CRT or unconventional split-course schedule of 5-fluorouracil and hydroxyurea)
Erlotinib (Martins 2013)	CRT ± concurrent erlotinib	No improvement in outcomes and increased toxicity
Lapatinib (Harrington 2015)	CRT ± concurrent lapatinib and maintenance in high-risk surgically treated HNSCC (stage III–IVa)	Lapatinib did not offer any efficacy/ safety benefit when compared to placebo
Afatinib (Burtness 2019)	Radiotherapy with either cisplatin or carboplatin ± concurrent afatinib	Addition of afatinib did not improve disease-free survival and increased toxicity

Table 73.3   Palliative use of tyrosine kinase inhibitors (TKI)

Treatment/Trial	Study info	Summary
Geftinib (Stewart 2009)	Recurrent or metastatic HNSCC treated with gefitinib (250 or 500 mg/day) or single-agent methotrexate	The data do not support the use of gefitinib as a palliative therapy in relapsed/metastatic HNSCC
Afatinib in LUX-Head and Neck-1 trial (Machiels 2015)	Methotrexate or afatininb for relapsed/metastatic HNSCC	Afatinib improved progression-free survival, but it did not improve OS. It also caused deterioration of global health status, pain, and dysphagia

Palliative TKI

Currently, there is no evidence that supports the use of TKI in the palliative setting (see Table 73.3), but there is continued research that may change this in the future.

Radiosensitisers

Radiotherapy is an extremely effective therapy for HNSCC. In tandem with the development of advanced radiotherapy techniques, a parallel track of studies has evaluated combinations of radiotherapy with cytotoxic drugs, in an attempt to enhance radiation-induced (RI) cyto-toxicity. Large meta-analyses demonstrate radiotherapy delivered with concomitant platin monotherapy as the standard-of-care for locally advanced HNSCC (Pignon 2009).

Cell Cycle

Cell division is an essential component of development, growth, and tissue repair. It is tightly regulated, and failure to copy the cellular DNA faithfully confers a risk of inheriting mutations.

Cells can also slow down or stop in the cell cycle when they experience DNA damage. There are four main cell cycle phases (Figure 73.2). Potentially the most lethal DNA lesions induced by ionizing radiation are double-strand breaks (DSB). Therapies that can prevent the repair of DSB are potentially profoundly radiosensitising.

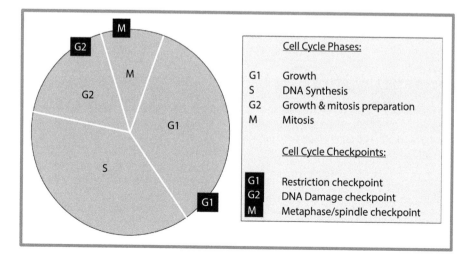

Figure 73.2   The cell cycle.

apoptosis occurs when cells attempt to divide with damaged DNA. The cell is unable to complete mitosis and dies, in a process known as mitotic catastrophe. The majority of HNSCC lack normal p53-mediated G1/S checkpoint and are dependent on S and G2/M arrest to allow repair of DNA damage after irradiation. Hence, G2/M checkpoint control is a particularly appealing target for cancer-specific radiosensitisation.

Radiosensitiser Drugs

The protein kinase ATR is involved in identifying DNA damage. ATR inhibitors can radiosensitise cancer cells through disruption of intra-S and G2 checkpoints. Inhibitors of ATR have been tested in pre-clinical studies. Thus far, there have been no publications on ATR inhibitors in cancer patients, but clinical trials have begun.

Chk1 is directly downstream of ATR in the DNA damage response signalling cascade. Chk1 inhibitors that have been tested include UCN-01, AZD7762, and SAR-020106, but all of them had severe toxicities and lacked clinical efficacy.

The Wee1 kinase regulates entry into mitosis, by negatively controlling CDK1 and Chk2. AZD-1775 is an agent shown to potentiate DNA-damaging agents in vitro and in vivo, and it is currently undergoing phase I trials.

Enhancing Antitumor Immune Responses

Recently, after decades of negative studies, immunotherapy has emerged as a major new modality for cancer treatment. Identification of immune checkpoints integral to normal immune responses has been pivotal in this progress. Checkpoints normally inhibit T-cells, preventing them from becoming chronically or aberrantly activated. This system functions as a negative regulator or 'the brakes' on the immune response. Many cancers subvert these inhibitory pathways in order to evade immunosurveillance and thereby escape immune detection and attack.

Proteins expressed on activated T-cells allow cancers to evade anti-tumour immunity by interfering with activation or effector phases of immune responses. CTLA4 is an important control mechanism that influences the immune response's activation phase, and it can switch off T-cells. MAbs that target CTLA4 are able to block this interaction and enhance T-cell activation against tumour cells. T-cells can be prevented from engaging with and/or killing a tumour cell if the tumour cell expresses PD-L1 on its surface. This negative interaction between T-cell and tumour cell can be interrupted by administration of specific MAbs that block PD-1.

Clinical Experience with Checkpoint Inhibitors

MAbs have demonstrated significant activity in a range of tumour types. It appears that the likelihood of a patient's benefiting from immunotherapy may correlate with the mutational burden and, hence, the neoantigenic load carried by their tumour. Head and neck cancers, especially human papillomavirus negative (HPV–) tumours, are also associated with a significant number of mutations.

There have been initial reports of single-agent activity in patients with relapsed/metastatic disease. For example, trials have used pembrolizumab (an anti-PD1 MAb). In the KEYN0TE-012 trial, patients with PD-L1-positive tumours were divided into HPV+ and HPV– cohorts and were treated with pembrolizumab. Overall, 26 of 51 patients had a reduction in tumour burden. There are several ongoing randomised phase II/III clinical trials with anti-PD1 agents (pembrolizumab, nivolumab, and durvalumab) in patients with relapsed/metastatic disease, and the results are likely to be reported in the next few years. The side effects of immune checkpoint inhibitors are autoimmune adverse reactions, such as skin rash, colitis, hepatitis, and endocrinopathy. In all instances, these treatments require specialist management because they can evolve into serious, even life-threatening, conditions. There is evolving work (both pre-clinical and clinical data) to demonstrate that immune checkpoint inhibition may enhance the effect of, and lead to systemic activity of, a local therapy, such as radiation. These observations, combined with the excitement over the efficacy of single-agent immune checkpoint inhibition, have led to a number of clinical studies that are combining immune checkpoint inhibitors with ionizing radiation.

KEY POINTS

- Understanding of fundamental biological processes involved in cancer cell formation has resulted in drug strategies to treat HNSCC.
- EGFR inhibitors, TKI, drugs which arrest the cell cycle, and radiosensitisers have been used in various treatment regimens.
- Knowledge about use of checkpoint inhibitors for treatment is evolving.

Further Reading

Bauml JM, Aggarwal C, Cohen B. Immunotherapy for head and neck cancer: where are we now and where are we going? *Ann Transl Med* 2019; 7(Suppl 3): S75.

Paleri V, Rollands NJ. (Eds.) Head and Neck Cancer United Kingdom National Multidisciplinary Guidelines, 5th edition, 2016.

Sim F, Leidner R, Bell RB. Immunotherapy for head and neck cancer. *Haematology/Oncology Clin* 2019; 36(2): 301–321.

---

74. QUALITY OF LIFE, SURVIVORSHIP, AND OUTCOMES IN HEAD AND NECK CANCER

Introduction

There are two million people living with or beyond cancer in the United Kingdom. It is a cause for celebration that more people than ever are surviving after diagnosis, but we know the impact of cancer does not suddenly stop when treatment is over. Survivorship focuses on the health and life of a person with cancer from the completion of treatment until the end of life. It covers the physical, psychosocial, and economic issues of cancer, beyond the diagnosis and treatment phases (Figure 74.1). It is recognised that family members, friends, and caregivers are also part of the survivorship experience.

Measurement of Treatment Outcomes

Survival Outcomes

Undoubtedly, survival is the cornerstone of outcome assessment for head and neck cancer (HNC). Analysis of survival has the advantages that there can only be two categories, alive or dead, and that this outcome cannot be misrepresented.

A 'time-to-event' analysis, such as the Kaplan-Meier survival curve, is commonly used, where a log-rank test is used to compare two or more survival curves. This is only appropriate where relative mortality does not change over time (proportional hazards assumption). Another limitation is that patients may not experience the outcome within the analysis time frame, so it can be insensitive for certain diseases. Other parameters besides overall survival are disease-free survival, progression-free survival, disease-specific survival rate, and median survival; therefore, it is important to clarify which parameter is being reported.

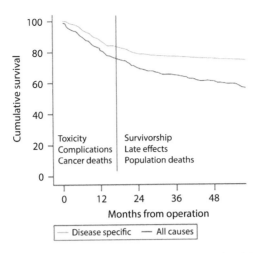

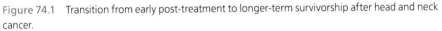

Figure 74.1   Transition from early post-treatment to longer-term survivorship after head and neck cancer.

Functional Outcomes

Currently, there are no outcome reporting standards for clinical practice or trials in HNC. The World Health Organisation (WHO) recommended as early as 1981 that, as a minimum standard, oncology clinical trials should measure tumour and metastasis response, duration of response, and adverse effects. Treatment for HNC affects speech, social interaction, swallowing, and breathing, with speech and eating having the most impact on well-being in a disease-specific quality of life (QoL) survey.

Measures of Voice, Speech, and Swallow Outcome

Voice and speech represent different ends of the same spectrum. The larynx serves as the source of phonation, thereby producing voice, while the vocal tract (oral cavity, oropharynx, nasopharynx, nasal cavity, and paranasal sinuses) act as a filter, altering the voice and shaping speech. Speech is the final outcome of voiced sound. Cancers or treatments involving the vocal tract sites will affect speech and not the voice. Voice is predominantly affected by laryngeal cancers or treatments affecting the larynx, directly or indirectly. Numerous tools are used for the evaluation of voice and speech (Box 74.1), but there is no widely accepted outcome measure.

Dysphagia assessments require a multimodality approach (Box 74.1b) and fall broadly into two categories: those that assess the severity of the swallowing disorder and those that try to establish its cause.

Adult Comorbidity Evaluation

Adult Comorbidity Evaluation-27 (ACE-27) is a modification of the Kaplan-Feinstein Index (KFI), validated and especially designed for patients with cancer. An overall score of 1, 2, or 3 is assigned according to the highest ranked single condition, except where two or more grade 2 illnesses occur in different organ systems, in which case a score of 3 is given. Other comorbidity indexes are available, but the National Cancer Intelligence Network in the United Kingdom recommends the use of ACE-27 for all cancer patients.

What is Health-Related QoL (HRQoL) and How is it Measured?

HRQoL involves four areas: physical functioning, psychological functioning, social functioning, and symptoms from the disease and treatment.

HRQoL has a major role in treatment decisions in several situations. For example, when different treatments have a good chance of cure, their HRQoL outcomes will influence treatment

BOX 74.1   ASSESSMENT TOOLS FOR MEASURING VOICE, SPEECH, AND SWALLOW IN HNC PATIENTS

a) Assessment of Outcome of Voice

Questionnaire-Based Measures
- Voice Handicap Index (VHI)
- Voice Symptom Scale (VoiSS)
- Voice Activity and Participation Profile (VAPP)
- Voice Prosthesis Questionnaire
- Vocal Handicap Index-10
- Vocal Performance Questionnaire (VPQ)

Perceptual Measures
- GRBAS rating scheme
- Perceptual evaluation of alaryngeal speech

Instrument-Based Measures
- Stroboscopy
- Acoustic analysis of voice using inverse filtering and linear predictive coding
- Electroglottography (EGG)
- Electromyographanalysis

b) Assessment of Outcome of Swallow

Questionnaire-Based Measures
- Sydney Swallow Questionnaire (SSQ)
- SWAL-QOL and SWAL-CARE
- MD Anderson Dysphagia Inventory (MDADI)

Perceptual Measures
- Blue dye test
- Water swallow test

Instrument-Based Measures
- Videofluoroscopy
- Functional endoscopic evaluation of swallowing (FEES)–score on the penetration-aspiration scale
- Flexible endoscopic evaluation of swallowing with sensory testing (FEESST)
- Electromyography

Performance Scales
- Performance Status Scale for Head and Neck
- The Functional Intraoral Glasgow Scale

c) Tools Available for the Assessment of Outcome of Speech

Questionnaire-Based Measures
- Speech Handicap Index (SHI)

Perceptual Measures
- The London Speech Evaluation (LSE) scale

Instrument-Based Measures
- Assessment of Intelligibility of Dysarthric Speech (ASSIDS)
- Acoustic analysis of speech signal using linear predictive coding

selection. The priority given to the best chance of cure often outweighs HRQoL outcomes for individual patients, treatment protocols, and trial designs. Patients set cure and survival as priorities. When cancer treatment is very unlikely to be curative or the intention of treatment is palliative, there is a strong focus on treatments that maintain HRQoL.

Studies show that long-term survivors of advanced HNC accept major surgical procedures, with over 90% of 273 patients stating that 'I would undergo the same treatment'. There is also strong agreement among patients, their companions, and members of the multidisciplinary team (MDT) about priorities in HNC outcomes, and there is low post-treatment regret among patients and their companions.

HRQoL is usually measured by a patient's self-completed questionnaire. Questionnaires can be complemented by objective measures of swallowing, speech, and shoulder movement. There is no gold standard questionnaire that is best. The British Association of Head and Neck Oncologists and the British Association of Otorhinolaryngologists Head Neck Surgeons both recommend that HRQoL should be longitudinally recorded. The most commonly used questionnaires are the European Organization for Research and Treatment for Cancer (EORTC) and the University of Washington Quality of Life (UW-QoL) questionnaires.

Treatment Decisions and Outcomes in the Context of HRQoL and Survivorship

The epidemiology of HNC in the United Kingdom is changing. The oral cavity is now the subsite most often involved, and there was a 51% increase in human papillomavirus (HPV)-related oropharyngeal cancers between 1989 and 2006. The HPV-related cancers appear to affect younger people and may respond better to chemoradiotherapy with or without surgery.

Shared decision-making improves patients' satisfaction with the consultation, leading to better QoL. Information supplied to the patient needs to be tailored to the individual patient. Giving patients too much information can result in anxiety and reduced recall, while too little information makes it unlikely that patients will fully understand.

Outcomes used in clinical trials of HNC treatment frequently focus on objective measures of function and survival rates. Mortality may not be the most important outcome to the patient, nor is it necessarily a good proxy for other outcomes. A range of outcome predictors should be considered, including the social and healthcare environment, psychosocial factors, and health behaviours, as well as biological factors.

HRQoL and Survivorship

The risk factors for poor HRQoL outcomes are given in Table 74.1. Poor HRQoL has been identified as an independent predictor of survival.

Total Laryngectomy (TL)

After laryngectomy, patients are more accepting of anticipated sequelae (such as sensory impairments, cough, and dyspnoea), than they are accepting of more general side effects (such as constipation and nausea/vomiting). Surprisingly, many patients who have undergone total laryngectomy (TL) maintain a good overall QoL, although they face potential difficulties in returning to work after TL. There is also evidence that both primary and secondary trachea-oesophageal puncture (TEP) affect HRQoL. Primary TEP provides almost immediate and satisfactory voice rehabilitation.

Treatment

In general, single-modality treatment (e.g. radiotherapy or surgery alone) confers much better HRQoL. Transoral robotic surgery offers a way to preserve functional anatomy without compromising surgical resection margins and could have a positive impact on HRQoL. The advantage of less-invasive surgery for HRQoL (e.g. transoral resection versus open resection and free flap reconstruction) is lost if primary surgery has to be followed by adjuvant radiotherapy. Avoiding radiotherapy after primary surgery has substantial benefits for HRQoL as long as optimal survival is maintained. There is also evidence that reducing the dosage of radiotherapy can make a substantial difference. In addition, IMRT has much better HRQoL outcomes than 3D-conformal radiotherapy (3D-CRT) has.

Table 74.1 Common factors associated with worse HRQoL outcomes

Alcoholism: Pre-existing comorbidity and poor coping mechanisms
Age: Young patients have much more to lose in terms of life expectancy and finances
Combined treatments: Surgery and radiotherapy, chemoradiotherapy
Deprivation: Lower socioeconomic background
Personality: Negative, nihilistic
Pre-existing distress: Anxiety-related conditions, mental health problems
Single: Lack of support
Site: Oropharynx and hypopharynx
Stage: Advanced disease
Unknown: Clinicians clinical experience

Although the short-term side effects of treatment may differ, long-term QoL is remarkably similar with either primary chemoradiation or surgery with post-operative radiation.

Osteoradionecrosis (ORN) of the mandible is a severe complication of radiation therapy and has a detrimental impact on HRQoL. Surgery for ORN can result in an improved HRQoL; however, lack of improvement despite the restoration of an intact mandible is related to the persistent effects of chemoradiotherapy.

Clinical Trials

In the literature, the evidence is limited concerning HRQoL with respect to clinical trials. HRQoL is often included as a secondary outcome of a clinical trial and is not explicitly driven by hypothesis. In the future, an increasing number of trials and interventions will specifically aim at evaluating HRQoL differences (such as a study to assess the effect of low-level laser therapy on oral mucositis and QoL in HNC patients receiving chemoradiotherapy). IMRT will also continue to be the subject of trials for until it becomes a standard of care.

HRQoL Issues

A diverse range of patient and carer needs and concerns arise after completion of HNC treatment. Significant HRQoL issues are reflected in Table 74.2. The issue that patients raise most frequently is fear of recurrence (FoR).

Carer Support

The benefit of carer support is a key issue in terms of patients' HRQoL. During the treatment phase and in the early period after interventions, a wide range of supportive care is needed, including dental hygienists, physical therapists, specialist dietitians, and speech therapists. Long-term supportive care focuses on dental hygiene, speech therapy, and physical therapy. Increased social isolation may be a risk factor for poorer physical recovery from, or adjustment to, treatment-related side effects. Carers see patients as they are, 'day to day', and not

Table 74.2   A summary of HRQoL issues after HNC treatment

Issues, in alphabetical order
Carer: Positive carer support is important
Coping: Seeking social support is good, avoidance is bad
Dental status: Eating, social interaction, and coping are affected by dental issues
Disfigurement: Appearance, body image, and intimacy are adversely affected
Emotion: Anxiety is common pre-treatment, and depression and mood disorders require treatment
Fatigue: Common in first year and is associated with poor sleep and low energy
Fear of recurrence: Does not lessen over time
Financial/work: Employment, benefits, and retirement are all affected by illness
Information: various amounts, in various ways, at various times
Nutrition: Weight loss, poor diet, and percutaneous endoscopic gastrostomy (PEG) feeding are concerns
Oral rehabilitation: Chewing/eating are subject to expectations vs trade-off with actual function
Pain: Causes need for opiates, poor sleep, and depression
Personality: optimism and HRQoL + survival, high neuroticism
Self-esteem: Low self-esteem is associated with poor QOL
Sociodemographic: children, social support, ethanol abuse
Speech: Laryngeal speech and isolation affect QOL
Swallowing: Presence of a feeding tube is most significant
Shoulder: Shoulder discomfort and neck tightness
Trismus: Difficulty with mouth opening affects diet, social life, and intimacy
Xerostomia: Profound impact on social function, intensity modulated radiotherapy (IMRT)
Unknown: clinical art of the individual not a precise science

just at the review clinic visit. Carers are often more able to identify needs than the patient themselves. Family caregivers also report significant stress and needs, including the need for more information and for healthcare services. There is merit in developing a tool to identify carer needs and caregiving training programs.

Interventions

As our understanding of the HRQoL outcomes of patients has increased, it has led to a focus on intervention, but evidence for interventions is limited by the small number of studies, methodological problems, and poor comparability. Even so, some interventions can be suggested. A nurse-led intervention around the time of discharge from hospital, based on informational needs, has potential benefits for HRQoL. Early provision of psychotherapy may reduce patients' post-traumatic stress disorder, anxiety, and depressive symptoms. Interviewing patients to allow them to express their concerns has merit. Acupuncture has been used in the prevention and treatment of radiation-induced xerostomia. There is scope for other interventions (e.g. interventions addressing secondary lymphoedema) to help in the management of associated symptom burden, functional loss, and psychosocial impact.

Conclusions and Future

HNC is biologically heterogeneous; therefore, tumour behaviour and response to treatment vary as well. Furthermore, the incidence and severity of adverse effects of treatments are also variable among patients. Consequently, the identification, selection, and reporting of disease-specific and appropriate endpoints have become a research priority. Advances in information technology and patients' familiarity with computers and the internet allow for a much more integrated approach to HRQoL assessment and intervention.

HRQoL is now an integral part of the management of the HNC patients and their carers. Also, as our understanding of the patient's perspective on outcome increases, treatment selection will become more refined and aftercare will be determined by the patient's needs.

KEY POINTS

- Outcome measures are integral to the management of patients with HNC and can relate to survival or function. Choice of appropriate outcome measures is essential.
- HRQoL is an essential component of outcomes after HNC.
- HRQoL is usually measured by questionnaires. The choice of questionnaire is an important consideration and depends on the reason for collecting the patient-reported outcomes.
- The many factors that affect HRQoL relate to the physical/functional, social, and emotional consequences of treatments.
- Advances in computer technology will make a substantial difference in collecting HRQoL outcomes and will allow the insights gained to be applied on an individual patient basis.

75. TEMPOROMANDIBULAR JOINT DISORDERS

Introduction

Temporomandibular joint (TMJ) problems are common and may affect around 30% of the population at some stage during their life. Differential diagnosis can be confusing, and patients are often referred to ENT services with 'earache'. TMJ disorders are a spectrum of disorders ranging from internal derangement (disc-related disorder) to masticatory myofascial pain (purely muscle disorder).

Epidemiology

Although TMJ disorders can present at any age, patients less than 40 years old are unlikely to have degenerative joint disease. In people over age 40, there is increased remodelling of the joint, with possible osteoarthritic changes.

Women are affected more commonly than men, and reported sex ratios range from 2:1 to 10:1. Predisposing factors include previous trauma, history of clicking joint, and clenching or grinding of teeth (nocturnal parafunction).

HISTORY

Clinical Examination

- Palpation of the joint for tenderness and noises/crepitus laterally and posteriorly with the mouth both open and closed.
- Palpation of the masseter and temporalis muscles for tenderness and areas of muscle tightness.
- Use of tongue spatula to assess bite between teeth on both sides.
- Measurement of interincisal opening in millimetres.
- Observation of the opening path of the mandible in relation to maxillary centreline.
- Interdigitation of teeth (dental occlusion).

Investigations

- Orthopantogram (OPG) plain radiograph is useful in screening for other pathology and dental causes.
- Computed tomography (CT) delineates bony anatomy of joint and surrounding structures.
- Magnetic resonance imaging (MRI) can highlight soft tissue but is difficult to interpret even for experienced radiologists.
- Isotope bone scanning (^{99m}Tc) is useful to show increased bone turnover (e.g. condylar hyperplasia).

Table 75.1 Primary symptoms of temporomandibular joint disorders

Pain	• In joint itself (TMJ pain), usually localised in front of tragus. Worsens on function • In muscles of mastication (myofascial pain), usually aching, poorly localized but often over ramus of mandible and temple. Worse in mornings
Joint noises	• Clenching usually relates to anteromedial displacement of the disc, repositioning it over the joint. No active intervention is required • Cracking or crepitus suggests degeneration within or around the joint. No active treatment required in isolation
Locking	• Inability to fully open (closed lock) or fully close • Related to disc displacement, muscle spasm, or trauma
Restriction of opening	• Normal interincisal opening between 35 and 55 mm • Can be caused by muscle spasm, disc displacement, ankylosis, trauma, infection, or spasm
Disturbance of bite	• Unilateral collapse of the joint will lead to premature contact and centreline deviation towards side of problem • Bilateral collapse will move chin back and cause anterior open bite
Alteration in facial appearance	• Collapse of the joint will cause retrusion or rotation of the chin
Other joint disorders	• Rheumatoid disease can lead to joint collapse or ankylosis • Ankylosing spondylitis may lead to restriction and ankylosis • Hypermobility may lead to dislocations

Differential Diagnosis

Internal Derangement
'Clicking joint' is common, and it is now accepted as a variation of normal. Clinical examination may elicit muscle tenderness or direct joint tenderness and reduction of interincisal opening. Physical limitation and lack of joint glide can indicate occlusion of the upper joint space. Muscle tenderness will guide to a diagnosis of myofascial pain.

Degenerative Disease of the TMJ (Osteoarthrosis)
Degenerative joint disease occurs when the reparative process is overtaken by wear and tear on the joint. It is much less common in the TMJ than in other major joints due to reduced load on the TMJ. Symptoms include pain, swelling, and restriction of movement. Clinical examination reveals tenderness of joint with palpable crepitus and restriction of movement with intermittent swelling. CT findings include sclerosis, loss of joint space, osteophytes, and erosions or cyst formation.

Inflammatory Disease of the TMJ
Rheumatoid disease can occur in the child, adolescent, or adult. It usually presents with signs and symptoms of synovitis, namely pain, swelling, heat, and restriction of movement. Progression can lead to joint collapse, resulting in malocclusion with anterior open bite and retrusive contact. Diagnosis is made in coordination with the rheumatology team and is guided by the presence of other affected joints.

Psoriatic arthropathy can lead to acute synovitis, joint collapse, or ankylosis. Classical skin changes can be difficult to identify in up to 50% of patients, but larger joint arthropathy is usually apparent. Patients who are HLA-B27 positive have a tendency to progress to ankylosis rather than a synovitis disease pattern.

Trauma
Unilateral or bilateral condylar fractures account for approximately 30% of mandibular fractures. Interpersonal violence is the most common cause. Occasionally, the fracture can involve the temporal bone, leading to hemotympanum or perforation of the external auditory canal. Symptoms and signs include pain at site of injury, swelling, malocclusion, and possible lateral open bite.

Fractures in children tend to occur within the joint capsule and are difficult to treat operatively. Initial management is often early mobilization and analgesia, but a short period of intermaxillary fixation with elastics and wires is sometimes required to reduce a malocclusion. Long-term follow-up is required to screen for growth abnormalities.

Adult fractures are more likely to be extracapsular and can be managed nonoperatively with soft diet and mobilization if there is no change in occlusion. Early surgical management is becoming more common practice but should only be performed in experienced hands. Early referral to oral and maxillofacial teams is advised for complex fractures.

Hemifacial Microsomia
Some TMJ findings are due to the failure of the condyle to develop, possibly secondary to inadequate blood supply in utero. This causes associated undergrowth of the ear, ear canal, joint, and fossa to varying degrees. Hemifacial microsomia is a complex craniofacial disorder and management should involve supraregional craniofacial centres.

Condylar Hyperplasia
Condylar hyperplasia is due to either overgrowth of the condyle centre on one side before or during puberty, or continued growth after completion of puberty but with cessation of growth on the affected side. Patients present with progressive malocclusion, usually with centreline deviation and associated chin point deviation (hemimandibular hyperplasia). They may also present with bowing of the mandible and downward cant of dental occlusion (hemimandibular hypertrophy).

Diagnosis is aided with OPG, and isotope bone scans can also be useful. Management is with removal of the growth plate, and when burnt out, orthognathic jaw realignment.

Infection of the TMJ

Infection of the TMJ is an uncommon occurrence in the developed world. It can be due to direct inoculation of the joint or distant spread. Primary infection can be bony (osteomyelitis) or involve the soft tissue (arthritis). The usual causative agent is *Staphylococcus aureus*. The most common cause is local spread from neighbouring structures—ear, brain, or oropharynx. Haematogenous spread is rare.

Management includes diagnostic aspiration, intravenous antibiotics, and systemic support if required. Repeated arthrocentesis may be required.

Neoplastic Disease of the TMJ

Primary benign and malignant tumours of the TMJ are rare and include chondroma, osteochondroma, and osteoma. Benign tumours tend to have slow growth and present with occlusal deformity, centreline deviation, and chin point changes.

Management includes excision and reconstruction, with or without orthognathic corrective surgery.

Iatrogenic/Idiopathic Disorders

The previous use of open surgery for pain, restriction, and joint noises has led to troublesome sequelae. Most of the problems include pain from local damage and are best managed in conjunction with the pain team.

Initial Management

The primary management of most TMJ disorders is reassurance that there is unlikely to be a significant underlying condition. The disorder is unlikely to precede arthritis, and the majority of patients can be managed with nonsurgical treatments. There is an underlying psychological component in a significant number of patients.

Explanation of the disease process will help empower the patient and reduces the risk of the patient's following misleading advice found on the internet.

Initial resting of the joint, with avoidance of sticky foods and restriction of wide mouth opening, will gradually improve most symptoms over a period of weeks. Use of a topical NSAID will give additional benefit.

A lower, soft, full occlusal coverage splint to wear at night helps reduce load on muscles and joint overnight and gives particular benefit to those with a clenching habit. Again, it takes several weeks for the benefit to be felt.

Following a 2-month trial, if there has been no significant improvement or if there is severe restriction, then referral to a specialist is warranted.

Referral for maxillofacial advice is indicated when there is:

- Acute severe restriction of opening
- Failure of conservative measures in conjunction with dental care over 2 months
- Associated rheumatological disease
- Recurrent dislocation of joint
- Disturbance of dental occlusion

Surgical Management

Surgery can be divided into open and closed procedures. Closed procedures are arthrocentesis and arthroscopy. Arthrocentesis is the washing out of the upper joint space with 200 ml of isotonic solution, most commonly under general anaesthesia. It gives 70–80% improvement in cases of locking, restriction, and pain. Arthroscopy is similar but allows visualisation of the internal joint anatomy. Both procedures carry a 1% risk of temporary temporal branch weakness.

Open joint surgery is approached by a pre-auricular incision, avoiding the facial nerve. Procedures include eminoplasty (modification of the articular eminence), condylar shave (modification of the condylar head), and full joint replacement. For full joint replacement, outcomes of >90% joint survival have been reported at 15 years.

Conclusion

TMJ disorders are a common cause of morbidity, although most can be managed with simple measures. Surgery should be considered a last resort.

Further Reading

1. Rajapakse S, Ahmed N, Sidebottom AJ. Current thinking about the management of dysfunction of the temporomandibular joint: a review. *Br J Oral Maxillofacial Surg* 2017; May(4): 351–356.

2. Connelly ST, Tartaglia G, Silva RG. (Eds.) Contemporary Management of Temporomandibular Disorders, 2019. ISBN 978-3-030-13328-3.

3. National Institute of Health and Care Excellence Guidelines: Temporomandibular Disorders (TMDs). (Last revised December 2016.)

---

76. BENIGN AND MALIGNANT CONDITIONS OF THE SKIN

Introduction

One in every three cancers is a skin cancer.

Common or important benign and malignant skin lesions that are discussed here are shown in bold in Table 76.1.

Benign and Premalignant Skin Lesions

Actinic Keratosis (AK)

Actinic keratosis is the most common premalignant lesion, with a low transformation rate into SCC. Found on sun-exposed areas (80% occur on the head and neck or hands). Asymptomatic, palpable, dry, scaly lesions. Biopsy is indicated if SCC is suspected. Nonsurgical options include topical treatments (e.g. 5-fluorouracil or imiquimod), cryotherapy, or photodynamic therapy (PDT). Surgery is either curettage and cautery (C&C) or excision with 2-mm margins.

Bowen's Disease (BD; A.K.A. Squamous Cell Carcinoma in situ)

Risk of progression to SCC is 3–5%. Occurs on sun-exposed areas (mainly head and neck and lower limb). Lesions are asymptomatic, long-standing, and slow-growing well-defined/demarcated scaly erythematous plaques. Biopsy excludes differentials (e.g. SCC). Nonsurgical and surgical management are similar to those for AK.

Keratoacanthoma (KA)

KA clinically and histologically resembles well-differentiated SCC. However, it enlarges rapidly over 6 weeks and then regresses. Management is either observation (because KA spontaneously involutes) or removal if there is concern about SCC. Associations include Ferguson-Smith and Muir-Torre syndromes.

Table 76.1 Examples of skin lesions

Main classification	Subclassification	Examples
Benign nonpigmented	Epidermal	**Actinic keratosis, Bowen's disease, keratoacanthoma,** keratin horn, viral wart, squamous papilloma, seborrheic keratosis
	Dermal	Hair follicle: Trichoepithelioma, pilomatrixoma Sebaceous gland: Sebaceous naevus Sweat gland: Cylindroma Neural tissue: Neurofibroma Miscellaneous: Cysts (e.g. dermoid)
Malignant nonpigmented	Common	**Basal cell carcinoma (BCC), squamous cell carcinoma (SCC)**
	Uncommon	**Merkel cell carcinoma, sebaceous carcinoma**
Benign pigmented	Naevus cell naevi	Congenital—Congenital melanocytic naevus Acquired—Junction naevus, compound naevus, intradermal naevus Special—Spitz naevus, spindle cell nevus, halo naevus
	Melanocytic naevi	Epidermal—Ephelis (freckle), lentigo, café-au-lait spot Dermal—Blue naevus
Premalignant pigmented		**Dysplastic/atypical mole** **Lentigo maligna/melanoma in situ**
Malignant pigmented		**Melanoma**
Soft tissue tumours	Cutaneous sarcoma	**DFSP,** MFX, AFX

Dysplastic/Atypical Nevi

Dysplastic/atypical naevi occur in 5% of the population. They contain atypical melanocytes but no invasion. There is a 5% risk of change to melanoma. They have unusual features: >5 mm diameter, irregular border, and pigment. FAMM syndrome (high risk of melanoma) is >50 moles, dysplastic on histology, and a 1st/2nd-degree relative with melanoma. Management is in an atypical mole clinic and includes full skin examination with dermatoscopy and photographs. If there is diagnostic uncertainty, then treatment is excision with 2-mm margins.

Lentigo and Lentigo Maligna/Melanoma in situ

Lentigo is an increased number of normal melanocytes, lentigo maligna is an increased number of abnormal melanocytes, and lentigo maligna melanoma is invasive. Assessment of lentigo is with dermatoscopy, and if there is diagnostic uncertainty, then treatment is excision. Lentigo maligna/melanoma in situ is managed by excision with 5 mm margins, although histology may show incomplete margins, as associated with 'field change,' and therefore require post-excision imiquimod or observation.

Non-Melanoma Skin Cancers (NMSC)

BCC and SCC are the main types.

Risk Factors

Risk factors are shown in Tables 76.2 and 76.3. Fitzpatrick types 1 and 2 have the highest risk.

Table 76.2 Risk factors for non-melanoma skin cancers

Risk factor	Examples
Radiation	Chronic sun exposure (e.g. UVA/B), ionising radiation
Premalignant conditions	AK, BD, KA, keratin horn, viral infection (e.g. HPV-related SCC), sebaceous naevus
Chronic wounds	Marjolin's ulcer (SCC)
Immunosuppression	Malignancy, drugs
Toxins	Smoking (SCC lip), soot, arsenic
Genetics	Xeroderma pigmentosum, albinism, Gorlin's syndrome (BCC)

Table 76.3 Fitzpatrick skin types

Type	Colour and response to sunlight
1	Pale white, never tan, and always burn
2	Fair skin, difficult tan, and usually burn
3	Light brown, gradual tan, and sometimes burn
4	Mediterranean, easy tan, and minimal burn
5	Indian, very easy tan, and rarely burn
6	Black, never burn

Staging

Points on BCC/SCC American Joint Committee on Cancer (AJCC) 8th edition TNM classification:

a. Tumuor (T): T1 <2 cm, T2 2–4 cm, T3 > 4 cm or deep (e.g. >6 mm, perineural invasion, beyond fat or minor bone), T4a gross bone involvement, and T4b skull base involved.
b. Node (N): Specific category for head and neck.
c. Staging: Stage 1 = T1, Stage 2 = T2, Stage 3 = T3 or T1–3N1, Stage 4a = T4, T1–3N2/3, Stage 4b = M1.

Basal Cell Carcinoma

Background
75% of NMSC. From epidermal keratinocytes. Locally invasive. Distant metastases are rare.

Clinical Features
Slow growing over months/years. Classically, pearly appearance with telangiectasia.

Classified as nodular (75%), superficial (15%), infiltrative/morpheaform (10%), other.

Diagnosis
Clinical, but punch biopsy to exclude differentials. Imaging (e.g. CT/MRI) if deep invasion.

Management
Principles
Decide if 'high risk' or 'fixed'. Risk factors: Macroscopic—Increasing size, poorly defined, location on central face. Microscopic—Infiltrative/morpheaform or perineural invasion. Systemic—Immunosuppression.

Nonsurgical
Superficial BCC: Topical treatment (e.g. imiquimod/5-fluorouracil), PDT, or cryotherapy.

Surgical

Options include:

1 Destructive treatments if small, well-demarcated/superficial: C&C, cryotherapy, CO_2 laser
2 Nondestructive treatment: Excision
   a. Margin for <2 cm and well-defined: 3 mm (85% clearance) or 4–5 mm (95%). Depth is cuff of fat.
   b. Margin for large/poorly defined: 5 mm (80% clearance) or 13–15 mm (95%).
   c. Mohs micrographic surgery (MMS) for high-risk lesions in cosmetically sensitive areas.
   d. Incompletely excised (5%) options: Observe, re-excise +/– frozen section, Mohs, radiotherapy.

Radiotherapy

Cure rates similar to surgery. First-line or adjuvant for incompletely excised tumours. Contraindicated for recurrent tumours in previously irradiated areas. Usually reserved for elderly.

Advanced disease

Vismodegib if locally advanced (e.g. Gorlin's syndrome). Electrochemotherapy if other treatment failed.

Follow-Up

Completely excised tumours: no follow-up. Incompletely excised tumours: observe (or treat) for recurrence.

Squamous Cell Carcinoma

Background

Second most common NMSC. Malignant neoplasm of keratinocytes. Arise de novo or from precursor lesion. Potential to metastasize. Metastatic risk is low (< 5%), but if there is metastasis, 25–40% 5-year survival.

Clinical Features

1 *History*: Lesion grows quickly (e.g. weeks/months), may ulcerate or bleed.
2 *Examination*: If well-differentiated, has everted nodule and keratin core; if poorly differentiated, may be ulcerated. Check lymph nodes.

Diagnosis

1 Punch or incisional biopsy. Key histologic features include keratin pearls.
2 Fine-needle aspiration for cytology, or radiology-guided core biopsy if there is an enlarged lymph node.
3 Staging CT if there is deep invasion (e.g. bone/parotid) or evidence of spread.

Management

Principles

High-risk lesions have increased risk of local recurrence and metastasis. Factors include:

1 *Macroscopic*: Size >2 cm, site, recurrent lesions. Sites include chronic/radiotherapy wounds, non-sun-exposed areas (e.g. sole of foot), sun-exposed areas (e.g. lip or ear). NB: Other sun-exposed areas are lower risk.
2 *Microscopic*: Histological differentiation (e.g. poor is worst), Broder grade (e.g. 3/4 worst), subtype (e.g. acantholytic/spindle/desmoplastic worst), depth (>4 mm or perineural invasion, etc.).
3 *Systemic*: Immunosuppression.

Key management: Decide if 'high risk', 'fixed', or 'regional/distant spread'. Then AJCC stage.

Surgical Treatment

1 Low-risk lesions (T1) have 4-mm margins, high-risk (T2 and above) have 6-mm margins minimum, ideally to fascia.
2 Consider MMS if high-risk or critical area.
3 Lymphadenectomy if there is regional disease.

Radiotherapy
SCC is radiosensitive. Radiotherapy is used as primary treatment or as an adjunct if there is incomplete surgical excision. However, radiotherapy does not give histology, is not curative if bone is involved, and over the long term can cause skin atrophy/telangiectasia, secondary cancer, or radionecrosis.

Melanoma
A malignant neoplasm of melanocytes. Accounts for 5% of skin cancers but 75% of skin cancer deaths.

Risk Factors
FPPARENTS mnemonic—Family history, Premalignant lesion (as above), Previous melanoma, Age (median 59), Race (Caucasian), Economic status, Nevus (>50), Fitzpatrick Types 1&2, Sunburn/sunbed.

Pathology

1 *V600E* gene codes for BRAF enzyme, if it is mutated, then there is BRAF mutation and cell proliferation.
2 Ultraviolet radiation (UVA/B) damage to DNA.

Clinical Features

1 (Dermatoscopy) assessment—ABCD mnemonic: Asymmetry, Border irregularity, Colour, Diameter >6 mm
2 Regional lymph nodes and systemic examination
3 Photography

Management
Initial
Excision biopsy with 2-mm margin to fat. Incisional (or punch) biopsies only performed if large lesion (e.g. lentigo) or subungual melanoma.

MDT
Discuss results with Specialist Skin multidisciplinary team (SSMDT). Biopsy helps give:

a. *Subtypes*: Superficial spreading melanoma (60%), nodular melanoma (30%), lentigo maligna melanoma (7%), acral lentiginous melanoma (2%), desmoplastic melanoma (1%).
b. *AJCC stage*: Staging system splits melanoma into cutaneous (Table 76.4) and head and neck mucosal, conjunctival, and uveal melanoma.

Investigation

1 Stages IIC and above need BRAF testing on primary or secondary lesion.
2 Stage IIC (if no sentinel lymph node biopsy [SLNBx]) or IIIB/C needs staging CT of head & neck/chest/abdomen/pelvis.
3 Stage IV needs serum lactate dehydrogenase (LDH) +/− PET CT.

Nonsurgical
Psychological support, vitamin D, inform colleagues (e.g. transplant team) if patient is on immunosuppressants.

Table 76.4 AJCC TNM staging for cutaneous melanoma

T: Primary tumour		
Tx	Thickness cannot be assessed	
T0	No evidence	
Tis	Melanoma in situ	
T1a	Breslow <0.8 mm thick without ulceration	
T1b	<0.8 mm with ulceration	
	0.8–1 mm	
T2a	1.1–2 mm	
T2b	1.1–2 mm with ulceration	
T3a	2.1–4 mm	
T3b	2.1–4 mm with ulceration	
T4a	>4 mm	
T4b	>4 mm with ulceration	
N: Regional lymph nodes		
Nx	Not assessed	
N0	No regional node metastasis	
N1a	1 occult node (i.e. SLNB)	
N1b	1 clinical node	
N1c	No nodes, presence of in-transits/satellites/microsatellite	
N2a	2–3 occult nodes	
N2b	2–3 nodes, at least 1 clinical	
N2c	1 lymph node with presence of in-transit, satellite, or microsatellites	
N3a	>4 occult nodes	
N3b	>4 nodes, at least 1 clinical	
N3c	>2 lymph node with presence of in-transit, satellite, or microsatellites. Matted nodes	
M: Distant metastasis		
M0	No metastasis	
M1a	Distant skin, soft tissue, or nonregional lymph nodes	
M1b	Lung	
M1c	All sites (not CNS) or raised LDH with any metastasis	
M1d	CNS metastasis	
Stage 5-year survival (%)		
0	TisN0M0	—
IA	T1aN0M0, T1bNoMO	97
IB	T2aN0M0	92
IIA	T2bN0M0, T3aN0M0	81
IIB	T3bN0M0, T4aN0M0	70
IIC	T4bN0M0	53
IIIA	T1a/b–T2a,N1/N2a,M0	78
IIIB	T0N1b/cMo, T1a/b–T2aN1b/cN2bM0, T2b/T3aN1a–N2bM0	59
IIIC	T0N2b/cN3b/cM0, T1a–T3aN2c/N3abcM0, T3b/T4a any N > 1M0, T4bN1a–cN2cM0	40
IIID	T4bN3a/b/cM0	—
IV	Any T/N M1	15–20

Table 76.5 WLE margins for melanoma

Thickness (mm)	WLE (cm)
In situ	0.5
<1	1
1.01–2	1–2
2.01–4	2–3
>4	3

Local Surgery

1 Wide local excision (WLE; Table 76.5) reduces micrometastases (i.e. WLE for local control).
2 MDT decision if there is to be MMS for indistinct margins (e.g. LM) or tumour in critical areas (e.g. eyes).

Lymph Node Surgery (Stage III)

1 SLNBx for IB–IIC and for pT1b if lymphovascular invasion/mitotic rate > 2. SLNBx is for staging/prognosis and guides adjuvant therapy but has no therapeutic/survival advantage. If positive SLNBx, follow up with examination +/– ultrasound of nodes +/– systemic treatment.
2 Indications for dissection (NB: Head and neck involve levels 1–5 +/– superficial parotidectomy):
   a. Post SLNBx:
       i.   If SLNBx shows features of risk of regional relapse (e.g. extracapsular spread or >3 nodes involved)
       ii. Dewar criteria
       iii. In head & neck and there is concern later surgical rescue would be complex
       iv. Failed first-line systemic treatment and node-only recurrence
   b. Palpable/imaged IIIB/C positive for melanoma following FNAC or image-guided core/open biopsy (if FNAC negative/equivocal)
3 NB: There is no evidence of survival benefit for 'elective' lymph node dissection.

Metastatic Disease (Stage III or IV)

1 Options:
   a. Immunotherapy (checkpoint inhibitors)—Pembrolizumab/nivolumab (anti-PDL1) or ipilumab (CTLA4 inhibitor)
   b. Targeted therapy if BRAF mutation—Vemurafenib/dabrafenib (BRAF inhibitor), or trametinib (MEK inhibitor), or imatinib (targets C-KIT gene)
   c. Interleukin-2
   d. Chemotherapy (e.g. dacarbazine)
2 Further locoregional recurrence options: Systemic therapy, surgical excision if isolated lesions, CO_2 laser or electrocautery if multiple small lesions, radiotherapy for symptoms, electrochemotherapy if larger area.

Rare Skin Cancers

Merkel Cell Carcinoma

Aggressive and rare—has special AJCC TNM. Dermal neuroendocrine carcinoma. Associations include polyomavirus, previous radiation, B-cell lymphoma. Immunosuppression is a risk factor. Rapid, painless, enlarging, dome-shaped solid nodule on head and neck (50%). Lymph nodes may be involved at presentation (15%). Need tissue biopsy. Subsequently, staging CT. Discuss in MDT. Wide excision with 2- to 3-cm margins to fascia, as well as SLNBx and adjuvant radiotherapy to primary site +/− regional nodes.

Sebaceous Carcinoma

Aggressive and rare. From sebaceous glands. Risk factors include Muir-Torres syndrome. Firm yellowish nodule, especially near eyelids (75%). Obtain tissue diagnosis. Discussion in MDT. Requires wide excision with minimal 5-mm margins or Mohs (33% risk of recurrence). If orbit involved, exenteration.

Dermatofibrosarcoma Protuberans

Most common skin sarcoma. Approximately 15% occur in head and neck. Incidence greatest in patients 20–40 years old. Intermediate malignancy, prone to local recurrence but not metastasis. Slow-growing, red/brown nodule fixed to dermis. Obtain tissue biopsy. Discuss in MDT. Requires ~3-cm margins to fascia or Mohs. If unresectable or there are metastases, consider radiotherapy or chemotherapy (imatinib).

Further Reading

1. Amin MB, Edge S, Greene F, et al. (Eds.) *AJCC Cancer Staging Handbook*, 8th ed., 2017. New York: Springer.

2. Motley R, Preston P, Lawrence C. Multiprofessional guidelines for the management of the patient with primary cutaneous squamous cell carcinoma. London: British Association of dermatologists. Available from: http://www.bad.org.uk/library-media/documents/SCC_2009.pdf

3. Peach H, Board R, Cook M, Corrie P, Ellis S, Geh J, King P, Laitung G, Larkin J, Marsden J, Middleton M, Moncrieff M, Nathan P, Powell B, Pritchard-Jones R, Rodwell S, Steven N, Lorigan P. Current role of sentinel lymph node biopsy in the management of cutaneous melanoma: A UK consensus statement. *J Plast Reconstr Aesthet Surg* 2020; 73(1): 36–42.

HEAD AND NECK ENDOCRINE SURGERY

77. ANATOMY AND PHYSIOLOGY OF HEAD AND NECK ENDOCRINE GLANDS

Anatomy of the Thyroid Gland

Macroscopic Anatomy

The thyroid gland, a bilobed butterfly-shaped endocrine organ, extends from the thyroid cartilage to the level of the fourth or fifth tracheal ring (Figure 77.1). Its lobes are connected by the isthmus overlying the second to fourth rings. The recurrent laryngeal nerve runs immediately posterior to the gland in the trachea-oesophageal groove.

The thyroid is held within the pre-tracheal fascia, which attaches superiorly to the hyoid bone, inferiorly to the mediastinum, and laterally to the carotid sheath. The fibres condense posteriorly to form the suspensory ligament of Berry, which attaches firmly to the cricoid cartilage and first tracheal ring.

The thyroid's blood supply is from paired superior and inferior thyroid arteries. The superior thyroid artery arises as the first branch of the external carotid, the inferior originates from the thyrocervical trunk. Less commonly, the isthmus receives blood from the brachiocephalic trunk via the thyroid ima artery.

Venous return occurs through a venous plexus, draining the paired superior and middle thyroid veins to the internal jugular vein, and the inferior thyroid veins to the brachiocephalic vein. The thyroid has an extensive lymphatic drainage, with peri-thyroid nodes draining to the pre-laryngeal, pre-tracheal, para-tracheal, and deep cervical nodes.

Common Anatomical Variants

A third 'pyramidal' lobe can arise from the upper poles or the isthmus; it is seen as a short stump or a process extending to the hyoid bone. Additionally, in approximately 60% of patients, the tubercule of Zuckerkandl is seen extending immediately lateral to the recurrent laryngeal nerve.

Developmental Anatomy

The thyroid gland is derived from the primitive pharynx (median anlage) between the first and second branchial arches and the lateral anlage. By week 7, these fuse and are pulled into position by descent of the heart, and they remain attached to the pharyngeal floor by a fibrous stalk. Typically, the stalk fragments, leaving the foramen caecum between the anterior and

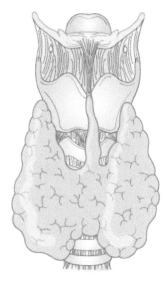

Figure 77.1   Relationship of the thyroid gland, larynx, and trachea.

posterior two thirds of the tongue. This tract can persist, forming a thyroglossal duct cyst, a midline swelling that may require excision.

Microscopic Anatomy

Thyroid cells are organised into functional lobules surrounding a lobular artery. Lobules contain 20–40 spherical follicles lined by a single layer of follicular cells around a collection of colloid. The basal and apical layers of the follicular cells are bound by tight junctions to allow control of the release of thyroid hormones. In response to thyroid-stimulating hormone (TSH), follicular cells adopt a columnar shape, and their apical surfaces protrude microvilli to facilitate reabsorption of colloid.

Follicles are located within a loose connective tissue stroma containing extensive capillary networks arranged into angiofollicular units. Parafollicular C cells can be found either individually or within small clusters throughout the stroma, and they are responsible for secretion of calcitonin.

Physiology of the Thyroid Gland

Thyroid hormones are vital to the regulation and stimulation of cell metabolism; thus, they have a number of significant systemic effects on bone, the cardiovascular system, and the central nervous system.

Synthesis of Thyroid Hormones

The thyroid produces two thyroid hormones, tetraiodothyronine (T_4) and triiodothyronine (T_3). Eighty percent of production comprises T_4. T_4 is converted to T_3 in the peripheral circulation. T_3 is more biologically active, with a fivefold greater potency and a shorter half-life (1.5 days for T_3 vs 7 days for T_4). Serum T_3 and T_4 concentrations are maintained peripherally by plasma thyroxine-binding globulins, with only a small volume of free hormones available to stimulate physiological effects.

Synthesis and release of thyroid hormones begin with absorption of iodine from the small intestine. Thyroid cells actively concentrate iodine at a level 20–50 times higher than plasma levels. Within the follicular cells, iodine is oxidised and bound to thyroglobulin. Thyroglobulin forms the polypeptide framework from which T_3 and T_4 are synthesised. Production of thyroglobulin is unique to the thyroid; it can therefore serve as a tumour marker following total thyroidectomy and radioiodine treatment for thyroid cancer.

When stimulated, follicular cells reabsorb thyroglobulin, breaking it down into diiodotyrosine (DIT) and monoiodotyrosine (MIT) using lysosomal proteases. DIT and MIT are then

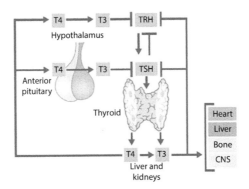

Figure 77.2 Feedback inhibition of thyroid hormones.

oxidised into T_3 and T_4 in a process mediated by thyroid peroxidase (TPO). The presence of TPO antibodies can result in autoimmune thyroiditis.

Control of Thyroid Hormone Synthesis
The negative feedback loop of the hypothalamic-pituitary axis (HPA) controls release of T_3 and T_4 (Figure 77.2). A low metabolic rate or a reduction in circulating T_3 stimulates the release of thyrotropin-releasing hormone (TRH) by the hypothalamus. TRH stimulates the anterior pituitary gland, releasing TSH, which binds to TSH receptors on follicular cells. This results in a cascade ending in release of T_3. Conversely, a high serum concentration of T_3 directly inhibits release of TRH and TSH.

Calcitonin
Calcitonin is produced by the parafollicular C cells. It counteracts parathyroid hormone action by reducing calcium reabsorption from bones and kidney tubules in response to hypercalcaemia and hypergastrinaemia. Its role in humans is thought to be negligible.

Anatomy of the Parathyroid Glands

Macroscopic Anatomy
The parathyroid glands are two small pairs of yellow-brown ovoid organs located posterior to the thyroid gland. The glands are surrounded by a thin capsule that is frequently continuous with the capsule of the thyroid, and they average 6 mm by 3–4 mm in size.

In 84% of patients, there are four parathyroid glands: two superior glands found 1 cm above the inferior thyroid artery, and two inferior glands within approximately 1 cm of the lower pole of the thyroid. The glands can have highly variable anatomy, and their number can vary between 2 and 12. The inferior parathyroid's embryological development from the third branchial arch and its descent with the thymus means they can have a variable location. Supernumerary and ectopic glands can be found within the thymus, posterior neck, retropharyngeal space, and mediastinum.

The inferior thyroid arteries supply blood to the parathyroid glands with anastomoses with the superior thyroid arteries, the parathyroid veins drain into the thyroid's venous plexus. Lymphatic drainage occurs via the deep cervical and paratracheal chains.

Microscopic Anatomy
Parathyroid lobules contain clusters of parenchymal cells surrounded by a fibrovascular stroma with a rich capillary network. The most prominent cell type is the chief (principal) cell; chief cells are responsible for production of parathyroid hormone (PTH). Larger and less prevalent are the oxyphil cells. The function of oxyphil cells is not well understood.

Physiology of the Parathyroid Glands
The parathyroid glands release PTH, which regulates calcium homeostasis. The concentration of PTH and calcium is governed by a negative feedback loop independent of the HPA.

Calcium Homeostasis

Over 99% of human calcium reserves (approximately 1.1 kg) are stored in bones and teeth. Around 50% of the remaining free calcium is ionised and is essential to the cell signalling pathways of the heart, blood, muscles, and central nervous system. The remainder is bound to proteins, such as albumin, which can change depending on the pH of blood.

The parathyroid glands release PTH when calcium-sensing receptors (CaSR) detect a reduction in extracellular calcium concentration. PTH release is inversely proportional to serum calcium levels. PTH acts via physiological effects on the bones and kidneys. PTH has a short half-life of just 3 min, and concentrations change within 1 min, peak in 4–10 min, and decline again within 60 min.

In the kidneys, PTH blocks the reabsorption of phosphate at the proximal tubule while increasing reabsorption of calcium within the ascending loop of Henle and distal and collecting tubules. Within the proximal renal tubules, PTH activates the enzyme 1-hydroxylase, which converts vitamin D to its active form calcitriol.

In bone, PTH stimulates calcium reabsorption in slow and fast phases. The slow phase results in proliferation, differentiation, and activation of osteoclasts over the course of several days. The fast phase occurs over a period of minutes, but its physiological mechanism is not well understood.

Vitamin D

Vitamin D regulates calcium homeostasis at a slower rate than PTH (Figure 77.3). Within the skin, UVB light changes 7-dehydroxycholesterol into vitamin D_3 (cholecalciferol), which undergoes 25-hydroxylation in the liver and 1-hydroxylation in the kidneys to form 1,25-dihydroxycholecalciferol (calcitriol). Calcitriol raises serum calcium levels through increased absorption from the small intestine and, in conjunction with PTH, increases the rate of renal and bone calcium reabsorption.

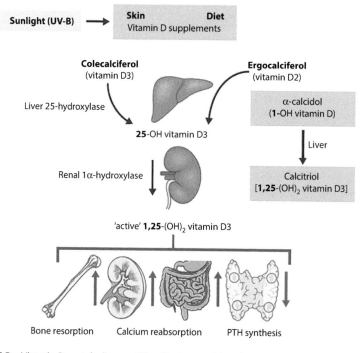

Figure 77.3   Vitamin D metabolism and its effects on calcium homeostasis.

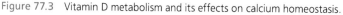

Post-Operative Hypoparathyroidism

Post-operative hypoparathyroidism can result in life-threatening hypocalcaemia. It occurs secondary to accidental devascularisation or excision of all four parathyroid glands. Early symptoms include finger, toe, and peri-oral numbness or tingling, with more acute symptoms including papilloedema, tetany, seizures, and death. Avoidance of life-threatening hypocalcaemia is achieved through monitoring of post-operative serum calcium and PTH, prompt replacement of falling serum calcium levels, and correction of pre-operative vitamin D deficiency.

KEY POINTS

- TSH is the best parameter for assessing thyroid function and monitoring replacement therapy.
- TSH reacts slowly to changes in hormone supply, especially after long-term dysfunction. Here, T_4 monitoring gives more timely information.
- Thyroid hormone replacement with levothyroxine (T_4) is standard. Replacement with T_3 is more likely to result in fluctuations of thyroid function tests and side effects.
- PTH concentrations alter within 1 min, peak in 4–10 min, and decline in 60 min.
- PTH deficiency after damage to the parathyroids can result in life-threatening hypocalcaemia.
- Vitamin D deficiency in patients with primary hypoparathyroidism may introduce additional (secondary) stimulation to the parathyroid glands.

---

78. THYROID AND PARATHYROID PATHOLOGY

The Normal Thyroid Gland

The thyroid gland is a bilobate structure, typically weighing between 15 g and 25 g. It is comprised of lobules of colloid-containing follicles lined by a monolayer of bland follicular epithelial cells, surrounded by a thin fibrous pseudocapsule. A subpopulation of parafollicular/C cells are present within the stroma.

Fine-Needle Aspiration Cytology (FNAC)

- FNAC is a useful first-line investigation of a thyroid mass (see Chapter 80, Evaluation and Investigation of Thyroid Disease).
- Some lesions can be confidently diagnosed (e.g. papillary thyroid carcinoma).
- Distinction between hyperplastic nodules and follicular neoplasms may not always be achievable on FNAC.
- It is not possible to distinguish between a follicular adenoma and carcinoma on FNAC.
- FNAC can induce histological changes that may modulate or obscure underlying pathology.

Thyroglossal Tract Abnormalities

Thyroglossal duct remnants (cysts, sinuses, and fistulae) are common and can occur at almost any site, from the base of the tongue to the suprasternal region.

Thyroid Gland Pathology

Thyroiditis

Thyroiditis can be autoimmune (e.g. Hashimoto's thyroiditis and Graves' disease) or non-autoimmune (e.g. subacute thyroiditis, drug-induced thyroiditis, infectious thyroiditis, and Riedel's thyroiditis). While there are recognised pathological features in each, the diagnosis is usually dependent on clinical, radiological, and serological findings.

Hyperplastic Nodules

Nodules in a multinodular goiter are designated hyperplastic nodules and are comprised of numerous follicles, often with a growth pattern similar to that in the adjacent gland. Bland papillary structures may be seen. They are sometimes surrounded by a thin capsule and often show secondary changes, such as fibrosclerosis, cystic degeneration, calcification, and haemorrhage.

Follicular Adenoma

Follicular adenoma classically occurs as a solitary, encapsulated tumour that shows follicular epithelial differentiation with no evidence of capsular/vascular invasion and no features of papillary thyroid carcinoma. An adenoma can show a variety of growth patterns, although the architecture tends to be uniform. Mitoses are few. Several distinct histological subtypes are recognised, although they do not differ in biological behaviour from a conventional adenoma.

Follicular Thyroid Carcinoma

Follicular thyroid carcinoma is a malignant tumour showing follicular differentiation, with no features of papillary thyroid carcinoma. It can be minimally or widely invasive. Meticulous examination of the tumour/capsule interface is required to make the diagnosis.

Minimally invasive follicular carcinoma is a follicular neoplasm showing capsular invasion and/or pericapsular vascular invasion (Figure 78.1). The presence of angioinvasion is associated with aggressive behaviour.

Widely invasive follicular carcinoma is an aggressive neoplasm with a high risk of metastases. Characteristically, there is infiltrative, destructive, or multinodular growth of tumour cells through the capsule. Extrathyroidal extension and vascular invasion are common.

Oncocytic (Oxyphil) Cell Tumours

Oncocytic change (swelling, with granular, mitochondrial-rich cytoplasm)

- Common in benign and malignant conditions in the thyroid.
- Masses with 75% or more oncocytic cells are designated oncocytic tumours.
- Oncocytic tumours are subclassified according to the same criteria as their non-oncocytic counterparts (e.g. oncocytic adenoma, carcinoma, etc.).
- More oncocytic tumours are malignant than standard follicular lesions are.

Papillary Thyroid Carcinoma

Papillary thyroid carcinoma (PTC) is the most common thyroid malignancy and has an excellent prognosis.

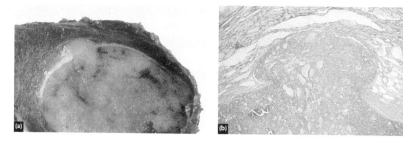

Figure 78.1 Macroscopic (a) and microscopic (b) capsular invasion.

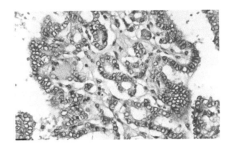

Figure 78.2 Characteristic nuclear features of PTC—nuclear crowding, overlap, and nuclear grooves.

The principal defining feature of PTC is its nuclear morphology. Distinctive appearances may be localised; therefore, adequate sampling is essential.

Characteristic nuclear features of PTC (Figure 78.2) are:

- Nuclear enlargement, crowding, and overlapping
- Margination of chromatin ('ground glass' nuclei)
- Longitudinal nuclear grooves and nuclear irregularity
- Intranuclear cytoplasmic inclusions

Other non-nuclear features include a papillary architecture, multinucleate giant cells, hypereosinophilic colloid, and psammoma bodies.

There are a number of recognised variants of PTC, some of which have a more aggressive behaviour (e.g. tall cell, diffuse sclerosing, diffuse follicular, solid, and trabecular variants). Other poor prognostic indicators are increased mitoses, necrosis, extrathyroidal extension, increasing size, and nodal metastases.

Papillary microcarcinomas are less than 10 mm and often an incidental finding. They are commonly multicentric, and while they may metastasise to local lymph nodes, they generally pursue an indolent clinical course.

Follicular-Patterned Tumours of Uncertain Malignant Potential
Encapsulated follicular-patterned lesions with equivocal capsular/vascular invasion and no features of PTC are termed follicular tumours of uncertain malignant potential (FT-UMP).

The follicular variant of papillary thyroid carcinoma (FVPTC) is the most common PTC and can be classified into invasive and encapsulated variants. A group of tumours exist that are classified as non-invasive follicular thyroid neoplasm with papillary-like nuclear features (NIFTP). These are associated with an excellent clinical outcome and can be managed more conservatively than malignant tumours. Stringent histological criteria are used to define a NIFTP, and they require careful assessment of the entire lesion.

Poorly Differentiated Thyroid Carcinoma
Poorly differentiated thyroid carcinoma shows limited evidence of follicular differentiation, with biological behaviour intermediate between differentiated thyroid carcinoma and undifferentiated/anaplastic carcinoma. The diagnosis is based upon growth pattern (typically insular), mitotic activity, and necrosis. Minor elements of classical PTC and/or follicular carcinoma may be recognised.

Undifferentiated (Anaplastic) Thyroid Carcinoma
Anaplastic carcinoma is a highly malignant tumour typically seen in elderly patients that has a high mortality. It can arise de novo or result from dedifferentiation of an existing neoplasm. It is usually widely invasive and inoperable at presentation. The pathology varies, with the two main patterns being epithelioid and sarcomatoid.

Medullary Thyroid Carcinoma (MTC)

MTC is a calcitonin-secreting malignant tumour arising from parafollicular/C cells. It can occur sporadically or in the context of a mutation of the *RET* proto-oncogene (seen in multiple endocrine neoplasia and familial MTC). Microscopically, tumours can be well demarcated or infiltrative and comprise solid sheets, nests, and trabecula of cells separated by fibrovascular septa. There is usually only modest nuclear pleomorphism, but necrosis may be a feature. Amyloid protein deposition is present in around 80% of cases.

Other Neoplasms and Tumour-Like Lesions

The thyroid is commonly affected by metastases, most often from the lung, breast, skin, and kidney cancers.

There are numerous other neoplasms that can occur in the thyroid, including hyalinizing trabecular tumour, squamous cell carcinoma, and mucoepidermoid carcinoma.

Thyroid Cancer Staging

Thyroid carcinomas are staged using the UICC/TNM8 system (Table 78.1). Stage is dependent upon tumour size and the amount of extrathyroidal extension. Anaplastic carcinomas are by definition pT4.

Table 78.1   TNM8 staging of thyroid carcinoma

TNM clinical classification		
T–primary tumour*		
TX	Primary tumour cannot be assessed	
T0	No evidence of primary tumour	
T1	Tumour 2 cm or less in greatest dimension, limited to the thyroid	
	T1a	Tumour 1 cm or less in greatest dimension, limited to the thyroid
	T1b	Tumour more than 1 cm but not more than 2 cm in greatest dimension, limited to the thyroid
T2	Tumour more than 2 cm but not more than 4 cm in greatest dimension, limited to the thyroid	
T3	Tumour more than 4 cm in greatest dimension, limited to the thyroid, with gross extrathyroidal extension invading only strap muscles (sternohyoid, sternothyroid, or omohyoid muscles)	
	T3a	Tumour more than 4 cm in greatest dimension, limited to the thyroid
	T3b	Tumour of any size with gross extrathyroidal extension invading strap muscles (sternohyoid, sternothyroid, or omohyoid muscles)
T4a	Tumour extends beyond the thyroid capsule and invades any of the following: subcutaneous soft tissues, larynx, trachea, oesophagus, recurrent laryngeal nerve	
T4b	Tumour invades prevertebral fascia or mediastinal vessels, or encases carotid artery	
Note: *Including papillary, follicular, poorly differentiated, Hürthle cell, and anaplastic carcinomas.		
N – regional lymph nodes		
NX	Regional lymph nodes cannot be assessed	
N0	No regional lymph node metastasis	
N1	Regional lymph node metastasis	
	N1a	Metastasis in Level VI (pretracheal, paratracheal, and prelaryngeal/Delphian lymph nodes) or upper/superior mediastinum
	N1b	Metastasis in other unilateral, bilateral, or contralateral cervical nodes (Levels I, II, III, IV or V) or retropharyngeal nodes
M – distant metastasis		
M0	No distant metastasis	
M1	Distant metastasis	

Normal Parathyroid Glands

Most individuals possess at least two pairs of parathyroid glands, AND each gland weighs approximately 0.03 g. Microscopically, they have a lobulated appearance and are composed of chief, oxyphil, and water-clear cells arranged in nests and trabeculae in a richly vascularised stroma interspersed with adipocytes.

Parathyroid Gland Pathology

Parathyroid Gland Adenoma

Parathyroid adenoma is the predominant cause of primary hyperparathyroidism. It can occur spontaneously or within the context of various syndromes. Excision of the abnormal gland is curative.

Pathological distinction between hyperplasia and adenoma can be difficult. Adenomas typically affect one gland and are well circumscribed, with a mean weight of 0.55 g. Microscopically, they are hypercellular, with a loss of intraglandular adipocytes and a peripheral rim of normal tissue. Most are composed of chief cells, which can be arranged in a number of patterns.

Several subtypes are recognised, including cystic adenoma, lipoadenoma, papillary variant, water-clear adenoma, follicular variant, and oxyphil adenoma.

An atypical parathyroid adenoma is a descriptive term applied to a tumour that displays suspicious/atypical features but falls short of a confident designation of malignancy.

Parathyroid Carcinoma

Parathyroid carcinoma is rare. It is slow-growing and tends to invade local structures and to metastasise late. Complete excision at first operation affords the best opportunity for cure, although it relies upon early recognition of malignancy.

Carcinomas can be encapsulated or infiltrative. Microscopically, the appearances can vary from deceptively bland to overtly malignant. Biological behaviour ultimately distinguishes carcinoma from adenoma.

Absolute histological criteria to diagnose carcinoma are local invasion and metastatic disease. In the absence of these, secondary criteria can be used, which include capsular/vascular invasion, broad intralesional fibrous septae, coagulative necrosis, increased mitotic activity, abundant macronuclei and diffuse growth/cellular atypia.

The proposed staging classification for parathyroid carcinoma is shown in Table 78.2.

Other Parathyroid Gland Tumours

Parathyroid cysts, branchiogenic cysts, amyloidosis, paragangliomas, and secondary neoplasms can occur in the parathyroid glands.

Table 78.2 Proposed TNM staging for parathyroid carcinoma

T – primary tumour	
TX	Primary tumour cannot be assessed
T0	No evidence of primary tumour
Tis	Atypical parathyroid neoplasm (neoplasm of uncertain malignant potential)
T1	Localised to the parathyroid gland with extension limited to soft tissue
T2	Direct invasion into the thyroid gland
T3	Direct invasion into laryngeal nerve, oesophagus, trachea, skeletal muscle, adjacent lymph nodes, or thymus
T4	Direct invasion into major blood vessels or spine
N – regional lymph nodes	
NX	Regional lymph nodes cannot be assessed
N0	No regional lymph node metastasis
N1	Regional lymph node metastasis
N1a	Metastasis to Level VI (pretracheal, paratracheal, and prelaryngeal/Delphian lymph nodes) or upper/superior mediastinal lymph nodes
N1b	Metastasis to unilateral, bilateral, or contralateral cervical nodes (Levels I, II, III, IV, or V) or retropharyngeal nodes
M – distant metastasis	
M0	No distant metastasis
M1	Distant metastasis
Stage	
There are not enough data to propose a formal staging system at this time.	

Source: Adapted from *AJCC Cancer Staging Manual*, 8th Edition, 2017.

KEY POINTS

- It can be difficult to distinguish primary parathyroid gland hyperplasia and a parathyroid adenoma histologically.
- Parathyroid carcinoma is rare, and the diagnosis requires clinicopathological correlation.

---

79. ENDOCRINE IMAGING

Introduction

In assessing patients with suspected endocrine pathology, imaging is a key investigative step that provides details of anatomy, morphology, and function.

Ultrasound, in general, is the simplest and quickest investigative modality for the head and neck and has the benefit of dynamic vascular assessment as well as guiding fine-needle aspiration (FNA) and core biopsies. Computed tomography (CT), magnetic resonance imaging (MRI), and nuclear medicine studies can provide additional anatomical or functional detail prior to surgical intervention.

Table 79.1   Ultrasound (U) classification of thyroid nodules as recommended by the British Thyroid Association

U classification	Nodule type	Ultrasound characteristics
U1	Normal	
U2	Benign	Vascularity, eggshell calcification, cystic change, isoechoic or mildly hyperechoic
U3	Indeterminate/equivocal	Homogeneous, hyperechoic, equivocal echogenic foci, mixed or central vascularity, solid or halo
U4	Suspicious	Solid, hypoechoic, peripheral calcification, lobulated outline
U5	Malignant	Solid, hypoechoic, lobulated outline, intranodular vascularity, taller > wide, lymphadenopathy

Source: From Table 61.16 in Scott Brown.

Thyroid

Ultrasound is the primary imaging modality for the assessment of the thyroid gland. It is key in identifying thyroid nodules and supports risk stratification in decision-making about sampling concerning nodules.

- Thyroid nodules are clinically palpable in up to 4% of patients.
- 60–70% of patients can be found to have nodules on imaging.
- Various ultrasound features of nodules are indicative of a potential malignancy. The U classification is recommended for assessment and reporting of ultrasound features in the United Kingdom (Table 79.1).
- Where an indeterminate/suspicious nodule is seen, FNA or core biopsy should be undertaken.
- While size of a nodule is often suggested as a criterion, nodule size correlates poorly with risk of malignancy.
- In practice, only nodules >1 cm are sampled.

Thyroid Malignancy

Papillary thyroid cancer (PTC) demonstrates four cardinal signs on ultrasound:

1 Solid and hypoechoic
2 Ill-defined margins
3 Microcalcifications
4 Taller than wide

If none of these four features is present, then the negative predictive value for PTC is more than 97%.

Medullary thyroid cancers (MTC) appear quite similar to PTC on ultrasound, although calcifications can be more globular.

Follicular carcinoma:

- Cannot be differentiated from adenoma on FNA or ultrasound and is diagnosed on pathology after excision.
- Follicular lesions tend to appear hyperechoic, with a low echogenic halo and increased internal blood flow.

Anaplastic thyroid cancer (ATC):

- Presents more commonly in the elderly and demonstrates a rapid, infiltrative progression.
- Ultrasound features are that of a large, solid, hypoechoic, ill-defined mass with evidence of extrathyroidal spread and nodal metastases.
- Core biopsy is superior to fine-needle aspiration cytology (FNAC) for confirming the diagnosis.

Thyroid lymphoma:

- While rare, lymphoma is a recognised thyroid pathology.
- Ultrasound features may be similar to those of ATC.
- Core biopsy is indicated to accurately categorise and differentiate from ATC.

In all cases of suspected or confirmed malignancy, CT will demonstrate nodal staging of disease and local anatomical spread. It won't, however, reliably differentiate malignancy from benign thyroid disease.

Benign Thyroid Disease
Multinodular goitre:

- Ultrasound is the primary tool in assessing for pathological nodules in a large thyroid.
- Targeted FNA should be performed if indicated (see above).
- CT is useful for providing anatomical assessment, particularly in relation to retrosternal extent and tracheal compression/deviation.

Graves' disease:

- On ultrasound, the thyroid appears hyper-reflective, without nodules, and with increased intrinsic blood flow on Doppler.

Hashimoto's thyroiditis:

- On ultrasound, the thyroid appears diffusely hypoechoic, with occasional hyperechoic fibrous bands, and with increased intrinsic blood flow on Doppler.

Parathyroid Glands
Imaging of the parathyroids is usually indicated in hyperparathyroidism to help identify an enlarged or hyperfunctioning gland and to aid targeted surgical excision.

All imaging modalities can be used to complement each other for targeted exploration and excision. While the superior parathyroid glands are fairly consistent in their position, the inferior glands are much more varied.

Ultrasound
Ultrasound is quick and can identify an abnormal gland of at least 10 mm. Abnormal parathyroid glands have low echogenicity compared to the thyroid. However, the sensitivity and specificity of ultrasound are user-dependent. In addition, ultrasound is less reliable when there is an overlying multinodular goitre or the gland is in the tracheo-oesophageal groove or the mediastinum.

Nuclear Imaging
Parathyroid scintigraphy is a common localisation scan technique using a radioisotope. Technetium-99m (^{99m} Tc) is a radioisotope tracer bound to methoxyisobutylisonitrile (MIBI) molecules. It is taken up by both thyroid and parathyroid glands, but clearance is slower with abnormal parathyroid glands. This property is taken advantage of by acquiring serial planar images after administration of tracer. Images can be subtracted from one another to highlight the abnormal gland. While this is useful for visualising all parathyroid glands, including ectopics, it does not provide spatial anatomical detail.

An alternate technique is SPECT (single-photon emission computed tomography), which captures images using a gamma camera. SPECT images can be fused with standard CT images (SPECT-CT) to provide useful anatomical localisation that surgeons can interpret for surgical planning.

Computed Tomography (CT)

On contrast-enhanced CT, parathyroid adenomas show arterial phase enhancement with subsequent rapid washout, whereas lymph nodes show gradual increasing enhancement. This is taken advantage of in multiphase '4D CT', a technique using serial CT sequences acquired at various intervals after contrast administration. However, use of this technique means the patient is exposed to a higher radiation dose.

Pituitary

High-resolution MRI is considered the best modality for pituitary-related diagnostic purposes. It uses a dedicated multiplanar protocol of at least 3-mm slices in both coronal and sagittal planes with pre- and post-contrast enhancement.

CT is usually used for pre-operative planning. The CT sinus protocol provides local nasal and paranasal sinus anatomy for transnasal endoscopic surgery.

Adenomas

Pituitary adenomas can be macroadenomas (>1 cm) or microadenomas (<1 cm), and they account for 10–15% of all intracranial tumours. They usually originate from the anterior pituitary, and macroadenomas often extend through the diaphragma sellae.

Microadenomas are usually seen on imaging done for investigation of hormone dysfunction. On T1-weighted MRI, they appear hypointense compared to normal gland, and they have a slow uptake of contrast. Therefore, serial post-contrast sequences can identify the slow contrast enhancement.

Macroadenomas are usually evident due to damage to local structures. Bony remodeling may be evident on CT if the macroadenoma is slow-growing, or the image may show invasion of bone. On MRI, macroadenomas usually appear isointense and enhance with contrast, with central necrosis appearing hyperintense on T2-weighted images.

There are several features to consider when differentiating sellar masses:

- Location: Is it intrasellar, suprasellar, infundibular, or in a combination of locations?
- Connection: Is the mass separate from the pituitary gland?
- Age of the patient

Meningiomas

Meningiomas mostly appear to arise from the parasellar areas and extend into the sella turcica. They are rare in children. They typically appear hypo- to isointense on T1- and T2-weighted images, with avid post-contrast enhancement. The hallmark sign is a 'dural tail' (Figure 79.1).

Metastases

Metastatic involvement of the pituitary is rare, but lung and breast cancers are the most likely sources. MRI findings can be nonspecific and appear to be adenomas. Metastases can appear as isointense lesions with local invasion of the cavernous sinus and sclerosis of the sella turcica.

Craniopharyngioma

Craniopharyngiomas are the most common suprasellar masses in children. There is a bimodal age distribution, with peaks at 5–10 years and 50–60 years of age. The most common presentation is that of a multilobulated, suprasellar, cystic mass with a solid component and enhancing calcification. Therefore, the mass appears hyperintense on T2-weighted MRI due to the cystic component, with patchy enhancement on T1-weighted post-contrast images. Rathke cleft cysts can appear similar to craniopharyngiomas; however, they do not calcify.

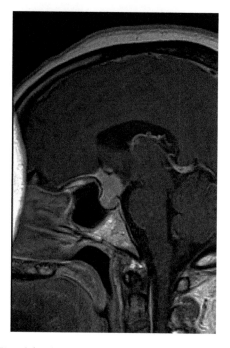

Figure 79.1   Sagittal T1-weighted post-contrast image demonstrates a sella/suprasellar meningioma. It enhances with contrast, and a 'dural tail' is seen as a linear enhancement extending anteriorly. The normal pituitary is visibly separate and non-enhancing within the sella.

KEY POINTS

- Ultrasound is the primary modality for assessing thyroid and parathyroid glands.
- CT helps to provide anatomical detail when used with ultrasound or nuclear imaging to aid surgical planning.
- Functional nuclear medicine imaging using ^{99m}Tc is useful to identify metabolically abnormal parathyroid glands.
- Primary imaging for pituitary glands is multiplanar MRI with pre- and post-contrast sequences.
- Differentiating pituitary masses depends upon their location, the age of the patient, and clinical signs and symptoms.

80.   EVALUATION AND INVESTIGATION OF THYROID DISEASE

CLINICAL EVALUATION OF THYROID DISORDERS

Functional Disorders

Functional disorders relate to the activity of the thyroid gland. They affect 2% of the population, and they are more common in females (M:F ratio is 1:10).

Functional disorders are further divided into reduced thyroid function (hypothyroidism) and increased thyroid activity (hyperthyroidism).

Hypothyroidism

The most common causes of hypothyroidism include chronic autoimmune thyroiditis (Hashimoto's thyroiditis) and iodine deficiency.

Secondary hypothyroidism is commonly a result of hypothalamic or pituitary insufficiency.

Symptoms

Patients usually present with a combination of symptoms that include fatigue, weight gain with poor appetite, feeling cold, poor concentration and memory, hoarseness, shortness of breath, abnormal sensation, constipation, dyspepsia, and altered menstruation.

Extreme hypothyroidism can result in coma, and congenital untreated hypothyroidism is the cause of cretinism.

Signs

Common signs on physical examination are dry coarse skin, cool extremities, hair loss, and bradycardia.

Rarer signs are Reinke's oedema, myxoedema, delayed tendon reflexes, carpal tunnel syndrome, pleural or pericardial effusion, and ascites.

Hyperthyroidism

The most common causes of hyperthyroidism are Graves' disease, toxic multinodular goitre, and toxic adenoma.

Symptoms

The common presenting symptoms of hyperthyroidism are weight loss, nervousness, anxiety, irritability, sweating, palpitations and tremor, thin skin, muscle weakness, and gastrointestinal and menstrual disturbances.

In extreme cases, the following symptoms can co-exist: tachydysrhythmia, pyrexia, vomiting, diarrhea, and mental agitation. This is a medical emergency known as thyroid storm and requires urgent attention because it has a 20–50% mortality rate.

In Graves' disease, eye symptoms can be evident due to thyroid ophthalmopathy; patients present with exophthalmos, diplopia (particularly on upward gaze) in adduction, and a staring appearance.

Signs

On examination, signs of hyperthyroidism include perspiration, agitation, tremor; palmar erythema, proximal muscle wasting, tachycardia, and/or atrial fibrillation.

In Graves' ophthalmopathy, eye signs include axial proptosis with lid lag (von Graefe's sign), lid retraction (Dalrymple's sign), conjunctival injection (Goldzeiher's sign), and optical neuropathy.

Thyroid dermopathy (pretibial myxoedema with waxy, indurated, itchy skin that can spread onto the foot and rarely other body parts) and thyroid acropathy (soft tissue swelling of hands, with occasional clubbing) are also signs of Graves' disease.

Structural Disorders

Structural disorders are disorders affecting the thyroid parenchyma, resulting in thyroid nodules.

They are palpable in only 3–7% of the adult population, but their prevalence increases up to 70% following ultrasonographic assessment.

Thyroid Nodules

Most thyroid nodules are solitary, but they may be part of a multinodular goitre, which can be focal, diffuse, or associated with thyroiditis. Thyroid nodules can be benign or malignant, with the latter being more common after radiation exposure and with a family history of a first-degree relative with thyroid cancer.

Underlying Systemic Disorders

Structural thyroid disorder can arise as part of an underlying systemic disorder. Medullary cancer exists as part of the multiple endocrine neoplasia syndrome type 2 (MEN 2) in 20% of cases. Thyroid lymphoma can occur in isolation or as part of a wider haematological malignancy.

Symptoms

Patients commonly present with a painless, sometimes incidental, neck lump. Pain and rapid increase in size are commonly associated with bleeding into a pre-existing cyst but can be also suggestive of malignancy, especially if hoarseness co-exists. Large goitres can cause compressive symptoms of dysphagia, dyspnoea, or stridor.

Signs

The most common examination finding is midline neck lump with elevation on swallowing. Lymphadenopathy and lump fixation to surrounding structures are worrying features. Retrosternal extension is suspected if the lower extent of the thyroid is impalpable. Tracheal deviation can be seen secondary to compression and superior vena cava obstruction is seen secondary to venous compression.

Venous congestion is elicited by raising both arms until they are touching the sides of the face, causing cyanosis and respiratory distress (Pemberton's sign).

Endoscopic signs include Reinke's oedema, tracheal deviation, and direct invasion of the upper aerodigestive tract.

Investigation of Thyroid Disorders

Biochemical Thyroid Function Tests

Serum Thyroid-Stimulating Hormone (TSH) Measurement

TSH is measured using antibody immunoassays. Generally, normal TSH rules out thyroid dysfunction, but an elevated or suppressed TSH level should be considered in association with the serum free thyroxine (FT_4) and free serum triiodothyronine (FT_3) levels. Primary hypothyroidism causes elevated TSH, whereas primary thyrotoxicosis causes TSH suppression (Table 80.1). The normal reference range for TSH is 0.4–4.5 mU/L, but it can be affected by pregnancy, age, genetic factors, obesity, and nonthyroidal conditions.

Table 80.1 Factors affecting the measurements of serum TSH, FT_3, and FT_4

	TSH	FT_4/FT_3
Primary hypothyroidism Subclinical Overt	↑	Normal ↓ FT_4, ↓ FT_3 in 25%
Primary hyperthyroidism Subclinical Overt	↓	Normal ↑ FT_3 earlier; ↑ FT_4 usually
Pituitary and hypothalamic disease TSH-secreting Destructive	↑ ↓	↑ ↓ FT_4; FT_3 normal or ↓
Nonthyroidal illness (including psychiatric disease)	Usually ↓	p
Pregnancy	↓ (1st trimester)	Normal (1st trimester) ↓ (by 30% in last trimester)
Drugs • Dopamine, somatostatin, glucocorticoid • Propylthiouracil, amiodarone	↓ -	Normal FT_3/FT_4 ratio <0.3
Thyroid hormone resistance	↑	↑
Activating TSH receptor mutations	↓	↑
Hydatidiform mole, choriocarcinoma	↓	↑
TSH assay interference	↑	Normal

FT_3 and FT_4 Measurement

FT_3 and FT_4 are measured using immunoassays. Subclinical hypo- or hyperthyroidism involves elevated/suppressed TSH levels with normal FT_4 and FT_3 findings. In subclinical disease, TSH and FT_4 should be retested after 3 months to assess for disease progression.

TSH, FT_4, and FT_3 are measured during assessment of symptomatic thyroid disorders.

Routine neonatal TSH screening is performed with a heel-prick test.

In patients taking antithyroid medication for hyperthyroidism, FT_4 monitoring is the test of choice, as TSH can remain suppressed even after treatment cessation. FT_3 is the more accurate measurement for patients taking propylthiouracil because its action blocks FT_4 di-iodination.

In treatment with radioiodine, TSH and FT_4 should be measured 6 and 12 weeks after the first treatment and then every 3 months for the first year, with annual measurements thereafter.

Monitoring of thyroxine replacement after thyroidectomy or for primary hypothyroidism evaluates TSH levels. TSH should be measured 2 months following initiation or adjustment in the treatment regime to allow TSH stabilisation. Once the patient has stabilised, annual TSH measurement will suffice.

For secondary hypothyroidism, FT_4 level is the only available monitoring measurement, aiming for levels in the upper third of the reference range.

Causes of Thyroid Dysfunction

Thyroid Antibodies

Thyroid antibodies are found in around 10% of the healthy, euthyroid population. Thyroid peroxidase (TPO) antibody immunoassays are usually used in isolation for diagnosis of autoimmune thyroid disease, including overt hypothyroidism and Hashimoto's thyroiditis.

Thyroglobulin antibody (TgAb) immunoassay is used for monitoring of differentiated thyroid cancer recurrence postoperatively (see below).

TSH-receptor antibodies (TRAb) are measured in the diagnosis of Graves' disease. They have a 95% sensitivity and 100% specificity for diagnosis of Graves' disease in patients presenting with hyperthyroidism.

High TRAb is a poor prognostic factor for development of Graves' ophthalmopathy and can be also used for diagnosing euthyroid Graves' ophthalmopathy as well as predicting neonatal Graves' disease.

Erythrocyte Sedimentation Rate (Esr) and C-Reactive Protein (Crp)

ESR and CRP can be high in subacute thyroiditis, acute suppurative thyroiditis, and occasionally in Hashimoto's thyroiditis.

Thyroglobulin (TG)

TG is a normal protein produced by thyroid follicular cells. The measurement of TG is only reliable in a patient who has negative TgAb. A low serum TG level before radioiodine ablation of any thyroid remnant has 94% negative predictive value for the absence of disease at future follow-up. There is no utility in measuring TG in the initial evaluation of a thyroid nodule.

Nature of Structural Thyroid Lesions

Scintiscanning

The use of radioiodine scintiscanning has declined because it less sensitive and specific than thyroid blood tests and ultrasound. ^{99m}Tc or ^{123}I were most frequently used for:

- Localisation of congenital anatomical thyroid defects
- Differentiating between destructive thyroiditis (subacute, postpartum) and hyperthyroidism (Graves' disease or nodular thyroid disease), in which the isotope is reduced ('cold'—nonfunctional) and increased ('hot'—functional), respectively

- Identifying solitary hyperfunctioning nodules (increased uptake)
- Monitoring of treated thyroid cancer (see Chapter 82, Management of Differentiated Thyroid Cancer)

Ultrasound (US)

US is recommended in the evaluation of all clinically significant thyroid nodules and incidental findings on other investigative modalities (see Chapter 79, Endocrine Imaging).

- Nodules with normal or benign US characteristics do not require further investigation.
- US is used for diagnostic purposes and to guide biopsies.
- During follow-up, US is used for detection of locoregional recurrent thyroid cancer.

Fine-Needle Aspiration Cytology (FNAC)

FNAC is the gold-standard investigation in the evaluation of thyroid nodules after US assessment.

The cytological classification of fine-needle aspiration findings introduced by the American Thyroid Association (ATA) is called the Bethesda System, and the classification used by the British Thyroid Association (BTA) is called the RCPath Thy System. Both systems are used to guide clinicians in the management of thyroid nodules.

Nodules of Thy3f-4-5 (or Bethesda IV–VI) require surgical resection for final diagnosis (Table 80.2).

Other Imaging Techniques

Computed tomography (CT) and magnetic resonance imaging (MRI) are used in conjunction with US assessment for the evaluation of substernal components in large goiters and for staging of thyroid malignancy. Positron emission tomography (PET) also has been used to localise thyroid cancer recurrence when TG levels are high with inconclusive CT scans, but its overall sensitivity and specificity are low.

Table 80.2 Cytological classifications of fine-needle aspirates and the corresponding management

Diagnostic category		Cytological diagnosis	Management
Thy classification	Bethesda system		
Thy1	I	Nondiagnostic	US assessment ± repeat FNA
Thy2	II	Benign	Correlate with US and clinical findings
Thy3	III	Neoplasia/atypia possible Thy3a—atypia Thy3f—atypia (possible follicular neoplasm)	Repeat US-guided FNAC Diagnostic hemithyroidectomy
Thy4	IV–V	Suspicious of malignancy	Diagnostic hemithyroidectomy
Thy5	VI	Diagnostic of malignancy	Total thyroidectomy

KEY POINTS

- Thyroid disorders are divided into functional and structural abnormalities.
- A nodule is the commonest presentation of thyroid malignancy.
- Normal TSH rules out thyroid dysfunction.
- The presence of TSH-receptor antibodies and thyrotoxicosis is diagnostic of Graves' disease.
- US ± FNAC is the investigation of choice of initial assessment of structural thyroid lesions.

81. BENIGN THYROID DISEASE

Introduction
Benign thyroid disease encompasses abnormal enlargement of the thyroid gland, thyroid hormone imbalance, and thyroid tenderness.

Hyperthyroidism
Hyperthyroidism is diagnosed by suppressed levels of thyroid-stimulating hormone (TSH) and increased thyroxine (T_4)/triiodothyronine (T_3). Thyrotoxicosis is driven by β-adrenergic overactivity and the intracellular action of thyroid hormone. Hyperthyroidism is ten times more common in females than in males, and the incidence increases with age. T_3 toxicosis accounts for 10% of thyrotoxicosis. The signs and symptoms of hyperthyroidism are shown in Table 81.1.

Graves' Disease
Graves' disease is the commonest cause of thyrotoxicosis in iodine-replete regions of the world. It is five times more common in females than in males, with a peak incidence in the twenties and thirties. It is characterised by a syndrome of hyperthyroidism, diffuse goitre, ophthalmopathy, and dermopathy. The pathogenesis is an autoimmune condition with IgG autoantibodies targeting TSH receptors (TRAb) and stimulating thyroid hormone synthesis and secretion. Increased expression of fibroblast growth factor, found in the majority of patients, leads to a diffuse goiter.

Onset of symptoms is usually gradual and insidious. Ophthalmopathy is found in half of patients and is due to swelling of the extraocular muscles, proliferation of periorbital fat, and muscle fibrosis leading to muscle tethering. Smoking doubles the risk of ophthalmopathy. Exophthalmos and eyelid retraction are common clinical findings, and in severe cases, corneal ulceration may develop.

Diagnosis is made in the hyperthyroid patient by measuring TRAb. Management is categorised into medical, radioiodine, and surgical options. Graves' disease is rarely self-limiting.

Antithyroid drugs are first-line medical management and are tried for 12–18 months, with a third of patients achieving lasting remission. Poor prognostic factors for relapse in patients treated medically initially are shown in Table 81.2.

Table 81.1   Signs and symptoms of hyperthyroidism

Symptoms	Signs
Weight loss	Sinus tachycardia
Anxiety	Atrial fibrillation
Agitation	Fine tremor
Irritability	Warm, moist skin
Palpitation	Palmar erythema
Fatigue and weakness	Onycholysis
Breathlessness	Hair loss
Heat intolerance	Proximal myopathy
Sweating	Muscle wasting
Increased appetite	High-output heart failure
Menstrual irregularity	Thyroid bruit
Hair loss	
Brittle nails	

Table 81.2 Poor prognostic factors for relapse of medically treated Graves' disease

Factor type	Prognostic factor
Demographic	Male sex
	Age <40 years
Clinical history	Repeated episodes of relapse
	Presence of a large goitre
Biochemical	Severe biochemical disease
	Greatly increased T_3:T_4 ratio
	High levels of TSH receptor antibodies

Radioiodine can exacerbate eye symptoms and is relatively contraindicated in patients with ophthalmopathy (steroid cover required), and it is absolutely contraindicated in pregnancy and breast-feeding. A total thyroidectomy offers cure with a low recurrence rate.

Toxic Multinodular Goitre

Toxic multinodular goitre is the most common cause of hyperthyroidism in the elderly in iodine-deficient regions. Atrial fibrillation is the principal sign. Definitive treatment is with radioiodine, resulting in permanent hypothyroidism in most patients. Surgery (total thyroidectomy/thyroid lobectomy) is reserved for patients with compressive symptoms, patients with large goitre and cosmetic concerns, or patients with contraindications to radioiodine.

Solitary Toxic Adenoma

Solitary toxic adenoma is a benign tumour that autonomously secretes thyroid hormone and that results from TSH receptor activation. It occurs commonly in the fourth and fifth decades and is an uncommon cause of thyrotoxicosis (5%). Many patients have a palpable nodule, although the autonomously functional thyroid tissue can be diffuse. Radionuclide scanning differentiates a solitary toxic adenoma from other causes by demonstrating a focus of isotope accumulation, a 'hot spot'. Radioiodine treatment is ideal because radioiodine is preferentially taken up in the hyperfunctioning nodule, sparing the rest of the gland.

Destructive Thyroiditis

Destructive thyroiditis is an inflammatory condition of the thyroid and is categorised into conditions that are painful and those that are not (Table 81.3).

Treatment of Thyrotoxicosis

Treatment strategies for thyrotoxicosis are categorised into medical, nuclear medicine, and surgical approaches. Medical management entails antithyroid drugs ± beta blockers. Thionamines are prescribed in a 'block and replace' or titration regimen. The most common side-effect is pruritic rash. The most serious side-effects are agranulocytosis and liver failure. Lugol's iodine solution is variably used as a second-line control in the work-up for surgery. Radioiodine is safe and effective and is considered first-line treatment in the elderly and those with cardiac dysfunction who may not tolerate physiological stress of surgery. Surgery is the preferred option in toxic multinodular goitre, in those with compressive symptoms, and in Graves' disease associated with eye disease.

Pre-Operative Preparation of Hyperthyroid Patients

Thyroid surgery can result in the liberation of preformed thyroid hormone, precipitating 'thyroid storm', which has a mortality of up to 50%. Avoidance by pre-operative preparation is paramount and involves antithyroid drugs to restore euthyroidism, beta-adrenergic blockade, and Lugol's iodine, which can reduce the vascularity of the thyroid.

Hypothyroidism

Hypothyroiidism is insufficient production and secretion of thyroid hormones. It affects females more frequently than males, with a peak incidence in the forties and fifties. The most common cause in iodine-replete regions is Hashimoto's thyroiditis, and iodine deficiency in nonreplete regions. Myxedema refers to accumulation of glycosaminoglycans in the dermis in the context of severe hypothyroidism. It is most easily identified in the lower leg, as pre-tibial myxedema.

The clinical effects of hypothyroidism can be categorised into generalised slowing of metabolic processes and an accumulation of glycosaminoglycans. The diagnosis is made by low serum T_4 concentrations in the presence of normal levels of TSH.

Management entails returning the patient to a euthyroid state clinically and biochemically with levothyroxine replacement.

Hashimoto's Thyroiditis (Chronic Autoimmune Hypothyroidism)

Hashimoto's thyroiditis is characterised by diffuse lymphocytic infiltration of the thyroid gland in the presence of circulating anti-TPO antibodies causing follicular destruction and fibrosis. Patients may have subclinical hypothyroidism at initiation but progress to hypothyroidism over the years.

Thyroid Disease in Pregnancy

Hyperthyroidism

Thyroid disease in pregnancy is associated with adverse outcomes; therefore, a euthyroid state is required throughout pregnancy to limit developmental risk to the fetus. High levels of HCG in pregnancy can cause a transient hyperthyroidism by stimulating TSH receptors.

In Graves' disease, untreated hyperthyroidism is associated with miscarriage, premature labor, low birthweight, and pre-eclampsia. Therefore, an endocrinologist, an obstetrician, and a pediatrician should jointly manage these patients. Management entails rapid return to a euthyroid state and symptom control. Propylthiouracil is the preferred antithyroid agent in the first trimester because it has fewer teratogenic effects; however, carbimazole is preferred in the second and third trimesters due to its causing fewer liver function abnormalities. At 20 weeks, TSH-receptor antibody concentrations should be measured, and patients with significantly raised levels should be closely monitored due to transplacental transfer leading to fetal thyrotoxicosis.

Hypothyroidism

Hypothyroidism is rare in early pregnancy and is associated with increased risk of spontaneous miscarriage, pregnancy-induced hypertension, pre-eclampsia, low birthweight, and perinatal mortality. Treatment entails preventing hypothyroidism, doubling thyroxine dose 2 days of the week in early pregnancy, and monitoring TSH in each trimester. Iron supplementation and antacids, commonly prescribed in pregnancy, may affect thyroxine absorption. Due to the significant risk of pre-eclampsia, prophylactic aspirin is advised.

Euthyroid Goitre

A goitre may be diffuse or result from the presence of one or multiple nodules. The lifetime risk of developing a thyroid nodule is 5–10%. The enlargement may be due to physiological factors (puberty and pregnancy), metabolic factors (endemic goitre), abnormal iodine metabolism, or inflammatory (Hashimoto's)/autoimmune disease (Graves' disease). The causes of thyroid nodular enlargement are listed in Table 81.4.

Most goitres are asymptomatic. However, mechanical compression of the trachea and/or the oesophagus may occur. Patients may notice a change in their shirt collar size or they may stop wearing necklaces.

Table 81.4 Causes of nodular thyroid enlargement

| Benign | Malignant | |
	Follicular or C-cell origin	Malignancy of other origin
Follicular adenoma	Papillary carcinoma	Thyroid lymphoma
Hürthle cell adenoma	Follicular carcinoma	Malignancy metastatic to the thyroid
Colloid cyst	Hürthle cell carcinoma	
Simple/haemorrhagic cyst	Medullary thyroid carcinoma	
Lymphocytic thyroiditis	Anaplastic carcinoma	
Granulomatous thyroiditis		
Infectious processes		

Thyroid enlargement because of malignancy is indistinguishable from benign causes in many cases.

Investigations

See Chapter 80.

Management

For benign goitre, surgery is indicated for compressive symptoms.

- Lobectomy is used when only one lobe is severely affected.
- Total thyroidectomy is appropriate if the gland is diffusely involved.
- Rarely, sternotomy is required for retrosternal goitre.

Radioiodine is an option in patients who refuse surgery or if age, frailty, or comorbidities preclude operative intervention.

For the solitary nodule, hemithyroidectomy is indicated for suspected malignancy or cosmesis.

Thyroid cysts, found in 10–15% of patients presenting with a thyroid nodule, are usually benign. Most resolve over time. Thyroid lobectomy is performed for symptomatic recurrent cysts, cysts associated with a solid nodule, or those with rapid nodular growth.

KEY POINTS

- Pre-operative preparation of the hyperthyroid patient is vital to prevent post-operative thyroid storm and should be managed in conjunction with an endocrinologist.
- All thyroid nodules over 1 cm should have assessment by ultrasound and FNAC.
- Surgery for benign disease is indicated for compressive symptoms, suspicion of malignancy, and cosmesis and for those who have contraindications to medical treatment of hyperthyroidism.
- Total thyroidectomy is required for thyrotoxic patients who fail medical management.
- A multidisciplinary team including an endocrinologist, an obstetrician, and a pediatrician should manage patients with thyroid disease in pregnancy.

Further Reading

1. Patel KN, Yip L, Lubitz CC, Grubbs EG, Miller BS, Shen W, et al. The American Association of Endocrine Surgeons guidelines for the definitive surgical management of thyroid disease in adults. *Ann Surg* 2020 Mar; 271: e21–e93.

2. Thyroid disease: assessment and management. NICE Guideline, 2019.

82. MANAGEMENT OF DIFFERENTIATED THYROID CANCER

Differentiated thyroid cancer (DTC), including the papillary and follicular subtypes, has an excellent prognosis, with 10-year survival rates exceeding 98% in stage I–III disease. TNM staging is used for classification (Table 82.1).

Surgery is the most common primary treatment, with some patients requiring adjuvant treatment, most frequently radioiodine ablation with TSH suppression. Individualised treatment has been introduced in recent years, to take into consideration patient and tumour factors and risk of recurrence.

Patients with thyroid cancer require a detailed clinical history, including previous radiation exposure and family history of thyroid cancer and Hashimoto's disease. Ultrasound scan and fine-needle aspiration cytology (FNAC) obtain the diagnosis in most cases. Cross-sectional imaging with computed tomography (CT) or magnetic resonance imaging (MRI) may be required to further assess locoregional disease (Table 82.2).

Thyroidectomy

Thyroidectomy is the mainstay of treatment in DTC.

A total thyroidectomy is recommended for patients with:

- Tumours >4 cm, bilateral disease
- Extrathyroidal spread or metastatic disease
- Adverse histopathological features
- Familial types of DTC
- History of radiation exposure

For patients with smaller tumours and no poor prognostic features, a hemithyroidectomy will suffice, but preoperative discussion in a thyroid cancer multidisciplinary team meeting is advised.

During surgery, if recurrent laryngeal nerve (RLN) involvement is encountered, the surgeon should aim to preserve the nerve if it was functioning pre-operatively. It is acceptable to leave a small amount of disease to preserve laryngeal function because no survival benefit is gained by RLN sacrifice. Tracheal or oesophageal involvement leads to a significant decrease in survival and may require partial resection. Cross-sectional imaging should be carefully examined pre-operatively.

Table 82.1 TNM staging for differentiated thyroid cancer

Age at diagnosis < 55 years			
Stage I	Any T	Any N	M0
Stage II	Any T	Any N	M1
Age at diagnosis ≥ 55 years			
Stage I	T1	N0 / NX	M0
	T2	N0 / NX	M0
Stage II	T1	N1	M0
	T2	N1	M0
	T3a/T3b	Any N	M0
Stage III	T4a	Any N	M0
Stage IVA	T4b	Any N	M0
Stage IVB	Any T	Any N	M1

Thyroid hormone replacement is required if there is an endogenous deficiency, to prevent stimulation of any remaining thyroid tissue and to reduce recurrence in high risk cases. TSH suppression is usually reserved for higher-risk cases.

Papillary Thyroid Carcinoma (PTC)

Papillary thyroid microcarcinoma (PTMC) is defined as PTC no greater than 1 cm in size.

- PTMC is rarely identified pre-operatively due to patient symptoms.
- PTMC tends to present incidentally during radiological examination.
- Post-operatively, PTMC can be identified during histological assessment.
- In some centres, monitoring is offered without active treatment.

These patients have an excellent prognosis following hemithyroidectomy. Cases identified on histological assessment are discharged without follow-up, whereas pre-operatively identified cases are monitored for 5 years because they may be higher risk. Any patient who has PTMC with aggressive features should be managed in the same way as a patient with non-low-risk PTC.

The majority of patients undergoing surgery for follicular thyroid cancer will be undiagnosed at the time of the initial surgery (Thy 3). Frozen-section histology cannot currently reliably differentiate benign follicular lesions from follicular thyroid cancer; therefore, a diagnostic lobectomy is recommended.

Low-risk patients with a diagnosis of minimally invasive tumour (<4 cm) do not require further treatment after hemithyroidectomy. Hürthle cell cancer (follicular oncocytic thyroid cancer) tends to be more aggressive and should be treated by total (completion) thyroidectomy

Management of Cervical Lymph Node Metastasis in DTC

In the presence of nodal disease, a compartment-oriented neck dissection is recommended, with dissection of Level VI for central disease and Levels IIa–Vb for lateral neck disease.

In DTC >4 cm and in patients with extrathyroid extension but without evidence of nodal disease, prophylactic central neck dissection should be considered—but there is no conclusive evidence of benefit. Involvement of Level I or VII nodes is rare in DTC, and these nodes should be dissected only if they are involved. Prophylactic lateral neck compartment dissection for node-negative patients is not recommended; however, ipsilateral Level VI dissection is advised in pre-operatively diagnosed PTC without imaging evidence of nodal disease, as Level VI ultrasound assessment is inaccurate.

Radioiodine

Radioiodine, ^{131}I, can be used for radioiodine remnant ablation (RRA) when a total thyroidectomy has been performed or for treatment of residual, recurrent, or metastatic disease. RRA may improve survival, reduce recurrence, and allow more effective monitoring with thyroglobulin in the long term.

Radioiodine is administered orally. Prior to administration, the total body iodine pool is depleted with a 2-week low-iodine diet and the TSH level is elevated by stopping thyroid hormone replacement; these steps encourage radioiodine uptake into thyrocytes. Administration of radioiodine requires care on an isolation ward and avoidance of contact with people for 14–25 days after treatment. There are short-term implications for pregnancy, breastfeeding, and fertility.

The indication for radioiodine has undergone radical change recently, and cases should be discussed on an individual basis in the thyroid cancer multidisciplinary setting. RRA is indicated in patients with tumours >4 cm and in those with gross extrathyroidal spread or distant metastasis. RRA is not indicated in patients with low-risk tumours. The intermediate group require discussion, and those with poorer prognostic features could be offered RRA.

Higher treatment doses are recommended in patients with gross residual disease after initial surgery (R_2 resection) in an adjuvant setting. Patients who develop distant metastases or who present with radioiodine-avid inoperable disease may receive therapeutic radioiodine, which can be repeated at 6- to 12-month intervals. An iodine scan 2–10 days after treatment allows assessment of radioiodine uptake in the neck and elsewhere.

Radioiodine can cause toxicity, which is generally mild and short-term. Early toxicity includes local reaction in the neck (especially if there is residual thyroid tissue), sialadenitis, xerostomia, gastrointestinal effects, bone marrow suppression, and lacrimal dysfunction. Late complications can include permanent bone marrow suppression, pulmonary fibrosis, and secondary cancers.

External-Beam Radiotherapy (EBRT)

EBRT may be used in patients with evidence of gross tumour invasion at surgery, in patients with residual or recurrent tumours that are not radioiodine avid, and for palliation of inoperable metastatic disease. Intensity-modulated radiotherapy (IMRT) reduces the dose to radiosensitive areas and allows better dose distribution to the target. Common toxicities include mucositis, skin erythema, skin desquamation, and laryngitis. Radiotherapy may reduce uptake of radioiodine into residual thyroid tissue.

Chemotherapy

No data are available to support adjuvant chemotherapy agents in the management of DTC, and it is not routinely used in recurrent or metastatic disease.

Targeted Therapies

Targeted treatments are indicated for patients with progressive, locally advanced, metastatic DTC (papillary, follicular, Hürthle cell), refractory to conventional treatments (such as surgery or RRA). The tyrosine kinase inhibitors sorafenib and lenvatinib have demonstrated the greatest clinical benefit to date.

Assessing Treatment Outcome

Evaluation of effectiveness of treatment is undertaken 9–12 months after treatment using stimulated thyroglobulin (TG) measurements and ultrasound scanning. When assessed together, these are more accurate than radioiodine scanning.

- TG is used as a tumour marker to assess treatment response (following total thyroidectomy and radioiodine therapy) and potential recurrence. It is a key substrate for biosynthesis and storage of thyroid hormones. Its release from both normal and malignant thyroid cells is TSH-dependent. If it is found to be increasing in a patient previously treated for thyroid cancer, it may indicate recurrence or metastases.
- Stimulated TG allows assessment of disease activity but can only be used in the absence of TG antibodies (TGAb). TG and TGAb are measured after a TSH increase induced by either recombinant TSH injection or thyroxine withdrawal.

Disease-free status can be predicted with 98–99% accuracy if stimulated TG is <0.5 mcg/L. A result of >2 mcg/L predicts persistent disease. Unstimulated TG can also be measured in low-risk patients, and a result of <0.1 mcg/L in the absence of TGAb, along with a negative ultrasound, has a high negative predictive value.

Cross-sectional imaging is only indicated where post-radioiodine-ablation scan shows uptake beyond the neck, or serum TG is unreliable.

Follow-Up

Low-risk patients managed with hemithyroidectomy may be monitored using neck ultrasound. For patients having undergone total thyroidectomy and RRA, ultrasound neck imaging and stimulated TG should be performed 9–12 months after RRA. Groupings of three treatment outcomes can be identified using dynamic risk stratification: patients with an excellent response, patients with equivocal or indeterminate response, and those with persistent disease (Table 82.3).

The excellent responders are patients who have been treated with surgery and RRA and at follow-up have a stimulated TG <1 mcg/L and a negative ultrasound scan. This group can undergo annual TG assessment, and their TSH should be maintained in the low-normal range. After 5 years, if they remain disease-free, they can be followed up in a less intensive clinic.

The equivocal or indeterminate group (those with stimulated TG of 1–10 mcg/L and nonspecific ultrasound changes) should be closely monitored with serial stimulated TG and ultrasound assessment. It is prudent to detect recurrence early. Low TSH should be maintained for 5–10 years.

The persistent disease group are those with rising TG, stimulated TG >10 mcg/L, or an ultrasound scan indicating local recurrence. Imaging to investigate the site of recurrence, such as FDG PET-CT or ^{131}I scan, is indicated if the ultrasound scan is negative. After further treatment, TSH suppression to <0.1 mU/L indefinitely and close follow-up are indicated.

Lifelong follow-up is indicated because DTC has a long natural history, late recurrences can occur, radioiodine can cause late side-effects, and supraphysiological thyroid hormone replacement can result in conditions that require monitoring.

Recurrence

Higher rates of recurrence are found in patients with

- Locally advanced disease or bulky nodal metastases
- Macroscopic extrathyroid extension
- Aggressive histological subtypes

PTC relapse occurs in 5–20% of patients and usually affects the thyroid bed or cervical lymph nodes.

When TG is detectable, imaging is utilised to localise the disease recurrence and to target it with further treatment.

For patients in whom extensive imaging fails to identify a site of recurrent disease, management involves continued monitoring until the site is symptomatically apparent or imaging identifies recurrence or treatment with empirical ^{131}I therapy.

The aim of treatment is to surgically remove recurrent disease and to prevent further recurrence, but morbidity and impact on quality of life should be considered.

- Lymph node recurrence may be monitored if it is small-volume and distant from the nerve and airway.
- Rapid enlargement or proximity to important central neck structures should prompt a more aggressive approach.
- Thyroid bed recurrence can present a significant challenge for further surgical resection. If complete resection is not possible, debulking can be beneficial to facilitate greater radioiodine uptake in the smaller residual volume. Distant metastases occur in 10–20% of cases, with pulmonary and bone spread accounting for the majority. Radioiodine-avid disease can be managed with repeat doses of radioiodine, and remission can be achieved in about one third of patients with distant metastases.

KEY POINTS

- An individualised approach to treatment for DTC is now the mainstay, taking into consideration patient and tumour factors and risk of recurrence.
- Surgery continues to be the first-line management in thyroid cancer.
- All thyroid cancer patients should be discussed in the multidisciplinary setting.
- Radioiodine remnant ablation and therapy doses should be personalised, depending on patient and tumour factors.
- Biochemical evaluation and ultrasound imaging detect most recurrences.

Further Reading

American Thyroid Association Management Guidelines for Adult Patients with Thyroid Nodules and Differentiated Thyroid Cancer, 2016.

British Thyroid Association Guidelines for Management of Thyroid Cancer, 2014.

Haugen BRM, Alexander EK, Bible KC, Doherty G, Mandel SJ, Nikiforov YE, et al. American Thyroid Association Management Guidelines for Adult Patients with Thyroid Nodules and Differentiated Thyroid Cancer. *Thyroid* 2016; 26:1–133.

Mitchell AL, Gandhi A, Scott-Coombes D, Perros P. Management of Thyroid Cancer: United Kingdom National Multidisciplinary Guidelines. *J Laryngol Otol* 2016; 130(S2): S150–S160.

Perros P, Boelaert K, Colley S, Evans C, Evans RM, Gerrard Ba G, et al. Guidelines for the Management of Thyroid Cancer. *Clin Endocrinol (Oxf)* 2014; 81(Suppl 1): 1–122.

UK National Multidisciplinary Guidelines: Management of Thyroid Cancer, 2016.

83. MANAGEMENT OF MEDULLARY THYROID CANCER

Incidence

Medullary thyroid cancer (MTC) is diagnosed in approximately 1,000 people each year in the United States and 25–50 people in the United Kingdom. It constitutes 5–10% of paediatric thyroid cancers.

Pathology

MTC is a neuroendocrine tumour arising from parafollicular C cells. C cells are of neural crest origin and produce calcitonin, calcitonin gene-related peptide (CGRP), and carcinoembryonic antigen (CEA).

C-Cell Hyperplasia

C-cell hyperplasia (CCH) is defined as a multifocal, quantitative increase in C cells. CCH can be neoplastic or reactive/physiological.

MTC

Sporadic tumours are usually solitary (90%) and unilateral. In familial disease, MTC is usually bilateral and multifocal. Variants of classical MTC include papillary, follicular, squamous, and oncocytic subtypes.

Genetic Basis of MTC

Genetically determined disease accounts for 25% of MTC cases, and its prevalence is estimated at 1 in 30,000. The three main clinical variants are all inherited as autosomal dominant disorders with 100% risk of developing MTC:

- Multiple endocrine neoplasia type 2A (MEN 2A): >50% of cases, associated with phaeochromocytoma and hyperparathyroidism
- Multiple endocrine neoplasia type 2B (MEN 2B): 5% of cases, biologically the most aggressive, with the highest propensity for metastasis, associated with phaeochromocytoma, marfanoid habitus, and ganglioneuromas
- Familial medullary thyroid cancer (FMTC): only MTC

Gain of function germline and somatic mutations of the *RET* proto-oncogene (chromosome 10q11.2) are implicated in the pathogenesis of MTC. *RET* encodes a plasma membrane-bound receptor-type tyrosine kinase that is expressed by thyroid C cells, cells of the adrenal medulla, autonomic nerve ganglia, colonic ganglia, and parathyroid cells.

Clinical Features of Sporadic and Hereditary MTC
Presentation:

- *Sporadic MTC*: fourth to sixth decade
- *MEN 2A*: first decade
- *MEN 2B*: first and second decades
- *FMTC*: adulthood
- Almost equal sex ratio

A thyroid mass is normally the first indication of disease (>75%), and cervical lymphadenopathy is a presenting feature in approximately 40–50% of patients. Around 10% of patients will have distant metastases.

Diagnosis of MTC
Fine-needle aspiration cytology (FNAC) produces a diagnosis in 50% of cases, and when it is coupled with calcitonin assays, it increases sensitivity and specificity for MTC diagnosis. Targeted core-needle biopsy avoids the need for open biopsy.

Routine measurement of basal calcitonin in patients presenting with nodular thyroid disease is not recommended by the British Thyroid Association.

Pre-Operative Investigations
Calcitonin and CEA
Serum calcitonin is a sensitive and accurate marker of MTC and should be measured in MTC patients pre-operatively because it can indicate disease extent. Lymph node involvement may be found in patients with calcitonin as low as 10–40 pg/mL; distant metastasis and extrathyroidal growth can be indicated by calcitonin levels of 150–400 pg/mL. False-positive serum calcitonin levels are recorded in patients with autoimmune thyroid disease, hypercalcaemia, foregut-derived neuroendocrine tumours, and renal failure. The positive predictive value of an abnormal basal calcitonin greater than 100 pg/mL is 100%. CEA should be measured in all patients with MTC.

Urinary or Plasma Catecholamines/Metanephrines
Biochemical testing for phaeochromocytoma (24-hr urine, or plasma free metanephrines and normetanephrines) is mandatory prior to surgery in all patients with a diagnosis of MTC. Phaeochromocytoma should be treated before treatment of the thyroid disease.

Calcium
Serum calcium and PTH levels should be obtained pre-operatively. Hypercalcaemia or inappropriate serum PTH will indicate the need for careful assessment of the parathyroid glands at the time of thyroidectomy and excision of enlarged glands.

Ret Mutation Analysis
RET mutation and genetic testing should be performed in all patients diagnosed with MTC, as they may represent the index case of a previously undiagnosed MEN kindred.

When a patient with MTC is identified as carrying a *RET* mutation, genetic screening should be offered to first-degree relatives. Family members identified as gene-positive can be offered therapeutic, risk-reduction, or prophylactic surgery for MTC (see below).

Imaging
A neck ultrasound can identify the extent of the tumour and cervical lymph node metastasis. Cross-sectional computed tomography (CT) of the neck, chest, and abdomen is essential to

Table 83.1   Medullary thyroid cancer staging

Stage I	T1a, T1b	N0	M0
Stage II	T2, T3	N0	M0
Stage III	T1, T2, T3	N1a	M0
Stage IVA	T1, T2, T3, T4a	N1b, Any N	M0
Stage IVB	T4b	Any N	M0
Stage IVC	Any T	Any N	M1

assess extrathyroidal spread into the trachea or oesophagus, mediastinal lymphadenopathy, phaeochromocytomas, and distant metastasis. The liver is the commonest site of distant metastasis. A high calcitonin (>400 pg/mL) is associated with distant metastasis.

Staging
MTC is classified according to the TNM staging system (Table 83.1).

Surgery for MTC
Depending on the MTC stage, a total thyroidectomy and selective neck dissection are required in most patients.

The aims of surgery are:

- Remove all disease in the neck
- Produce biochemical and clinical cure
- Minimise the risk of locoregional relapse that might compromise the airway, oesophagus, or recurrent laryngeal nerves

Rationale for Lymph Node Dissection in MTC

- Node metastases are common (>75%) in patients with palpable MTC, occurring early and in medullary microcarcinoma (<1 cm).
- Ipsilateral lateral neck nodes may be involved in over 80% of cases and contralateral lateral nodes in over 50% of cases.
- Approximately 20% of patients will have skip metastases (negative central compartment and positive lateral or mediastinal compartments).
- Positive cervical nodes and extrathyroidal extension increase the risk of mediastinal and distant metastases.

A reasonable approach to the primary surgical treatment of MTC without distant metastases includes the following:

Procedure	Indication
Total thyroidectomy and central compartment neck dissection	• MTC greater than 5 mm • *RET*-positive family members • Known distant metastases at diagnosis (to reduce disease burden)
Above + Ipsilateral Level IIa–Vb selective neck dissection	Ipsilateral lymph node involvement Positive central neck nodes (which imply 70% risk of ipsilateral metastasis and 35% risk of contralateral nodal metastasis)
Mediastinal lymph node dissection (thoracotomy)	Infrabrachiocephalic mediastinal nodal disease and no evidence of distant metastases

Completion thyroidectomy is not required in incidental micro MTC <5 mm (*RET*-negative) with normal post-operative basal calcitonin.

Surveillance

MTC requires lifelong follow-up with a combination of serum calcitonin, CEA, and neck ultrasound. Specialist thyroid cancer multidisciplinary team input is required.

Post-operative monitoring includes the following considerations:

- If serum calcitonin is undetectable and CEA is normal at 2 months, consider annual calcitonin and CEA (and biochemical screening for primary hyperparathyroidism and phaeochromocytoma for MEN 2A/2B, namely serum calcium, PTH, and plasma free normetanephrines and metanephrines).
- If calcitonin is detectable and CEA is abnormal, the patient requires a neck ultrasound to look for structural evidence of disease. If there is no structural disease, measure calcitonin/CEA every 3 months to check doubling times and examine with neck ultrasound every 6 months. If there is structural evidence of disease, locoregional or systemic therapy should be considered (see the section on adjuvant therapy below).

Persistent/Recurrent Hypercalcitonainemia and Recurrent MTC

Residual/recurrent disease is diagnosed (usually within the first 5 years) on the basis of clinical symptoms, signs, or an elevated/rising calcitonin or CEA. Radiological evidence of metastases is best detected when serum calcitonin levels are greater than 800 pg/mL.

Consider:

- Was the initial surgery less than that recommended according to best practice?
- Is the source of calcitonin in the neck (residual thyroid or lymph nodes) or in the mediastinum?
- Will further surgery result in cure or improved survival?

Surgery aims to cure or significantly reduce the disease bulk as well as to relieve or prevent future compression of surrounding structures. The presence of distant disease should not in isolation preclude surgery.

Outcome and Prognosis

- 10-year survival range is 56–96%.
- Biochemical cure after surgery is associated with a 97.7% survival at 10 years.
- Children with MTC have 5-year survival rates of 95%.
- Rate of 6-month post-thyroidectomy calcitonin/CEA doubling correlates with prognosis (<1 year is poor, >2 years is better).

Adjuvant Therapy

External-beam radiotherapy can reduce local relapse in high-risk patients and in those with advanced disease. There is no survival benefit. It should be considered for controlling local symptoms in patients at high risk of locoregional recurrence or with inoperable disease.

Clinical benefit from the use of tyrosine kinase inhibitors, such as vandetanib and cabozantinib, is seen in over half of patients with progressive/metastatic MTC. Toxicity is considerable and side effects are common.

Risk Reduction Surgery for Hereditary MTC

Timing of Thyroidectomy

The timing of the intervention and the extent of surgery should be based on the affected *RET* codon, the age of the patient, and the calcitonin level.

- Children with *RET* codon 918 and 883 mutations (MEN 2B) should have prophylactic thyroidectomy performed within the first year of life, preferably in the first 6 months.
- Children with a *RET* codon 634 mutation have a high risk for MTC in the first decade. Prophylactic thyroidectomy should be performed at 5 years of age, or earlier if the calcitonin level is elevated above 40 pg/mL.

- Children with other *RET* codon mutations should undergo clinical examination every 6 months, with measurement of serum calcitonin and neck ultrasound until age 5 years. Thyroidectomy may be delayed until later in childhood or the teenage years if calcitonin levels do not rise above the normal range.

Need for, and Timing of, Lymph Node Surgery

Risk-reduction surgery should be performed before the onset of MTC to reduce the need for lymph node dissection.

- Children from a known *RET* kindred with highest-risk mutations (codons 918, 883) should be considered for lymph node dissection at the time of surgery.
- Children with MEN 2A with a mutation of codon 634 should undergo central neck dissection at the time of surgery if the calcitonin level is greater than 40 pg/mL or if there is evidence of nodal metastasis on imaging.

KEY POINTS

- MTC care should be provided by a specialist multidisciplinary thyroid cancer service.
- Preoperative investigations must include serum calcitonin, CEA, plasma free normetanephrines and metanephrines, serum calcium, and parathyroid hormone.
- All MTC patients should be offered *RET* gene mutation analysis. In confirmed cases of genetically determined disease, first-degree relatives should be offered genetic screening.
- Staging should include cross-sectional CT imaging of the neck, chest, and abdomen.
- Risk-reduction/prophylactic surgery should be offered to *RET*-positive family members.
- A phaeochromocytoma should be excised prior to MTC treatment.
- Patients with MTC and an elevated basal calcitonin should undergo at least a total thyroidectomy and central neck lymph node dissection.
- MTC requires lifelong follow-up.

Further Reading

Ceolin L, Duval M, Benini AF, Ferreira CV, Maia AL. Medullary thyroid carcinoma beyond surgery: advances, challenges, and perspectives. *Endocr Relat Cancer* 2019; 26(9): R499–R518.

Maia, AL, Wajner SM, Vargas CV. Advances and controversies in the management of medullary thyroid carcinoma. *Curr Opin Oncol* 2017; 29(1): 25–32.

Wells, SA Jr, Asa, SL, Dralle H, Elisei R, Evans DB, Gagel RF, Lee N, Machens A, Moley JF, Pacini F, Raue F, Frank-Raue K, Robinson B, Rosenthal MS, Santoro M, Schlumberger M, Shah M, Waguespack SG, American Thyroid Association Guidelines Task Force on Medullary Thyroid Cancer. Revised American Thyroid Association guidelines for the management of medullary thyroid carcinoma. *Thyroid* 2015; 25(6): 567–610.

---

84. MANAGEMENT OF ANAPLASTIC THYROID CANCER AND LYMPHOMA

Introduction

Anaplastic thyroid cancer and thyroid lymphoma are two rare malignancies of the thyroid gland. They are similar in that for most patients, surgery is limited to diagnosis and airway management. Unfortunately, most anaplastic thyroid cancers present at an advanced stage with complete surgical resection impossible. In the majority of thyroid lymphomas, surgery is not curative, and radiotherapy with or without chemotherapy is the optimum treatment.

Table 84.1   Staging of anaplastic thyroid cancer

Stage IVA	T1, T2, T3a	N0	M0
Stage IVB	T1, T2, T3a	N1	M0
Stage IVB	T3b, T4a, T4b	N0, N1	M0
Stage IVC	Any T	Any N	M1

Anaplastic Thyroid Cancer

Anaplastic thyroid carcinoma (ATC) is rare, accounting for only 2% of all thyroid cancer. It is more common in females (F:M, 3:2) and occurs in older patients (median age 65). It is at the extreme end of a continuum of dedifferentiation of differentiated thyroid cancer (DTC). Unlike DTC and thyroid lymphoma, ATC has one of the poorest prognoses of any cancer, with a median survival of only 3–5 months.

Patients commonly present with an enlarging neck mass within a background of pre-existing goitre. Hoarseness, dysphagia, and stridor are other presentations. Local pain is a less common presentation (15% patients). Extrathyroid extension is usual, with local invasion occurring in up to 90% of cases and distant metastases at presentation in 30–50%. Lung metastases are common (35%). ATC is classified according to TNM staging (see Table 84.1).

Poor prognostic factors are presence of metastasis, male sex, age over 60, and a large primary tumour size (>5–7 cm).

Radiology for staging should include computed tomography (CT) of the head, neck, chest, and abdomen. FDG-PET can be performed to assess for distant disease. Ultrasound-guided fine-needle aspiration (FNA) or core biopsy can give a histological diagnosis. Flexible nasoendoscopy is essential to assess vocal cord movement, airway patency, and intraluminal tumour extension. Once a diagnosis is made, a timely multidisciplinary discussion about further management or best supportive care is imperative.

Treatment

Management of anaplastic thyroid cancer is evolving, with new treatments and trials ongoing.

Surgery for Potentially Resectable Locoregional Disease

Of patients with ATC, 10% have ATC confined to the thyroid at the time of diagnosis. In this situation, the goal of surgery is gross tumour resection, not debulking. Aggressiveness of surgery must be balanced with quality of life; given the prognosis, total laryngectomy should be avoided. Current guidelines recommend total thyroidectomy and neck dissection only if R_0 (microscopically negative resection) or R_1 (grossly negative, microscopically positive) resection is achievable. Pre-operative evaluation is paramount to determine tumour extent before undertaking surgical resection.

Adjuvant Therapy

A large Surveillance, Epidemiology and End Results (SEER)-based population study demonstrated that multimodality therapy (surgery + radiotherapy) gives a survival advantage in resectable disease. Several single-institution studies have also demonstrated the survival benefit of multimodality treatment in the form of surgery + radiotherapy/chemoradiotherapy.

Unresectable Locoregional Disease

Patients who present with unresectable disease have a better outcome following high-dose radiotherapy ± chemotherapy. Hyperfractionated and accelerated radiotherapy regimes, with two fractions a day, have been used to try to overcome the rapid growth and potential for tumour cell repopulation. Radiosensitisation with chemotherapy may also be used. Doxorubicin has been used historically, but recent evidence supports the use of more common head and neck agents, such as cisplatin and taxanes.

Toxicity from treatment must be taken into consideration when decisions are being made about management of patients with ATC. A study assessing a hyperfractionated protocol with a larger fraction size did not demonstrate any survival advantage but did show significant toxicity. The use of intensity modulated radiotherapy (IMRT) allows more concave dose distribution with sparing of normal structures. However, hyperfractionated radiotherapy and chemoradiotherapy can have significant treatment-related toxicity for the patient. Enteral feeding and tracheostomy may be required. In patients with a poor performance status, low-dose radiation may be of palliative benefit in helping with pain and obstructive symptoms.

Metastatic Disease

Patients who present with metastatic ATC have a very poor life expectancy. The key for these patients is to ensure that quality of life is optimised for as long as possible. Short courses of radiotherapy, as mentioned above, may help control local symptoms. Systemic therapy response rates are usually poor, with the taxanes, doxorubicin, and cisplatin having the best clinical response. More recently, the multikinase inhibitors (MKIs) have been used.

KEY POINTS

- Anaplastic thyroid cancer is a very rare disease.
- It has a very poor survival (3–5 months).
- Multimodality treatment is required.
- Surgery is for diagnosis, airway management, and resection if R_0 or R_1 is possible.
- Newer taxanes can stabilise disease.
- Palliative care and quality of life are important considerations.

Lymphoma

Several different lymphoma subtypes can present in the thyroid, but thyroid lymphoma is very rare, occurring in only 1–2% of patients diagnosed with lymphoma. Management is dictated by the acuteness of presentation, the histology, and the Ann Arbor stage. There are two stages; IE, when only the thyroid gland is involved, and IIE, when cervical or superior mediastinal lymph nodes are involved. The 'E' label is an indication that an extranodal site (in this case, the thyroid) is involved as a primary site. Histological diagnosis is critical and ideally involves immunophenotypic and special molecular studies. A fine-needle aspirate may give a suggestion of lymphoma, but ideally a core-needle biopsy or open biopsy is performed. Fresh tissue, rather than fixed, is required. Staging investigations should include a full lymphoma-protocol CT of the neck, chest, abdomen, and pelvis, and FDG-PET. Blood tests required include a full blood count, liver function tests, urea and creatinine, and lactate dehydrogenase (LDH). A bone marrow aspirate and biopsy are also part of routine staging. For stage I and II disease, the treatment is a curative approach with radiotherapy or combined radiotherapy and chemotherapy.

Indolent Lymphoma

Extranodal marginal lymphomas (MALT) are the most common indolent lymphomas of the thyroid gland, with follicular lymphoma being the second most common. There is almost always pre-existing Hashimoto's thyroiditis. Patients typically present with a nodule within the gland or diffuse enlargement of the gland. Cervical lymphadenopathy occurs in a third of cases. Females are more commonly affected than males (3:1). Treatment of stage I and II is with low-dose radiotherapy (24–30 Gy, fractionated over 2–4 weeks), covering the thyroid and draining cervical nodes. Prognosis is excellent, with local control rates greater than 95% and long-term disease-free survival >90%. If lymphoma is confined to the thyroid, then surgical resection is also a treatment option.

Lymphoma with Aggressive Histology

Thyroid lymphoma with aggressive histology is the most common, accounting for 65–70% of cases. Patients are more often female, with the mean age at presentation being 65. Patients typically present with a rapidly enlarging mass that is often as much as 10 cm+ when diagnosed. Cervical lymph nodes are frequently involved. Aggressive lymphoma can arise de novo or in pre-existing Hashimoto's thyroiditis. Diffuse large B-cell lymphoma is the most frequent histology, for which there is a well-established treatment, combining chemotherapy and radiotherapy. Systemic treatment is used, given the high rate of occult systemic disease. Patients will typically receive the CHOP-R regimen (cyclophosphamide, doxorubicin, vincristine, prednisone, and rituximab), with chemotherapy given for 3–6 cycles followed by radiotherapy (30–40 Gy) 3–6 weeks later. This systemic treatment can achieve cure rates of 70–85%. Radiotherapy coverage and volume are dependent on the stage at presentation; stage IE patients can have radiotherapy limited to the primary thyroid disease only, without cover of the cervical lymph nodes, while stage IIE patients will typically have radiotherapy coverage of the thyroid primary site and the draining lymph nodes (Levels III–VI). Long-term cure is 75%.

Toxicity of Treatment

Patients treated with the CHOP-R regime have a standard pre-assessment to minimise toxicity of treatment, which would include the use of premedication, echocardiography, and the use of growth factor support. Toxicities patients must be warned about when undergoing the regime include nausea and vomiting, alopecia, mucositis, myelosuppression, increased risk of infection, and neuropathy. Total radiotherapy doses are low for lymphoma (30–40 Gy), so toxicity is mild. Xerostomia is not encountered because the treatment volume falls below the salivary glands.

KEY POINTS

- Thyroid lymphoma represents 1–2% of lymphoma patients.
- Surgery is for diagnosis and airway management.
- Indolent lymphomas can be treated with local therapy (radiotherapy or surgery) and have an excellent prognosis.
- Lymphoma with aggressive histology requires combined chemotherapy and radiotherapy and has a long-term cure rate of 75%.

Further Reading

Ferrari SM, Elia G, Ragusa F, Ruffilli I, La Motta C, Paparo SR, Patrizio A, Vita R, Benvenga S, Materazzi G, Fallahi P, Antonelli A. Novel treatments for anaplastic thyroid carcinoma. *Gland Surg* 2020; 9(Suppl 1): S28–S42. doi: 10.21037/gs.2019.10.18.

Glaser SM, Mandish SF, Gill BS, Balasubramani GK, Clump DA, Beriwal S. Anaplastic thyroid cancer: prognostic factors, patterns of care, and overall survival. *Head Neck* 2016; 38(Suppl 1): E2083–2090. doi: 10.1002/hed.24384.

Sharma A, Jasim S, Reading CC, Ristow KM, Villasboas Bisneto JC, Habermann TM, Fatourechi V, Stan M. Clinical presentation and diagnostic challenges of thyroid lymphoma: a cohort study. *Thyroid* 2016; 26(8): 1061–1067. doi: 10.1089/thy.2016.0095.

85. THYROIDECTOMY

Introduction
Thyroid surgery is associated with Theodore Kocher, the father of modern thyroid surgery, whose techniques are still largely used today.

Indications for Thyroid Surgery
Up to 30% of thyroid nodules investigated have an indeterminate pre-operative diagnosis.

Thyroid lobectomy (TL) is recommended for:

- Compressive or autonomously functioning solitary nodules
- Indeterminate uninodular disease
- Uninodular differentiated thyroid cancer (DTC) without extrathyroidal extension (ETE) or metastases

Surveillance of the remaining lobe and regular thyroid function tests are required, as up to 33% of patients develop hypothyroidism.

Total thyroidectomy (TT) is recommended for:

- Bilateral multinodular goitre (MNG)
- Multinodular disease or global dysfunction (e.g. Graves' disease)
- ≥T3 DTC, medullary thyroid carcinoma, poorly differentiated thyroid cancer, multi-focal cancer, evidence of ETE, or overt nodal metastases

Subtotal thyroidectomy is no longer recommended.

Pre-Operative Considerations

- Findings from clinical examination, cytological or histopathological analysis, and adequate imaging should be available.
- Laryngeal examination and pre-operative voice assessment with fibreoptic laryngoscopy should be performed.
- Patients should be euthyroid. In thyrotoxic patients, adequate precautions should be taken to reduce the possibility of thyroid storm (a life-threatening condition associated with elevation of heart rate, blood pressure, and body temperature).

Risks

- Hypertrophic/keloid scar
- Infection
- Haemorrhage
- Injury to external branch of the superior laryngeal nerve (EBSLN) and/or recurrent laryngeal nerve (RLN)
- Hypocalcaemia
- Hypothyroidism
- Tracheostomy
- With intrathoracic goitre requiring sternal split or lateral thoracotomy, risks include injury to pleura, phrenic nerve, or pericardium; pneumothorax; and pneumonia

Sternotomy carries a 25% risk of respiratory complications (2% with cervical approach). Risk of deep sternal infection is 1–5%, with sternal dehiscence carrying a 50% mortality rate.

Anesthetic Considerations

- Massive goitre can cause intubation difficulties; intravenous induction or awake fibreoptic intubation is effective.

- Tracheomalacia due to goitre may require prolonged intubation, supporting sutures, tracheal stenting, or tracheostomy.
- Sudden, post-induction cardiorespiratory collapse is a risk, necessitating cardio-pulmonary bypass. This risk is greater with posterior mediastinal goitre and with extremely low tracheal compression.

Key Goitre Considerations

- Posterior mediastinal extension and relationship to neighbouring structures.
- ETE due to malignancy.
- Most retrosternal goitres are deliverable cervically.
- Cardiothoracic input is necessary with primary intrathoracic goitre and in malignant disease with ETE into the chest.

Surgical Technique

Under general anaesthesia with a north-facing neuromonitoring endotracheal tube, position the patient supine, with a soft shoulder support and head ring for neck extension. Via a transverse cervical incision, divide the subcutaneous fat and platysma. Raise subplatysmal flaps from the thyroid cartilage down to the suprasternal notch and protect the anterior jugular veins.

For large goitre, it may be necessary to extend the incision to the membranous insertion of the sternocleidomastoid muscle (SCM) and raise subplatysmal flaps laterally beyond the SCM. Division of the most inferior tendinous insertions of the SCM and strap muscles may improve access.

Incise the cervical fascia in the midline from the thyroid cartilage to the suprasternal notch, to reveal the isthmus. Dissect out the superior pole and lateral aspect of the gland first, before defining Joll's triangle (lateral border—the upper pole of the thyroid gland and its vessels; superior border— the attachment of the strap muscles and deep investing layer of fascia; medial—the midline; and the floor—cricothyroid muscle), within which the EBSLN is located. Ligate and divide the superior pedicle vessels on the gland to minimise damage risk to the EBSLN.

Dissect off the strap muscles, then ligate and divide the middle thyroid vein. Dissect the gland's fascial layer and mobilise the thyroid to visualise the tracheo-oesophageal groove. With a large goitre, the carotid sheath may lie anterior, posterior, or lateral to the thyroid. Extending a finger along the goitre into the mediastinum allows extension assessment and usually delivery from the chest.

Develop a plane to dissect the inferior pole without jeopardizing the RLN. Identify the RLN; most are single, but 30% branch before entering the larynx.

- Lateral approach: In Beahr's triangle within the tracheo-oesophageal groove, the RLN forms the third side of a triangle made up of the common carotid artery laterally and the inferior thyroid artery superiorly.
- Superior approach: At the cricothyroid junction as the RLN enters the larynx (Figure 85.1).
- Inferior approach: For large goitres and revision surgery.

In posterior mediastinal goitre, the nerve can lie anterior to the retrosternal portion (Figure 85.2). Therefore, identify the nerve prior to lobe delivery. Early identification of the vagus nerve through dissection of the carotid sheath is extremely helpful during goitre surgery. This allows reflection of the carotid sheath's contents off the lateral surface of goitres as well as vagal monitoring. Ongoing passive vagal monitoring and intermittent stimulation can be used during goitre surgery to test the ipsilateral vagus and RLN and to ensure that the RLN is intact during manoeuvres on the goitre that risk neural stretch.

The RLN is at greatest risk at Berry's ligament. Carefully dissect and divide using bipolar diathermy on the thyroid away from the nerve down to the tracheal perichondrium. A low

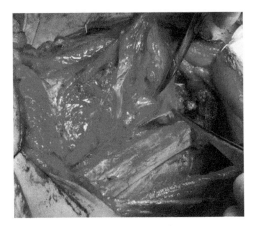

Figure 85.1   Recurrent laryngeal nerve identified at the cricothyroid joint.

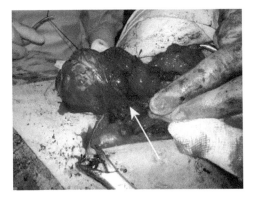

Figure 85.2   Delivery of right posterior mediastinal goitre through a cervical incision. The recurrent laryngeal nerve lies anterior to the goitre (arrow).

ligament sits posteriorly on the trachea, with the nerve close to the gland. Therefore, carefully trace and mobilize the gland off the nerve. With a high ligament, the nerve is often laterally placed and minimal dissection is required. Mainly on the right, 2% of nerves are not RLNs. Pre-operative imaging identifying situs inversus or retro-oesophageal subclavian arteries increases suspicion. A non-RLN runs inferomedially from the vagus nerve (Figure 85.3).

The integrity and function of the RLN can be assessed with intermittent intra-operative RLN monitoring, which has been shown to avoid RLN injury.

Parathyroid Glands

The superior parathyroids normally lie posterior to the RLN, and inferior parathyroids lie anterior. Carefully dissect them off the thyroid, preserving the blood supply. The superior glands' positions are relatively uniform. Inferior glands can be ectopic, due to their embryological path, and 1% of all parathyroids are intrathyroidal. If a parathyroid is excised or is considered nonviable, auto-implantation into the SCM should be considered.

Pyramidal Lobe

Dissect the thyroid off the anterior tracheal wall and remove any pyramidal tissue. Left in situ, it may reduce the efficacy of ablative radioiodine.

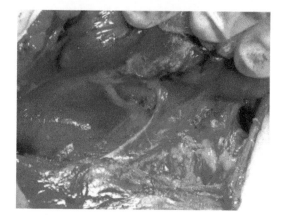

Figure 85.3   Non-RLN arising directly from the right vagus nerve.

Closure

- Wash out the thyroid bed.
- Ensure haemostasis with Valsalva manoeuvres.
- Check the RLN signal.
- Prospective randomised controlled trials have demonstrated drains do not reduce haematoma or seroma rates.
  - However, drainage may be considered in high-risk patients.
- Approximate the strap muscles with one absorbable suture.
  - This prevents tracheo-cutaneous adhesions.
  - Allows a connection between the deep and superficial spaces, reducing the risk of supraglottic oedema in the event of hematoma.
- Approximate the platysma with absorbable sutures and meticulously close the skin.

Post-Operative Care

- Position the patient with head up at 45°, allow patient to resume oral intake, and mobilise as soon as possible.
- Pharmacological venous thromboembolism prophylaxis in high-risk patients only.
- Identification and management of potential hypocalcaemia:
  - Supplementation typically includes oral calcium carbonate (or intravenous calcium gluconate if the patient has severe hypocalcaemia) and/or a vitamin D analogue (typically alfacalcidol).
  - Each unit will have an algorithm to follow, but advice from endocrinologists should be sought in challenging cases.

Etiology and Management of Goitre

- Intrathoracic goitre usually extends into the right anterior mediastinum, because the great vessels impede extension into the left.
- 10–15% grow into the posterior mediastinum.
- Primary intrathoracic goitres are supplied by intrathoracic vessels.
- Primary intrathoracic goitres represent <1% of all goitres, but up to 12% of all mediastinal tumours.
- The risk of spontaneous intragoitre haemorrhage leading to acute respiratory compromise is extremely low. With asymptomatic, euthyroid, benign cervical goitre, conservative management may be appropriate.

- In symptomatic patients who decline or are unsuitable for surgery, radioiodine therapy is an option. In 80% of patients, radioiodine reduces nontoxic goitre size by 30–45% after 1–2 years. This effect diminishes with goitre size and 10% will continue to grow. ^{131}I is inappropriate for compressive goitres because it can induce an acute increase in size. Complications include radiation-induced thyroiditis, transient hyperthyroidism, and long-term hypothyroidism (up to 58%).

Minimally Invasive and Robotic Thyroid Surgery

Introduction
Surgical scars are a significant concern for patients. Of patients from a thyroid clinic who were surveyed, 71% preferred an extracervical scar given the choice, and results were independent of sex and skin colour.

Minimally invasive thyroidectomy (MIT) is synonymous with minimally invasive video-assisted thyroidectomy (MIVAT) or Miccoli technique, endoscopic-assisted thyroidectomy (EAT), and Henry technique. Radford's meta-analysis demonstrated complications were no higher than with conventional thyroidectomy and cosmetic outcomes were superior, but surgery was more time consuming.

Miccoli Technique
A 2- to 3-cm midline incision facilitates endoscopic dissection of the superior pole, with completion thyroidectomy performed once the thyroid is delivered.

Advantages:

- No complications from insufflation
- Total thyroidectomy (TT) is possible
- Excellent visualisation of nerves and parathyroids

Disadvantages:

- Requires two assistants and video stacks
- Limited by the lesion (solitary nodules ≤3 cm, total thyroid lobe ≤20 mL)
- Steep learning curve
- Unsuitable for thyroiditis, cancer, or re-operative surgery

Henry Technique
Three ports are created along the anterior border of the SCM, two for instrumentation and one for the CO_2 insufflator endoscope. Dissection takes places intracervically and the thyroid is delivered through the endoscope port. Indications replicate those for the Miccoli technique, but TTs are not possible.

Extracervical Techniques
Axillo-bilateral-breast and bilateral axillo-breast approaches were pioneered in the Far East. Although the techniques are technically demanding, total thyroid lobectomy (TL) and TT can be achieved safely.

Robotic-Assisted Thyroidectomy (RAT)
Data support superior cosmetic outcomes, better post-operative swallowing function than with conventional thyroidectomy, and safety with thyroid microcarcinomas (<1 cm). Investigation into the safety in treating thyroid cancers >1 cm is required.

Risks of bleeding, infection, vocal cord palsy, parathyroid dysfunction, inpatient stay, and time off work are equal to those for conventional thyroidectomy. However, RAT can potentially cause brachial plexus dysfunction. Airway obstruction does not occur following RAT because blood can disseminate in a larger space than is available after conventional thyroidectomy.

Indications:

- Nodules ≤6 cm for TL
- TT, provided the contralateral lobe is near normal

Contraindications:

- BMI >30
- Degenerative shoulder pathology
- ASA >2

KEY POINTS

- Surgery (TL/TT +/– central and/or lateral neck dissection) is the mainstay of thyroid cancer management, accompanied by adjuvant therapies (^{131}I +/– external beam radiotherapy).
- Surgery is performed on goitre to manage:
  - compressive/obstructive symptoms
  - thyroid overactivity
  - cancer or suspicious goitre
- For large retrosternal goitres, for those with mediastinal extrathyroidal extension, or for those with primary intrathoracic goitre, cardiothoracics should be involved.
- With posterior mediastinal goitre, the RLN may pass anterior to the thoracic portion of the goitre.
- If parathyroid glands are excised or considered nonviable, consider auto-implantation into the SCM muscle.

Further Reading

Chang EHE, Kim HY, Koh YW, Chung WY. Overview of robotic thyroidectomy. *Gland Surg* 2017; 6(3): 218–228.

Hobbs CGL, Watkinson JC. Thyroidectomy. *Surgery* (Oxford), 2007; 25(11): 474–478.

Randolph GW, Clark OH. Principles in thyroid surgery. In: Surgery of the Thyroid and Parathyroid Glands, 2nd edition. Philadelpia: Elsevier Saunders; 2012

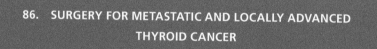

86. SURGERY FOR METASTATIC AND LOCALLY ADVANCED THYROID CANCER

Introduction

Differentiated thyroid cancer (DTC) has an excellent prognosis. Nonetheless, tumour breaching the thyroid capsule may be more challenging. Treatment should be preceded by discussion at an appropriately constituted multidisciplinary team (MDT) meeting. Surgery is the main treatment modality for both primary and recurrent disease.

Risk stratification, particularly after primary index surgery, is important in managing risk of locoregional recurrence, which is often predictable.

Patients with residual disease frequently live many years with minimal symptoms. Balancing complication morbidity with the natural history of the disease requires a personalised approach that considers the patient's age and the tumour biology. A balanced decision on treatment is important in the paradigm of patient care.

Advanced Thyroid Cancer

Surgical management of advanced thyroid cancer includes:

- Extrathyroidal spread (ETE)
- Recurrent or residual disease in the thyroid bed and neck
- Extracapsular nodal disease
- Surgery for distant metastases

Extrathyroidal Spread

Cancer breaching the thyroid capsule is associated with increased morbidity and mortality. ETE is present in 25% of patients and varies between minimal extension into surrounding strap muscles (T3) to invasion of the larynx, recurrent laryngeal nerve, oesophagus, and prevertebral muscles (T4a/b). Residual disease can result in local recurrence, and disease clearance is associated with improved survival.

Factors associated with an increased risk of extracapsular spread include:

- Older patients
- Larger tumours (>4 cm)
- Advanced nodal disease
- Presence of distant metastases

Voice and swallowing symptoms necessitate appropriate clinical and radiological assessment. Examination of the vocal cords is mandatory, and for large tumours, cross-sectional imaging by contrast-enhanced computed tomography (CT) is strongly recommended. Tracheoscopy and oesophagoscopy may be selectively required before primary index surgery. Pathological factors associated with a higher risk of ETE include insular, tall cell, and undifferentiated subtypes of thyroid cancer.

Involvement of Nonvital Structures Around the Thyroid Bed

If ETE involves strap muscles only, simple excision produces no morbidity.

Involvement of the Recurrent Laryngeal Nerve

In up to 60% of locally advanced disease, the recurrent laryngeal nerve (RLN) can be involved. Radiology cannot predict involvement in the functioning RLN, but it aids discussion for informed consent related to the likelihood of nerve injury, resection, and the need for reconstruction.

In an ipsilateral cord palsy with the nerve encased in tumour, resection is advised, with primary reconstruction if feasible. With a functioning nerve, particularly in the young patient (<55 years old), nerve resection is not advised, because the morbidity and mortality from a nerve palsy counterbalance those of the index disease.

If both nerves are functional but involved with disease, or if one nerve is involved in a preexisting contralateral palsy, nerve preservation to avoid tracheostomy is advised.

Involvement of the Trachea and Larynx

Up to 50% of mortality from DTC is due to direct invasion of the airway. However, the prognosis for those with locoregional recurrence is better than that for distal disease. When locoregional control is achieved, disease-specific mortality arises from metastatic tumour burden.

Intraluminal tumour extension is fundamental to surgical planning, and when it is suspected, laryngoscopy and tracheoscopy are mandatory. Although poorly sensitive, contrast-enhanced CT is specific in detecting airway invasion. Magnetic resonance imaging (MRI) may also help define disease if laryngeal cartilage invasion is present.

If there is superficial invasion of the trachea with no intraluminal extension, tracheal shaving is sufficient. In the trachea, local control rates as high as 95% have been reported

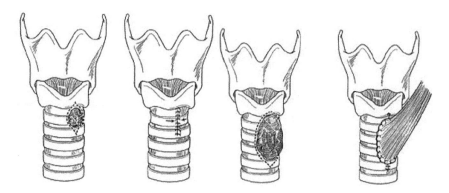

Figure 86.1   Options for tracheal resection and repair: a small defect can be closed primarily, and a larger defect can be reconstructed with a local muscle flap.

using this method, irrespective of microscopically involved margins. Adjuvant treatment with radioiodine may reduce recurrence, but radiotherapy should seldom be given, if at all, particularly in the young. With intraluminal tumour extension, tracheal resection is advised.

With laryngeal invasion, the same principles apply, but laryngectomy is seldom necessary and is usually reserved for elderly patients with undifferentiated disease. In the young, intra-luminal disease can be controlled by other techniques, such as laser surgery, and again radio-therapy rarely should be considered, particularly in young patients. These decisions should be made on a personalised and shared basis in a central unit.

Options for segmental tracheal and laryngeal resection are shown in Figures 86.1–86.4.

Involvement of the Pharynx and Oesophagus

Pharyngeal and oesophageal invasion are rare, because muscle, unlike cartilage, acts as a good biological barrier to invasive thyroid cancer. When seen pharyngeal or oesophageal invasion is commonly associated with airway involvement. Most patients are asymptomatic, because invading tumour is often restricted to the muscularis layer and does not penetrate intraluminally. For this reason, endoscopy of the pharynx and oesophagus is often not pre-dictive. A history of true dysphagia, however, should prompt a thorough examination of the aerodigestive tract. MRI is both sensitive and specific in detecting invasion.

With intraluminal breach, which is exceedingly rare, segmental resection will be required, with the assistance of an oesophageal surgeon.

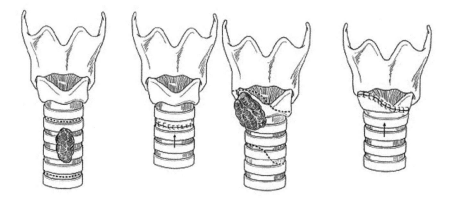

Figure 86.2   Segmental tracheal resection: *Left,* an end-to-end primary anastomosis; *Right,* a stepped closure involving partial resection of the cricoid cartilage.

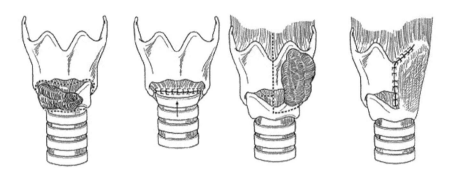

Figure 86.3 Total cricoid resection: *Left,* trachea to cricothyroid membrane anastomosis; *Right,* vertical hemilaryngectomy.

Involvement of the Vascular Compartment

Clinical signs of arterial involvement are often minimal, but major venous involvement should be suspected in the presence of facial flushing, oedema, or unexplained headaches.

Both the internal jugular vein (IJV) and common carotid artery can be involved by direct primary tumour spread, although IJV compression and thrombosis is more commonly caused by extensive nodal disease.

Where vascular involvement is suspected, pre-operative evaluation is essential. Combination imaging, including Doppler ultrasound, MRI, magnetic resonance angiography (MRA), and/or CT angiography, can evaluate intraluminal tumour and distinguish it from thrombus.

Ipsilateral IJV involvement can be resected without reconstruction of the venous system. In bilateral IJV involvement, due to the associated morbidity, vein graft reconstruction will usually be required.

A completely encased carotid constitutes inoperable disease and is usually associated with undifferentiated tumour biology. The literature details ad hoc cases of carotid resection; in these cases, formal angiography is required to assess the arterial supply to the circle of Willis. Encasement up to 270° is usually amenable to resection if there is no direct invasion, although surgical morbidity should be given careful consideration in discussion with a vascular surgeon.

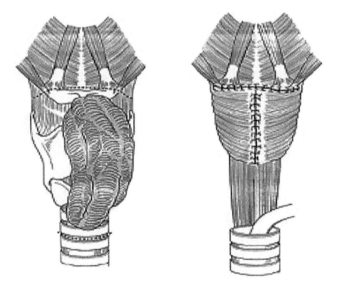

Figure 86.4 Total laryngectomy, for advanced disease extending across the midline.

Surgery for Locoregional Recurrent Disease

Local recurrence is commonly seen in the thyroid bed, with lateral neck disease being less common. Patients with high-risk tumour biology have recurrence associated with higher mortality. Surgery is the primary modality of treatment. In low-volume and low-risk disease, surveillance may be preferable and is appropriate for many patients. If there is evidence of structural disease progression, the approach can be re-evaluated and clearance of the central compartment can be performed.

In treating the lateral compartment, full clearance of Levels IIa, III, IV, and Vb is the treatment of choice. Where extranodal extension affects vascular or neural structures, the surgical strategy should balance surgical morbidity with patient age and tumour biology. Where nodal disease recurs after previous surgery, revision surgery can be considered, following similar principles. In general, unless nodal disease is over 10 mm, a surveillance strategy is advised. Radiotherapy should seldom if ever be considered, and adjuvant treatments, such as radioiodine, alcohol injection, and radiofrequency ablation, can be considered for low-volume recurrence

Surgery for Distant Disease

Distant metastatic spread to lung, bone, soft tissues, and brain reduces life expectancy by 50%. Disease progress can be slow and often is without symptoms. In addition to radioiodine, radiotherapy should be considered for bony metastases. However, bony metastases trap radioiodine in only 30% of patients. For lung, radioiodine is recommended. Sorafenib, a tyrosine kinase inhibitor, can be considered, and opportunities to participate in clinical trials should be sought by the MDT.

Surgery for isolated cerebral metastasis has demonstrated improved long-term survival in patients with good performance status. It should be considered regardless of radioiodine uptake, and the decision should be made in consultation with a neurosurgical team.

KEY POINTS

- Risk stratification should be included in decision-making in advance of the primary index surgery.
- Treatment should be patient-focused and personalised.
- Patient age and tumour biology have critical importance in management.
- Microscopic residual disease does not adversely affect long-term survival.
- The extent of surgery must be a balanced decision, weighing morbidity, patient age, and tumour biology.
- Advanced disease should be treated at a cancer centre.

87. INVESTIGATION OF HYPERCALCAEMIA

Introduction

Most patients with hypercalcaemia are asymptomatic. Very high calcium (more than 3 mmol/L) is uncommon. Primary hyperparathyroidism (PHPT) and malignancy account for 90% of cases of hypercalcaemia. Distinguishing between these two causes is integral in evaluating hypercalcaemia.

Interpretation of Serum Calcium

- 45% of serum calcium is bound to serum proteins, mostly albumin.
- Biologically relevant hypercalcaemia is due to an elevated ionised (free) calcium concentration—This is referred to as the adjusted calcium (most labs will report this).
- Fluctuations in protein binding can affect total calcium concentration without affecting ionised calcium. Increased binding can result from hyperalbuminaemia caused by dehydration. Alternatively, total calcium concentration can be low when albumin is low in conditions like chronic illness, severe malnutrition, or liver disease. In each of these cases, ionised calcium remains unchanged.

It is important to observe the trends in calcium concentration to determine whether it is an acute or chronic problem. Chronic, stable, and asymptomatic hypercalcaemia is usually due to PHPT or familial hypocalciuric hypercalcaemia (FHH). FHH is an autosomal dominant condition associated with mildly elevated calcium and parathyroid hormone (PTH) with low urinary calcium. The degree of hypercalcaemia can be useful diagnostically. Mild hypercalcaemia (adjusted calcium <2.75 mmol/L) is usually found in patients with PHPT. Values above 3.25 mmol/L are uncommon in PHPT and are more common in patients with malignancy-associated hypercalcaemia.

Clinical Evaluation

Mild to moderate hypercalcaemia is usually asymptomatic. Symptoms of hypercalcaemia are nonspecific, and other conditions may account for the patients' symptoms. Symptoms include weakness, lethargy, intellectual weariness, and depression.

- Patients with hypercalcaemia due to PHPT are frequently asymptomatic. A history of kidney stones and osteoporosis, both suggesting chronicity and end-organ dysfunction, may provide reassurance that the cause of hypercalcaemia is not neoplastic.
- Malignancy-associated hypercalcaemia occurs in patients with advanced disease, and the underlying disease is the initial presenting complaint, with hypercalcaemia detected during investigation. Breast, lung, colon, and prostate cancer are the commonest solid organ tumours that metastasise to bone.

A thorough medical and drug history is also important in assessing patients with hypercalcaemia. Clinical evaluation should include examination of the respiratory system, breast examination in women, and prostate examination in men to exclude occult malignancies.

Laboratory Evaluation

Once hypercalcaemia is confirmed, the next step is to determine whether it is PTH-driven (Table 87.1). PTH-driven hypercalcaemia occurs in both HPT and FHH, but all other causes of hypercalcaemia suppress PTH (Table 87.2).

Serum Parathyroid Hormone

Elevated or Higher End of Normal Range

Hypercalcaemia with elevated PTH is likely to be PTH-driven and is most likely due to PHPT.

Physiologically, high calcium levels should suppress PTH production. Elevated PTH or PTH within the upper range of normal (inappropriately elevated) with hypercalcaemia should raise the possibility of PHPT. PTH concentration also increases with age, and one should bear this in mind when measuring PTH in the elderly population. FHH is also a possible diagnosis in patients with elevated calcium and PTH. A 24-hr urinary calcium/creatinine clearance ratio should routinely be calculated to differentiate between the two.

In chronic kidney disease, the characteristic biochemical picture is elevated PTH in response to high phosphate and low calcitriol, with or without low serum calcium. Hypercalcaemia is

Table 87.1   Causes of hypercalcaemia

PTH-dependent	PTH-independent
PHPT	Neoplastic
• Adenoma	• Osteolytic skeletal metastases
• Parathyroid hyperplasia	• Multiple myeloma
• Parathyroid cancer	• Paraneoplastic syndrome (PTHrP)
Ectopic hyperparathyroidism (HPT)	Chronic granulomatous disease (sarcoidosis)
Lithium therapy	Endocrine disorders
Secondary HPT due to renal failure Tertiary HPT as a result of chronic renal secondary HPT	• Hyperthyroidism • Acromegaly
FHH	
Hypovitaminosis D	Medications (thiazides, hypervitaminosis A&D)
	Excessive calcium intake (TPN)
	Immobilisation

Table 87.2   Differential diagnosis of hypercalcaemia with associated changes in blood values

Condition	Ionised serum calcium	Phosphate	PTH	Urinary Ca^{2+}	Vitamin D
PHPT	↑	⇔ or ↓	↑ or high-normal	High-normal or ↑	⇔ or ↓
FHH	↑	⇔ or ↓	↑	Ca/Cr excretion ratio < 0.01	⇔
Osteolytic skeletal metastases	↑↑	or ↑	↓↓	↑	⇔
Multiple myeloma	↑	⇔ or ↑	↓	⇔ or ↑	⇔
Paraneoplastic syndrome	↑	⇔ or ↑	↓	⇔ or ↑	⇔
Vitamin D excess (oral ingestion, granulomatous disease, lymphoma)	↑	↑ or ⇔	↓	⇔ or ↑	⇔ or ↑

relatively rare until the later stages of chronic kidney disease. Hypercalcaemia in this situation may occur as a progression of compensatory parathyroid hyperplasia to an autonomous overactivity of parathyroid glands. This is known as tertiary HPT. Most patients who develop tertiary HPT also have end-stage renal failure. Hypercalcaemia may be absent in those patients if they are on haemodialysis.

Suppressed PTH

PTH-independent causes of hypercalcaemia should be considered if the PTH is low or within the lower half of the reference range. If the hypercalcaemia is of a short duration and very high (>3.00 mmol/L), then malignancy should be suspected. Lung, breast, colon, kidney, and prostate cancer can metastasise to bone and cause hypercalcaemia. In the absence of overt bony metastases, some tumors (squamous cell carcinoma of the lung and skin and renal cell carcinoma) can secrete PTH-related protein (PTHrP). This protein does not react with PTH assays, and PTH in these conditions is usually suppressed.

With multiple myeloma, 30% of patients are hypercalcaemic, with associated impaired renal function and anaemia but suppressed PTH.

24-Hr Urinary Calcium and Urine Calcium/ Creatinine Excretion Ratio

In patients with suspected PHPT, 24-hr urinary calcium excretion should be routinely measured to confirm the diagnosis (>10 mmol/day) but also exclude FHH. FHH has a biochemical profile similar to that of PHPT apart from urinary calcium—excretion is very low in patients with FHH. The calcium/creatinine (Ca/Cr) excretion ratio should be calculated and is preferable in helping to exclude FHH:

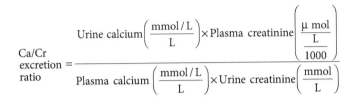

$$\text{Ca/Cr excretion ratio} = \frac{\text{Urine calcium}\left(\dfrac{\text{mmol}/\text{L}}{\text{L}}\right) \times \text{Plasma creatinine}\left(\dfrac{\mu\,\text{mol}}{\dfrac{\text{L}}{1000}}\right)}{\text{Plasma calcium}\left(\dfrac{\text{mmol}/\text{L}}{\text{L}}\right) \times \text{Urine creatinine}\left(\dfrac{\text{mmol}}{\text{L}}\right)}$$

A ratio less than 0.01 is present in 80% of patients with FHH, while the ratio is greater than 0.02 in patients with HPTH. It also important to exclude other causes of low urinary calcium, such as low vitamin D and use of thiazide diuretics, because they can affect the sensitivity of the ratio. Patients with low vitamin D should have the vitamin replaced before their Ca/Cr excretion ratio is calculated.

Vitamin D Metabolites

Testing for vitamin D metabolites is useful in patients with PTH-independent hypercalcaemia. Elevated 25-hydroxycholecalciferol, 25(OH)D, is indicative of excessive ingestion of vitamin D.

PTH catalyses the conversion of 25(OH)D to 1,25-dihydroxycholecalciferol (1,25-DHCC). With long-standing PHPT, it is common for the substrate 25(OH)D to become depleted. Serum calcium may drift lower with coexisting vitamin D deficiency, and the true extent of the hypercalcaemia is revealed only after the vitamin D deficiency has been corrected.

PTH-independent hypercalcaemia associated with normal or low vitamin D metabolites may result from unsuspected stimulation of bone resorption (as in multiple myeloma, thyrotoxicosis, prolonged immobility, hypervitaminosis A), or unrecognised high calcium intake, especially in the face of milk-alkali syndrome.

Serum Phosphate

PTH is phosphaturic, and low serum phosphate levels are found in PHPT. Vitamin D increases phosphate reabsorption from the kidney. Hypercalcaemia that occurs in association with vitamin D excess or in granulomatous diseases is associated with high phosphate levels. Phosphate levels are variable in FHH.

Other Tests of Endocrine Function

Thyroid Function Tests

Hypercalcaemia occurs in 15–20% of patients with thyrotoxicosis. If it persists after control of thyrotoxicosis, then the cause of hypercalcaemia should be investigated to exclude concomitant PHPT.

Adrenal Function

Hypercalcaemia can occur in patients with adrenal insufficiency. Possible explanations include increased bone resorption, extracellular fluid volume contraction, haemoconcentration, and increased reabsorption of calcium. Administration of steroids reverses the hypercalcaemia. Patients with phaeochromocytomas may also have hypercalcaemia, which is PTHrP driven.

88. MANAGEMENT OF HYPERPARATHYROIDISM

Introduction

Hyperparathyroidism (HPT) means excess secretion of parathyroid hormone (PTH). The classification of HPT into primary, secondary, and tertiary allows an aetiology-based approach to management. As the terms imply, primary HPT (PHPT) involves excess PTH secretion due to overactivity of the parathyroid gland(s), and secondary HPT involves excess PTH secretion due to a stimulus external to the glands (Table 88.1). Therefore, removal of the secondary stimulus should return the patient to the euparathyroid state. If this does not occur, by definition, tertiary HPT exists. The commonest example of tertiary HPT is the existence of HPT after renal transplantation in a renal failure patient who previously had renal HPT.

PHPT represents a biochemical syndrome of inappropriate or unregulated hypersecretion of PTH by one or more of the four parathyroid glands in the absence of a recognised stimulus, leading to hypercalcaemia. Most cases are sporadic and are caused by a single parathyroid adenoma (85–95%). Other cases are caused by multigland disease, either multiple adenomas or four-gland hyperplasia (5–10%), with parathyroid carcinoma accounting for <1%. Rarely, the condition is genetic.

With the generalised introduction of the serum autoanalyser in the 1970s, the clinical profile of PHPT has shifted from a symptomatic disorder with hypercalcaemia-related symptoms, kidney stones, and overt bone disease to a symptomatically milder condition.

The annual incidence of PHPT is around 20 cases per 100,000 population. Classical skeletal complications (osteitis fibrosa cystica) are present in less than 5% of newly presenting patients, and the incidence of renal stones has fallen to around 15–20%. Neuromuscular manifestations tend to be vague and include fatigue and subjective weakness, as opposed to a definable myopathy. Reduction in neurocognitive function that sometimes ameliorates following successful parathyroidectomy has been described. Peptic ulcer disease and pancreatitis are associations of classical PHPT. Pancreatitis is rarely seen nowadays because most

Table 88.1 Causes of secondary HPT

Renal failure
Hypovitaminosis D
Rare causes
Malabsorption (e.g. inflammatory bowel disease, post small bowel resection)
Pancreatic insufficiency
Chronic lithium therapy
Hypermagesaemia
Malnutrition

PHPT is 'mild'. Peptic ulcer disease may be seen in patients who have PHPT in association with multiple endocrine neoplasia type 1 (MEN 1). Cardiovascular risk is increased in PHPT, particularly with respect to increased vascular stiffness. There is an increased incidence of hypertension with PHPT, although the underlying mechanisms are not fully understood.

A number of large population-based cohort studies have demonstrated that patients with PHPT appear to be at risk of premature death, predominantly due to cardiovascular disease. A matched cohort study, using hospital episode statistics and mortality data, demonstrated that patients with mild PHPT had significantly worse cardiovascular outcomes, in terms of mortality and nonfatal events. The risk of other comorbidities was also increased. The adverse outcomes were subsequently shown to be linked to high baseline PTH concentration but not baseline calcium.

Primary Hyperparathyroidism

PHPT is sporadic in the majority of cases. Parathyroidectomy is the only curative treatment for PHPT, with first-time cure rates exceeding 95%. Parathyroidectomy should be recommended in all patients with symptomatic PHPT or evidence of end-organ damage, such as low bone mineral density (BMD) or kidney stones.

In asymptomatic patients, controversy exists about the need for surgery, but guidelines exist for conservative follow-up (Table 88.2). Studies vary in outcome, although surgery does seem to lead to some increase in BMD and a decrease in vascular stiffness that positively affects cardiac risk.

The National Institutes of Health (NIH) have developed consensus guidelines, updated in 2014, giving specific indications for when to recommend surgery in patients with asymptomatic PHPT (Table 88.3).

In patients who decline or are unsuitable for surgery there are medical options. Bisphosphonates and hormone replacement therapy (HRT) are treatment options for individuals with PHPT for whom the primary goal is skeletal protection, while the calcimimetic cinacalcet effectively lowers serum calcium and PTH levels in PHPT. However, there are few data demonstrating positive end-organ outcomes. The NHS advises cinacalcet be used

Table 88.2 Monitoring guidelines for patients with asymptomatic PHPT

Check serum calcium annually.
Estimate eGFR annually and serum creatinine
If renal stones are suspected, undertake 24-hr biochemical stone profile, renal imaging by x-ray, ultrasound, or computed tomography (CT)
Every 1–2 years (3 sites), x-ray or vertebral fracture assessment (VFA) of spine if clinically indicated (e.g. height loss, back pain)

Source: Bilezikian 2014.

Table 88.3 National Institutes of Health consensus guidelines for surgery in asymptomatic PHPT

• Age <50
• Serum calcium >0.25 mmol/L above upper limit of normal
• Renal A. Creatinine clearance <60 mL/min B. 24-hr urine for calcium >400 mg/day (>10 mmol/day) C. Presence of nephrolithiasis or nephrocalcinosis on x-ray, ultrasound, or CT
• Bone mineral density (by DXA): A. T-score <−2.5 at lumbar spine, total hip, femoral neck, or distal third of radius B. Vertebral fracture on x-ray, CT, magnetic resonance imaging (MRI), or VFA
• Medical follow-up undesired or impractical

Source: Bilezikian 2014.

in renal failure patients with secondary HPT refractory to standard treatments in whom surgery is contraindicated.

Inherited Disease

Inherited PHPT occurs in familial isolated HPT or as part of the MEN syndromes. Germline mutations in the *MEN1* tumour suppressor gene form the commonest cause of inherited PHPT. Additionally, *CDC73* mutations lead to another autosomal dominant inherited form of PHPT, the HPT jaw-tumour syndrome, which is associated with HPT, mandibular osseous tumours, and a higher incidence of parathyroid carcinoma. Furthermore, *RET* proto-oncogene mutations are associated with MEN 2a, which carries a risk of inherited PHPT.

Inherited PHPT characteristically presents at a younger age than sporadic HPT. Again, the treatment of choice is surgical, but controversy exists about the surgical approach. MEN 2a is generally mild and only enlarged glands need removal during thyroidectomy for prevention or cure of medullary thyroid cancer. In familial isolated PHPT and MEN type 1, the decision rests between pre-operative localisation and removal of only the largest gland(s) to minimise surgical scarring and to reduce the risk of morbidity at later second surgery, or total parathyroidectomy (TP) with thymectomy and autotransplantation in an attempt to avoid further surgery.

Renal Parathyroid Disease

Renal HPT is managed medically with a low-phosphorus diet, vitamin D analogues, phosphate binders, and calcimimetics. In many patients, these modalities fail to control the condition and surgery is performed (Table 88.4). Once again, there is debate about the optimal surgical intervention, and different centres will offer procedures ranging from TP, TP with autotransplantation, to subtotal parathyroidectomy (3.5 gland removal), with each option including or excluding transcervical thymectomy.

Tertiary Hyperparathyroidism

Tertiary HPT is most frequently encountered after renal transplantation. Increased filtering of calcium through the donor kidney is thought to increase the risk of donor loss. The most frequent surgical option in this scenario is 3.5 PT.

Parathyroid Cancer

Parathyroid cancer is rare, presenting with severe PHPT in 90% of cases. A palpable neck mass with a serum calcium of 3 mmol/L or greater should arouse suspicion of the diagnosis. The management of parathyroid cancer is surgical. In 25% of cases, the diagnosis is often made intra-operatively or post-operatively through histopathological analysis. Even then, the diagnosis can be difficult, and diagnosis is sometimes made years later when metastases appear. If parathyroid cancer is suspected, an en bloc resection involving all adherent tissues should be performed. Nodal involvement occurs in only 8% of cases, so level 6 clearance is usually all that is required.

Chemotherapy has no proven additional survival benefit and the tumours are relatively radioresistant; however, in tumours with aggressive characteristics, adjuvant radiotherapy

Table 88.4   Indications for surgical referral in renal HPT

Medical management of renal HPT for >6 months with persistant hypercalcaemia or hyperphosphataemia
PTH > 800 pg/mL
Calciphylaxis with documented PTH elevation
Osteoporosis (T-score −2.5 or worse) or pathological bone fracture

Symptoms/signs:
    Pruritus
    Severe vascular calcifications
    Bone pain
    Myopathy

is advised. Surgical removal of metastases is also worth considering for management of hypercalcaemias and symptom relief. Survival rates are 85% at 5 years and 35–75% at 10 years.

KEY POINTS

- PHPT is caused by unregulated hypersecretion of PTH by one or more of the four parathyroid glands. Rarely, it may be genetic.
- The clinical profile of PHPT has shifted to a symptomatically milder condition.
- Skeletal complications, renal stones, neuromuscular manifestations, peptic ulcer disease, and pancreatitis are now rarely seen in the context of PHPT.
- Parathyroidectomy is the only curative treatment for PHPT, and if no contraindications exist, it should be performed in all patients with symptoms or end-organ disease.
- Medical treatments can improve bone mineral density and normalise serum calcium, but they have not been shown to improve long-term outcomes.
- Asymptomatic PHPT may have clinical sequelae, and specific indications exist for when surgery is recommended.
- Structured follow-up is required for patients with asymptomatic PHPT who do not fulfill criteria for surgery.
- Criteria exist for the timing of surgical intervention in secondary HPT.
- The primary management of parathyroid cancer is surgical, because adjuvant therapies have limited utility
- Although the diagnosis of parathyroid cancer may be challenging, suspect it in the patient with a palpable neck mass and serum calcium > 3 mmol/L.

---

89. PARATHYROID SURGERY

Introduction

Surgery provides the only cure for patients with primary hyperparathyroidism (PHPT) and is also an option for select patients with secondary/tertiary hyperparathyroidism. Historically, patients with PHPT underwent bilateral neck exploration (BNE) and examination of all four parathyroid glands, with removal of macroscopically abnormal glands. However, with improvements in pre-operative localisation and intraoperative monitoring, including technetium-99m sestamibi single-photon emission computed tomography (SPECT), 4-dimensional computed tomography (4D CT), and intra-operative assays of parathyroid hormone (ioPTH), patients can now be offered minimally invasive parathyroidectomy (MIP), reducing morbidity and facilitating same-day surgery.

Some patients still require BNE and examination of all four parathyroid glands; therefore, parathyroid surgeons should have expertise in both techniques.

Surgical Anatomy and Embryology

A thorough knowledge of the embryology and anatomy of the parathyroid glands is essential to aid identification and successful removal of abnormal glands.

- Parathyroid glands are usually four in number.
- *Embryologically*:
  - Superior parathyroids arise from the fourth pharyngeal pouch.
  - Inferior parathyroids, as well as the thymus, arise from the third pharyngeal pouch. (The shared origin of the thymus and inferior parathyroids accounts for the occasional finding of an inferior parathyroid within the thymus.)
- Superior parathyroids usually lie on the posterior surface of the thyroid gland.

- Inferior parathyroids can be found near or within the thyrothymic tract, which extends from the lower pole of the thyroid gland into the superior mediastinum.
- The intersection of the inferior thyroid artery and the recurrent laryngeal nerve is a useful anatomical landmark.
  - Most parathyroid glands will lie within a 2.5-cm area either above or below this point.
- Other locations are seen, with the inferior parathyroids having a wider distribution due to their longer descent. These anatomical locations are discussed in detail below.

Bilateral Neck Exploration

With the introduction of imaging in parathyroid disease, there has been a shift towards more minimally invasive approaches, but subsets of patients still require BNE, including those with:

- Suspected multigland disease
- Parathyroid cancer
- Failed pre-operative localisation
- Failed MIP

Current guidelines from the National Institute for Health and Care Excellence (NICE) on the management of primary hyperparathyroidism (NG132) recommend that patients with negative or equivocal imaging (ultrasound and sestamibi scan—up to 20% of patients) should be offered four-gland exploration and referral to a surgeon with expertise in BNE.

A failed minimally invasive approach will often require a second operation for suspected multigland disease or a double adenoma. Suspected multigland disease may occur in patients with hyperplasia (up to 15% of patients with PHPT), double adenomas (4% of patients with PHPT), or familial hyperparathyroidism, as in multiple endocrine neoplasia (MEN 1, MEN 2A), familial isolated HPTH, and hyperparathyroidism-jaw tumour syndrome.

Technique

Ideally, patients give informed consent before the day of surgery. The procedure is normally performed under general anaesthesia. The patient is placed in a supine position with 30 degrees of head elevation. The neck is extended using a sandbag placed under the shoulders, with the head stabilised on a head ring. Local anaesthetic with or without epinephrine may be infiltrated as a superficial cervical block or directly into the site of the incision. A 5-cm curvilinear incision is placed 1–2 cm above the sternal notch. A subplatysmal flap is raised superiorly to a point just above the cricoid cartilage. The strap muscles are then separated in the bloodless midline plane. Haemostasis is important, because blood in the surgical field can make visualisation of the parathyroid glands difficult.

The left or right side of the neck is opened by raising the strap muscles off the thyroid, with lateral retraction of the carotid sheath and medial retraction of the thyroid. This manoeuvre ensures that the area directly surrounding the dorsal thyroid and tracheo-oesophageal gutter may be explored.

The thyroid lobe is rotated medially into the wound to allow inspection of the posterior aspect (Figure 89.1).

The search should proceed in a methodical way. Ideally, no gland should be removed until all have been visualised.

Superior glands are more constant in position and generally lie on the posterior surface of the thyroid gland, within 1 cm of the cricothyroid joint, posterior to the recurrent laryngeal nerve.

- Enlarged superior glands often migrate downward and inferiorly into a retropharyngeal/retro-oesophageal position by the combined effects of gravity and swallowing.
- Superior glands can be found by identifying the inferior thyroid artery laterally and the recurrent laryngeal nerve inferomedially and by entering the retropharyngeal space by delicate dissection.

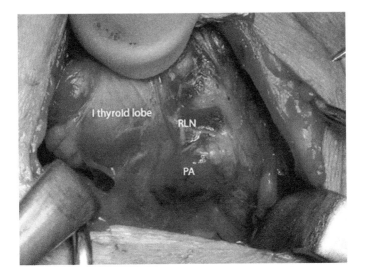

Figure 89.1 The inverted relationship between the left superior parathyroid (PA) and the left recurrent laryngeal nerve (RLN) when the left thyroid lobe is retracted onto the trachea.

The inferior thyroid gland is found near or within the thyrothymic tract, which extends from the inferior pole of the thyroid gland into the superior mediastinum, usually anterior to the recurrent laryngeal nerve.

- Dissection into the thyrothymic tract will usually identify the gland.
- An inferior parathyroid gland can sometimes lie within the thymus and its delivery should only be performed if an adenoma is not found on either side of the neck, to avoid devascularising a normal but suppressed gland.
- Thymic delivery is facilitated by dissection inferiorly, anterior to the carotid artery but medial to the recurrent nerve and lateral to the trachea at the level of the clavicle. The thymus continues as an extension of the thyrothymic tract, and progressive traction on its capsule will aid delivery from the chest (Figure 89.2).

If a superior parathyroid gland is not found, exploration of the retropharyngeal/retro-oesophageal compartment and posteromedial surface of the superior thyroid pole is

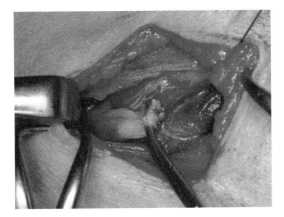

Figure 89.2 Left thymic remnant being delivered from the mediastinum and containing an ectopic inferior parathyroid adenoma.

> ### BOX 89.1 CONTRAINDICATIONS TO MIP
>
> - Negative imaging
> - Multigland disease
> - Family history of MEN or familial hyperparathyroidism
> - Chronic renal insufficiency
> - Hyperparathyroidism from lithium therapy
> - Suspected parathyroid cancer

warranted; then, inspection behind the hyoid and larynx and within the carotid sheath at the level of the inferior thyroid artery is performed.

If an inferior parathyroid is not identified, the carotid sheath is explored from the level of the superior thyroid artery down to the sternoclavicular joint.

One should remember the law of symmetry in parathyroid surgery:

> In 80% of cases, a parathyroid gland located on one side of the neck will have a corresponding gland in the same location on the other side.

If, after a meticulous search, no abnormal parathyroid glands are identified, then one should reconsider the diagnosis and carefully document the location of identified glands. If abnormal or suspect parathyroid glands are identified, then frozen section and ioPTH are useful adjuncts to decision-making.

Minimally Invasive Parathyroidectomy

The MIP approach to the parathyroid glands is facilitated by accurate pre-operative localisation via scans. See Endocrine imaging (Chapter 79). Contraindications to MIP are listed in Box 89.1.

Technique

The patient is positioned similarly to positioning for BNE. The procedure can be performed under local or general anaesthesia. The initial incision can be either a medial or a focused lateral approach.

Lateral Approach

- Incision is made in the medial border of the sternocleidomastoid muscle (SCM) over the pre-localised adenoma.
- The incision is deepened and a subplatysmal plane is developed.
- The medial border of the SCM is identified and a plane is developed.
- Lateral retraction of the SCM and jugular vein with medial traction on the strap muscles allows the thyroid gland to be identified.
- These simple manoeuvres allow most pre-localised parathyroid adenomas to be identified.

Medial Approach is Like the Approach for BNE

- This approach also allows identification of the other parathyroid gland to ensure they both are normal.

Wounds are closed with absorbable sutures in the strap muscles/platysma and Monocryl sutures for the skin.

Complications

Complications are rare following parathyroid surgery and are listed below in Box 89.2.

> **BOX 89.2   COMPLICATIONS OF PARATHYROIDECTOMY**
>
> - Bleeding
> - Wound infection
> - Recurrent laryngeal nerve palsy (<1%)
> - Hypoparathyroidism (rare and more common in BNE)
> - Failure to cure (2–5%)

KEY POINTS

- Surgery provides the only cure for patients with primary hyperparathyroidism (PHPT).
- Bilateral neck exploration is reserved for patients with suspected multigland disease, patients with negative imaging, or those undergoing revision surgery.
- Knowledge of embryology and anatomy is important to ensure successful identification of parathyroid glands.
- The intersection of the recurrent laryngeal nerve and inferior thyroid artery is a key landmark for identifying parathyroid glands.
- Enlarged superior parathyroid glands tend to migrate posteriorly and inferiorly while inferior glands tend to migrate anteriorly.
- Intra-operative PTH assay and frozen section are useful adjuncts in parathyroid surgery.

Further Reading

Glaser SM, Mandish SF, Gill BS, Balasubramani GK, Clump DA, Beriwal S. Anaplastic thyroid cancer: prognostic factors, patterns of care, and overall survival. *Head Neck* 2016; 38(Suppl 1): E2083–E2090. doi: 10.1002/hed.24384.

National Institute for Health and Care Excellence (NICE). Hyperparathyroidism (primary): diagnosis, assessment and initial management. NICE guideline NG132, published May 2019.

90.   MEDICOLEGAL ASPECTS OF THYROID AND PARATHYROID SURGERY

Introduction

Thyroid and parathyroid operations offer unique challenges that are reflected in the complications and litigation that can arise. Surgery-related legal claims (see Box 90.1) have decreased since 2011—with ENT representing about 2.5% of claims—and a higher proportion are being defended. Thirteen to fourteen claims per year pertain to thyroid disease.

- 44% of claims are resolved without payment.
- <5% of all cases are decided in court.
- 79% of court cases are successfully defended.

Diagnosis

Delayed and incorrect diagnosis cause approximately one third of all thyroid-related claims in the United Kingdom. Internationally, 6–8% of cancer-related claims and 6% of all thyroid-related claims arise from delayed diagnosis, with the requirement for a second operation increasing the chance of a successful claim.

> ## BOX 90.1 THE LEGAL DEFINITION OF MEDICAL NEGLIGENCE
>
> A successful claim of medical negligence must prove:
>
> - *Breach of duty of care*: Treatment below the reasonable/accepted standard
> - *Damage*: Patient injury or loss
> - *Causation*: The injury would not have occurred or would have been less severe with appropriate treatment
>
> The claim must be brought within a specific period of limitation. Successful damages awards reflect two elements:
>
> - *Pain, suffering and 'loss of amenity'* (i.e. nonfinancial impact)
> - *Financial loss* and extra expenses
>
> NHS Resolution (formerly called the NHS Litigation authority) manages NHS-related claims.

False-negative thyroid fine-needle aspiration (FNA) rates are <3–10.2%, and suspicious features on ultrasound are reported in 90% of patients with false-negative FNA.

- *Inadequate or incongruous cytology indicates repeat FNA.*
  Evidence on the effect of delayed thyroid cancer diagnosis is limited. A small Korean study found mortality was lowest for patients who had thyroid surgery 1–4 weeks after diagnosis but there was no increased risk with longer delays. An older retrospective study found that cancer mortality was 4% in patients who underwent initial therapy within a year, compared to 10% in others who waited longer. The 'delayed' group had twice the 30-year cancer mortality (6% vs. 13%).
- *It is difficult to attribute negative outcomes to delayed diagnosis.*
  Pre-operative thyroid function, calcium levels, and vitamin D status are predictive of post-operative complications. Studies rarely separate these claims.
- *Guidelines recommend pre-operative biochemistry in at-risk patients.*

Pre-Operative Consent

Historically, a legal test (*Bolam*) determined whether the conduct of a doctor could be supported by a responsible body of U.K. medical opinion. The *Sidaway* judgement that followed required doctors to decide how much risk information to disclose to patients. However, since an early 2015 Supreme Court judgement (*Montgomery v. Lanarkshire Health Board*), doctors must now take 'reasonable care to ensure that the patient is aware of any material risks involved in any recommended treatment and of any reasonable alternative or variant treatments'. A material risk is one to which a reasonable person would be likely to attach significance (i.e. a risk that might alter a decision).

The importance of adequate informed consent cannot be overstated, mainly for best patient care and, secondly, for avoidance of undesired consequences if a claim of negligence is submitted. In the United States, 19% of vocal cord palsy, 7–9% of recurrent laryngeal nerve injury, and 21% of spinal accessory nerve injury claims relate to consent.

- *Inadequate consent is a recognised major factor in legal claims being upheld.*
  Unfortunately, patients have poor retention of consent information, and there is a discrepancy between what surgeons and thyroid cancer patients feel is important. In the United Kingdom, providing information whilst checking and facilitating the patient's understanding are overriding duties defined by the General Medical Council and Royal College of Surgeons. Risk explanation should be tailored to

patient-specific factors, such as thyrotoxicosis, age, previous surgery, and pre-existing vocal cord palsy.

- *Patient information leaflets (e.g. ENT UK website) are recommended but do not replace thorough discussion because they do not improve understanding.*

Intra-Operative Factors

Experience of the Surgeon

High-volume thyroid surgeons have better outcomes. Despite variability in what constitutes high volume, current evidence suggests that high volume means 35–40 thyroidectomies per surgeon and 90–100 thyroidectomies per centre per year. This exceeds the British Association of Endocrine and Thyroid Surgeons recommendation of 20 per year. However, it mirrors the figures for paediatrics, where experience is thought particularly important.

- *Surgeons performing less than 30 relevant operations per year have approximately double the endocrine complications.*

Recurrent Laryngeal Nerve (RLN) Injury

RLN palsy is the major motivator of surgery-related claims in U.K. thyroid surgery. Risk factors include Graves' disease, post-operative bleeding, retrosternal, malignant, recurrent benign, malignant goitre and failure to identify the RLN.

- *Vocal cord movement should be documented pre-operatively.*

Due to the extremely high number of cases required to power a definitive study, it remains uncertain whether intra-operative nerve monitoring (IONM) reduces RLN injury rates, although for temporary RLN palsy, evidence seems to be amassing in favour of IONM.

- *It is imperative that IONM be carried out in the recommended manner, and failure to do so can expose surgeons to litigation.*

Another IONM debate is whether bilateral thyroid surgery should be stopped and staged in the event of loss of signal on the first side. To settle this, surgeons and patients will need to define what is safe and acceptable. In the meantime, studies report that a staged approach in the event of first-side signal loss can eliminate occurrence of bilateral vocal cord palsy. Regardless of approach, the local management algorithm should be pre-operatively discussed with patients.

Parathyroid Preservation

The preservation or removal of the correct parathyroid gland(s) is implicit to diligent surgery. Recent American Thyroid Association (ATA) guidelines support the use of loupes and the identification of at least two parathyroid glands.

Documentation

Documentation of relevant findings, including the results of intra-operative investigations that guided decision-making (e.g. parathyroid hormone biochemistry or frozen-section pathology), should be completed.

- *The location and preservation of the RLN should be clearly documented on a legible (preferably typed) operation note that would stand up to scrutiny by an expert third party in the event of a claim.*

Post-Operative Factors

Post-operative care is as important as all other factors. Recent U.K. claim analysis showed eight of fifteen claims related to post-operative care were upheld. The issues in these cases included hypocalcaemia management, diagnosis of vocal cord paresis, and haematoma development.

- *German experience suggests that claims are more likely to be successful if related to faulty post-operative care.*

Diagnosis of Vocal Cord Palsy

German and British guidelines recommend all thyroid patients have pre-and post-operative laryngeal examinations. Their timing, although significant in terms of detecting neuropraxia, is not prescribed.

- *The failure to recognise a problem motivates 36% of U.S. vocal cord palsy-related claims (and 20% of spinal accessory-related claims).*

Hypocalcaemia

Assessment of parathyroid function after completion or total thyroidectomy is mandatory. National specialist databases record post-operative hypocalcaemia rates of 21% after total thyroidectomy for multinodular goitre (MNG) and, in Scandinavia, 6.4% of patients required intravenous calcium after total thyroidectomy. Serum calcium or parathyroid hormone biochemistry and routine calcium supplementation are all strategies to manage significant hypocalcaemia. Recommendations differ between North America and Europe regarding the choice and timing of these tests.

- *There is consensus that a robust protocol for management of post-operative hypocalcaemia be in place.*

Duration of Inpatient Stay

A patient's attorney may question the safety of a <24-hr inpatient stay for a patient who developed neck haematoma after surgery. Risk factors for post-operative bleeding, which occurs in 0.6–2.1% of cases, include re-operation and bilateral procedures. Although most haemorrhages occur within 6 hours of surgery, 20–37% will occur after 6–24 hours, and 0–10% after 24 hours. Notably, the lowest serum calcium level can occur after the second post-operative day:

- *If discharged too soon, patients may develop severe, untreated hypocalcaemia.*

When Things Go Wrong

Since 2014, the U.K. duty of candour has placed a legal duty on care providers to inform and to apologize to patients or their families regarding mistakes in care that led to death or severe or moderate harm. This adds to a doctor's ethical duty to disclose when an incident has occurred.

- *Patients should be informed as soon as possible of any harm, with an apology and relevant reassurance provided.*

A Claim Arises

Medical negligence cases that go to court are generally civil prosecutions. The plaintiff's/defendant's attorneys will instruct an expert witness to provide a report on possible breach of duty and/or condition and prognosis. An expert witness should provide an independent, balanced opinion for the court (not the lawyers) on the facts of a case, an explanation of technical issues, a view on what is considered 'reasonable', and matters of causation (symptoms or condition) that have arisen as a result of damage.

Litigation Rates and Costs

Three U.K. analyses including nearly 400 cases between 1971 and 2016 were analysed. Diagnostic delay (40 cases, 51.4% closed claims successful), incorrect diagnosis (22 cases, 85% closed claims successful), and recurrent laryngeal nerve injury (33 claims, 54.5% closed claims successful) robustly emerged as principal factors.

91. EVALUATION AND INVESTIGATION OF PITUITARY DISEASE

Introduction

The pituitary gland sits within the sella turcica of the sphenoid bone, inferior to the hypo-thalamus and optic chiasm. It is surgically accessible transnasally via the sphenoid sinus. The gland is composed of two lobes. The anterior pituitary (adenohypophysis) secretes luteinising hormone (LH), follicle-stimulating hormone (FSH), growth hormone (GH), adrenocortico-tropic hormone (ACTH), thyroid-stimulating hormone (TSH), and prolactin. The posterior pituitary (neurohypophysis) is not a gland in itself, but a projection of the hypothalamus, and it releases antidiuretic hormone (ADH) and oxytocin. It is connected to the hypothalamus above by the pituitary stalk (infundibulum), which passes through the diaphragm that forms the roof of the sella. The function of the anterior pituitary is controlled chiefly by hypotha-lamic hormonal control; the hypothalamic-pituitary-peripheral axis is regulated by multiple feedback loops.

Clinical Features of Pituitary Disease

Pituitary disease may manifest clinically due to:

- Hormone hyposecretion
- Hormone hypersecretion
- Mass effect
- Pituitary apoplexy
- A combination of the above

Not all functionally significant pituitary tumours are visible radiologically; conversely, inci-dental pituitary lesions are common.

Hormone Hyposecretion

One or multiple hormones may be reduced, leading to the clinical syndrome of hypopituitarism. Deficiency of GH is most common, leading to lethargy, decreased muscle mass, central adiposity, and reduced bone density. LH and FSH hyposecretion results in reproductive dysfunction (low libido, infertility, erectile dysfunction in men, oligomenorrhoea in women, and delayed puberty in adolescents). ACTH hyposecretion leads to failure to produce an appropriate level of cortisol. This leads to lethargy, postural hypotension, and hyponatraemia when the person is under physiological stress (Addisonian crisis). Hypothyroidism is less common but may manifest with typical symptoms of lethargy, dry skin, constipation, etc. Hyposecretion of ADH from the posterior pituitary is rare, but it may lead to diabetes insipidus (polyuria and polydipsia with hypernatraemia).

Hormone Hypersecretion

Hormone hypersecretion occurs due to the proliferation of secretory cells within an adenoma. The most common functioning pituitary adenoma is a prolactinoma, leading to low libido, infertility, galactorrhoea in women, and gynaecomastia in men. Hypersecretion of GH leads to acromegaly, with an insidious onset of tiredness, sweating, and bony and soft-tissue overgrowth. Hypersecretion of ACTH, and thus cortisol, leads to Cushing's disease, which includes central obesity, striae, diabetes, hypertension, cardiovascular disease, hirsutism, bruising, and proximal myopathy. Hypersecretion of TSH, FSH, or LH is very rare.

Mass Effect

A pituitary macroadenoma may exert mass effect on surrounding structures. Pressure on the optic chiasm due to suprasellar extension of the tumour initially leads to a bitemporal superior quadrantanopia, followed by bitemporal hemianopia. The visual field defect may be asymmetrical. The patient may be unaware of the visual field defect or may complain of nonspecific symptoms, such as clumsiness. Less commonly, lateral expansion into the cavernous sinus may lead to diplopia and ophthalmoplegia. Large pituitary adenomas may cause headaches and rarely hydrocephalus due to obstruction of the third ventricle. Headache is a common presenting symptom in pituitary disease but cannot always be attributed to the tumour.

Pituitary Apoplexy

In a minority of patients, pituitary apoplexy can be the first presentation of a pituitary adenoma. The classical presentation is severe, sudden headache and acute visual field deficit. The patient may present with a triphasic abnormality of ADH secretion: initially, diabetes insipidus, followed by a period of a syndrome of inappropriate ADH secretion (SIADH), followed by a return of diabetes insipidus.

Anterior Pituitary Function Testing

The presenting symptoms of a patient with a known sellar mass may guide the endocrine investigations. Symptoms in many cases are nonspecific or non-existent. In such cases, the laboratory tests are conducted to screen for either pituitary hormone hypersecretion or hypopituitarism (Table 91.1).

Testing for Hypersecretion

Hyperprolactinemia is diagnosed with basal morning prolactin levels. Repeated tests or serial cannulated prolactin levels are necessary to make the diagnosis confidently, as levels can be falsely elevated due to a stress response. Prolactin levels can be increased in hypothyroidism,

Table 91.1 Tests for pituitary hormone hypersecretion

Hormone	Initial test(s)	Confirmatory test(s)
Prolactin	Morning serum prolactin level	–
GH	IGF-1 level	Oral glucose suppression test
ACTH	24-hr urinary cortisol	High-dose dexamethasone suppression test
TSH	Serum free T_4 and TSH	Alpha-subunit levels
ADH	Urine/serum Na & osmolalities	—

in polycystic ovarian syndrome, with the use of some medications (e.g. metoclopramide and some antidepressants), and with some nonfunctioning macroadenomas, due to stalk compression.

Acromegaly (GH hypersecretion) is screened for by checking levels of insulin-like growth factor (IGF-1), a downstream product of GH. The diagnosis is confirmed by a 75-g oral glucose load that fails to suppress the GH level to <1 during the test.

Cushing's disease (Cushing's syndrome due to pituitary ACTH hypersecretion) can be challenging to diagnose, as many ACTH-secreting tumours are not visible on MRI. A detailed endocrine workup is essential. Excess cortisol (hypercortisolism) must be demonstrated first, and subsequently, an adrenal or ectopic source of ACTH must be ruled out to confirm a pituitary cause. As a screening test for hypercortisolism, 24-hour urinary cortisol is measured first. Obesity, pregnancy, alcohol dependency, and poorly controlled diabetes should be ruled out as potential physiological causes of high cortisol. Cushing's disease is then confirmed by:

- Dexamethasone suppression and measurement of serum ACTH. Failure of cortisol suppression to <50% after dexamethasone suppression suggests Cushing's. Plasma ACTH levels will be elevated with a pituitary cause of Cushing's but suppressed with adrenal ACTH hypersecretion.
- A reduction in serum cortisol after high-dose dexamethasone administration favours a pituitary source over an ectopic one. Salivary cortisol can be measured instead of serum cortisol.
- Inferior petrosal sinus (IPS) sampling is used to confirm the source and lateralisation of excessive ACTH in pituitary Cushing's. If the ACTH source is a pituitary adenoma, samples from the IPS will demonstrate high ACTH levels, a differential between IPS and peripheral blood levels, and an exaggerated spike in ACTH levels following the administration of corticotropin-releasing factor (CRF).

Elevated free T_4 *and* TSH levels suggest the rare diagnosis of a TSH-secreting adenoma. High alpha-subunit levels can be used to distinguish this from thyroid hormone resistance.

Testing for Hypopituitarism

Hypopituitarism is suggested where both the target hormone (e.g. T_4) and the tropic hormone (e.g. TSH) are low. In most cases, dynamic testing is also required to prove that pituitary reserve is affected. Multiple dynamic tests can be performed simultaneously.

GH deficiency and ACTH hyposecretion can be demonstrated by an inadequate response to the insulin tolerance test or glucagon stimulation test. The glucagon stimulation test can be performed when insulin is contraindicated (adrenal insufficiency, coronary artery disease, or seizure disorders). Basal LH, FSH, and sex hormone levels can be measured and are sufficient to establish the diagnosis of hypogonadism. The GnRH stimulation test is now rarely used. Thyroid function tests (TSH, T_4, T_3) can confirm secondary hypothyroidism, and the TRH test is generally not required.

Posterior Pituitary Function Testing

SIADH

Hyponatraemia has numerous causes and SIADH is an important one. SIADH is a diagnosis of exclusion. SIADH can be confirmed with paired urine and serum sodium osmolalities. Hyponatraemia demonstrated by reduced serum osmolality and associated with inappropriately high urinary sodium and osmolality confirms the diagnosis.

ADH Deficiency—Diabetes Insipidus

ADH deficiency leads to the production of large volumes of inappropriately dilute urine. This results in compensatory polydipsia, urinary frequency, nocturia, and enuresis. A 24-hr urine collection is performed to confirm excessive urine volume (>50 mL/kg/day) and low osmolality (<300 mOsmol/L). A water deprivation test, with close monitoring of plasma and urinary sodium and osmolalities, will confirm the inability to appropriately concentrate the urine in severe diabetes insipidus (DI).

A central cause of DI (such as the pituitary) can be differentiated from a nephrogenic cause by using desmopressin (DDAVP). With central causes, urine becomes concentrated 1-2 hr after the administration of desmopressin (DDAVP), whereas in nephrogenic DI, the patient is resistant to treatment with DDAVP.

Imaging

The pituitary is typically visualised via magnetic resonance imaging (MRI) with gadolinium, in pre- and post-contrast 3-mm images. The normal pituitary gland and stalk enhance intensely on post-contrast images. Macroadenomas (>1 cm) are visualised by merit of their size and can extend beyond the sella, most often superiorly. They are usually isointense with cortical tissue and may have hyperintense foci on T2-weighted images, findings indicating focal necrosis and often a more readily excised tumour. Microadenomas take up contrast less quickly than the surrounding gland and are visualised as a filling defect within the normal gland on post-contrast images.

The posterior pituitary usually emits a hyperintense signal on T1-weighted images. This 'bright spot' is almost always reduced or absent in diabetes insipidus.

Small, incidentally discovered pituitary lesions are common. In the absence of evidence of hormone hypersecretion, they can be monitored with serial MRI.

Ophthalmological Investigations

Tumours with suprasellar extension may lead to peripheral visual field defects. The classical bitemporal hemianopia is not always seen; however, some degree of visual field defect is frequently observed even in patients who do not complain of visual symptoms. Perimetry is the preferred method of visual field testing. Testing should be conducted in all patients with sellar lesions that are in contact with the optic chiasm.

KEY POINTS

- Pituitary adenomas can lead to hypersecretion or hyposecretion of pituitary hormones, and/or local mass effects on surrounding structures. Many pituitary tumours present incidentally on imaging performed for other indications.
- Tumours are classified by size (greater or less than 10 mm in diameter), and by whether or not they are 'functioning.'
- All patients with lesions involving the pituitary fossa should undergo an endocrinology assessment.
- Thin section, multiplanar MRI with pre- and post-contrast sequences should be performed, although some functioning microadenomas may not be visualised, despite there being evidence of hormonal disturbance.
- Patients should have an assessment of their visual fields using perimetry techniques if the tumour abuts the optic chiasm. Macroadenomas may not produce a classical bitemporal field defect.

Further Reading

Freda PU, Beckers AM, Katznelson L, Molitch ME, Montori VM, Post KD, Vance ML, Endocrine Society. Pituitary incidentaloma: an endocrine society clinical practice guideline. *J Clin Endocrinol Metab* 2011; 96(4): 894–904.

Schwartz TH, Anand VK. *Endoscopic pituitary surgery*. New York: Thieme; 2012.

92. PRIMARY PITUITARY DISEASE

Introduction
Consisting of both an anterior and a posterior portion, termed the adenohypophysis and the neurohypophysis, respectively, the pituitary lies immediately below the hypothalamus.

Anterior Pituitary (Adenohypophysis)
The anterior pituitary secretes thyroid-stimulating hormone (TSH), adrenocorticotropic hormone (ACTH), growth hormone (GH), prolactin (PRL), and the gonadotropins follicle-stimulating hormone (FSH) and luteinising hormone (LH). Pituitary hormone secretion is subject to marked cyclical rhythms and varies widely among the different hormones. Loss of a recognisable rhythm may indicate disease. Secretion of hormones is controlled by the hypothalamus. Active hormones influence pituitary hormone production both by direct feedback on anterior pituitary cells and, more significantly, by inducing the synthesis of neurohormones from hypophysiotropic neurohormones. See Table 92.1.

Table 92.1   Principal pituitary hormones and their regulators, secreting cells, and action

	Pituitary hormone	Secreting cells	Downstream target	Positive feedback	Negative feedback	Effects
Anterior pituitary	Adrenocorticotropic hormone (ACTH) hormone	Corticotrophs	Adrenal gland	CRH	Cortisol	Corticosteroid secretion
	Growth hormone (GH)	Somatotrophs	Liver Adipose tissue	GHRH	IGF-1 Somatostatin	Growth Modulation of lipid/ carbohydrate metabolism (effects modulated by insulin-like growth factor 1; IGF-1)
	Luteinising hormone (LH)	Gonadotrophs	Gonads	GnRH Oestrogen	Sex steroids Inhibin (FSH)	Reproductive system development Gametogenesis
	Follicle-stimulating hormone (FSH)					
	Prolactin (PRL)	Lactotrophs	Breast	TRH	Dopamine	Lactation
	Thyroid-stimulating hormone (TSH)	Thyrotrophs	Thyroid	TRH	T_4 and T_3	Thyroid hormone (T_4 and T_3) synthesis and release
Posterior pituitary	Oxytocin	Supraoptic and paraventricular nuclei in hypothalamus	Myoepithelial cells (uterine) Prefrontal cortex	Cervical stretch Suckling		Supports lactation Uterine contraction Emotional bonding
	Antidiuretic hormone (ADH)		Liver Kidney Brain Vasculature	Reduced plasma volume/ os-molality Angioten-sin II Cholecyst-okinin	Atrial natriuretic peptide	Regulates water retention Induces vasoconstriction

Note: CRH = corticotropin-releasing hormone; GHRH = growth hormone-releasing hormone; GnRH = gonadotropin-releasing hormone; IGF-1 = insulin-like growth factor 1; T_3 = triiodothyronine; T_4 = thyroxine; TRH = thyrotropin-releasing hormone.

Posterior Pituitary (Neurohypophysis)

The posterior pituitary sits in continuity with the hypothalamus and secretes oxytocin and antidiuretic hormone (vasopressin).

Congenital Primary Hypopituitarism

Mutations seen in genes encoding specific cell types or hormone subunits generally give rise to isolated pituitary hormone deficiencies, while mutations in genes responsible for early pituitary development result in combined hypopituitarism.

Congenital Combined Pituitary Hormone Deficiency

Combined hypopituitarism may occur as part of a syndrome or independently. Mutations in *PROP1* and *POUIFI* are responsible for most nonsyndromic cases. Syndromic causes include septo-optic dysplasia, holoprosencephaly, and Rieger's syndrome.

Congenital Isolated Pituitary Hormone Deficiency

Isolated Gonadotropin Deficiency (Hypogonadotropic Hypogonadism)

- May be sporadic or X-linked, with autosomal dominant or autosomal recessive inheritance.
- It is characterised by hypogonadism, which may occur alone or in association with anosmia (Kallmann's syndrome).
- Treatment is targeted towards stimulating gametogenesis with pulsatile GnRH or combined gonadotropins and inducing secondary sexual characteristics with gonadal steroids.

Isolated GH Deficiency

- Congenital GH deficiency occurs in 1 in 4,000–10,000 births.
- There are four distinct forms of GH deficiency
  - Type la: Autosomal recessive, GH undetectable, anti-GH antibodies raised against exogenous GH
  - Type lb: Autosomal recessive, GH low, but no anti-GH antibodies raised
  - Type II: Autosomal dominant, short stature (effectively managed with GH replacement)
  - Type III: X-linked, associated with agammaglobulinaemia, causative gene not yet known

Isolated TSH Deficiency (Central Hypothyroidism)

- Rare: occurs in 1 in 50,000 births.
- Both sporadic and familial cases are described.
- Routine neonatal screening with 'blood spot' test.
- Infants may present with nonspecific symptoms and failure to thrive.
- In cases of established central hypothyroidism, hormonal assays reveal low free thyroxine (FT_4) with inappropriately normal or low TSH levels.

Isolated ACTH Deficiency

- Very rare.
- Symptoms may vary from failure to thrive to signs of acute adrenal insufficiency.

Acquired Primary Hypopituitarism

The causes of acquired primary hypopituitarism are summarise in Table 92.2.

Table 92.2 Causes of acquired hypopituitarism

Category	Examples
Neoplasia	Nonfunctioning pituitary adenomas Functioning pituitary adenomas Parapituitary tumours Craniopharyngioma Meningioma Metastatic deposits Chordoma Glioma
Iatrogenic	Radiotherapy Pituitary procedures Cranial procedures Nasopharyngeal Surgery (see Trauma)
Systemic disease	Sarcoidosis Haemochromatosis Langerhans cell histiocytosis Granulomatosis with polyangiitis (Wegener's disease) Lymphocytic hypophysitis
Infection	Tuberculosis Pituitary abscess
Vascular	Subarachnoid haemorrhage Pituitary apoplexy Sheehan's syndrome
Trauma	Traumatic brain injury Direct pituitary trauma (e.g. surgery)

Pituitary Apoplexy

- A medical emergency in which infarction of the pituitary gland occurs.
- It should be considered in all patients with sudden-onset headache, meningism, reduced consciousness, and visual impairment.
- Pituitary hormones should be assayed.
- Urgent MRI or focused pituitary CT should be undertaken in all patients suspected of pituitary apoplexy.
- Use empirical steroid therapy if the patient is haemodynamically unstable.
- Early decompressive surgery may support recovery in patients with severe or progressive symptoms.

Pituitary infarction due to postpartum haemorrhage is termed Sheehan's syndrome.

Lymphocytic Hypophysitis

- Autoimmune disease that most commonly presents in late pregnancy or first postpartum year.
- Oedema and fibrosis of the pituitary parenchyma result in mass effects and hypopituitarism.
- Corticosteroids may play a role in management.
- Spontaneous recovery has been reported.

GH Deficiency

Adult-onset GH deficiency occurs in 1 in 10,000 people. It is associated with poor skeletal health, impaired quality of life, and increased cardiovascular disease. In paediatric patients, replacement therapy is initiated. In adults, there is no absolute evidence for a reduction in mortality after GH replacement.

- Current NICE guidelines advocate treatment if quality of life is impaired.
- Dose titration is required.
- GH replacement may be contraindicated in certain circumstances.

TSH Deficiency and Replacement

Once-daily thyroxine is sufficient for hormone replacement in central thyroid hormone deficiency.

Gonadotropin Deficiency and Replacement

Oestrogen and testosterone replacement are the usual method of sex hormone replacement for males and females, respectively, with gonadotropin deficiency. Gonadal steroid replacement will not, however, induce fertility. Patients who are seeking to conceive must therefore receive gonadotropin therapy.

ACTH Deficiency and Replacement

Glucocorticoids are generally required in ACTH deficiency.

Empty Sella Syndrome (ESS)

- Rare.
- Occurs because of the herniation of the suprasellar subarachnoid space into the intrasellar space, causing compression of the pituitary gland.
- Primary ESS—Weakness of the diaphragma sella or increased intracranial pressure is thought to promote arachnoid membrane herniation. This most commonly occurs in obese women, and both hypertension and headache are common concomitant features. Hypopituitarism is uncommon and management is supportive.
- Secondary ESS follows pituitary radiation, surgery, infection, or infarction.

Pituitary Adenomas

Pituitary adenomas are classified by whether they produce hormones (functioning versus nonfunctioning) and by size (tumours <1 cm are classified as microadenomas, and tumours >1 cm are macroadenomas). They are invariably benign. The majority produce a single hormone, but 1–30% express more than one hormone (plurihormonal).

Functioning Pituitary Adenomas

Prolactinoma

- Prolactin has an important role in preparing for lactation.
- Mild hyperprolactinaemia may occur in stress, with use of antidopaminergic drugs, and in pituitary stalk compression.
- Prolactinomas can cause very high levels of prolactin and may result in galactarrhoea or amenorrhoea.
- Dopamine agonists are first-line treatment.

Somatotroph Adenomas (GH)

- Acromegaly results from GH excess occurring after closure of the epiphyseal plate.
- Profound changes in physical appearance occur in untreated GH excess.
- Long-term consequences include the metabolic syndrome and increased risk of colonic polyposis.

Corticotroph Adenomas

- Cushing's disease results from a functioning corticotroph adenoma.
- Hypercortisolaemia results in mood disturbance, loss of libido, change in facial appearance, proximal myopathy, weakened skin, easy bruising, and a raft of other signs.

TSH-Secreting Adenomas

TSH-secreting adenomas are rare and represent only a very small percentage of functioning adenomas. They will cause features of hyperthyroidism, but investigation will reveal inappropriately normal or elevated TSH levels.

Gonadotropinomas

Gonadotropinomas seldom present as functioning tumours.

FSHOMA

- More common in men and premenopausal women
- Usually asymptomatic
- The clinical features vary according to gender:
  - Males—tumour mass effect and the development of hypogonadism.
  - Females—In a premenopausal woman, FSHoma can result in ovarian hyperstimulation syndrome (abdominal bloating secondary to increased ovarian size or the accumulation of ascites). Postmenopausal women are invariably asymptomatic.

Nonfunctioning Pituitary Adenomas

Of pituitary adenomas, 30% are nonfunctioning. They may be associated with partial or complete hypopituitarism. Classically, there is a progressive loss of pituitary hormone secretion, with gonadotropins (LH and FSH) affected first, followed by GH, TSH, and ACTH. Children may present with cessation of growth or delayed puberty.

Pituitary Carcinoma

Pituitary carcinoma accounts for <0.1% of all tumours, and it is most commonly ACTH- or prolactin-secreting. Metastases are more likely to be systemic than craniospinal. Mass effects predominate, and surgery forms the mainstay of management. There is some evidence for the use of chemotherapy. Palliation for malignant prolactinomas is provided through medical management with dopamine agonists and radiotherapy. Prognosis is poor, and most patients die within a year.

Familial Pituitary Tumour Syndromes

Familial syndromes account for less than 1 in 20 pituitary adenomas.

Multiple Endocrine Neoplasia Type 1

MEN 1 (Wermer's syndrome) is characterised by dermal tumours in addition to tumours of the parathyroid, pancreas, and pituitary. MEN 1 is the result of mutations in the *MEN1* gene.

Multiple Endocrine Neoplasia Type 4

MEN 4 is due to mutations in the *CDKN1B* tumour susceptibility gene. It is rare, and there are no current guidelines for treatment. Hyperparathyroidism is the most common feature, and pituitary adenomas are the second most common tumour in this syndrome.

Carney Complex

Pituitary adenomas are seen in approximately 1 in 5 patients with Carney complex, a rare autosomal dominant condition.

Familial Isolated Pituitary Adenomas (FIPAS)

FIPAs represent 2% of all pituitary adenomas. Gigantism is a feature of *AIP* mutations.

KEY POINTS

- The pituitary gland plays an important role in regulating reproduction, metabolism, and growth.
- Production of pituitary hormones is subject to cyclical rhythms, necessitating dynamic testing.
- Hypopituitarism may be congenital or acquired and may feature isolated or combined hormone deficiencies.
- Benign pituitary adenomas are common.
- With functioning adenomas, the clinical characteristics are determined by the effects of the excess hormone.
- Extrinsic growth of a pituitary adenoma can result in visual field impairment or, rarely, CSF rhinorrhoea and meningitis.

Further Reading

Melmed S. The Pituitary. Academic Press; 2017.

93. MANAGEMENT OF PITUITARY DISEASE

Surgical Management of Pituitary Disease

One third of pituitary adenomas require surgical intervention. Pituitary adenoma is the third most common intracranial tumour requiring surgical intervention.

First-line treatment for adenomas that hypersecrete or cause mass effect is transsphenoidal decompression/excision, except for prolactinomas.

The current gold standard approach is fully endoscopic transnasal surgery.

Endoscopic surgery requires two surgeons, one to hold the endoscope, the second surgeon to perform dissection bimanually. Ideally, the team is formed by a neurosurgeon and a skilled endoscopic sinus surgeon.

For pre-operative assessment, see Chapter ##, 'Evaluation and Investigation of Pituitary Disease.'

History and Examination

- Visual acuity and visual fields examination.
- Cranial nerves that pass through the cavernous sinus.
- Nasal endoscopy.
- Endocrinological status assessment is paramount.

Imaging

- Computed tomography (CT) will give detailed sinus bony anatomy and anatomical variations.
- Magnetic resonance imaging (MRI) provides information about tumour morphology.
- MRI should be used for intra-operative image-guided navigation.

Endoscopic Transsphenoidal Approach to Sella

Optimising the nasal cavity for an endoscopic approach is an important first step. The patient is catheterised to enable monitoring of fluid balance, broad-spectrum antibiotics are given, and the nose is decongested. The abdomen may be prepared for the harvest of fat and rectus abdominis fascia; in addition, the right thigh can be prepared for fat and fascia lata harvest if the potential defect is larger. The patient should be in reverse Trendelenburg position. Image guidance should be set up.

Surgical Technique

If an extended pituitary approach is required, a nasoseptal flap (NSF) should be raised.

Generally, the vascular pedicle of the potential flap should be preserved on one side by placing an incision from the lower edge of the natural ostium of the sphenoid and carrying the incision anterior and horizontal for about 3–4 cm. A suction Freer is used to mobilise the flap to the level of the posterior bony choana, allowing the anterior face of the sphenoid to be widely opened. A flap can then still be raised and utilised if required.

Bilateral access to the sella is required. The middle corridor is widened by lateralising the middle turbinates, and the inferior half of the superior turbinate is resected. The sphenoid ostium is identified, visually or with palpation. The ostium is entered with a blunt Freer elevator or a sinus mushroom punch. The ostium is widened from the septum to the lamina laterally and from the roof of the sphenoid to the floor. The mucosa of the sphenoid is elevated medially to laterally, leaving the lateral aspect still attached for further reconstruction potential. A posterior septectomy is performed, and a diamond drill or rongeur is used to take down the intersinus septum. These septations frequently veer towards the carotid artery or optic nerve (Figure 93.1). The medial and lateral opticocarotid recesses are identified with the optic nerves and anterior genu of the carotid artery (image guidance is used to confirm the structures). These define the limits of the bony exposure of the sella.

The bone of the sellar face, if not already thin due to tumour expansion, should be 'eggshelled' using a diamond burr. This bone is gently fractured and removed. A Kerrison punch is used to remove bone off the dura, allowing exposure from one cavernous sinus to the other and from just below the tuberculum sella to the pituitary fossa floor (Figure 93.2).

The dura is opened with a U-shaped incision placed a few millimetres medial to each cavernous sinus and meeting at the floor of the sella. Macroadenomas should be visible, and tissue should be taken for histology. With microadenomas, image guidance and MRI help identify the tumour.

Attempted complete extracapsular resection of the tumours improves the chances of complete resection. Tumours have varying consistency, and the best instruments for removal will depend on the consistency.

Once the tumour has been removed, haemostasis is secured using Gelfoam® paste, made from Gelfoam® powder (Pfizer Inc., New York, NY) and saline. The pituitary fossa is gently

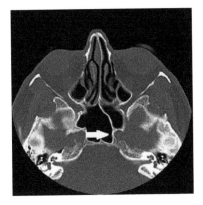

Figure 93.1 CT of the intersinus septum carotid artery. (Taken from Chapter 115, Figure 115.3(b), in *Surgical management of pituitary and parasellar disease*. Philip G. Chen and Peter-John Wormald.)

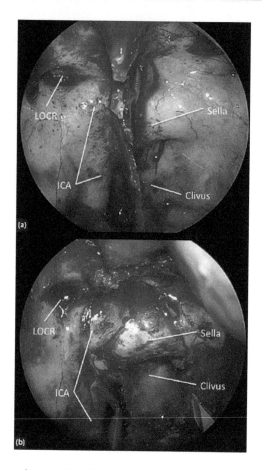

Figure 93.2 Exposure for resection of a pituitary microadenoma. (a) The sphenoid sinus has been entered; observe the bony landmarks and the relation between the septation and the right ICA. (b) The face of the sella has been removed, from ICA to ICA and from superior to inferior intercavernous sinuses. Note the proximity of the ICAs, narrowing the operative corridor. ICA = internal carotid artery; LOCR = lateral opticocarotid recess. (Taken from Chapter 85, Figure 85.2, in *Surgical management of recurrent pituitary tumours*. Mihir R. Patel, Leo F.S. Ditzel Filho, Daniel M. Prevedello, Bradley A. Otto, and Ricardo L. Carrau.)

filled with the paste and the dura is replaced. The sphenoid mucosal flaps are placed over the dura and are secured with Surgicel® (Ethicon, Somerville, NJ), fixed with a layer of fibrin glue. No packing is placed in the sphenoid sinus.

Management of a cerebrospinal fluid (CSF) leak depends on the leak size.

- Small CSF Leak.
- The defect is identified, and a small triangle of fat is placed, ensuring cessation of the leak. Fat can be placed in the sella and a multilayer repair can be completed using the dura and sphenoid mucosa, Surgicel®, and fibrin glue.
- Large CSF Leak (or an extended approach with a defect in the arachnoid mater).
- The NSF is raised. Fascia is placed as an underlay intracranial graft with the pedicled septal flap placed over onto the bone of the defect. Flap edges are secured with Surgicel® and fibrin glue, and the repair is covered with Gelfoam® and the sinus is packed with ribbon gauze soaked in bismuth iodoform paraffin paste (BIPP) for 3 to 7 days depending on the defect size.

Complications

CSF leak is the most common complication. Tumour resection should not be compromised due to fear of CSF leaks because they can be dealt with during the procedure. A post-operative CSF leak is a complication. Post-operative CSF leaks should occur at a rate of 5% or less. If post-operative CSF leak occurs, strict bed rest and a lumbar drain are recommended. If the leak persists, surgical closure is indicated.

Other complications include vision damage and both venous and arterial bleeding, with the latter being potentially devastating.

Revision Surgery

Recurrence rates for pituitary adenomas vary between 7% and 21%. Surgical indications for recurrent tumours are mass effect or persistent symptomatic hormonal hypersecretion. Small recurrences confined to the lateral cavernous sinus must be considered for radiotherapy.

- Identify factors that lead to recurrence and possible problems that might arise during the revision procedure.
- Identify the sequelae of the previous procedure that may hinder the efficient creation of a sinonasal corridor.
- Reconstruction plan may need to include an alternative to nasal septal flap.
- Identify contraindications.
- Determine whether recurrent tumour is secreting or nonsecreting. This identifies the goal of surgery—total removal or debulking.
- Identify sequelae of the previous procedure that may increase the risk of the subsequent procedure (e.g. pseudoaneurysm).

Meticulous radiological assessment is crucial. MRI of the sellar and parasellar regions is required with a CT angiogram. A vascular study to evaluate the ICAs and to rule out a pseudoaneurysm due to previous cavernous sinus manipulation, should be considered.

Hypopituitarism requires hormone replacement to avoid peri-operative complications. Diabetes insipidus must be ruled out and should be addressed properly if present.

Reconstruction options include the NSF and/or free tissue grafts. Prior surgery may have used a NSF. This can be carefully taken down and reused.

Adjuvant Treatment of Pituitary Disease

- Complete excision is not commonplace.
- 30% of nonfunctioning pituitary adenomas increase in size 5–10 years after the original surgery.
- 20% of cases show some clinically significant tumour after resection.
- 60% of functioning pituitary macroadenomas remain biochemically active after primary treatment.
- Watchful waiting is now commonplace due to the availability of high-quality MRI.
- If an adenoma extends laterally into a cavernous sinus, proximal to the carotid siphon and cranial nerves, without any danger of impingement on the optic apparatus, other treatments are likely to be the first line.

Prolactinoma

- 90% of macroprolactinomas shrink with dopamine analog drug treatment.
- First-line treatment for prolactinomas is dopaminergic drugs, such as cabergoline or bromocriptine.
- Surgery can be used for a microprolactinoma if drug side-effects or costs are an issue.
- Watch for CSF leak if the sphenoid bone has been eroded by previous large tumour that subsequently shrank.

Somatotropinoma (Growth Hormone Excess)

Somatotropinoma has a 50% chance of achieving biochemical remission from surgery. One third of patients have persistent disease. Persistent disease is associated with an approximately fourfold increased risk of colorectal carcinoma and with widespread arthralgia and arthritis, impaired glucose tolerance, hypertension, carpal tunnel syndrome, sweating, obstructive sleep apnea, and dysmorphophobia, all of which contribute to a 30% increase in all-cause mortality

- First-line adjuvant treatments are somatostatin analogs, which can normalise circulating growth hormone (GH) levels within 5 years. GH antagonist (pegvisomant) can reduce GH levels by 75%, and dopamine agonists (cabergoline) may be successful in a third of acromegaly patients.
- Conventional fractionated and stereotactic radiosurgery can be considered.

Corticotropinoma (ACTH Excess)

Corticotroph adenomas are typically microadenomas.

- Surgery fails in 10–30% of patients.
- Persistent disease can be addressed with further radical transsphenoidal clearance.
- If preservation of pituitary function is a priority, laparoscopic bilateral adrenalectomy can be considered.
- Drugs used in Cushing's disease include metyrapone, ketoconazole, mitotane, etomidate, sodium valproate, and mifepristone.

Even in remission, patients with a history of corticotroph adenoma have an increased standardised mortality ratio.

Thyrotroph Adenoma (TSH Excess)

Debulking of thyrotroph adenoma is the primary treatment. Due to the chance of recurrence, radiotherapy is strongly recommended as an adjuvant treatment.

Craniopharyngioma

Aggressive attempts to resect craniopharyngiomas are associated with significant morbidity; therefore, radiotherapy can be considered as an adjuvant therapy.

KEY POINTS

- The management of pituitary disease requires a multidisciplinary team approach.
- The endoscopic transsphenoidal approach to the pituitary is the gold standard surgical approach and has many advantages over previous techniques.
- Correct patient selection and workup are vital.
- The surgical team should include a neurosurgeon and otolaryngologist, and a four-handed technique is recommended.
- Revision surgery should be done cautiously by an experienced surgical team.
- Adjuvant treatment should be considered where pathology, anatomy, or persistent disease makes it a more suitable option.

Further Reading

Schwartz TH, Anand VK. Endoscopic pituitary surgery: endocrine, neuro-ophthalmologic, and surgical management. Thieme; 2011.

Stamm AC. Transnasal Endoscopic Skull Base and Brain Surgery: Surgical Anatomy and its Applications. Thieme; 2019.

Wormald P-J. Endoscopic sinus surgery: anatomy, three-dimensional reconstruction, and surgical technique, Fourth Edition. Thieme; 2017.

PAEDIATRIC OTOLARYNGOLOGY

94. THE PAEDIATRIC CONSULTATION

Introduction
It is best practice to see children in dedicated paediatric ENT clinics separate from adult clinics. Paediatric consultations work best when as much information as possible is known about the patient before the consultation starts.

The Consultation
Good communication skills are central to any paediatric consultation. Introduce oneself, and greet the child by name. Make eye contact and use a combination of open and direct questions avoiding jargon. Listen well and talk less until you have the full picture and ensure the child gets an opportunity to speak, if able.

The following are important:

- The birth, perinatal and postnatal history.
- Special care baby unit admission.
- History of airway intervention.
- Child's growth chart.
- Record of doctor visits.
- Diary entries, photographs, or short video clips may also provide useful information.

Examination
Note the child's gait, breathing pattern, and state of alertness when they come into the room. Allow the child time to settle and explain in an age-appropriate way what is going to happen. The parent/guardian can gently but firmly hold a baby or toddler to facilitate examination. It is inappropriate to restrain an older child for the purpose of an elective clinical examination.

Otoscopy
The biggest speculum that will comfortably fit in the ear canal gives the best view. Wax and debris may be removed by suction using the microscope in a cooperative child. Otoendoscopes are useful for recording findings that can facilitate better explanations of pathology to parents.

Nasal Examination

Assess nasal airway patency using a cold metal spatula to identify condensation. Elevating the tip of the nose and using a good light source provide a good view of the nasal cavity and are better tolerated than a Thudicum's speculum. Use a nasoendoscope if the child tolerates it.

Pharynx

Examine the pharynx with a standard headlight. A good view of the nasopharynx is achieved using an endoscope with an angled lens, carefully placed between the tonsils.

Larynx

Flexible transnasal laryngoscopy depends on cooperation from the child and is not always possible. It is usually possible in babies if they are supported appropriately.

Neck Examination

Neck examination should focus on lumps, bumps, sinuses, and asymmetry, with gentle palpation to assess for lymph nodes. 'Lymphadenopathy' is probably a misnomer in children, because some degree of lymph node enlargement is physiological and should cause no alarm.

Investigations and Management Plan

Investigations are based on clinical assessment. Explanations of diagnosis and management options are given to the parent/guardian and child where appropriate, in an open and honest manner using models, diagrams, and printed and audiovisual material as necessary.

Recognition and Management of the Sick Child

Introduction

The sick child is best assessed using a standardised approach, such as the Advanced Paediatric Life Support (APLS) system. The APLS teaches a structured and reproducible set of skills applicable across specialty, language, and cultural and geographical boundaries. The APLS concentrates on different body systems and prioritises assessing and managing life-threatening problems first before others. These body systems are:

A– Airway
B– Breathing
C– Circulation
D– Disability (central neurological system)
E– Exposure (temperature, rash, bruising)

Sick children can deteriorate rapidly, and an awareness of normal parameters in children (Table 94.1) and fluid requirements (Table 94.2) is critical to early recognition and management. Paediatric Early Warning Scores' (PEWS) guide the need for a rapid response and can help monitor improvement.

Table 94.1 Normal range at different ages for children's weight, respiratory rate, pulse rate, and systolic blood pressure (adapted from APLS manual)

Age	Weight (kg)	Respiratory rate (RR) (breaths/minute)	Pulse (bpm)	Systolic blood pressure (mmHg)
Birth	3.5	25–50	120–170	65–105
1 year	9.0	20–40	110–160	70–95
4 years	16.0	20–30	80–135	70–110
10 years	32.0	15–25	70–120	80–120

Table 94.2   Fluid requirements in normal healthy children (adapted from APLS manual[1])

Body weight	Fluid per day (mL/kg)
First 10 kg	100
Second 10 kg	50
Each subsequent kg	20

Airway and Breathing (A, B)

A compromised airway has to be addressed as a matter of extreme urgency because it quickly affects all the organ systems. Airway compromise leads to an increase in the work of breathing. The key signs of increased work of breathing include:

- Stertor (snoring sound)
- Stridor (high-pitched sound—can be inspiratory or expiratory)
- Wheeze (usually expiratory)
- Use of accessory muscles of breathing
- Tracheal tugging
- Nostril flaring
- Fatigue
- Silent chest
- Decreased level of consciousness
- Opisthotonic position (sign of severe obstruction)

Chest expansion and auscultation inform on the amount of air passed during inspiration and expiration. A silent chest is a late sign and portends cardiopulmonary arrest, while asymmetry may indicate a pneumothorax or foreign body. Pulse oximetry gives a measure of arterial oxygen saturation but its accuracy is vulnerable to factors like hypovolaemia, hypothermia, and anaemia.

Suctioning of secretions, removal of intraoral foreign bodies or debris, and a chin lift and jaw thrust manoeuvre are immediate measures likely to overcome any oropharyngeal obstruction. If obstruction is not improved, a nasopharyngeal airway (NPA), oropharyngeal airway, or laryngeal mask airway (LMA) is considered.

Orotracheal or nasotracheal intubation should be considered if the above adjuncts are inadequate, with tracheostomy or cricothyroid puncture reserved for dire emergencies. If an airway foreign body is likely and the child is in extremis, then immediate transfer to an operating theater for removal of the foreign body is mandated. Oxygen should be given early, using an age-appropriate device. Heliox, nebulised epinephrine, and intravenous steroids, such as dexamethasone, may all help to improve upper airway obstruction.

Circulation (C)

Tachycardia and prolonged capillary refill time are early signs of circulatory compromise. Capillary refill is best assessed centrally: digital pressure is applied on the sternum for 5 sec to blanch the skin and then the pressure is released, and colour should return to normal within 2 sec. Pulse rate is best assessed by manual palpation of the central vessels, such as the carotid or femoral arteries, in conjunction with pulse oximetry, accepting the limitations outlined above. Bradycardia and hypotension are late signs and may signify an impending cardiac arrest.

Prompt fluid replacement through intravenous canulae or via the intraosseus route (in cases of severe shock) is critical to correct circulatory losses. In the presence of significant blood loss, replacement of blood may also be needed. Blood pressure readings can be misleading, because children can maintain a normal systolic blood pressure in the presence of significant volume loss.

> **BOX 94.1   THE 'SEPSIS SIX' (NICE GUIDELINES)**
>
> 1. High-flow oxygen via face mask
> 2. Blood investigations, including blood culture (ideally before antibiotics) and blood gas analysis
> 3. Antibiotics—broad-spectrum, intravenous (or parenteral) according to local guidance and taking account of patient's microbiology, given at maximum recommended dose within an hour of recognition of sepsis
> 4. IV fluid bolus—if signs of fluid depletion (including raised lactate)
> 5. Lactate measurement—repeated regularly if raised (> 2 mmol/L)
> 6. Fluid balance monitoring

Disability (D)

Using the acronym AVPU is a quick way of assessing the consciousness level in a child and to signal progressively decreasing consciousness level and need for intubation:

- **A**lert
- Responds to **V**oice
- Responds to **P**ain
- **U**nresponsive

A child who only responds to painful stimulus (P) or is unresponsive (U) needs intubation. Any patient with a neurological deficit must have their glucose level checked (**D**on't **E**ver **F**orget **G**lucose —**DEFG**). Signs of raised intracranial pressure require computed tomography (CT) and specialist input from neurology or neurosurgical teams. Adequate analgesia is an important part of the early management of the sick child.

Exposure (E)

The child should be stripped down so that the skin can be examined for bruising related to injury or rashes related to infection or allergy.

Whenever a patient presents with symptoms or signs raising the possibility of infection, sepsis should be considered. Sepsis is a time-critical emergency and warrants immediate intervention with completion of the 'sepsis six' within an hour, as shown in Box 94.1.

Conclusion

The assessment and management of a sick child rely on a systematic and structured approach. Ongoing assessment, monitoring, and accurate documentation are critical to early detection of change and to prompt life-saving intervention.

Further Reading

1. National Institute for Health and Care Excellence. *Fever in under 5s: assessment and initial management*. NICE Clinical Guideline (NG143). London: NICE; 2020.
2. World Health Organization. *Updated guideline: paediatric emergency triage, assessment and treatment*. Geneva: WHO; 2016.

95. PAEDIATRIC ANAESTHESIA

Anaesthesic Considerations: Patient Factors
Table 95.1 lists patient-related factors that affect anaesthesia in children.

Anaesthesic Considerations: Institutional Factors

- Team experience, case type, case complexity
- Peri-operative facilities—Nursing care, ventilatory support
- Multidisciplinary team
  - Discuss complex cases with team members (e.g. surgeons, anaesthetists, intensivists, specialist nurses, and other disciplines).
  - Identify and book PICU/HDU beds in advance and plan ward and anaesthetic staffing rosters.
- Other disciplines
  - For example, in major airway reconstructions or where the patient has significant comorbidities, assistance from other disciplines may be needed.

Pre-Operative Assessment
Ideally, pre-operative assessment occurs on the same day as the surgeon's review (convenient, less disruptive for the child) and is undertaken by an experienced, suitably trained children's nurse.

- History and examination
- Information (e.g. leaflets) to help the child prepare for surgery
- Detection of potential problems requiring advance planning and communication of them to the anaesthetist and surgeon

Table 95.1 Patient factors affecting anaesthesia

Problems from the Condition Itself		
Obstructive sleep apnea: special nursing care, challenges for post-operative management Stridor/Airway obstruction: potential problems on induction/difficult airway (risk of CICV (cannot intubate cannot ventilate))		
Problems from Associated Conditions		
C O N G E N I T A L	Directly affecting airway: laryngotracheal obstruction	Problems may change with age:
	Affecting general health: myotonic, neurological, or cardiac conditions	• Micrognathia improves in Pierre Robin sequence or Goldenhar's syndrome
	Multiple coexisting conditions (e.g. Down syndrome—abnormal tissues, neck instability, cardiac anomalies)	• Some can worsen (e.g. Treacher Collins' syndrome, the mucopolysaccharidoses, such as Hurler's syndrome)
	Behavioural (e.g. attention deficit hyperactivity disorder) Patients with autistic spectrum disorder may struggle with disturbance of their routine—plan for same-day procedure, preferably first on the list and with early discharge to the child's normal routine and surroundings	
Acquired	Subglottic stenosis, laryngeal webs, respiratory papillomatosis. Find out as much information as possible on cause and previous management to aid anaesthesia	
Drug History	Effect on cardiorespiratory or nervous system	
	Inquire about drugs that directly affect anaesthetics, including beta-blockers, vasodilators, and diuretics	

Table 95.2 Fasting guidelines

Food/drink	Fasting time (hours)
Clear fluids*	2
Breast milk	4
Formula or cow's milk	6
Pastes and solids	6

* Clear fluids include diluted juice but NOT natural fruit juices.

Day of Surgery

Admission type: Same-day or inpatient, as per local policies, geography, and operation

Nursing: Measure patient's weight and temperature

Surgeon review: Consent, marking

Anaesthetic Review:

- General health, anaesthetic suitability, appropriate fasting (Table 95.2), evidence of respiratory infection (if active, delay surgery for 2 weeks)
- Explain induction and post-operative period, including analgesia, to the patient and family
- *Premedication*: sedatives to reduce anxiety (mostly contraindicated in obstructed airway)
- *Anticholinergics*: dry secretions, mitigate the bradycardia from volatile anaesthesia, but can be problematic post-operatively if patient has difficulty clearing sticky secretions

Team Briefing:

- Follow WHO surgical safety recommendations (Figure 95.1).
- All staff must be briefed at the beginning of the theater session to ensure they are fully informed about emergency planning and everything required for full pre-, peri- and post-operative care.

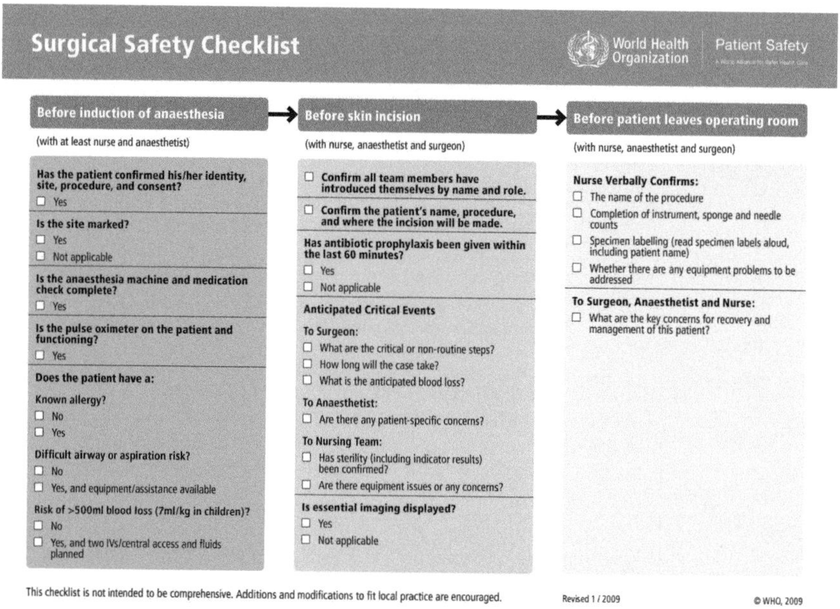

Surgical Safety Checklist

World Health Organization | Patient Safety

Before induction of anaesthesia (with at least nurse and anaesthetist)

Has the patient confirmed his/her identity, site, procedure, and consent?
☐ Yes

Is the site marked?
☐ Yes
☐ Not applicable

Is the anaesthesia machine and medication check complete?
☐ Yes

Is the pulse oximeter on the patient and functioning?
☐ Yes

Does the patient have a:

Known allergy?
☐ No
☐ Yes

Difficult airway or aspiration risk?
☐ No
☐ Yes, and equipment/assistance available

Risk of >500ml blood loss (7ml/kg in children)?
☐ No
☐ Yes, and two IVs/central access and fluids planned

Before skin incision (with nurse, anaesthetist and surgeon)

☐ **Confirm all team members have introduced themselves by name and role.**

☐ **Confirm the patient's name, procedure, and where the incision will be made.**

Has antibiotic prophylaxis been given within the last 60 minutes?
☐ Yes
☐ Not applicable

Anticipated Critical Events

To Surgeon:
☐ What are the critical or non-routine steps?
☐ How long will the case take?
☐ What is the anticipated blood loss?

To Anaesthetist:
☐ Are there any patient-specific concerns?

To Nursing Team:
☐ Has sterility (including indicator results) been confirmed?
☐ Are there equipment issues or any concerns?

Is essential imaging displayed?
☐ Yes
☐ Not applicable

Before patient leaves operating room (with nurse, anaesthetist and surgeon)

Nurse Verbally Confirms:
☐ The name of the procedure
☐ Completion of instrument, sponge and needle counts
☐ Specimen labelling (read specimen labels aloud, including patient name)
☐ Whether there are any equipment problems to be addressed

To Surgeon, Anaesthetist and Nurse:
☐ What are the key concerns for recovery and management of this patient?

This checklist is not intended to be comprehensive. Additions and modifications to fit local practice are encouraged.

Revised 1 / 2009

© WHO, 2009

Figure 95.1 WHO Surgical Safety Checklist (from http://whqlibdoc.who.int/publications/2009/9789241598590_eng_Checklist.pdf6) (Courtesy of the World Health Organization, copyright © 2009.)

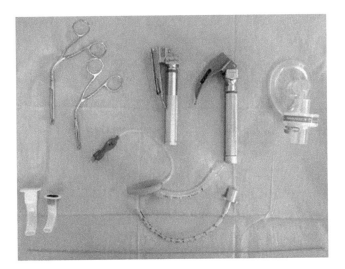

Figure 95.2   Basic set of equipment for paediatric airway anaesthesia.

- Ensure the list is correct, finalise plans, confirm and check availability and operability of any specialised equipment, check completion of WHO checklist for patient.

General Anaesthesia

Basic Principles

Shared Airway: The anaesthetist needs instant and full access if the patient deteriorates. The surgeon provides assistance; in life-threatening circumstances, this may include an emergency surgical airway (surgical cricothyrotomy or tracheostomy). Therefore, any surgeon undertaking an operation with this potential risk must be capable of performing such procedures.

Can't intubate, can't ventilate: NEVER FORGET the option of waking the patient up and rearranging the case.

Technique: The anaesthetic triad of anaesthesia, analgesia, and relaxation can be obtained in various ways. A planned approach to complications should be in place, with adequate training of all staff involved.

Equipment **(Figure 95.2)**: Included are a face mask with a soft seal, different laryngoscopes, endotracheal tube and laryngeal mask, Guedel airways, Magill forceps, and an intubating bougie.

Additional Equipment: Additional equipment (e.g. videolaryngoscope, etc.) should be chosen and used in routine cases, so that its use is familiar in an emergency. A difficult intubation trolley should be available in every theater suite (with duplication in elective airway centres).

Trained Anaesthetic Assistant: The assistant must be familiar with local policies and guidelines, have knowledge of the equipment including its use, and must be present at the pre-operative briefing.

Post-Operative Care

Only start a case if there are facilities to finish it. In emergency cases without appropriate facilities, the anaesthetic team must oversee the patient's recovery. **NEVER** start a new case until the last patient is safe.

- Post-anaesthesia care unit (PACU)—trained competent staff, emergency equipment (drugs, anaesthetic machine).
- High-dependency unit or intensive care unit.

- Patients should only be discharged when fully conscious, appropriately hydrated, and pain-free with appropriate analgesia prescribed, and with full handover of the post-operative care to the ward.
- On discharge, patients should be given information sheets about their procedure that contain contact details should they have any problems.

Anaesthetic Considerations: Specific Operations

Airway examination and treatment	The ideal situation for both diagnosis and treatment of airway problems is the spontaneously breathing patient maintaining their own airway. Basic principle = keep the patient breathing, with a **controlled and gradual** anaesthesia, and constant airway observation. Either use a volatile anaesthetic agent in oxygen (sevoflurane or halothane) • Simple: patient-controlled depth—if 'light', the patient breathes and gets deeper; if 'deep', the respiratory rate slows down, thereby lightening the anaesthetic. Or use total intravenous anaesthesia (TIVA). • Adjusting infusion rates can be labour-intensive. May distract the anaesthetist's attention from the airway. **Procedure**: • Gas induction with volatile agent in oxygen: high safety, preferred method. • Constant airway observation, establishment of intravenous access. • Ensure anaesthetised enough to spray the larynx with lidocaine (avoids laryngospasm and lessens the response to instrumentation) and the nose with xylometazoline. • Maintenance via nasal airway with spontaneous respiration using insufflated volatile with oxygen: additional benefits are that the anaesthetic won't alter the airway appearance and instrumentation is minimised. • Tracheo- or laryngomalacia may not be seen if there are pressure effects of insufflated gas. • An endotracheal tube may squash pathology, such as tracheal haemangiomata. **Remember**: • All anaesthetic agents depress respiration and reduce muscle tone, so any anaesthetised patient promptly loses their airway. • Some pathology may be impossible to intubate in an emergency (e.g. mediastinal tumours). • Dexamethasone may reduce postoperative airway oedema (scanty evidence for this). • If ventilation is required, intubation is better. Jet ventilation carries significant risk of barotrauma in small children, although it is used successfully in some centres. • Waking the patient up if the airway cannot be adequately secured is always an option.
Tonsillectomy and adenoidectomy	Endotracheal tube is more secure and easier for placing a Boyle Davis gag. Laryngeal mask airway is quicker and easier for the anaesthetist to place. Antiemesis with dexamethasone ± ondansetron: there is risk of vomiting after surgery from intra-operative swallowing of blood. Effective analgesia post-operatively.

Microlaryngoscopy and bronchoscopy	Airway examination is essential in diagnosis and treatment, including suspension laryngoscopy, examination with a Hopkins rod, and bronchoscopy. *Suspension laryngoscopy* is used for detailed examination of the larynx and associated structures. Risk: neck overextension with a pre-existing instability (e.g. in Down syndrome). *Bronchoscopy:* The bronchoscope has a side-arm attachment for the anaesthetic gas circuit T piece (Figure 95.3), and side holes for ventilation of both lungs with the instrument down one bronchus. The bronchoscope in the figure is prepared for laser surgery, with a Hopkins rod and YAG laser fibre in situ, which reduces the bore of the system considerably, making it even more important to keep gas leakage as low as possible. 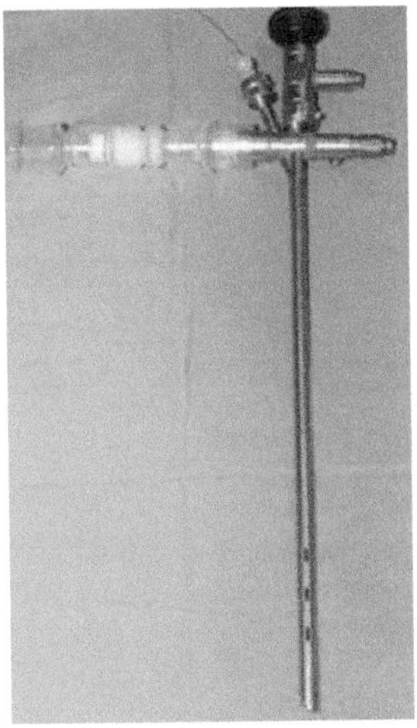 Figure 95.3 Bronchoscope. **Communication is key:** The anaesthetist ensures there is no positive airway pressure from the anaesthetic circuit, which may distend the trachea/bronchi and mask airway collapse. However, positive pressure on demand aids assessment of how much a collapsed airway can open.
Removal of airway foreign body	Approach as above, with grasping forceps, possibly aided with a Hopkins rod or through a bronchoscope. Spontaneous breathing is preferred, positive-pressure ventilation may force the object further into the airway. Periods of apnoea occur when examination and retrieval are taking place. Jet ventilation can be used as long as the anaesthetist is aware of potential problems.
Laser surgery	Safety is paramount. Laser is used only by trained staff with all appropriate precautions in place.
Airway reconstruction	Encompasses a spectrum of procedures (cricoid split to full tracheal reconstruction under cardiopulmonary bypass). With the same principles as above: scrupulous attention to the airway and good communication with the surgeon. For example, an anterior laryngotracheal graft may be approached as follows: Pre-operative examination finds normal, albeit partially obstructed, breathing. Oral intubation with smaller size endotracheal tube (ETT). Tracheostomy is performed for the majority of ventilation through the procedure, with nasal ETT placed at the end.

Airway reconstruction (continued)	The ETT tip is positioned under direct vision by the surgeon before the tracheal incision is closed. The patient remains intubated for some days post-operatively, with the head in a neutral position to allow time for the trachea to heal.	
Tracheostomy	Clear communication when withdrawing the endotracheal tube and inserting the tracheostomy tube, and for postoperative management of stay sutures (taped down left and right).	
Ear operations	Simple ear surgery: grommets	Laryngeal mask airway is often used. Beware: myringotomy is highly stimulating—the patient's suddenly moving as the incision is made could be disastrous.
	Middle and major ear operations	No induced hypotension in children (lower resting blood pressure), positioning with the head up reduces venous pressure. Nitrous oxide is controversial: surgeon preference should be discussed with the anaesthetist beforehand.
Nasal surgery	Adenoidectomy	Surgeon/anaesthetist choice
	Reduction of nasal fracture	Laryngeal mask airway + throat pack: rarely results in haemorrhage
Head and neck	Endotracheal tube	

KEY POINTS

- The airway must be protected at all times—the anaesthetist must instantly be given as much access as required if any problems occur.
- Good communication is crucial. Never start a procedure until there has been a full briefing of all involved staff. Never forget, the patient can always be woken up again to come back another day. Do not persist in the face of adversity.
- Finally, if in any doubt, discuss the case with the anaesthetist.

96. HEARING TESTING

Introduction

Accurate assessment of suspected hearing loss in young children is fundamental to diagnosis, investigation, and rehabilitation. Assessment techniques differ between children and adults. Considerations include learning disabilities and test environment.

Terminology and Definitions

Hearing impairment is based on hearing threshold in dB HL (hearing level) averaged over the frequencies 0.5, 1.0, 2.0, and 4.0 kHz for the better-hearing ear as follows:

- Mild 21–39 dB
- Moderate 40–69 dB
- Severe 70–95 dB
- Profound > 95 dB

Risk Factors for Hearing Loss

- Treatment in neonatal intensive care unit (NICU) or special care baby unit (SCBU) for more than 48 hr
- Family history of early childhood deafness
- Craniofacial anomaly (e.g. cleft palate) associated with hearing impairment

Acquired and Late-Onset Permanent Bilateral Hearing Impairment

Acquired hearing impairment is one that was not present and detectable using appropriate tests at, or very soon after, birth. Meningitis is the most common cause of acquired hearing impairment in children.

Auditory Neuropathy Spectrum Disorder

Children with auditory neuropathy spectrum disorder (ANSD) have normal outer hair cell function, normal otoacoustic emissions (OAEs) and/or the cochlear microphonic response, and absent or severely abnormal auditory brainstem response (ABR). Up to 10% of children with confirmed permanent childhood hearing impairment (PCHI) have auditory neuropathy. ANSD is more common in the NICU population but rare in the well-baby population.

Surveillance

Surveillance is recommended for babies who pass the screen but have the following risk factors:

- Syndromes with associated hearing loss (other than Down syndrome)
- NICU with fail in both ears at OAE and pass in both ears at AABR
- Craniofacial anomaly
- Down syndrome
- Congenital infection

School-entry hearing screening is widely implemented, with coverage of around 90% (in state schools).

Electrophysiological Testing

Key developmental age: 0–6 months up to adult if appropriate

Electrophysiological techniques include OAE, ABR, and cortical evoked response audiometry (CERA). These methods are used in a child's first 6 months and in any child when behavioural testing has failed to produce reliable results (e.g. a child with learning difficulties). Accurate assessment may require sedation or general anaesthesia.

Behavioural Observation Audiometry (BOA)

Key developmental age: 0–6 months

- The child is observed for a response to a sound stimulus.
- Response behaviours include eye widening, eye blink (auropalpebral reflex), alteration in sucking response, arousal from sleep, startle or shudder of the body, or definite movement of the arms, legs, or body.
- In children age 4–7 months, lateral inclination of the head toward the sound, listening attitude, or stilling may be observed.
- BOA is a subjective test requiring tester judgement.

Test Method

- Child's attention is engaged by a distractor while the child is on a parent's lap.
- Sound stimulus is presented for <2 seconds, 15 cm from the child's ear, out of peripheral vision, or it is delivered via insert earphones.
- Distractor observes response.
- Sound stimuli are calibrated, narrow-band, warble tones or ling sounds.

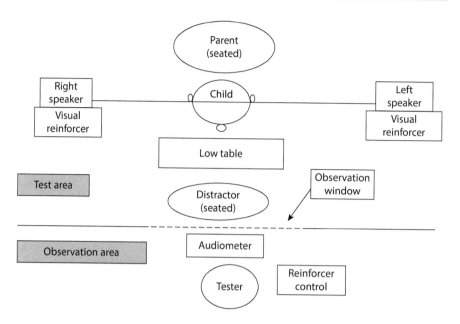

Figure 96.1   Test arrangement for visual reinforcement audiometry.

Visual Reinforcement Audiometry (VRA)
Key developmental age: 5–36 months

- Young children can be trained by operant conditioning to turn toward a visual stimulus in response to a sound stimulus.
- VRA is suitable for infants once they are able to sit unsupported or with minimal support.

Test Method

- Loudspeakers are placed at 90° from the child and at the child's head height, at least 1 m away from the child (Figure 96.1).
- Calibrated, frequency modulated (warble) tones, ling sounds, or narrow-band noise (NBN) stimuli are employed via soundfield, insert earphone, headphone, or bone conductor.
- The distractor draws the child's attention with gentle play.
- Sound stimulus duration is 2–3 seconds, initially with a concurrent visual reward. Then the stimulus is presented alone and the reinforcer is activated only after the child produces a turning response.
- Operant conditioning is achieved if correct response occurs 2–3 times. Then a minimal response level (MRL) is established for each frequency.
- MRL is the quietest level at which two of three clear responses were recorded for each sound stimulus.

The Distraction Test
Key developmental age: 6–18 months

- The test is based on the normal response observed when sound is presented to an infant, which is a head turn to locate the source of sound.
- Distraction testing largely has been discontinued in favour of VRA.

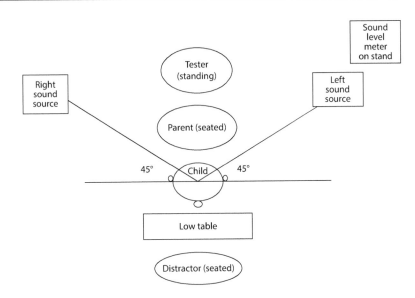

Figure 96.2 Test arrangement for the distraction test.

Test Method

- The test environment (Figure 96.2) is similar to that for VRA.
- The distractor directs the child's attention to an item covered by their hands.
- Sound stimulus is presented by the tester, half a second after the item is covered.
- Distractor observes the child's response.
- Sound stimulus (of up to 10 sec) should be presented in the horizontal plane to the ears at an angle, set back 45° between 1 m and 15 cm from the child's ear.
- Normal response is a full head turn in the direction of the sound, which is rewarded by the tester.
- Sound stimuli include voice (e.g. unforced 'S' = high frequency, or hum = low frequency), musical toys, calibrated high-frequency rattle, NBN, or warble tones.

Performance Testing (Play Audiometry)

Key developmental age: 2–5 years

The child is conditioned to wait for a sound and then to respond with a play activity (Figure 96.3).

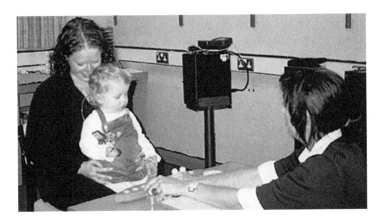

Figure 96.3 The performance test.

Test Method

- Once conditioned, a flexible descending/ascending technique, as described for pure-tone audiometry, can be applied to determine the MRL.
- Frequency-modulated warble tones with stimulus duration of 1–3 sec are the sound stimulus and can be delivered by portable soundfield noise generators, loudspeakers, insert earphones (using the child's own ear molds if available), or bone conductor.

Pure-Tone Audiometry

Key developmental age: 3 years and up

The techniques employed in play audiometry lead into pure-tone audiometry. This progression should be adapted to the individual child's ability to cooperate and to clinical priority. Masking techniques may not be reliable until the child being tested is 7 years old.

Auditory Speech Perception Tests

The ability to discriminate speech is a valuable measure of functional hearing in children with normal to moderate degrees of impairment, and auditory speech perception tests are increasingly used in evaluation of more severely affected children supplied with hearing aids or cochlear implants.

The Cooperative Test

Linguistic developmental level: 18–30 months

Cooperative testing requires the child to discriminate three different simple instructions (e.g. having been handed a small toy, the child is asked to give it to Mommy, or give it to the teddy bear, or give it to the baby doll). Starting at a suprathreshold level, the voice is dropped and visual clues are removed by covering the mouth. A child with normal hearing may discriminate the instruction at 35–40 dB(A). This technique has been superseded by VRA and speech discrimination tests.

Speech Discrimination Tests

Linguistic developmental level: 30 months and up

A wide range of speech discrimination assessments exist. They verify hearing thresholds and assess the effectiveness of hearing aids or auditory implants. The choice of test depends on the child's age, stage of linguistic development, and home language. Toy and picture tests have been developed and refined for the younger child, including the Stycar test, the Word Intelligibility by Picture Identification test (WIPI), Northwestern University Children's Perception of Speech test (NU-CHIPS), the Manchester picture test, and the McCormick toy test, which is widely used in the United Kingdom. This employs seven pairs of similar sounding nouns, such as spoon/shoe or cup/duck, each represented by a small, easily recognisable toy, placed on a table in front of the child in a quiet room (i.e. a closed-set assessment). Using live voice, the tester asks the child to 'Show me the … spoon', etc. Having established an understanding, the tester drops their voice level and removes visual clues by covering their mouth. The word discrimination threshold (WDT) is taken as the quietest level at which the child correctly identifies 80% of the toys including the paired consonants. For a child with normal hearing, this would be expected to occur at ≤40 dB(A).

Older children who have acquired appropriate linguistic skills, from around 6–8 years may be compliant with formal speech audiometry using open-set tasks whereby they listen and repeat a word or sentence presented at a calibrated level in quiet or in noise to a single ear or binaurally. Original examples include: AB word list (Arthur Boothroyd) and BKB (Bamford-Kowal-Bench) sentence list.

Hearing Assessment in Children with Complex Needs

Approximately 30% of hearing-impaired children have an additional disability. For a child with complex needs, the test must suit their developmental level rather than chronological age. The test should be adapted to suit the abilities of the child. If behavioural hearing assessment for a child with complex needs is inconclusive, electrophysiological measurement, which may require sedation or anaesthesia, is considered.

KEY POINTS

- Newborn hearing screening of all babies is the most effective and cost-effective way to identify congenital hearing loss.
- Numerous tests are available that account for the child's age, the availability of expertise, and the purpose of the test.

Further Reading

1. Public Health England. *NHS Newborn Hearing Screening Programme standards 2016 to 2017*. Available from: https://www.gov.uk/government/publications/newborn-hearing-screening-programme-quality-standards

2. British Society of Audiology. Practice guidance: *Auditory brainstem response testing in babies*, 2013. Available from: http://www.thebsa.org.uk/resources/guidance-auditory-brainstem-response- testing-babies/

3. British Society of Audiology. Practice guidance: *Visual reinforcement audiometry*, 2014. Available from: https://www.thebsa.org.uk/wp-content/uploads/2014/06/OD104-37-Recommended-Procedure-Visual-Reinforcement-Audiometry-2014-1.pdf

---

97. MANAGEMENT OF THE HEARING-IMPAIRED CHILD

Introduction

Permanent childhood hearing impairment (PCHI) is defined as permanent bilateral hearing impairment ≥40 dB HL (hearing level) averaged over 0.5, 1, 2, and 4 kHz in the better-hearing ear. One infant per thousand is born with permanent deafness or significant hearing impairment. A further one infant per thousand develops permanent deafness during childhood.

Onset may be prenatal, perinatal, or postnatal, and aetiology may be congenital or acquired (Figure 97.1). Most children with PCHI have sensorineural hearing loss (SNHL), but the hearing loss can be conductive or mixed. Those with pure conductive hearing loss may have a congenital middle ear abnormality.

Congenital PCHI

Genetic Causes

In the Western world, genetic factors are responsible for over half the cases of congenital SNHL, and 70% of cases of PCHI are nonsyndromic and 30% are syndromic (Table 97.1). Hearing loss is genetically very heterogeneous, involving mutations in many genes, making screening and prediction challenging.

Nonsyndromic Congential Hearing Impairment

In autosomal recessive nonsyndromic hearing impairment (ARNSHI), 50% of patients have mutations in the *GJB2* gene on chromosome 13. This gene encodes the gap junction protein connexin 26, which helps to maintain appropriate levels of endolymph intracellular potassium. The other 50% of cases are attributed to mutations in a wide variety of genes. Among 300 documented *GJB2* mutations, .35delG is responsible for 70%. The carrier rate in the general population for *GJB2* mutation is 1 in 33.

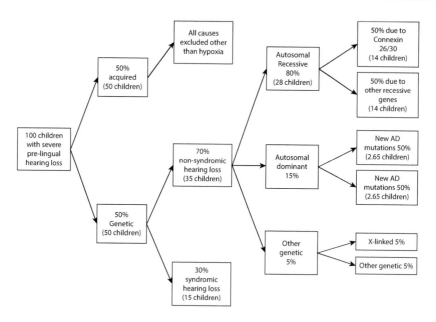

Figure 97.1 Aetiology of hearing loss in children.

Autosomal dominant nonsyndromic hearing impairment (ADNSHI) is more heterogeneous, with no single identifiable gene responsible for the majority of cases.

Another class of mutations affect the 12S RNA of mitochondria. These mutations (*1555A>G* and *1494C>T*) alter binding sites for aminoglycosides, resulting in a maternally transmitted predisposition to aminoglycoside toxicity (15% of all aminoglycoside-induced deafness).

Syndromic Hearing Impairment

Table 97.1 Syndromes associated with PCHI

Syndrome	Implicated genes	Clinical features
Autosomal Recessive		
Pendred's syndrome	*SLC26A4* pendrin gene—Chr 7	Most common syndromal deafness, 7–8% of congenital hearing loss: • Severe SNHL. • Euthyroid goitre develops in puberty. • Widening of vestibular aqueduct (Mondini dysplasia) can cause vestibular disturbance, also in branchio-oto-renal syndrome (BOR) and nonsyndromic deafness.
Usher's syndrome (USH)	15 loci and 12 genes— *MY07A/CDH23*	50% of deaf-blind children in the United States. Three major types are distinguished by severity of deafness, vestibular dysfunction, and age of onset. Type 1 patients have: • Congenital severe-to-profound SNHL • Vestibular dysfunction • Retinitis pigmentosa
Jervell and Lange-Nielsen syndrome	*KVLQT1* gene • Chr 11 • *KCNE1* gene–Chr 21	Elongation of QT interval on ECG causing fainting and sudden death. Highly associated with consanguinity.

Autosomal Dominant		
Waardenburg syndrome (WS)	Multiple genes— WS1&3 - *PAX3* WS2 - *MITF, SNAI2*	2–3% of all congenital hearing impairment. Primary phenotypes include: <ul><li>SHNL.</li><li>Pigmentation abnormalities (skin, white forelock, heterochromia iridis).</li><li>Dystopia canthorum or hypertelorism.</li><li>Hirschsprung's disease, limb anomalies, and constipation can be present.</li></ul>
Branchio-oto-renal syndrome (BOR)	*EYA1* (40%)	<ul><li>Hearing loss (conductive, sensorineural, or mixed)</li><li>Branchial cleft cysts or fistulae</li><li>Ear deformities</li><li>Renal malformations</li></ul>
Stickler syndrome	*COL2A1* (STL1), *COL11A1* (STL2), *COL11A2* (STL3)	Major features: <ul><li>Progressive SNHL</li><li>Cleft palate</li><li>Vertebral and epiphyseal abnormalities, osteoarthritis</li></ul> Three types: STL1 and STL2 have severe myopia, which predisposes to retinal detachment and is absent in STL3.
Neurofibromatosis 2 (NF2)	*'Merlin'* gene–Chr 22	Bilateral vestibular schwannomas, associated with meningiomas, ependymomas, and pre-senile cataracts. Mean age of vestibular schwannoma symptom onset is 20 years. 50% of NF2 patients have no family history.
X-linked		
Alport's syndrome	80% X-linked *(COL4A5)* 15% Autosomal recessive *(COL4A3/4)* 5% Autosomal dominant	<ul><li>50% develop progressive, bilateral SNHL, beginning in the second decade.</li><li>Renal disorder (glomerulonephritis, haematuria, renal failure).</li><li>Eye problems (lenticular and macular abnormalities).</li></ul>

Congenital Middle Ear Abnormalities

Conductive hearing loss in children is usually acquired, predominantly otitis media with effusion (OME) or chronic otitis media. Rare congenital deformities of the middle ear occur, and surgical intervention may be possible. Abnormalities are ossicular or nonossicular.

Ossicular Abnormalities

Ossicular abnormalities are relatively common in severe congenital deformity of the external ear, but rare in isolation, where diagnosis is often delayed. Children with bilateral ossicular abnormalities often present at similar ages as children with OME, hence they are often misdiagnosed. A conductive hearing loss with a normal tympanic membrane and normal middle ear pressure should raise suspicion. High-resolution computed tomography (CT) pre-operatively helps to assess ossicular abnormality and any accompanying middle ear abnormalities.

Using Cremers' classification, minor malformations can be categorised into four main groups:

1 Isolated stapes ankyloses (30.6%)
2 Ankylosis with other ossicular anomaly (38.2%)
3 Isolated ossicular anomaly with mobile stapes footplate (21.6%)
4 Aplasia or severe dysplasia of the oval or round windows (9.7%)

In general, unilateral hearing loss can be managed conservatively, and bilateral moderate hearing loss requires auditory rehabilitation (e.g. hearing aid). Surgery should only be undertaken by dedicated otologists with experience of complex middle ear reconstruction and should be preceded by an adequate trial of amplification.

Nonossicular Abnormalities

- **Persistent stapedial artery (PSA)**

  The stapedial artery usually atrophies in utero at around 10 weeks, leaving behind the obturator foramen of the stapes. Occasionally, the artery does not involute, leading to a PSA.

- **High jugular bulb (HJB)**

  The jugular bulb is 'high' if it reaches the level of the inferior bony annulus, is covered by thin bone, or is dehiscent. Usually asymptomatic and an incidental finding on otoscopy or middle ear surgery (with heavy bleeding). It can be associated with hearing loss. Differential diagnosis includes aberrant internal carotid artery (ICA), a PSA, or a glomus tympanicum tumour.

- **Aberrant ICA**

  Associated with vascular abnormalities (e.g. PSA). Symptoms include pulsatile tinnitus and hearing loss. Bilateral in 20%. Use CT/MRA imaging to avoid the high morbidity associated with unintended vascular injury.

- **Anomalous course of the facial nerve**

  The facial nerve canal may show dehiscence or have an anomalous course. It is more common with microtia or labyrinthine dysplasia, and there should be a high index of suspicion with surgery for congenital conductive hearing loss (facial nerve monitor recommended).

- **Congenital perilymphatic fistula (PLF)**

  PLF is an abnormal communication between the middle and inner ear that allows escape of perilymphatic fluid with no antecedent traumatic event. PLF is associated with microfissures around the oval and round windows or labyrinthine dysplasia. Management is based on the suggestive diagnosis of a child presenting with fluctuating SNHL, possibly associated with vertigo. Surgical treatment is packing with fat graft or temporalis muscle around the oval and round windows in suspected cases.

Nongenetic Causes

The nongenetic causes of congenital hearing impairment including maternal substance abuse, maternal endocrine disorders, birth complications, hyperbilirubinaemia, and maternal infections. The key maternal infections are outlined below.

- **Cytomegalovirus (CMV)**

  Congenital CMV is the most common cause of non-hereditary SNHL in the developed world. Infection occurs in 1% of pregnancies and 40% of affected mothers pass the virus on to the baby. The greatest risk accompanies first trimester infection. The hearing loss can be delayed, which challenges diagnosis.

- **Congenital rubella syndrome (CRS)**

  In countries with no rubella vaccination program, CRS is probably the most important cause of congenital hearing loss due to first trimester infection. CRS causes deafness, ocular defects (cataracts, glaucoma), cardiac anomalies (patent ductus arteriosus, pulmonary artery stenosis (PAS), ventricular septal defects), central nervous system problems (microcephaly, global retardation), and characteristic skin changes.

- **Syphilis**

  Caused by the bacterium *Treponema pallidum*. Syphilis is a common infection in the developing world and recently has been re-emerging in the developed world. During primary syphilis, the rate of vertical transmission in untreated women is 70–100%. Hearing loss is late feature of congenital syphilis. Hutchinson's triad is interstitial keratitis (visual impairment), peg-shaped upper incisors (Hutchinson's teeth), and VIIIth cranial nerve deafness.

- **Toxoplasmosis**
  There is growing evidence of correlation between congenital toxoplasmosis and hearing disorders.

Acquired PCHI

The following environmental factors are known risk factors for acquired permanent hearing loss:

- *Admission to a neonatal intensive care unit (NICU):* Improved survival rates of pre-term babies has increased the proportion of babies with hearing loss related to perinatal events. NICU admission significantly increases the risk of developing permanent hearing loss.
- *Hypoxia:* Known to be associated with neurodevelopmental deficits.
- *Hyperbilirubinaemia:* High levels of unconjugated bilirubin are associated with neuronal damage, preferentially involving the auditory nuclei and inferior colliculi.
- *Ototoxics:* Drugs causing hearing loss (cochlear level) are aminoglycosides (especially gentamicin and tobramycin), chemotherapeutic agents (platinum derivatives, cyclophosphamide, and methotrexate), antimalarials (chloroquine), diuretics (especially furosemide), and iron chelators (desferrioxamine).
- *Meningitis:* Bacterial meningitis is the commonest cause of acquired PCHI. There is a 10% risk of significant sensorineural impairment after bacterial meningitis. *Haemophilus influenzae* type b and meningococcus C vaccinations have significantly reduced these infections. All patients need early audiological assessment after meningitis, and those with severe loss should be fast-tracked for assessment by a cochlear implant centre.
- *Measles:* Incidence of measles has been significantly reduced in developed countries since measles vaccine introduction in 1968. Measles usually occurs after 6 months of age. Measles is reported as a major aetiological factor for mild to moderate bilateral hearing loss and causes both conductive and sensorineural impairment.
- *Mumps:* May cause profound, usually unilateral, SNHL.

Newborn Hearing Screening

Since 2005, all U.K. babies have been screened for congenital hearing loss. The median age of detection of PCHI is now 10 weeks. In England, all children are screened with automated otoacoustic emissions (AOAE) as soon after birth as possible. If there is no clear response after two trials of AOAE, then automated auditory brainstem response (AABR) is tested. Failure of AABR triggers audiology referral for further testing. All NICU babies have an AABR screen in addition to AOAE screen as standard.

The Newly Diagnosed Deaf Child and Family

Most deaf babies (95%) are born to hearing families. An ENT surgeon's primary aims include:

- Investigating the cause of hearing loss
- Developing a support plan along with other multidisciplinary team (MDT) members (parents, audiologists, paediatricians, speech therapists, teachers of the deaf)
- Considering surgical intervention for conductive loss
- Evaluating suitability for bone-anchored hearing aids or cochlear implantation

In the United Kingdom, national guidelines for investigating PCHI were developed by the British Association of Audiological Physicians and British Association of Paediatricians in Audiology. Core investigations (Table 97.2) are offered to parents of all children with a newly diagnosed hearing impairment. Additional investigations are dictated by individual circumstances and findings and may include serological tests for congenital rubella, immunological tests, metabolic screening, renal ultrasound, and chromosomal analysis.

Early identification of PCHI has led to routine fitting of hearing aids in the first few months of life and implantable devices in the first year of life. The earlier the device provision, the more effective it is in the long term.

Table 97.2 Core investigations for all cases of bilateral severe to profound sensorineural hearing loss

Investigation	Details
Paediatric history	Detailed history of pregnancy, delivery, and postnatal period. Developmental milestones, pre- and postnatal noise exposure, ototoxic medications, head injuries, ear disease, meningitis, viral illness, and immunisation status.
Family history	Deafness or risk factors associated with hearing loss in first- and second-degree relatives.
Clinical examination	Inspection and measurement of craniofacial region (skull and face shape, cleft palate), assessment of eyes (colour, position, intercanthal distance, cataracts), hair (white forelock), ears (pits, shape and size of pinna, ear canal, tympanic membranes), neck (branchial abnormalities, goitre), skin (café-au-lait spots), limbs, chest, and abdomen.
Audiology	Age-appropriate assessment, including tympanometry. Audiometry for first-degree relatives.
Imaging	MRI of internal acoustic meatus and CT of petrous temporal bones are preferred where there is a conductive component.
Electrocardiogram	Long QT interval in Jervell and Lange-Nielsen syndrome
Urine for microscopic haematuria and for CMV DNA PCR	Proteinuria and haematuria can be found in Alport's syndrome.
	Families of all children with bilateral PCHI are offered genetic screening for these two mutations.
Referral to clinical geneticist	
Ophthalmic assessment	20–60% of children with PCHI have ophthalmic abnormalities.
Vestibular investigations	
CMV serology	Laboratory testing must occur for neonate within 3 weeks of life to diagnose congenital CMV. After 3 weeks, virus isolation could be due to acquired infection (which usually has no adverse outcomes).
Routine blood tests	FBC, TFTs, ESR, U&Es, syphilis blood tests, cholesterol, and triglyceride levels. Abnormal results rarely relate to the cause of the hearing loss.

KEY POINTS

- One infant per thousand is born with permanent hearing impairment and an additional 1 per 1,000 develops permanent deafness during childhood.
- Early identification and rehabilitation lead to better life chances for the child.
- Progressive hearing loss is missed unless surveillance is carried out during childhood.
- Optimal initial management of PCHI is early fitting of binaural hearing aids. If aids are not appropriate, referral is made for assessment for implants.
- In autosomal recessive nonsyndromic hearing impairment, 50% of patients have mutations in the GJB2 gene (chromosome 13).
- Congenital abnormalities of the middle ear may occur in association with major malformations, such as microtia.

Further Reading

British Association of Audiovestibular Physicians. Guidelines for aetiological investigation into progressive permanent childhood hearing impairment, 2018. https://www.baap.org.uk/uploads/1/1/9/7/119752718/guideline_progressive_hl_final.pdf

British Association of Paediatricians in Audiology. Documents and Guidelines. http://www.bapa.uk.com/documents

Genetics Home Reference. https://ghr.nlm.nih.gov/

98. OTITIS MEDIA

Acute Otitis Media

Definition
Acute otitis media (AOM) is inflammation of the middle ear cleft of rapid onset and infective origin, associated with a middle ear effusion and a varied collection of symptoms and signs.

Epidemiology
The incidence of AOM peaks between 6 and 12 months of life. AOM affects 60% of children under 1 year old, 50–70% by age 3 years, and 75% by 9 years.

Risk Factors
Environmental factors that increase the risk of AOM include day-care attendance, seasonal upper respiratory tract infections (URTIs), bottle feeding, use of a pacifier, lower socioeconomic class, overcrowding at home, passive smoke inhalation, and dietary factors, such as cow's milk allergy. There are also genetic and immunological factors, as well syndromic associations (e.g. Down syndrome and cleft palate) that increase risk.

Aetiology
Viruses
Respiratory syncytial virus, influenza A, parainfluenza virus, human rhinovirus, and adenoviruses are associated with AOM.

Bacteria
Streptococcus pneumoniae, Haemophilus influenzae, Moraxella catarrhalis, Streptococcus pyogenes, and *Staphylococcus aureus* are implicated in AOM.

Routes of Spread of Infection
Infection spreads via the Eustachian tube, tympanic membrane perforations or grommets, and haematogenous spread.

Symptoms
Symptoms include rapid-onset otalgia, hearing loss, otorrhoea, fever, excessive crying, irritability, coryzal symptoms, vomiting, poor feeding, ear pulling, and clumsiness. AOM commonly develops 3–4 days after coryza.

Signs
The tympanic membrane (TM) is opaque and yellow or red, hypomobile, and bulging. Perforation results in otorrhoea. The child may appear unwell and may tug on the affected ear.

Investigations
AOM is largely a clinical diagnosis. A pus swab of otorrhoea may be taken for microbiology. A full blood count is indicated in cases of recurrent AOM.

Clinical Diagnosis
A typical history depicts crescendo otalgia in a coryzal child followed by rapid symptomatic relief associated with TM perforation and otorrhoea.

Differential Diagnosis
Nonotological differentials are caused by referred otalgia. Otological causes include bullous myringitis, otitis externa, trauma, otitis media with effusion (OME), Ramsay Hunt's syndrome, and acute mastoiditis.

Management Options

- Conservative treatment
  Simple analgesia is sufficient for most cases of AOM.
- Medical treatment
  Antibiotics for healthy children should be given after 3–4 days of symptoms during which conservative management has failed. Antibiotics are indicated immediately in children who have comorbidities (e.g. immunodeficiencies, craniofacial abnormalities, Down syndrome), are systemically unwell, or are < 2 years old with bilateral AOM, recurrent AOM, or TM perforation.
- Surgical management
  Myringotomy is performed where a complication is present or suspected, to relieve severe pain, or when microbiology is necessary.

Management of Recurrent Acute Otitis Media (RAOM)

- Alteration of risk factors
  - Reduce exposure to other children (e.g. in day-care nursery setting)
  - Avoid passive smoking
  - Sit the child semi-upright for bottle-feeding
  - Avoid pacifier use
  - In future, breastfeed the infant for at least 6 months
  - In pregnancy, avoid alcohol and increase vitamin C intake in the third trimester
- Medical prophylaxis
  The modest benefit of antibiotic prophylaxis may not outweigh the risks of antibiotic resistance, side-effects, and costs. Vaccinations, xylitol, zinc, and immunoglobulins are still under study.
- Surgical prophylaxis
  Grommets and adenoidectomy may decrease the frequency of RAOM.

Outcomes of AOM
An episode of AOM may resolve rapidly with or without antibiotics or progress to a complication. OME may follow an episode of AOM but will resolve spontaneously in most cases. An air–bone gap greater than 20 dB may occur after AOM but may reduce over time. OME may significantly affect expressive language development in the early years of life, and speech problems may persist through early school years.

Complications
Complications of AOM include TM perforation, acute mastoiditis, petrositis, facial nerve palsy, labyrinthitis, meningitis, extradural abscess, subdural empyema, sigmoid sinus thrombosis, focal otitic encephalitis, brain abscess, and otitic hydrocephalus.

Chronic Otitis Media

Definition

Chronic otitis media (COM) involves chronic inflammation within the middle ear (ME). COM can be active or inactive and with or without cholesteatoma. The active type involves ongoing inflammation, whereas the inactive type involves fibrosis and scarring.

COM with Cholesteatoma

Cholesteatoma is a mass of keratinising squamous epithelium in the ME and/or mastoid. Paediatric cholesteatoma (PC) can be congenital or acquired.

- *Congenital cholesteatoma (CC)*: CC is an expanding cystic mass with keratinising squamous epithelium located medially to an intact tympanic membrane, and 10–28% of cholesteatomas are congenital.
- *Acquired cholesteatoma (AC)*: AC is classified into primary and secondary types. Primary AC is explained by the retraction theory, where a retracted or atrophic TM secondary to Eustachian tube dysfunction (ETD) and negative ME pressure leads to ingrowth of TM squamous epithelium and invasion of the ME. Secondary AC is due to ingrowth of keratin epithelium through a TM perforation or iatrogenic implantation during surgery.

Epidemiology

PC is a rare disease but is more common in Caucasians and Africans, and 7–10% of children have bilateral disease at presentation or will develop contralateral symptoms during follow up. The mean age for surgery is 10 years.

Diagnosis

AC typically presents with a long history of otorrhoea and conductive hearing loss, along with a TM retraction filled with keratin.

CC may present with hearing loss alone. Presentation may be late if the contralateral hearing is normal. An examination under anaesthesia (EUA) is often needed to perform diagnostic myringotomy.

Microbiology

Proteus mirabilis, Pseudomonas aeruginosa, and *Staphylococcus aureus* are most frequently cultured.

Imaging

Computed tomography (CT) identifies temporal bone anatomy and extent of disease.

Magnetic resonance imaging (MRI) allows soft-tissue differentiation and assessment of dural plate erosion, intracranial spread, or an associated complication, as well as residual cholesteatoma post-operatively.

Treatment

Nonsurgical

Antibiotic/steroid drops and microsuction may be appropriate for children unfit for general anesthesia and for those awaiting surgery.

Rationale for Surgery in Pediatric Cholesteatoma

- Primary aims are
  - To remove all disease to prevent further erosion and complications
  - To provide a dry and watertight ear
  - To provide an ear that will be self-cleaning
  - To prevent the occurrence of recurrent cholesteatoma
- Secondary aims are to improve hearing

Surgical Approaches for Pediatric Cholesteatoma

1. Canal wall down (CWD) surgery includes modified radical mastoidectomy ± subtotal petrosectomy ± obliteration/closure of external ear canal (EAC).
2. Canal wall up (CWU) surgery includes tympanotomy/tympanoplastic surgery, atticotomy ± reconstruction and CWU mastoidectomy.

CWD Surgery

In CWD surgery, the ear canal wall and attic scutum are excised. This provides better intra-operative access to the ME, mastoid, and attic to clear keratin.

CWU Surgery

CWU surgery retains the canal wall and a closed ME at the level of the original TM. It may include an atticotomy or bony marginectomy followed by reconstruction of the defect and TM repair or a combined approach tympanoplasty (CAT).

COM with Cholesteatoma in Children with Other Syndromes

Down syndrome, craniofacial syndrome, and DiGeorge syndrome are associated with an increased incidence of PC, and patients with microtia may be difficult to diagnose due to abnormal external ear anatomy.

KEY POINTS

- Pediatric cholesteatoma presents with otorrhea, hearing loss, and keratin within a TM retraction pocket.
- Investigations may include microbiology swabs and CT and MRI.
- The mainstay of treatment is surgical with either a canal wall up or canal wall down approach.

Further Reading

1. Leung AKC, Wong AHC. Acute otitis media in children. *Recent Pat Inflamm Allergy Drug Discov* 2017; 11(1): 32–40.
2. Luu K, Chi D, Kiyosaki KK, Chang KW. Updates in pediatric cholesteatoma: minimizing intervention while maximizing outcomes. *Otolaryngol Clin North Am* 2019; 52(5): 813–823.
3. Jackson R, Addison AB, Prinsley PR. Cholesteatoma in children and adults: are there really any differences? *J Laryngol Otol* 2018; 132(7): 575–578.

99. EMBRYOLOGICAL DEVELOPMENT DISORDERS

External Ear
The pinna reaches adult size by 8-10 years.

Embryology
The external ear forms from the first two pharyngeal arches. The external auditory canal (EAC) develops from the first pharyngeal cleft.

The middle ear and the inner layer of the tympanic membrane are derived from first pharyngeal pouch. (Malleus and incus are from first pharyngeal arch, stapes from the second arch.)

Developmental Anomalies of the External Ear

Preauricular Sinus

- Opening anterior to helix, lined with squamous epithelium, and adherent to helix cartilage.
- Occurrence is sporadic (generally unilateral) or inherited (especially bilateral).
- Associated with syndromes (e.g. branchio-oto-renal syndrome).
- Acute infections require antibiotics and needle aspiration if severe.
- Wide local incision has lowest recurrence rates.

Preauricular Appendages
Occur on a line from tragus to angle of the mandible. Excision for cosmesis and facial symmetry.

Microtia

- Malformed or underdeveloped pinna (Table 99.1), may be associated with congenital canal atresia or canal stenosis.
- Incidence 1 in 10,000.
- Patients usually have conductive hearing loss.
- Cosmetic management options: no intervention, bone-anchored auricular prosthesis (BAAP), and autologous ear reconstruction using cartilage.

Cleft Lip & Palate

- Cleft lip (CL) and cleft palate only (CPO) are the commonest forms of orofacial clefting, with an overall incidence of 1 in 600–750.
- Associated with airway, hearing, speech, and nasal issues.
- Distribution: cleft lip and palate (46%), CPO (33%), and CL alone (21%).
- Classified by laterality and extent of the defect (Veau's classification).
- CL:
  - Cleft of structures anterior to incisive foramen
  - Unilateral or bilateral
  - Complete (involving alveolus), incomplete, or microform
- Cleft palate:
  - Defect of secondary palate
  - May be incomplete, complete, bilateral, unilateral, or submucous

Table 99.1   Marx classification of microtia

Grade 1	Smaller but recognisable normal pinna
Grade 2	Some features of normal pinna recognisable
Grade 3	Rudiment of soft tissue and cartilage
Grade 4	Absent pinna and ear canal

- Orofacial clefts are non-syndromic or syndromic; commonest is del(22)(q11.2), which is associated with a wide spectrum, including Di George and velocardiofacial phenotypes.
- Nonsyndromic clefting is multifactorial (i.e. genetic and environmental factors).
- Syndromes associated with CPO: 22q deletion, Treacher Collins', Stickler's, Apert's, Down (trisomy 21), Goldenhar's.
- Syndromes associated with CL ± P: Van der Woude syndrome, Down (trisomy 21).
- Risk factors for CL/P: maternal factors (age, smoking, obesity, first-trimester heavy alcohol consumption, pre-pregnancy diabetes, and medications).

ENT Issues

- **Airway**
  All children with craniofacial disorders need overnight oximetry started within their first 4 weeks because there is increased risk of obstructive sleep apnoea due to nasopharyngeal narrowing.
- **Hearing loss**
  Otitis media with effusion (OME) is almost ubiquitous with CL ± P (~97% of children have OME by age 2 years).

Insufficient evidence to determine benefit of early ventilation tubes.

Routine hearing tests are required at age 6 months and at 1, 2, 3, 4, 5, 10, and 15 years.

Management

Prenatal diagnosis is made with ultrasound.

Surgical management depends on the patient's age (Table 99.2).

Velopharyngeal insufficiency (VPI) can occur in children with a repaired cleft palate, submucous cleft, post-adenoidectomy (1:1500–3000), or children without any obvious palatal abnormalities.

KEY POINTS

- Clefts of the lip and palate are common congenital birth anomalies.
- Aetiology is multifactorial.
- Prenatal screening for cleft lip and palate is available and effective.

Craniofacial Surgery

Craniofacial conditions have no universal classification system.

Craniosynostosis

Craniosynostosis is premature fusion of one or more skull sutures, which can be primary or secondary (differentiation is important because treatment options differ) (Table 99.3).

Table 99.2 Surgical management of cleft lip and palate by patient age

Age	Procedure
3–6 months	Primary lip ± nose repair ± hard palate
9–12 months	Palate repair ± ventilation tubes
4–5 years	Secondary speech surgery (if required)
8–10 years	Alveolar bone graft (if required)
15–18 years	Secondary rhinoplasty
16+ years	Orthognathic surgery (if required)

Table 99.3 Single-suture nonsyndromic craniosynostosis

Shape of skull	Suture affected	Name	
	Sagittal	Scaphocephaly	• Most common • Frontal bossing • Elevated hairline • Bitemporal pinching with a posterior excessive occipital bullet
	Metopic	Trigonocephaly	• Wedge-shaped forehead • Supraorbital recession and often hypotelorism • Decreased interorbital and intercanthal distances
	Unilateral coronal	Frontal plagiocephaly	• Most varied • Facial and nasal twist toward affected side with resultant strabismus
	Bilateral coronal	Brachycephaly	8–15% family history
	Unilateral lambdoid	True posterior synostotic plagiocephaly	Trapezoid head

The brain grows rapidly in the first 2 years of life and this stimulates growth of the cranium.

Premature fusion aetiology:

Secondary craniosynostosis: uncommon, seen in microcephaly (lack of underlying brain growth), haematological disorders (polycythaemia, thalassaemia), and metabolic abnormalities (rickets, hyperthyroidism) or drug-induced disorder (retinoic acid).

Primary craniosynostosis: more common, classified based on number of sutures involved (single, multiple, total), site of involved suture (metopic, sagittal, coronal, lambdoid), and whether nonsyndromic (isolated) or syndromic (with other malformations).

- *Nonsyndromic:* 60% are sagittal, with a 4:1 male predominance.
- Commonest syndromic craniosynostosis is in Crouzon's syndrome, followed by Apert's syndrome.

Single-Suture Nonsyndromic Craniosynostosis

- Radiology assessment of suture patency and skull morphology
- Raised intracranial pressure (ICP) with craniosynostosis more common (up to 20%) in syndromic patients
- Indications for surgery: prevention and/or treatment of raised ICP, correct cosmetic deformity, and prevent future skull-shape deformity
- Treatment principles: remove cause (excise affected suture), correct deformity (reshape affected area)
- Note: Excised suture may re-ossify

Syndromic Craniosynostosis

Over 500 different syndromes include craniofacial anomalies (Table 99.4).

Management aims to avoid raised ICP and to normalise skull shape and morphology.

ENT comorbidities:

- Airway
  - Central apnoeas (Chiari malformation/raised ICP), obstructive sleep apnoea (40–83% children)

Table 99.4   Syndromic craniosynostosis

Syndrome	Features
Crouzon's syndrome (1:25,000 live births)	• Craniosynostosis (bicoronal) and maxillary hypoplasia • Proptosis from exorbitism • Ear canal atresia and middle ear anomalies
Apert's syndrome (1:60,000)	• Craniosynostosis (bicoronal) and abnormal midfacial development • Syndactyly • Cleft soft palate or bifid uvula (30%) • Fixation of stapes footplate
Pfeiffer's syndrome	• Craniosynostosis (coronal) and midfacial hypoplasia with shallow orbits • Broad thumbs and great toes • Solid cartilaginous trachea • Choanal stenosis/atresia

- Multilevel airway obstruction (choanal atresia, nasopharyngeal narrowing, narrow oropharynx, subglottic and tracheal stenosis)
  - Compromised neuromuscular control
- Visual considerations
  - Exorbitism (decreased orbital volume) with midfacial hypoplasia
  - Papilloedema, optic atrophy with raised ICP
- Intracranial pressure
  - Without treatment, visual and neurological deterioration
  - Influenced by craniocerebral disproportionation and hydrocephalus
  - Ventricular dilatation common (nearly 50%)

Complications of Craniofacial Surgery

- Blood loss (75–85% of patients require a blood transfusion)
- Air embolism
- Cerebral oedema
- Dural tear
- CSF fistula
- Infection
- Intracerebral/subdural haematoma
- Blindness
- Restenosis (more common in syndromic cases)

Hemifacial Microsomia/Oculoauriculovertebral Spectrum (OAVS)

- Combined definition encompassing hemifacial microsomia, first and second branchial arch syndrome, otomandibular dysostosis, facioauriculovertebral syndrome, and Goldenhar's syndrome.
- OAVS is classified by OMENS mnemonic (orbit/orbitozygomatic, mandible, ear, nerve, soft tissues).
- Most striking feature is facial asymmetry.
- Extracranial features can occur in OAVS.

Treacher Collins' Syndrome (Mandibulofacial Dysostosis)

- Absence or hypoplasia of zygomatic bones, eyelid abnormalities, mandibular hypoplasia, and microtia (usually normal intelligence).
- Autosomal dominant but 50% of cases have no family history.
- Cleft palate affects 35% of cases and bilateral ear abnormalities are common.

- High incidence of airway problems with syndromic craniosynostosis.
- Some patients require long-term tracheostomy.
- Microtia is an important feature of many craniofacial disorders, particularly OAVS/hemifacial macrosomia and Treacher Collins' syndrome.

Congenital Disorders of the Larynx, Trachea, and Bronchi

Congenital laryngeal, tracheal, and bronchial disorders are summarised in Table 99.5.

- Congenital airway anomalies tend to present in the first few weeks of life with stridor and/or feeding difficulties.
- Congenital airway disorders are often associated with underlying syndromes.
- Laryngomalacia is the most common congenital disorder.
- Propranolol is the first choice for subglottic haemangiomas.
- Slide tracheoplasty is the treatment of choice for long-segment congenital tracheal stenosis.

Haemangiomas and Vascular Malformations

Vascular anomalies may be classified as follows.

- **Vascular tumours** include infantile haemangiomas, congenital haemangiomas, tufted angiomas, kaposiform harmangiomas, pyogenic granulomas, etc.
- **Vascular malformations** are described according to flow (slow, fast, or complex) and include slow-flow malformations (capillary malformation and venous malformation), fast-flow malformations (arterial malformations, arterial fistula, and arteriovenous malformation), and complex combined-flow malformations.

Haemangiomas

- Most common tumour in Caucasian infants (10–12%), with female preponderance, mostly solitary, and two thirds are found in the head and neck region.
- Glucose transporter-1 (GLUT-1) is a marker (97% positive).
- Types: congenital (CH; present at birth) and infantile (commoner, proliferate from pink macules during first 2 months).
- Usually solitary; if there are multiple hemangiomas, there is a higher chance of visceral involvement.
- Natural history is proliferation and rapid growth that plateaus by 4–8 months. Involution begins at around 1 year and continues for 5–7 years.
- Permanent skin changes occur in over 50% of patients.
- Majority have no genetic basis. Large cervicofacial haemangiomas are seen with other malformations in 10% (e.g. PHACES syndrome: Posterior cranial fossa malformation, Arterial anomalies, Cardiac anomalies, Eye anomalies, Sternal anomalies, bifid or cleft).
- Treatment is usually conservative or propranolol administered 1–3 mg/kg/day in three divided doses.
- Surgical excision and laser treatment are indicated if there is poor response to propranolol.

Table 99.5   Congenital laryngeal, tracheal, and bronchial disorders

Site	Congenital disorders	Key points
Larynx— Supraglottis	Laryngomalacia • Collapse of supraglottis on inspiration • Epiglottis omega-shaped • Aryepiglottic folds short and tightly tethered to the epiglottis • Redundant mucosa of aryepiglottic folds	• Most common cause of congenital stridor • Usually present at, or shortly after, birth (worse with distress/activity) • Stridor severity increases during first 9 months, diminishes by 2 years • 90% need no intervention • Severe cases have respiratory obstruction, feeding difficulty, reflux, failure to thrive • Treatment: aryepiglottoplasty (each aryepiglottic fold divided and redundant mucosa excised)
	Saccular cysts *Mucus filled*	• Rare • Type 1 (internal) contained within laryngeal framework, type 2 (external) if pierces thyrohyoid membrane
	Laryngocoele *Air-filled dilatation of laryngeal ventricle*	• Rare • Treatment: endoscopic marsupialisation, consider lateral cervical approach for recurrence
	Vascular malformations *Lymphatic, venous, and arteriovenous*	Microcystic lymphatic malformations may extend into the tongue base, valleculae, and supraglottis causing airway obstruction.
	Bifid epiglottis *Midline fusion failure*	• Rare • Pallister-Hall syndrome • Feeding difficulties (aspiration and stridor)
Larynx— Glottis	Laryngeal webs *Failure of laryngeal canalisation*	• Respiratory obstruction and dysphonia • Inspiratory stridor, weak, high-pitched, squeaky voice • Associated 22q11 deletion • Treatment: endoscopic division (cold steel or laser) ± keel with covering tracheostomy
	Laryngeal atresia	• Incompatible with life unless associated tracheo-oesophageal fistula • If recognised antenatally needs ex utero intrapartum treatment (EXIT) tracheostomy
	Cri-du-chat syndrome *Posterior glottis remains open, giving diamond-shape appearance*	• Cat-like mewing cry • Microcephaly
	Vocal cord paralysis • Unilateral (50%) *Mostly injury to recurrent laryngeal nerve secondary to cardiac surgery* • Bilateral (50%) *Congenital abductor paralysis (cords lie in paramedian position)*	• Second commonest cause of congenital stridor • Up to 45% have coexisting airway pathology • Stridor, dysphonia, aspiration • Treatment: conservative, with recovery or compensation • Stridor • Associated with hydrocephalus and Arnold-Chiari malformation • Most cases idiopathic, half recover • Treatment: tracheostomy (50% cases), endoscopic laser cordotomy or arytenoidectomy at age >11 if no recovery

Site	Congenital disorders	Key points
Larynx— *Subglottis*	Congenital subglottic stenosis *Defective canalisation of the cricoid cartilage ± conus elasticus*	• Third most common congenital anomaly • Stridor or recurrent croup • Myer-Cotton grading (4 grades) • Treatment: conservative, tracheostomy, laryngotracheal reconstruction
	Subglottic haemangioma *Compressible, pear-shaped, red swelling in the subglottis on one side (more commonly left)*	• Gradually worsening stridor • Proliferative phase lasts 6–12 months followed by complete involution over 1–5 years • 1–2% patients with cutaneous lesion have subglottic lesion; 50% patients with subglottic lesion have coexisting cutaneous lesion • Treatment: propranolol (1–3 mg/kg for minimum 12 months before weaning), surgical excision, tracheostomy
	Laryngeal and laryngotracheo-oesophageal cleft	• Benjamin & Inglis classification (4 types) • Cyanotic attacks with feeding, recurrent infections, stridor, abnormal cry, incipient cardiorespiratory failure • 25% have tracheo-oesophageal fistula • Other associated congenital abnormalities: dextrocardia, situs inversus, congenital heart disease • Associated Opitz-Frias syndrome, Pallister-Hall syndrome
Trachea and Bronchi	Agenesis	• Long-term survival not possible • If only one main bronchus is compatible, associated with other congenital abnormalities
	Congenital tracheal stenosis (CTS) *Membranous web or thicker congenital fibrous stenosis with normal underlying cartilaginous ring structure*	• Endoscopic balloon dilatation ± laser • Mitomycin C may reduce restenosis • End-to-end anastomosis if short • 60% with long-segment CTS (LSCTS) have associated malformations (pulmonary artery sling, right-sided aortic arch, subglottic stenosis, tracheo-oesophageal fistula) • Respiratory distress within first year (symptoms when >50% stenosis) • Sometimes stenosis is too narrow for endoscope so contrast bronchography is needed.
	Tracheomalacia and Bronchomalacia	• Clinically significant when >50% obstruction • Primary (idiopathic) tracheomalacia is intrinsic wall abnormality. Secondary is due to external compression. • High-pitched expiratory stridor • Treatment: mild (<75% collapse) spontaneously resolve by 2 years; severe needs treatment if failure to thrive, treat cause (i.e. correct vascular anomaly, tracheo-oesophageal fistula), alternatively, CPAP (± tracheostomy for laryngotracheal ventilation (LTV))
	Tracheo-oesophageal fistula (TOF)	• 50% of TOF have additional congenital malformations and 10–20% have tracheomalacia • H-type fistula presents with recurrent minor aspiration • Treatment: ligation and division of the fistula

(continued)

Table 99.5 (continued)

Site	Congenital disorders	Key points
Trachea and Bronchi (continued)	Vascular compression • Vascular ring *Completely encircles trachea and oesophagus* • Vascular sling	• Surgical treatment necessary • Commonest is double aortic arch with compression of trachea and oesophagus. • Less common is right-sided aortic arch and descending aorta with an aberrant left subclavian artery • Commonest is aberrant innominate artery. • On bronchoscopy, a sloping, pulsatile compression of trachea is seen 1–2 cm above carina.
	Anomalous bifurcations (Porcine/pig bronchus)	• Tracheal bronchus for right upper lobe (normal arrangement in a pig) • Usually asymptomatic

Slow-Flow Malformations: Capillary Malformations

- Affect 0.1–0.3% of live births, and occur mostly in head and neck.
- Flat, pink areas that darken with age.
- Majority are isolated, but associated syndromes include Sturge-Weber and Klippel-Trenaunay.
- Treatment depends on vessel diameter but includes pulsed dye laser.
- Recurrence rate is 50% at 5 years.

Slow-Flow Malformations: Venous Malformations (VM)

- Abnormal collection of veins, typically without a uniform smooth muscle layer.
- Usually solitary and sporadic; multiple inherited subtype—multiple glomangiomas (autosomal dominant).
- All VMs are congenital and grow with the child.
- Management includes reassurance, monitoring, aspirin, compression, sclerotherapy, and laser.
- Friable vascular tissue makes surgical excision difficult.

Slow-Flow Malformations: Lymphatic Malformations (LM)

- Abnormal embryological development of the lymphatic system.
- 75% found in head and neck.
- LM represent 6% of all pediatric soft-tissue masses.
- LM grow with the child and 90% are diagnosed by 2 years.
- Several classifications exist, but two main types are common: slow, lateral disease (below mylohyoid) is usually macrocystic and managed by surgery or sclerotherapy; high (above mylohyoid) and medial disease is typically microcystic and may require tracheostomy and long-term multimodality treatment.

Fast-Flow Malformations: Arteriovenous Malformations (AVM)

- Less common than slow-flow malformations in head and neck.
- Early imaging is imperative.
- Treatment includes embolisation (not curative, as new vascular channels develop) or complete surgical excision (curative but challenging and sometimes impossible).

KEY POINTS

- Vascular anomalies, comprising vascular tumours and vascular malformations, are congenital lesions.
- A comprehensive understanding of these lesions is fundamental to accurate diagnosis and successful management.

100. IMBALANCE

Introduction

Young children do not usually complain of vertigo, but vestibular disorders are not uncommon. History and diagnosis can be elusive. Specific diagnoses may be unique to young children, but in older children, adult causes of vertigo may be seen. Reassurance that the prognosis is favourable and simple therapeutic measures are often effective.

The Vestibular System and the Developing Child

The otic capsule develops early, between 4 and 12 weeks of gestation. At this stage the vestibular system is always further developed and therefore less at risk than the primitive auditory system.

Assessment of the Dizzy Child

Childhood vertigo results from a mismatch of information from the three different sensory systems: vestibular, visual, and proprioceptive. However, vertigo is much more difficult to recognise in infants than in adults. Symptoms of vertigo in children can include:

- Sudden crying out and dropping to floor
- Sudden clinginess, particularly to the legs of adults
- Pallor
- Sweating
- Vomiting
- Screaming
- Lying face down in bed, reluctant to move
- Torticollis
- General poor balance
- Falling
- Fear of the dark

Table 100.1   Key in utero developmental milestones of the vestibular system

Development	Vestibular milestone
10 weeks	Semicircular canals form
11–12 weeks	Cochlear duct has two and a half coils
16 weeks	Myelination of the vestibular nerve
24 weeks	Primitive vestibulo-ocular reflex present
Full term	Doll's eye reflex Moro reflex

Table 100.2 Causes of childhood vestibular symptoms

Conditions with hearing loss	Conditions with normal hearing
Otitis media with effusion (OME)	Motion sickness
Chronic suppurative otitis media (CSOM) • Mucosal • Squamous if causing fistula	Benign paroxysmal vertigo (BPV) of childhood
Barotraumatic perilymph fistula	Migraine (Basilar)
Ménière's disease	Benign paroxysmal positional vertigo (BPPV)
Trauma	Trauma
Enlarged vestibular aqueduct syndrome	Viral labyrinthitis or neuronitis
Congenital temporal lobe anomalies (e.g. CHARGE association)	Posterior fossa tumours
Dehiscent superior semicircular canal syndrome (SSCS)	Cardiac causes
Ototoxicity	Poisoning
Congenital infections: • Herpes zoster oticus • Congenital syphilis • Congenital CMV	CNS infections: • Cocksackie A/B • Echovirus • HIV • Meningitis
Metabolic disorders • Hurler's syndrome • Hypothyroidism	Chiari malformation
Usher's syndrome	Hereditary cerebellar ataxia
	Acute cerebellar ataxia

Congenital causes of vertigo tend to present with motor delay and not with vertigo. The exception to the rule is where congenital vision and vestibular failure occur in tandem. This is due to children's reliance on visual stimuli to maintain balance.

Approach the history with the most likely diagnoses in mind. The principal conditions to consider in the pediatric population are highlighted in Table 100.2, which classifies causes of vestibular symptoms depending on their association with hearing loss.

History

Attempt to establish the nature of the dizziness (i.e. true vertigo, loss of balance, or light-headedness). The duration and periodicity can be useful guides. Other salient points in the history are noted below:

Associated factors may indicate specific etiologies:

- Trauma head and neck—post-traumatic vertigo
- Headaches occurring with vertigo or at other times:
  - Migraine
  - Tumours
  - CNS infections
- Vomiting may indicate vertigo or raised intracranial pressure
  - Migraine
  - Tumours
  - CNS infections
- Hearing loss
- Hallucinations—temporal lobe seizures
- Preceding viral illness

Developmental History

- Motor milestones, progress, and regression.

History of Toxicity

- Drugs
- Poisons

Family History

- Maternal migraine
- Familial sensorineural deafness
- Neurofibromatosis type 2 (NF2)

Examination of the Dizzy Child

Much of the examination of a dizzy child is the same as examination of adults. Specific examinations must include:

- Otoscopy
- Facial nerve
- Tongue movements
- Gag reflex
- *Eye examination*:
  - Movements
  - Strabismus
- *Specific vestibular tests*:
  - Smooth pursuit, saccades, opticokinetic nystagmus
  - Romberg test, Unterberger test, and heel–toe gait
  - Head thrust
  - Dix-Hallpike test
- Neurological examination

Investigations

The only mandatory investigations are age-appropriate audiometry and tympanometry, which provide vital insights into common causes of dizziness. Other diagnostic tests include:

- Blood tests
  - Inflammatory markers—infective process
  - Specific serological markers
- Vestibular tests—depend on the history and level of concern
  - Rotation testing
  - Bithermal calorics (earliest 6 months)
  - Vestibular evoked myogenic potential (VEMP) (children and babies)
  - Ocular VEMPs (over 2 years)
- Electroencephalography (EEG) to rule out epilepsy
- CT and/or MRI
  - Space-occupying lesion
  - Enlarged vestibular aqueduct
  - Perilymph fistula
  - CSOM

Causes of Childhood Vestibular Symptoms

The diagnostic flow chart (Figure 100.1) summarises the diagnostic process in managing the child with vestibular symptoms. The conditions causing vestibular symptoms are summarised in Table 100.3.

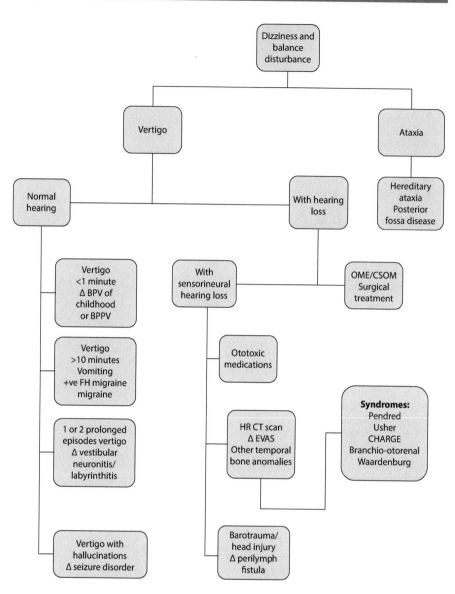

Figure 100.1 Diagnostic flow chart for childhood vestibular symptoms.

Treatments for Vertigo

The causative condition should be treated directly if possible. Reassurance of the child and parent is most likely all that is required.

Symptoms can be treated with a variety of vestibular sedatives:

1 Antihistamines for acute-on-chronic vertigo
2 *Dopamine antagonists*:
   a. Not to be used in children <10 kg
   b. Extrapyramidal side effects can be treated with procyclidine.
3 HT_3 *antagonists*:

   a. Powerful antiemetics
   b. Highly effective in acutely vertiginous child

Table 100.3   Causes of vestibular symptoms in children

Conditions with associated hearing loss	
Condition	**Features**
OME	See Chapter
Ménière's	• Uncommon—3–9% of cases begin in childhood • Clinical features are the same as in adult disease

Temporal bone abnormalities	• Temporal bone abnormality, vestibular failure, and sensorineural hearing loss (SNHL)—Presentation is usually with motor developmental delay
	• Conditions include:
	  • Usher's syndrome
	  • CHARGE association
	  • X-linked hereditary deafness
	  • Noonan's syndrome
	  • Down syndrome

Enlarged vestibular aqueduct syndrome	• Rare syndrome and presents rarely (4%) with vestibular disturbance
	• Presents with fluctuant progressive bilateral SNHL—variable hearing prognosis
	• Diagnosis with CT ± MRI
	  • >1.5 mm at midpoint
	  • >2 mm at operculum
	• Seen in:
	  • Waardenburg syndrome
	  • Pendred's syndrome with Mondini deformity
	  • Branchio-otorenal syndrome
	  • Also seen in non-syndromic patients
	• Management
	  • Symptomatic
	  • Head injury avoidance
	  • No current role for surgery

Perilymph fistulae	• Associated with temporal bone abnormalities and severe or complete hearing loss
	• Present with recurrent meningitis and CSF leak behind the tympanic membrane™
	• Causes
	  • Trauma
	  • Postoperative complication
	  • Barotrauma
	• Treatment is surgical patching of fistula

Drug-induced vertigo	Patients usually present with acute vertigo at the time of the exposure. Over time, chronic decline in vestibular function can develop. Drug causes include aminoglycosides and platinum-based chemotherapy.
Conditions without associated hearing loss	
Condition	**Features**
Motion sickness	• Conflict of kinetic and vestibular input • Occurs in girls more than in boys • Settles at puberty

Benign positional vertigo (BPV)	1 Children >4 years old
	2 35% of children with dizziness
	3 Attacks 30-60s, variable frequency
	4 Acute symptoms—falls, clutching adult legs, vomiting
	5 Rapid resolution to normality
	6 Examination—normal between attacks but nystagmus present during an attack
	7 Prognosis—favourable, settles in later childhood
	8 Associations:
	  • 50% develop migraine in adolescence
	  • Family history of migraine
	  • Associated with benign paroxysmal torticollis

(continued)

Table 100.3   (continued)

Conditions with associated hearing loss	
Condition	**Features**

Migraine	• Common, multifactorial
	• 7.7% lifetime prevalence
	• Found in 25% of children presenting with dizziness
	• More likely to be bilateral headaches, shorter than those in adults
	• Headaches not present in all attacks
	• Vestibular type—vertigo is prominent feature
	• Basilar type—associated posterior circulation symptoms
	• Treatment:
	  • Known trigger avoidance
	  • Encourage regular meals
	  • Medication:
	    • Prophylaxis
	    • Symptom relief for headaches, anxiety, nausea

Vestibular neuronitis	• Similar to adult disorder, but children recover faster • Acute, severe vertigo and nausea/vomiting • Nystagmus during the attack • Prognosis is favourable • 50% have a further attack (reduced severity) • Treatment is symptomatic during an attack and vestibular rehabilitation after an attack
Benign paroxysmal positional vertigo (BPPV)	• BPPV in children likely follows head trauma or whiplash injury • Prognosis is good

Post-traumatic vertigo	• Dizziness and headaches are common after trauma
	• Organic/functional causes are difficult to distinguish
	• An association with psychogenic dizziness:
	  • F > M
	  • Seen in children put under parental pressure
	  • Present with fainting in adolescence
	  • Treatment requires psychiatric referral if vertigo is affecting day-to-day life

Seizure disorders	• Vestibular symptoms:
	  • Aura as part of grand mal seizure
	  • Vertiginous epilepsy
	  • Vestibulogenic epilepsy
	  • Temporal/occipital lobe can cause a hallucination described as feeling of movement
	• Tonic-clonic/generalised seizures are simple diagnostically

Central disorders causing imbalance	
Ataxia	• Common mode of presentation of cerebellar, posterior column, and vestibular disease in children • Importance is due to the reversibility of some causes of ataxia (vitamin E deficiency and Refsum's disease) *Hereditary cerebellar ataxia* • Slowly progressive ataxia • 20 genetic causes *Refsum's disease* Disorder of lipid metabolism resulting in: • Pigmentary retinopathy • Demyelinating neuropathy • Ataxia presenting between 4 and 7 years • Hearing loss

Central disorders causing imbalance (continued)	

Ataxia (continued)	*Charcot-Marie-Tooth disease*
	
	 • Most common hereditary degenerative condition
	 • Autosomal dominant inheritance
	 • Clinical features:
	   • Sensorineural hearing loss
	   • Vestibular degeneration
	
	 Acute cerebellar ataxia
	
	 • Presents <3 years
	 • Previously normal children following a febrile illness
	 • Good prognosis and likely resolution over months

Chiari malformation	*Type 1* Cerebellar tonsil herniation through foramen magnum results in: • Positional vertigo • Central nystagmus • Treatment is surgical decompression of the foramen magnum

Infectious disease	• Infections include:
	   • Parasitic
	     • Lyme disease
	   • Viral
	     • Meningitis
	     • Coxsackie A and B
	     • Echovirus
	     • HIV
	   • Bacterial
	     • Meningitis
	     • Tertiary or congenital syphilis

In addition to vestibular sedatives, vestibular migraine may be treated with an array of adjuncts:

- Domperidone, cinnarizine, and cyclizine are used for associated nausea during acute attacks.
- $5HT_{1B/1D}$ receptor agonists are used for headaches.
- Propranolol and pizotifen are preventive treatments.
- If the above fail, seek pediatric neurology input to consider the full complement of adult pharmacological therapy.

Epley maneuver is used to treat BPPV but is age dependent. Vestibular rehabilitation can help in vestibular insufficiency where central compensation is delayed.

Further Reading

1. Davitt M, Delvecchio MT, Aronoff SC. The differential diagnosis of vertigo in children: a systematic review of 2726 cases. *Pediatr Emerg Care* 2017.

2. Devaraja K. Vertigo in children: a narrative review of the various causes and their management. *Int J Pediatr Otorhinolaryngol.* 2018; 111: 32–38.

3. NICE Guidelines: Suspected neurological conditions: recognition and referral recommendations for children under 16.

101. NASAL OBSTRUCTION

Congenital Nasal Obstruction

The causes of congenital nasal obstruction are listed in Box 101.1, and the causes of acquired nasal obstruction in the neonate are listed in Box 101.2.

Choanal Atresia

- Complete obstruction of the posterior choanae due to persistence of nasobuccal membrane. Can be bony (30%), membranous, or mixed (70%).
- Bilateral involvement presents as acute respiratory distress with cyclical cyanosis relieved by crying and oral airway placement.
- Cyanosis during feeding occurs due to loss of the respiratory channel between the nose and larynx formed by the uvula and epiglottis. McGovern nipples can be used as a temporary measure.
- CHARGE association—mutation *CHD7* gene of chromosome 8.
- *Investigations*:
  - Negative metal spatula misting test
  - Nasal endoscopy
  - Nasal computed tomography (CT)
  - Cardiac echocardiogram
  - Renal ultrasound (US)
  - Ophthalmology and audiology review
- Repair techniques are mainly transnasal and transpalatal, but no definitive evidence has been found favouring either approach.
- Some use mitomycin C or KTP laser to reduce granulation and fibrosis by inhibiting fibroblasts and angiogenesis.

BOX 101.1 CAUSES OF CONGENITAL NASAL OBSTRUCTION

Structural	Inflammatory
Osseocartilaginous nasal deformity	Neonatal rhinitis

BOX 101.2 CAUSES OF ACQUIRED NASAL OBSTRUCTION IN NEONATES

Anatomical/Skeletal anomalies	Congenital nasal cysts	Nasal masses
Choanal atresia	Dermoid cysts	Glial heterotopia
Piriform aperture stenosis	Nasolacrimal duct cysts	Meningocele or encephalocoele
Midnasal stenosis	Tornwald's cysts	Haemangioma
Nasal agenesis	Nasoalveolar cysts	Teratoma
Craniosynostosis	Dentigerous cysts	Hamartoma
'Cleft palate' nose	Mucous cysts	Chordoma

Piriform Aperture Stenosis

- Bony overgrowth of maxillary nasal process at the narrowest part of nasal airway.
- Similar symptoms to choanal atresia, with epiphora due to bony involvement of naso-lacrimal ducts.
- Axial CT: <11-mm aperture at level of inferior meatus ± mega-incisor when associated with holoprosencepaly.
- Treatment: nasal steroid or decongestants and saline irrigation.
- Transnasal or sublabial surgery is reserved for severe obstruction (<5 mm), respiratory distress, or failure to thrive.

Midnasal Stenosis

- Overgrowth of nasal bones halfway along nasal cavity, usually associated with midfacial hypoplasia (e.g. Apert's syndrome).
- CT: isolated bony narrowing of midpart of nasal cavity or rest of nasal cavity stenosis.
- Treatment is mainly conservative, allowing midface to grow until 6 months. Dilatation ± stents is reserved for significant respiratory problems.

Nasal Agenesis

- Failure of nasal placode to canalise to form passages during the fifth week in utero.
- Presents with acute respiratory distress at birth and is treated initially with oral airway and tube feeding ± tracheostomy.
- Definitive treatment involves two-stage nasal cavity and delayed external reconstruction.

Congenital Nasal Cysts

- Dermoid cysts
  - Most common midline mass over nasal dorsum; associated with pit and hair at its opening.
  - Early surgical excision recommended to avoid infection or further expansion.
  - 4–45% have intracranial component, so preoperative CT and magnetic resonance imaging (MRI) are required.
- Dacryocystocoele
- Tornwaldt's cyst
  - Cystic transformation of pharyngeal recess midline of posterior nasopharyngeal wall.
  - Inflammation can cause nasal obstruction, occipital pain, aural fullness, and discharge.
  - Endoscopy is diagnostic, while CT/MRI is used to assess cervical vertebral adhesion.
  - Rarely cause significant obstruction. Tornwaldt's cysts can be incised or excised, but need palatal approach for total clearance.
- Nasoalveolar cyst
  - Non-odontogenic lesion arising from incisive canal during maxillary development and causing asymmetrical alar flare
  - Excision via sublabial or transnasal approach
- Dentigerous cyst
  - Odontogenic cyst arising from nasal floor or maxillary sinus
  - Treatment: endoscopic marsupialisation or transnasal excision
- Mucous cyst
  - Commonly on nasal floor
  - Congenital or complication of rhinoplasty

Nasal Masses

- Encephalomeningocoele is a meningeal herniation (with or without associated brain) through bony defects of calvarium.

BOX 101.3   DIFFERENTIATING FEATURES OF GLIOMA AND ENCEPHALOCELE

Glioma	Encephalocele
Probe can be passed medially	Probe can be passed only laterally
Negative Furstenberg's sign	Positive Furstenberg's sign
Brain discontinuity (MRI)	Continuity with brain via skull base defect

- Meningocoele contains meninges only; encephalocoele contains nervous tissue.
- Frontoethmoidal encephalocoele is associated with craniofacial deformity because it arises at or anterior to the foramen caecum, whereas basal encephalocoele arises intranasally through skull base defects, causing nasal obstruction and widening of nasal bridges.
- Glioma (glial heterotopia) is a benign midline mass containing glial cells and fibrous and vascular tissue; 15% are attached to brain via a fibrous stalk and have no associated brain abnormality. They are also choristomas—aggregation of structurally normal tissue in an abnormal location. Glioma presents early as firm, noncompressible, reddish swelling. Box 101.3 shows the differentiating features of glioma and encephalocele.
- Surgical excision is indicated when nasal mass is causing significant problem and may require preoperative ventriculoperitoneal (VP) shunting.

Nasal Haemangioma

- Vascular anomalies (haemangiomas, AVMs, vascular and lymphatic malformations) are classically absent or flat at birth, grow rapidly from 6 weeks to 6 months, then gradually involute, disappearing by 6 years.
- US and MRI are used to exclude intracranial connection.
- Majority are treated conservatively or with propranolol. Surgery is indicated in cases of orbital encroachment with visual compromise.

Teratoma

- A true neoplasm consisting of all three germ layers
- Associated with polyhydramnios, stillbirth, prematurity
- Firm mass with raised alpha-fetoprotein and beta-HCG

Acquired Neonatal Nasal Obstruction

Osseocartilaginous Septal Deformity

- Thought to be due to intrauterine positioning or birth trauma
- Treatment:
  - Closed reduction under local anaesthesia in first few days of life for severe deviation
  - Delayed formal repair to avoid damage to main nasal growth centre

Neonatal Rhinitis

- Mucoid rhinorrhoea with mucosal oedema in an afebrile newborn without significant structural abnormalities.
- Treatments: nasal bulb suction with saline drops and short course of steroid drops.
- Consider chlamydial infection acquired in birth canal if associated with conjunctivitis.
- Congenital syphilis can present as thin, clear secretions between the second week and third month of life, progressing to mucopurulent discharge with significant obstruction and crusting. Antibiotic is needed to prevent chronic cartilaginous infection resulting in saddle nose deformity.

Fibrous Dysplasia

- Radiolucent 'ground glass' craniofacial bones with diffuse margins, endosteal scalloping of inner cortex, and smooth, nonreactive periosteal surface.
- Pain, with progressive facial deformity between 10 and 30 years of age.
- Treatments include surgical excision to preserve function-limiting disability and bisphosphonates to increase bone density.
- McCune-Albright syndrome—polyostotic involvement, hyperthyroidism, adrenal disorders, diabetes, hyperpituitarism, hypercalcaemia, café-au-lait spots, and mainly dormant by adulthood but has 1% malignant transformation.

Neoplasms

- Juvenile ossifying fibroma (JOF) presents as painless, radiolucent, expansile, well-defined lesion with variable calcification, cortical thinning, and possible perforation.
- Subtypes: trabecular and psammomatoid.
- Treatment is radical surgical excision due to high recurrence rates (30–50%) because of its propensity to perforate cortical bone.

The Adenoids

- The adenoids form part of Waldeyer's ring of lymphoid tissue by producing B-cells (IgG and IgA), and they play a role in development of immunological memory.
- Adenoids are located within mucous membrane of the roof of the nasopharynx and posterior nasopharyngeal wall. Enlargement can cause nasal obstruction rarely in neonates, more commonly in young children.
- Growth starts in the fourth to sixth gestational week; there is rapid growth in infancy to 2 years of age, and then growth plateaus until 14 years and regresses after 15 years.
- Unsuspected neoplasia of adenoids is rare. Non-Hodgkin's lymphoma should be considered with asymmetric adenoids and post-transplantation lymphoproliferative disorder.
- Some evidence supports use of intranasal steroid sprays for adenoid size reduction and improvements in nasal obstruction. Surgical option is adenoidectomy (curettage, suction diathermy, Coblation, microdebrider, KTP laser).

102. RHINOSINUSITIS AND LACRIMAL DISORDERS

Paediatric Rhinosinusitis (Box 102.1)

- Paranasal sinuses are lined by type 2 pseudostratified columnar ciliated epithelium.
- *Development*:
  - At birth, only maxillary, sphenoid, and ethmoid sinuses are present.
  - Frontal sinuses develop from cranial extension of ethmoid cells at 5 years old, reaching full size by 19 years.
  - Maxillary sinuses expand to reach the nasal floor level by 8 years, reaching full size by 16 years.
  - Sphenoid sinuses extend posteriorly over the first 7 years, reaching completion by 15 years.

BOX 102.1   CLINICAL ASSESSMENT—HISTORY

Current symptoms	Past history and risk factors
• Onset • Duration • Precipitants (viral URTI, nasal foreign body) • Improvement and deterioration in clinical picture ('double sickening') • Nasal/paranasal symptoms (congestion, mucopurulent discharge) • Facial/orbital pain or swelling • Headaches and neurological sequelae • Cough • Fever (severity and duration) • Hyposmia • Oral/dental/pharyngeal symptoms	• Similar episodes of sinusitis and RTI • Previous use of antibiotics • Comorbidities • Prior hospitalisation and sinonasal surgery • Allergy history • Day-care arrangements • Exposure to cigarette smoke • Immunisation history

- *European position paper on rhinosinusitis*:
  Nasal and paranasal sinuses inflammation characterised by two or more symptoms, one of which should be either nasal obstruction or discharge:
  ± facial pain/pressure, ± cough
  and either:
  endoscopic signs of polyps and/or middle meatal mucopurulent discharge and/or oedema/mucosal obstruction
  and/or:
  CT-proven mucosal changes within the osteomeatal complex and/or sinuses
- Inflammation of <12 weeks' duration is **acute rhinosinusitis** (with symptom-free intervals if it is recurrent).
  - Severity can be assessed by rating on a visual analogue scale from 1 (not troublesome) to 10 (worst): 1–3 is mild, 4–7 is moderate, and 8–10 is severe.

Acute Rhinosinusitis (ARS)

- The majority of cases of ARS are precipitated by viral upper respiratory tract infections (URTIs), and nasal symptoms usually last <10 days.
- More common in younger children, in Autumn/Winter, and in children in day care.
- *Bacterial causes*:
  - Most common: *Streptococcus pneumoniae, Haemophilus influenzae,* and *Moraxella catarrhalis*
  - Less common: *Staphylococcus aureus, Strep. pyogenes, Strep. viridans, Peptostreptococcus,* and *Fusobacterium*
- Gold standard for diagnosis is antral puncture and aspiration, but more commonly cultures from middle meatus (endoscopically) are taken instead.
- *According to EPOS, acute bacterial rhinosinusitis (ABRS) is diagnosed by presence of (3 or more)*:
  - Purulent, discoloured rhinorrhea
  - Severe local pain
  - 'Double sickening'
  - Elevated ESR/CRP
  - Fever >38°C

- *Examination*:
  - General observations (including neurological status)
  - ENT, as well as head and neck examination
  - Anterior rhinoscopy ± nasal endoscopy
- *Indications of culture and computed tomography (CT)*:
  - Severe symptoms and toxic presentation
  - No improvement after 48–72 hr of medical treatment
  - Immunocompromise
  - Complications
- *Treatments*:
  - Mainly symptomatic, with intranasal steroids, decongestants (<10 days), and saline spray.
  - Antibiotics to be reserved for severe and recurrent episodes, because they showed limited efficacy over placebo and routine prescribing does not prevent ABRS complications in the latest evidence reviewed in EPOS 2020.

Complications of ARS
Periorbital Complications

- Can be either from direct spread across lamina papyracea or via venous drainage
- Most commonly due to ethmoid involvement, followed by (in decreasing frequency) maxillary, frontal, and sphenoid involvement
  Chandler classification:

(i) Preseptal cellulitis
  - Eyelid and conjunctival inflammation anterior to orbital septum
  - No proptosis or ophthalmoplegia
(ii) Orbital cellulitis
  - Ophthalmoplegia, pain on eye movements, diplopia, chemosis, and proptosis
(iii) Subperiosteal abscess
  - Extraconal abscess between periorbita and sinuses
(iv) Orbital abscess (intraconal)
(v) Cavernous sinus thrombosis
  - Multidisciplinary approach involving pediatric, ophthalmology, neurosurgery and microbiology
  - First-line investigation is CT of the orbit, paranasal sinuses, and brain with contrast
  - Medical treatment consists of IV antibiotics, analgesia, IV fluids, and intranasal steroids
  - Surgical drainage (modified Lynch Howarth incision or endoscopic) is indicated when:
    - ➢ Progression or no clinical improvement of orbital signs and/or systemically after 24–48 hr of medical therapy
    - ➢ Subperiosteal and intraorbital abscess on CT or magnetic resonance imaging (MRI)
    - ➢ Reduced colour vision, reduced visual acuity, affected afferent pupillary reflex, or inability to assess vision
  - Sequelae of inadequate treatment: retinal artery occlusion, prolonged venous congestion, optic neuritis, corneal ulceration, intracranial spread, etc.

Endocranial Complications

- Epidural or subdural empyema, brain abscess, meningitis, encephalitis, superior sagittal and cavernous sinus thrombosis (Table 102.1).
- Usually associated with frontoethmoidal or sphenoidal ARS by direct erosion of sinus walls or via diploic veins.

Table 102.1   Cavernous Sinus Thrombosis

Thrombophlebitis of paranasal sinus veins, particularly associated with ethmoidal or sphenoidal ARS	
MR venography shows absence of flow in the thrombosed sinus.	
Treatment: anticoagulants, endoscopic drainage, high-dose IV antibiotics	
Clinical features:	
• Bilateral ptosis	• Complete ophthalmoplegia
• Proptosis and chemosis	• Papilloedema
• Ophthalmic nerve neuralgia	• Meningeal irritation
• Retro-ocular headache	• Altered mental state

- Associated with high fever, nausea, vomiting, neck stiffness, altered mental state, and focal neurological deficits (CN III, VI, VII).
- MRI is a useful adjunct (after CT) when considering neurosurgical intervention.
- Treatment: high-dose long-term IV antibiotics, burr hole drainage, craniotomy, or image-guided aspiration with paranasal sinuses drainage.
- Mortality is usually due to cortical vein thrombosis and cerebral vascular infarction.

Osseous Complications

- Subperiosteal abscess of bony sinus walls and osteomyelitis of surrounding bone causing avascular necrosis and venous congestion.
- Most common is osteomyelitis of maxillary (infants) and frontal bones.
- Pott's puffy tumour (PPT)—subperiosteal abscess of frontal sinus walls due to erosion of anterior table causing soft-tissue swelling and pitting oedema.
- Spread via posterior table can lead to concomitant meningitis and other intracranial complications.
- Treatment includes IV antibiotics with either surgical debridement and drainage or endoscopic/minimal external drainage in uncomplicated PPT.

Chronic Rhinosinusitis (CRS) (BOX 102.2)

- Most patients are 10 to 15 years old.
- Limited evidence of viral infection's role in paediatric CRS.
- Tobacco smoke exposure inhibits mucociliary clearance and epithelial regeneration.
  - Those exposed to passive smoking present with more severe disease and higher rates of revision surgery.
- Immunoglobulin deficiency and poor response to vaccines are the most common immunodeficiencies in children with refractory CRS.

BOX 102.2   CONTRIBUTING FACTORS IN PEDIATRIC CRS

Local factors	Inflammatory and infective factors	Systemic conditions
Sinus obstruction: anatomical (e.g. concha bullosa) Septal deviation Nasal polyps Adenoidal inflammation Trauma/ iatrogenic factors Foreign body	Viral URTI Bacterial infection Allergy Gastroesophageal reflux disease (GERD) Tobacco smoke exposure	Immunodeficiency Cystic fibrosis Primary ciliary dyskinesia

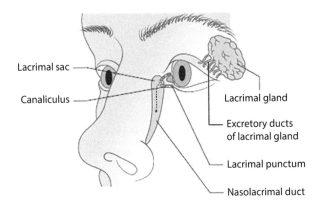

Figure 102.1 Anatomy of the lacrimal system.

- High index of suspicion for cystic fibrosis must be maintained in children with poor weight gain, respiratory disease, and gastrointestinal disease.
- Treatments are mainly with saline nasal irrigation and intranasal steroids.
- Antihistamines and proton pump inhibitors (PPI) are indicated only for concomitant allergic rhinitis and GERD, respectively.
- There is no evidence to support the use of antibiotics or prolonged macrolide therapy.
- Adenoidectomy with/without antral irrigation is the recommended first-line surgical treatment in young children refractory to medical therapy.
  - Adenoids act as a reservoir for pathogenic bacteria, rather than as a source of obstruction.
- Functional endoscopic sinus surgery (FESS) is likely to be beneficial in older children with CRS refractory to medical therapy, after adenoidectomy, and after other underlying pathologies have been excluded.

Further Reading

Fokkens et al. (2020). European position paper on rhinosinusitis and nasal polyps. *Rhinology* 2020; 58(Suppl S29): 1–464. https://www.researchgate.net/publication/339410718_European_Position_Paper_on_Rhinosinusitis_and_Nasal_Polyps_2020

Lacrimal Disorders in Children

Figure 102.1 shows the anatomy of the pediatric lacrimal system.

- The lacrimal glands, accessory lacrimal glands, Meibomian glands, and goblet cells secrete tear film, which is drained via lacrimal puncta, canaliculi, the lacrimal sac, and the nasolacrimal duct sequentially to the inferior nasal meatus (Hasner's valve).

Dry Eyes

- Reduced tear meniscus with punctate keratopathy; normally presents as irritable, gritty, and diffusely injected eyes.
- Congenital alacrima (rare) can be due to lacrimal gland absence or ectopy.
  - Associated with Allgrove syndrome, anhidrotic ectodermal dysplasia, Riley-Day syndrome
- *Acquired causes*:
  - Epstein-Barr virus infection
  - Sjögren's syndrome
  - Side-effect of isotretinoin (acne treatment)
- *Treatment*: artificial tears ± temporary or permanent punctal occlusion.
- Watery eyes (Box 102.3).

BOX 102.3   CAUSES OF WATERY EYES IN CHILDREN

Excess tear production (lacrimation)	Drainage failure (epiphora)
Allergic rhinitis	Congenital nasolacrimal duct obstruction
Upper respiratory tract infection Epiblepharon	Skeletal and sinus abnormalities
Subtarsal foreign body	Lid malposition
Iritis	Punctal malposition
Corneal abrasion/ulceration	Punctal occlusion
Conjunctivitis	
Glaucoma	Anomalous drainage system

Lacrimal Tumours and Granulomas

- Idiopathic orbital inflammatory disease is noninfective, involves the orbit, and responds well to steroids.
- Dacryocystocoele is a congenital swelling at medial canthus due to trapped fluid inside the lacrimal sac and nasolacrimal duct. It is tense, blue, and not pulsatile.
  - MRI is helpful in excluding other pathology.
  - Surgery is reserved if there is lack of spontaneous improvement in 2 weeks or the patient develops acute dacryocystitis or respiratory difficulties.
- *Other differentials*:
  - Malignancy (mixed cell adenocystic carcinoma)
  - Gland enlargement associated with sarcoidosis and leukaemia
  - Gland prolapse in craniofacial anomalies

Congenital Nasolacrimal Duct Obstruction (CNLDO)

- CNLDO occurs in 20% of infants, and it presents as epiphora with increased tear meniscus and lash stickiness or crusting ± mucocele.
- Most CNLDO spontaneously resolves during the first year of life.
- Lacrimal drainage system maturation delay causes persistent membranous obstruction or Hasner's valve stenosis.
- Associated with EEC (ectrodactyly, ectodermal dysplasia, clefting) syndrome, branchio-oculo-facial syndrome, Down syndrome, LADD (lacrimo-auriculo-dentodigital) syndrome, and CHARGE association
- Fluorescein disappearance test is diagnostic.
- Probing ('blind' or endoscopic) is recommended after first year of life, followed by dacryocystorhinostomy for persistent epiphora despite probing.

Punctal and Canalicular Abnormalities

- Punctal stenosis/atresia may result from failure of lacrimal drainage system canalisation and is only symptomatic when both puncta are involved.
- Treatment includes dilation ± needle to membranous obstruction.

Acquired Conditions

- Acute dacryocystitis is treated with IV antibiotics to prevent retrobulbar abscess.
- Probing and skin incision are not recommended to avoid false passage and fistula.
- Needle aspiration ± endonasal dacrocystorhinostomy (DCR) is reserved for pyocoele and residual mass following resolution.

103. ADENOTONSILLAR CONDITIONS AND OBSTRUCTIVE SLEEP APNOEA

Pathological Effects of Adenoids

- *Upper airway obstruction*: The prevalence of severe sleep disturbance in children due to upper airway obstruction is estimated to be approximately 1%, with a peak incidence between 3 and 6 years of age.
- *Otitis media*: Evidence from the MRC TARGET study supports consideration of 'adjuvant' adenoidectomy in children undergoing grommet insertion for otitis media with effusion (OME). This contrasts a Cochrane review that concluded that adenoidectomy could not be recommended for management of recurrent acute otitis media (AOM).
- *Rhinosinusitis*: In childhood, adenoids are implicated in rhinosinusitis, acting as a reservoir for pathogenic bacteria.
- *Neoplasia*: Unsuspected neoplasia of the adenoids (and tonsils) in childhood is rare. Consider lymphoma of the adenoids, a post-transplantation lymphoproliferative disorder, when symptoms of nasal obstruction develop.

Disorders of the Tonsils

Acute Tonsillitis

The causative organism usually is Group A beta-haemolytic *Streptococci*, although a range of other organisms have been implicated. Both viral and bacterial tonsillitis usually resolve quickly without treatment. Corticosteroids, in addition to antibiotics, expedite the resolution of pain.

Complications of Acute Tonsillitis

- *Peritonsillar abscess*: Peritonsillar abscess is a collection of pus lateral to the tonsil. Symptoms include unilateral sore throat, trismus, and lymphadenopathy. The treatment is antibiotics, needle aspiration, or incision and drainage.
- *Deep neck space abscess (DNSA)*: Retropharyngeal abscesses are rare and are seen mainly in infants and children <5 years old. Occasionally, peritonsillar and retropharyngeal abscess may spread to the parapharyngeal space. Computed tomography (CT) is the investigation of choice and facilitates treatment planning. Initial treatment of retropharyngeal and parapharyngeal abscess is high-dose intravenous antibiotics. For DNSA >2.5 cm in diameter, incision and drainage under a general anaesthetic should be considered to minimise the risk of mediastinitis or retroperitoneal sepsis.
- *Lemierre's syndrome (LS)*: LS is a rare but potentially fatal complication of acute oropharyngeal (or ear) infection. It is characterised by suppurative thrombophlebitis of the internal jugular vein and metastatic abscesses (due to septic emboli). The causative organism is usually *Fusobacterium necrophorum*. LS should be suspected in patients with antecedent oropharyngeal infection, septic pulmonary emboli and pyrexia unresponsive to antimicrobials. Treatment is with antibiotics for 6 weeks and anticoagulation may be considered.

Infectious Mononucleosis (IM)

Caused by Epstein-Barr virus (EBV), IM is diagnosed with the Monospot test (sensitivity <50% in children). Diagnosis is confirmed by specific antibody titres. Ampicillin is avoided if IM is suspected because 90% of patients develop a significant rash as a result of transient immunostimulation.

Neoplasia

Asymmetrical tonsils arouse suspicion of neoplasia, especially if the surface of one of the tonsils is irregular or ulcerated. Difference in size is not always an indication for biopsy in children, but any unusual appearances should be investigated.

Management

The Adenoids

Topical nasal steroid sprays reduce adenoid size, with related improvements in the presence of middle ear fluid, audiometric thresholds, nasal obstruction, rhinorrhea, and sleep apnoea.

Adenoidectomy techniques include:

- Curettage
- Suction diathermy
- Coblation®
- Microdebrider
- KTP laser (high risk of nasopharyngeal stenosis)

Pre-operative assessment should identify blood clotting history, Down syndrome (consider potential atlantoaxial instability), and a bifid uvula, which can be a marker of a submucous cleft, which is present in 59% of cases and is a high risk for developing velopharyngeal insufficiency (VFI) post-operatively. Partial adenoidectomy is an alternative technique that reduces the risk of VFI in these patients. Nontraumatic atlantoaxial subluxation (Grisel syndrome) is an uncommon risk associated with adenoidectomy and tonsillectomy. Post-operative torticollis should raise suspicion.

The Tonsils

Tonsillectomy as part of the treatment of an otherwise healthy child with obstructive sleep apnoea is the treatment of choice. SIGN guidelines have been developed for the management of recurrent throat infections.

The National Prospective Tonsillectomy Audit found cold steel dissection and ties had a significantly lower bleed rate and less post-operative pain than any other technique.

Tonsillotomy, a technique associated with lower secondary haemorrhage rates and postoperative pain levels than extracapsular tonsillectomy, involves removing a part of the tonsillar tissue, leaving the capsule intact. This can be achieved using microdebrider, laser, or Coblation®.

Obstructive Sleep Apnoea (OSA)

There are three groups of children in whom sleep-disordered breathing may occur, with some degree of overlap:

- Otherwise healthy children with adenotonsillar hypertrophy
- Slightly older children with obesity
- Children in whom OSA has multifactorial causes (Table 103.1)

Neurobehavioural clinical findings result from the disturbance to sleep and arousal patterns seen in children with OSA. This can have a profound impact on preschool children, who are in a critical period for neurodevelopment. OSA has an underlying inflammatory basis, and several biomarkers are elevated. C-reactive protein and endothelin-1, amongst others, are associated with an increased cardiovascular risk.

Clinical History

Symptoms of OSA are listed in Table 103.2.

Clinical Examination

ENT examination should include evaluation for any craniofacial abnormalities, mouth breathing, and audible stertor. Tonsil size can be graded using the Brodsky or Friedman scores.

Table 103.1   Conditions associated with OSA

Associated conditions	OSA prevalence	Clinical features predisposing to OSA
Obesity	45%	Mechanical obstruction (adenotonsillar hypertrophy, increased adipose tissue) and decreased activity of pharyngeal dilator muscles
Down syndrome	50–100%	Macroglossia, adenotonsillar hypertrophy, midface hypoplasia, obesity, hypothyroidism, hypotonia and gastroesophageal reflux
Treacher Collins' syndrome	54%	Hypoplastic mandible and zygomatic complex, cleft palate, and choanal atresia
Prader-Willi syndrome	80%	Hypotonia, morbid obesity, hypothyroidism, viscous secretions, and scoliosis

Table 103.2   Symptoms of OSA

Nighttime symptoms	Daytime symptoms
• Snoring • Restless sleeping • Frequent awakening • Pauses in breathing • Sleeping with an extended head • Hyperhidrosis • Nocturnal enuresis	• Behavioural or concentration problems • Mouth breathing • Feeding difficulty • Delayed growth milestones

The nose should be examined for coexisting rhinitis and adenoid hypertrophy. Examination of videos on mobile devices can be helpful in establishing the presence of snoring and obstruction.

Other conditions predisposing to OSA include CHARGE, achondroplasia, syndromic craniosynostosis, cleft palate, neuromuscular disease, and sickle-cell disease (due to upper aerodigestive tract lymphoid hyperplasia).

Investigations

Non-syndromic healthy children with a history suggestive of OSA along with enlarged tonsils could reasonably proceed to adenotonsillectomy in a nonspecialist unit without further investigations. Further investigations are indicated for patients in whom there is diagnostic uncertainty or residual symptoms following adenotonsillectomy (Table 103.3).

Polysomnography (PSG) is currently the gold standard for investigating OSA. An apnoea-hypopnoea index (AHI) > 1 is significant in children.

Oximetry is useful if PSG is unavailable. It carries a high positive predictive value (97%) but, because not all apnoeas result in decreased saturations, the negative predictive value is low (53%).

Table 103.3   Indications for paediatric respiratory investigations

• Age <2 years • Weight <15 kg • Failure to thrive • Down syndrome • Cerebral palsy • Neuromuscular disorders • Craniofacial anomalies • Mucopolysaccharidosis • Obesity • Significant comorbidity, such as congenital heart disease or chronic lung disease

Nonsurgical Management of Sleep-Disordered Breathing

Obesity should be addressed. Continuous positive airway pressure may be required in children with mild to moderate OSA in whom surgical treatment is not feasible or in whom treatment has failed.

Surgical Management of Sleep-Disordered Breathing

The Childhood Adenotonsillectomy Trial randomized children to early adenotonsillectomy or watchful waiting. Neuropsychological outcomes showed no difference; however, PSG findings and quality of life were significantly improved for the treatment arm.

Bilateral mandibular distraction osteogenesis and rapid maxillary expansion are reliable techniques for patients with symptomatic micrognathia. In patients with Beckwith-Wiedemann syndrome and other selected syndromes with macroglossia, tongue reduction may be indicated.

Postoperative Care for OSA

Children who have OSA are at increased risk of peri-operative respiratory complications. This may be due to hypersensitivity to opiates and inhalational anaesthetic agents. While the majority of patients with OSA can be managed safely in a standard paediatric ward, children identified as high risk (Table 103.3) or with severe OSA should be treated in a centre with paediatric intensive care facilities and anaesthetic support. Pre-operative PSG in this group allows an improved diagnostic certainty and facilitates risk stratification. Surgery can be avoided in those who do not have OSA, while those who have moderate to severe OSA can have appropriate arrangements made for post-operative care.

Further Reading

Medical Research Council Multicentre Otitis Media Study Group. Adjuvant adenoidectomy in persistent bilateral otitis media with effusion: hearing and revision surgery outcomes through 2 years in the TARGET randomised trial. *Clin Otolaryngol* 2012; 37: 107–116.

Redline S, Amin R, Beebe D, et al. The Childhood Adenotonsillectomy Trial (CHAT): rationale, design, and challenges of a randomized controlled trial evaluating a standard surgical procedure in a pediatric population. *Sleep* 2011; 34(11): 1509–1517.

Scottish Intercollegiate Guidelines Network. *Management of sore throat and indications for tonsillectomy.* SIGN 117. Edinburgh: SIGN, 2010. Available at: https://www.sign.ac.uk/assets/sign117.pdf

104. ACQUIRED LARYNGOTRACHEAL STENOSIS

Acquired subglottic stenosis (SGS) remains the most frequent cause of laryngeal stenosis. The typical patient is likely to be premature or to have birth defects. The primary aim of intervention is decannulation or prevention of tracheostomy.

Anatomy

- The paediatric larynx lies high in the neck.
- The hyoid may override the superior larynx.
- The narrowest point is the cricoid—as the only complete ring within the airway, it is most vulnerable to damage by intubation.

Presentation

History

- Laryngotracheal stenosis may present with stridor, failed extubation, or tracheostomy dependency.
- Voice change suggests supraglottic/glottic disease.
- Comorbidities are common, such as gastro-oesophageal reflux disease (GERD), aspiration, and pulmonary or cardiac disease.
- Symptoms: acute or chronic, stable or progressive, and time of onset.
- Impact on quality of life: poor exercise tolerance, evidence of obstructive sleep apnoea (OSA).
- Intubation history, because intubation causes stenosis, or history of previous airway surgery.
- In a tracheostomy-dependent child, the indication, age at cannulation, and tube size are important.

Examination

- *Stridor*: inspiratory, expiratory, or biphasic.
- Increased work of breathing.
- Flexible endoscopy if possible.
- Exclude nasal stenosis, choanal atresia, adenoid hypertrophy, and glossoptosis.
- Laryngeal examination should assess supraglottic stenosis/collapse, posterior glottic stenosis (PGS), and anterior webbing, which are often iatrogenic.
- Vocal cord paralysis must be identified, particularly if reconstructive surgery is required.
- Assess for SGS.
- In children with a tracheostomy, their ability to tolerate a speaking valve or finger occlusion indicates clinical severity.

Diagnosis

- Radiograph of neck to evaluate laryngeal and tracheal stenosis is occasionally useful.
- Chest radiograph for lung disease.
- Barium swallow assesses aspiration and excludes laryngeal cleft or tracheo-oesophageal fistula.
- Cross-sectional imaging with contrast can rule out a vascular ring.
- In complex patients, consider polysomnography, oesophagogastroduodenoscopy, and flexible bronchoscopy.
- Rigid microlaryngobronchoscopy (MLB) is the gold standard for airway evaluation. Perform MLB in a medically optimised patient who is spontaneously ventilating. MLB is superior to flexible endoscopy for excluding tracheal pathology (stenosis, malacia, complete tracheal rings, and tracheo-oesophageal fistula). It can prevent misdiagnosis of PGS as bilateral vocal cord palsy. SGS and tracheal stenosis are categorised in the Myer-Cotton classification (Figure 104.1) based on endotracheal tubes' producing an air leak at 20 cm of water pressure.

Treatment

- Always treat inflammation first.
  - *GERD*: H_2 antagonists and proton-pump inhibitors, with fundoplication considered for severe cases
  - *Eosinophilic oesophagitis*: oral fluticasone
- Anterior cricoid split is an option for the neonate who fails extubation.

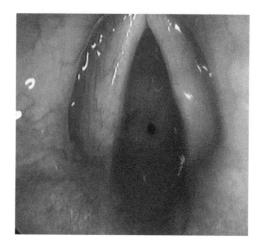

Figure 104.1   Endoscopic view of subglottic stenosis.

- *Supraglottic stenosis*: typically arytenoid or petiole prolapse. Endoscopic partial arytenoidectomy can be successful; however, ongoing continuous positive airway pressure (CPAP) may be required. Epiglottic petiole prolapse is difficult to treat and may require laryngofissure to reattach it to the inner thyroid ala.
- *Anterior glottic web*: requires a keel to prevent reformation of scar. In an older child, this is possibly done endoscopically with a Silastic sheet; however, a two-stage open approach may be needed.
- *Posterior glottic web*: A simple web can be divided endoscopically with good outcomes, whilst thick interarytenoid PGS must be managed with posterior augmentation.
- Tracheostomy as treatment is appropriate in the child with an unsafe, unstable airway in whom laryngotracheal reconstruction (LTR) is not advisable. Tracheostomy through tracheal rings 2–4 is recommended. Tracheostomy is often necessary, but it places a physical and emotional burden on child and family.

Subglottic and Tracheal Stenosis

- Subglottic and tracheal stenosis are the most common acquired stenoses.
- Endoscopic management is appropriate for grade I/II stenoses where scar is soft and immature. Thin stenoses have the best outcomes.
- Serial balloon dilation is undertaken with a high-pressure, noncompliant balloon exerting a radial force over the circumference of the narrowing. Incising the stenosis and steroid injection in conjunction with dilation may confer additional benefit.
- Because balloon catheters are thin and flexible, they can navigate tight stenoses.
- Complications are rare; however, they include airway rupture and pulmonary oedema.
- Where there is limited success after repeated dilations, LTR is considered.

Open Surgery

- Not all children are appropriate for airway reconstruction. Aspiration is a relative contraindication to LTR, and it is likely that children with neuromuscular or pulmonary disease will still require ventilation.
- Open LTR consists of incision or excision of the stenosis and placement of an anterior +/− posterior graft (Figure 104.2). An endoscopic LTR is appropriate in some, but laryngofissure is more reliable.
- Costal cartilage is the most widely used graft, but thyroid ala can suffice if a small graft is required.

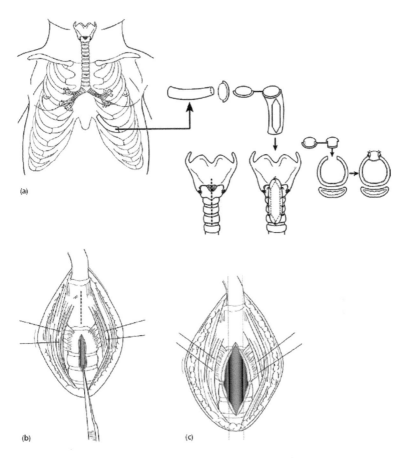

Figure 104.2 Subglottic stenosis repair using rib graft.

- For PGS and SGS, open LTR with posterior rib grafting is indicated. Laryngofissure and then posterior cricoid split are followed by graft insertion. In many cases, anterior grafting is also performed. This operation can be done in one or two stages.
  - *Single-stage procedure*: Children with good pulmonary function undergoing a simple LTR. At surgery, an age-appropriate endotracheal tube stents the airway, with extubation at 1–2 weeks.
  - *Two-stage procedure*: Requires tracheostomy and stenting. A stent maintains the lumen and prevents graft prolapse. Silastic stents are favoured because they are soft, minimise granulation, and can be left longer than 6 weeks. Teflon stents were formerly commonplace.
- With either endoscopic or open surgery, LTR complications can be significant, and restenosis occurs in 10–20% of patients.
- *Cricotracheal resection*: For grade IV stenosis, the anterior cricoid ring and proximal trachea are resected, and then thyrotracheal anastomosis is performed. This procedure removes disease, restores lumen diameter, and anastomoses healthy mucosa. Complications include anastomotic breakdown, vocal cord palsy, and loss of vocal range.
- *Tracheal stenosis*: Short-segment tracheal stenosis can be resected and primarily repaired with end-to-end anastomosis. Longer-segment stenosis requires slide tracheoplasty, in which the stenosis is transected and the proximal and distal ends are incised longitudinally and then overlapped for repair. Severe disease may require hyoid or pulmonary release, which reduces anastomotic tension but increases morbidity.

Juvenile-Onset Recurrent Respiratory Papillomatosis

Recurrent respiratory papillomatosis (RRP) is a potentially life-threatening disease characterised by papillomata anywhere in the respiratory tract, most commonly in the larynx. Juvenile-onset RRP (JORRP) occurs in children 3–4 years old; adult-onset RRP peaks at age 20–30 years and is less aggressive.

Etiology

- HPV is a double-stranded DNA virus with over 200 known subtypes.
- HPV 6 and 11 typically cause RRP, and HPV type 11 is more aggressive.
- HPV enters traumatised epithelium and resides in the basal layer.

Epidemiology

- Prevalence 4 per 100,000 children.
- HPV DNA is found in up to half of aerodigestive tract swabs of children born to affected mothers, but the majority of these children do not develop disease. Risk factors include maternal genital warts, prolonged labour, host immunology, and genetics.

Presentation

- Laryngeal RRP can mimic other airway pathologies, such as asthma, laryngitis, bronchitis, and croup.
- Children commonly present with hoarseness and stridor. May have chronic cough, choking, recurrent infections, or failure to thrive.

Diagnosis

- *Flexible nasendoscopy*: Look for sessile or pedunculated lesions of the endolarynx.
- Rigid endoscopy (under anaesthesia with spontaneous ventilation) permits biopsy and evaluates extent of disease (Derkay score).
- Pulmonary disease in up to 4%.
- Bronchial RRP predisposes the patient to recurrent pneumonia, with greater risk of malignant transformation.
- *Histology*: Exophytic projections of keratinised squamous epithelium overlying a fibrovascular core.

Treatment

- RRP is a surgical disease; papilloma removal restores a safe, patent airway. Good surgical technique, GERD prophylaxis, and the use of adjuvant therapies may minimise complications like dysphonia and airway stenosis.
- Tracheostomy is reserved for severe cases.
- Tracheobronchial disease is managed similarly to proximal disease, but with greater surveillance for malignancy. Remission may occur in teenage years.
- Surgery
  - Powered microdebrider—Most commonly used for papilloma removal. Good surgical technique is required to prevent subepithelial injury.

- CO_2 laser—Previously the mainstay of surgical treatment, yet thermal injury can lead to long-term complications, such as fibrosis and webbing.
- Other—KTP and Nd:YAG lasers can be delivered through a fibre, permitting management of tracheobronchial disease. Pulsed-dye laser in the paediatric population is being evaluated. Photodynamic therapy has significant side effects due to photosensitivity. Coblation® is not widely used for RRP.
- Adjuvant therapy
  - Inteferon-α—Administered systemically. Some studies demonstrate remission of disease. Risks include pancytopaenia, hepatorenal failure, and cardiac dysfunction.
  - Bevacizumab—Anti-VEGF monoclonal antibody. Both systemic and intralesional therapy have shown promise in RRP.
  - Cidofovir—Antiviral that inhibits viral DNA polymerases. Intralesional injection can be effective.
  - Other antiviral agents—Ribavirin and acyclovir; however, evidence is anecdotal.
  - Indole-3-carbinol and cimetidine are other adjuvant therapies with variable efficacy.

Vaccination

- *Quadrivalent vaccine*: Used in many countries, recommended for RRP. Studies demonstrated vaccinated patients had increased intersurgical interval and reduced disease burden.

KEY POINTS

- JORRP can affect any part of the respiratory tract.
- The mainstay of treatment is surgical debulking.
- In the majority of patients, the disease goes into spontaneous remission.
- Tracheobronchial disease carries a worse prognosis and greater risk of malignant transformation.

Further Reading

Derkay CS, Faust RA. Recurrent respiratory papillomatosis. In: Lesperance M, Flint P, eds. *Cummings Pediatric Otolaryngology*, 1st ed. Philadelphia, PA: Elsevier Saunders; 2015.

Rutter MJ, Cohen AP, de Alarcon A. Laryngeal stenosis. In: Johnson JT, Rosen CA, eds. *Bailey's Head & Neck Surgery Otolaryngology*, 5th ed. Philadelphia, PA: Lippincott Williams & Wilkins; 2014.

Smith MM, Cotton RT. Diagnosis and management of laryngotracheal stenosis. *Expert Rev Respir Med* 2018; 12(8): 709–717.

---

105. STRIDOR

Introduction

Stridor is a symptom that may indicate significant underlying pathology. In the acute situation, the paediatric airway can deteriorate rapidly, requiring urgent intervention.

Anatomy and Physiology

Children develop upper airway obstruction more readily than adults. Mucosal swelling results in greater obstruction in a smaller airway. Poiseuille's law states that airway resistance

Table 105.1   Clinical presentation according to level of obstruction

	Airway noise	Voice/cry	Cough
Nasopharynx/oropharynx	Stertor	Muffled	Typically absent
Supraglottis/glottis	Stridor— inspiratory	Hoarse	Barking
Subglottis/upper trachea	Stridor—biphasic	Unchanged	Brassy
Lower trachea	Stridor—expiratory	Unchanged	Wet-sounding

is inversely proportional to the fourth power of the radius. Therefore a 50% reduction in airway diameter results in a 16-fold increase in resistance.

Increased airflow velocity creates negative pressure on the walls (Bernoulli's principle), leading to collapse and vibration.

Characteristics of Stridor

Stridor is typically high-pitched, originating in the larynx or trachea. Stertor is a low-pitched snoring noise from naso- and oropharyngeal obstruction (Table 105.1). Obstruction of the small airways is called wheeze.

Causes of upper airway obstruction are shown in Table 105.2. Typically, inspiratory stridor is due to extrathoracic obstruction (larynx or upper trachea). Bronchial or lower tracheal obstruction produces an expiratory stridor. A prolonged expiratory phase may also indicate an intrathoracic obstruction. Biphasic stridor can occur with obstruction anywhere in the tracheobronchial tree.

Evaluation of the Child with Stridor

The aim is to determine the obstruction site and the stridor cause and severity. Rapid progression typically occurs in acute infection and foreign body inhalation.

History

- *Perinatal history.* Neonatal intubation may result in subglottic stenosis; instrumented delivery may cause vocal cord palsy.
- *Onset and progression.* Stridor at birth suggests a fixed narrowing (laryngeal web, subglottic/tracheal stenosis, bilateral vocal cord palsy). Laryngomalacia presents in the first few weeks of life.

Table 105.2   Common causes of upper airway obstruction

	Congenital	Acquired
Nasopharynx/ oropharynx	Choanal stenosis Craniofacial abnormalities Micrognathia—glossoptosis	Neonatal rhinitis Allergic rhinitis Adenoiditis Adenotonsillar hypertrophy Foreign body
Larynx	Laryngomalacia Vocal cord palsy	Intubation trauma Foreign body Croup Epiglottitis Bacterial tracheitis Recurrent respiratory papillomatosis
Trachea	Primary tracheomalacia Secondary tracheomalacia (vascular compression)	Post-intubation tracheal stenosis Croup Foreign body Bacterial tracheitis

- *Pattern of stridor.* Laryngomalacia improves at rest and is worse when the infant is crying or feeding. Pharyngeal obstruction worsens during sleep. Tongue base occlusion (e.g. micrognathia) worsens when the child is supine. Nasal obstruction improves with crying.
- Associated features, such as apnoeas, cyanosis, cough, and respiratory distress.
- Feeding history (growth charts). Aspiration suggests vocal cord palsy, tracheo-oesophageal fistula, neuromuscular pathology, or laryngeal cleft.
- Medical and surgical history.

Examination

Observe the child at rest for respiratory distress and stridor. Wheeze, cough, and abnormal voice are localising signs. The carer may have recorded a stridulous episode.

Subcostal, intercostal, and suprasternal recession are good indicators of severity. Younger children, who depend on diaphragmatic movement, do not employ accessory muscles of respiration. Nasal flaring, head bobbing, and abnormal posturing are concerning signs. The volume of stridor can paradoxically reduce with increased obstruction due to diminishing airflow. Cyanosis is a very late event and suggests obstruction is severe or prolonged.

Examine the ears, nose, throat, and neck. Avoid instrumenting the throat in suspected epiglottitis. Observe the child attempting to feed.

History and examination can give a working diagnosis and avoid progression to immediate endoscopy (e.g. mild laryngomalacia). Up to 20% of laryngomalacia patients may have a second pathology, though few will require treatment.

Investigations

May be inappropriate in the acute setting.

- AP and lateral neck x-rays for bulky soft-tissue lesions or subglottic narrowing in croup
- Chest x-ray for mediastinal shift due to foreign body
- Contrast swallow for vascular ring or tracheo-oesophageal fistula
- Bronchography for tracheobronchial stenosis
- Laryngeal ultrasound: vocal cord palsy and structural lesions
- Computed tomography (CT) and magnetic resonance imaging (MRI): thoracic vasculature, tracheal compression (usually following endoscopy)
- Lung function tests to differentiate between intra- and extrathoracic obstruction and between fixed and variable pathologies
- Sleep studies: rarely used

Endoscopy

Two principal concerns in paediatric upper airway endoscopy are safety and diagnostic accuracy. Outpatient flexible laryngoscopy is a useful tool in a cooperative child or neonate, and it is complementary to direct laryngotracheobronchoscopy (DLTB).

DLTB is the gold standard diagnostic procedure. Surgeon and anaesthetist must work closely together. Numerous anaesthesia techniques may be used: most centres achieve spontaneous ventilation with oxygen delivery to the supraglottis using a nasopharyngeal airway, a supraglottic airway device, or an endotracheal tube that is subsequently partially withdrawn.

- Equipment checked
- Head extended with sandbag
- Laryngoscopy with suspension, protecting the teeth and lips
- Hopkins rod endoscopy
- Probe used to assess arytenoid mobility and look for laryngeal cleft
- Assessment of subglottis, trachea, carina, and main bronchi
- Dynamic assessment of vocal cords

In some cases, spontaneous ventilation without endotracheal intubation is not possible. In these cases, a ventilating bronchoscope attached to an anaesthetic circuit should replace the endoscope.

Management of Acute Airway Obstruction

Medical Management

Oxygen therapy (e.g. nasal cannula), can improve oxygen saturation levels but will not aid carbon dioxide clearance. There is no evidence that humidified air is beneficial in upper airway obstruction.

Low-density helium and oxygen (Heliox) reduces turbulent flow and is beneficial in moderate to severe croup.

Steroids reduce the work of breathing in croup. Options include nebulised budesonide (2 mg) or oral or intramuscular dexamethasone (0.15–0.6 mg/kg). Nebulised adrenaline (0.4 mL/kg of 1:1000, maximum 5 mL) should be considered in inflammation.

Consider transfer to a specialist paediatric centre.

Surgical Management

Paediatric tracheostomy is associated with significant morbidity and has largely been superseded by intubation in acute airway obstruction. Nasotracheal intubation is preferred for prolonged periods: it is better tolerated than orotracheal intubation, less sedation is required, the tube can be secured more reliably, and nursing care is easier.

Intubation may not be possible due to the underlying pathology. An ENT surgeon (and appropriate equipment) should be available if a child with airway obstruction of unknown aetiology requires intubation. If intubation fails, a ventilating bronchoscope or an endotracheal tube mounted on a Hopkins rod may be passed. Emergency tracheostomy may be required.

Acute Laryngeal Infections

Croup is the most common (90%) cause of acute airway obstruction in children in the developed world. Epiglottitis occurs rarely due to the *Haemophilus influenzae* type b (Hib) vaccine.

Croup

- *Presentation*: hoarseness and a barking cough progressing to inspiratory/biphasic stridor (due to laryngeal/tracheal mucosal oedema), following upper respiratory tract symptoms. Diagnosis is clinical.
- *Causative organisms*: parainfluenza virus types I and II, respiratory syncytial virus (RSV) virus types A and B, rhinovirus.
- *Peak age*: 2 years (range: 6 months to 3 years).
- *Risk factors for severe croup*: subglottic stenosis, chronic lung disease, allergic airway reactivity. Recurrent croup should be investigated with endoscopy.
- *Treatment*: systemic steroids and supportive care.

Bacterial Laryngotracheobronchitis

- *Presentation*: worsening stridor not responding to steroids and nebulised epinephrine, high fevers, sepsis. Rare but life-threatening airway obstruction due to profuse mucopurulent secretions and epithelial sloughing not cleared by coughing.
- *Age*: 4 to 8 years.
- *Risk factors*: Down syndrome, immunodeficiency, ventilated newborns (neonatal necrotising tracheobronchitis).
- *Causative organisms*: *Staphylococcus aureus, Haemophilus influenzae, Moraxella catarrhalis, Streptococcus pneumoniae, Pseudomonas aeruginosa*. Viral cultures are also frequently positive.
- *Diagnosis*: endoscopy reveals subglottic and tracheal pseudomembrane with mucopus extending into the bronchi.

- *Treatment*: broad-spectrum antibiotics, intubation, DLTB to remove secretions, intensive nursing to prevent obstruction of the endotracheal tube.
- *Complications*: airway stenosis, acute respiratory distress syndrome, respiratory failure, toxic shock syndrome, anoxic encephalopathy, death.

Diphtheria

- *Presentation*: sore throat, fever, and malaise with grey tonsillar pseudomembrane. May progress to inspiratory stridor, barking paroxysmal cough, and life-threatening airway obstruction if it involves the larynx.
- *Causative organisms*: *Corynebacterium diphtheriae* and *Corynebacterium ulcerans*. Both produce an exotoxin that can cause myocarditis and peripheral neuritis.
- *Treatment*: urgent high-dose benzylpenicillin and antitoxin. Airway management: oxygen, humidification, removal of laryngeal membrane, and systemic steroids. Intubation may be necessary.
- Rare in countries with an immunisation programme.

Acute Epiglottitis

- *Presentation*: short history of sore throat, inspiratory stridor, muffled voice, drooling, and sepsis. Classical tripod position: using the arms to support the shoulders and maximise accessory muscle use.
- *Age*: 2 to 8 years. Mortality is up to 3%.
- *Examination (only to be attempted in theatre)*: gross oedema and erythema of the supraglottis.
- *Causative organisms*: *Haemophilus influenzae* type b (Hib), meningococcus, group A streptococcus, pneumococcus, *Haemophilus parainfluenzae,* and *Staphylococcus aureus*.
- *Treatment*: intubation or tracheostomy. IV penicillin if patient has been vaccinated against Hib. If patient is unvaccinated, treat with IV third-generation cephalosporins for 5–7 days (chloramphenicol or clindamycin if allergic).

KEY POINTS

- Stridor results from a narrowed airway.
- Assessment determines the diagnosis and the severity of the obstruction.
- Assessment and treatment occur together in the acute presentation.
- Hypoxemia is a late feature of airway obstruction.
- Improvement in stridor may paradoxically be due to worsening obstruction.
- Intubation is preferable to tracheostomy.
- Rapid progression of airway obstruction occurs in acute infection and foreign body inhalation.
- Croup should be treated with oral dexamethasone on presentation.
- Bacterial laryngotracheobronchitis should be considered in children presenting with croup who fail to respond to steroids and epinephrine.

Further Reading

Boudewyns A, Claes J, Van de Heyning P. Clinical practice: an approach to stridor in infants and children. *Eur J Pediatr* 2010; 169(2): 135–141.

Oshan V, Walker RWM. Anaesthesia for complex airway surgery in children. *Contin Educ Anaesthesia Crit Care Pain* 2013; 13: 47–51.

Stroud RH, Friedman NR. An update on inflammatory disorders of the pediatric airway: epiglottitis, croup, and tracheitis. *Am J Otolaryngol* 2001; 22: 268–275.

106. FOREIGN BODIES IN THE EAR, NOSE AND THROAT

Introduction
Foreign body (FB) is a common presentation seen by ear, nose, and throat specialists.
Risks:

- Extremes of age
- Impaired behavioural development
- Neurological condition
- Psychological condition
- Poor dentition
- Alcohol consumption

Incidence
The largest active registry of nonfood FB incidents is the Susy Safe project. The number of FB incidents in the European Union in children 0–14 years old is 50,000 per annum, and 1% are fatal. Up to 22% have a repeat of the FB incident; therefore, education is essential.

The frequency is higher in the ear and nose than in the throat, forming around half of the incidents recorded, with the tracheobronchial tree affected in ~11–12% of incidents.

Children with neurological disorders present later, with FB in the aerodigestive tract; they remain in hospital longer, and they may have a more complicated management. Among healthy children, the majority (96%) do not require supplementary oxygen support beyond 2 hours. FB inhalation is potentially life threatening, but in most cases removal is without complication. Immediate post-operative chest radiographic features are predictive of pulmonary complications. However, the mortality for FB inhalation is still high.

Ear Foreign Bodies
Inert FBs in the ear may be found incidentally. Delayed removal of certain items (e.g. button batteries) may have serious consequences. Many aural FBs will migrate out of the ear. The urgency of removal of FBs is based upon the nature of the FB. Potentially corrosive and organic FBs should be removed without delay.

The removal technique depends on FB characteristics, FB position, and cooperation from the patient. Non-graspable FBs (e.g. beads) are better removed by otolaryngologists, with fewer complications than with removal by emergency department staff.
Methods include:

- Microsuction
- Wax hook
- Irrigation

Nasal Foreign Bodies
A nasal FB must be considered in any child with unilateral nasal discharge. The most common age of presentation is 2–4 years. A nasal FB usually requires a minimum of 4 days before discharge occurs, unless it is a button battery, when discharge is immediate. Inert nasal FBs may be present for a considerable number of years, leading to granulation and potential rhinolith formation.

Techniques for removal include:

- Hook
- Bent Jobson-Horne probe behind FB
- 'Mother's kiss': gently blowing into the child's mouth with the unaffected nostril held closed

Nasal FBs can be inhaled, especially by patients with an impaired gag reflex.

Inhaled Foreign Bodies

Most inhaled FBs occur in males under 3 years old.

- *Under age 3*: FB usually organic
- *Over age 5*: FB usually inorganic

Mortality from FB inhalation is near 1% and is the most common cause of accidental death in children under 3 years old.

Symptoms and signs:

- Choking
- Coughing
- Hoarseness
- Shortness of breath
- Wheeze
- Increased effort
- Cyanosis
- Stridor

Delayed presentation can occur in children and may be treated as asthma. Delayed diagnosis (over 24 hours) occurs in about 40% of cases. The longer the duration of retention of the inhaled FB, the more there is probability of long-term complications, including chronic cough, wheeze, and bronchiectasis.

Laryngeal FB presents with either partial or complete airway blockage.

Symptoms and signs:

- Hoarseness
- Stridor
- Dyspnoea
- Atypical croup
- Odynophagia (hence misdiagnosis)

The Heimlich manoeuvre expels laryngeal FBs.

Complications include:

- Oesophageal-gastric rupture
- Diaphragmatic hernia
- Emphysema

Radiographic findings on chest films will often be normal (11–26%) unless there is a radiopaque FB. Additional radiographic features include:

- Atelectasis
- Hyperinflation
- Mediastinal shift
- Pneumonia
- Pneumothorax

Classically, the image shows ipsilateral lung hyperinflation due to a ball-valve effect. On inspiration, air enters the bronchus because the intrathoracic pressure is decreased. On expiration, the air is trapped in the lung because the bronchus is compressed around the FB (Figure 106.1).

Sensitivity and specificity of radiographs for airway FBs are 73% and 45%, respectively; therefore, radiographs are only an aid to airway endoscopy.

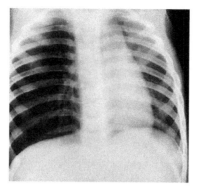

Figure 106.1   Chest X-ray showing hyperinflated right lung due to a foreign body in the right main bronchus.

Computed tomography virtual bronchoscopy is highly sensitive in identifying a FB within the airway but requires a general anaesthetic; therefore, most examiners opt for rigid bronchoscopy.

Direct microlaryngoscopy-tracheobronchoscopy (MLTB) is required to diagnose and remove the FB. The level of urgency depends on the clinical condition of the patient and resources available. Controversy remains around the hour of night FB removal should occur. Generally, if the child is stable, removal should be done during daylight hours (even if that is the following morning). Exceptions include:

- Unstable symptoms
- FB that could cause oil release (e.g. peanut) and granulation formation or FB that could swell (e.g. dried beans)
- Batteries

MLTB and removal of the FB is best in a spontaneously breathing non-intubated child, because there is a small risk that the FB may be lodged at the larynx or immediate subglottis. The rigid bronchoscope should be ready for use. Paralysis is best after the airway has been assessed and secured. Topical anaesthetic on the larynx prevents laryngospasm.

Topical epinephrine will decongest the area immediately around the FB. Post-operative steroid reduces oedema caused by airway instrumentation, and the patient should be under observation until the next day. Flexible bronchoscopy via a laryngeal mask or endotracheal tube has also been described and can sometimes help with a different angled approach.

Life-threatening complications following endoscopic removal occur in 4% of patients. The complications include:

- Pneumothorax
- Tracheal laceration
- Pneumonia
- Bleeding
- Cardiac arrest due to hypoxia
- Delayed pneumothorax

The risk of hypoxia during removal increases in the child <1 year of age and with a prolonged procedure. Death during endoscopy for FB removal is reported at 0.42–1.8%. A negative MLTB is not a failure, because the threshold for suspecting FB inhalation must be low. The negative rate is reported to be 60%.

In some circumstances, it may be impossible to remove a FB using endoscopy. Alternatives include tracheal fissure or thoracotomy for bronchial sites.

Ingested Foreign Bodies

Peak incidence of FB ingestion occurs in children <4 years old (up to 75%). The most common item ingested is a coin. Symptoms include:

- Drooling
- Odynophagia
- Dysphagia

Foreign bodies that contain bones may stick in the tonsil, tongue base, cricopharyngeus, and pharyngeal wall (in decreasing order of occurrence). Larger items typically stick at the cricopharyngeus or upper oesophagus above the aortic arch.

For food-related impaction, medical management is often attempted. Agents include hyoscine (Buscopan) and diazepam (evidence inconclusive).

Flexible nasendoscopy may identify the FB in the pharynx or saliva pooling in the piriform fossae. Metallic FBs may be detected by radiography (Figure 106.2).

Retained FBs may migrate into the soft tissue of the neck. Controversy remains around the choice of flexible or rigid oesophagoscopy. The latter has a significantly higher perforation rate (0.2–1.2) than the flexible type (0.02–0.05), yet both methods have similar success rates. For sharp FBs (bones and pins), early intervention results in reduced complications. Complications include:

- Perforation
- Mediastinitis
- Retropharyngeal abscess
- Oesophageal stenosis

Special consideration needs to be given to batteries. There has been a significant and increasing rise in battery ingestions, with a 6.7-fold increase between 1985 and 2009.

Batteries cause harm in a variety of ways:

1. Soft tissue forms an electrical circuit, and tissue is hydrolysed by hydroxide at the negative terminal.
2. Leakage of alkaline from the battery occurs when it is in a saline environment.
3. Pressure necrosis can form around the battery.
4. The battery can release toxic compounds.

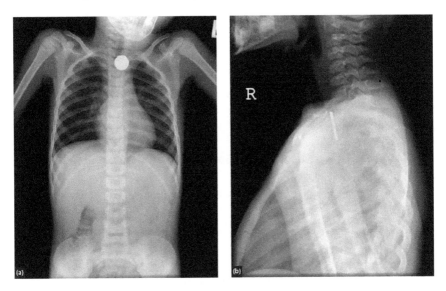

Figure 106.2 Radiograph of metallic foreign body (coin) lodged in the oesophagus.

The majority of batteries are alkaline. Burns occur within 2–2.5 hours. Cases of battery ingestion require urgent x-ray and removal (54% of cases with a fatal outcome were misdiagnosed). The x-ray feature of button batteries is a double contour. Complications of button batteries in the oesophagus include:

- Oesophageal perforation
- Tracheo-oesophageal fistula
- Tracheal granulation
- Haemorrhage
- Vocal cord palsy
- Ulceration
- Death

Post-operative management includes a chest x-ray, which may identify a pneumothorax (0.8%) or pneumomediastinum. Possible options include nasogastric tube, proton pump inhibitors, repeat endoscopy, or contrast swallow a few days to a week later. Steroids have not been shown to confer a clinical benefit following caustic ingestion.

Caustic Agent Ingestion

Caustic ingestion is important in young children because caustic liquids typically have no flavour or odour. Strong alkalis cause injury by tissue liquefaction and necrosis. A significant proportion of caustic ingestions in older teenagers and adults are due to a suicide attempt. Detergents in the home are regulated by legislation. Liquitabs (liquid detergent parcels/tablets) are responsible for 1,500 incidents each year in the United Kingdom. Caustic ingestion injury to the oesophagus is graded 1–4 based on the depth of injury. Grade 1 is erythema and oedema, which can be managed conservatively. Grade 4 is perforation. Most strictures occur within 8 weeks of caustic ingestion and the subsequent dilatations may result in perforation. Furthermore, the risk of subsequent carcinoma is significantly higher, and it can occur at the stricture site.

KEY POINTS

- Incidents related to foreign bodies are common.
- Battery-related incidents are increasing in frequency and can be fatal.
- Batteries require removal without delay.
- A history of possible foreign body inhalation despite a comfortable patient should prompt investigation.

107. CHILDHOOD MALIGNANCIES, CYSTS, AND SINUSES OF THE HEAD AND NECK

Childhood Malignancies

Of primary childhood malignancies, 12% occur in the head and neck. In order of decreasing frequency, they are:

1 Lymphoma, thyroid tumours, and neural tumours
2 Sarcomas and salivary gland tumours
3 Squamous cell carcinoma (rare)

Primary childhood malignancies have a bimodal age distribution: they are most common in patients 15–18 years old, but they can occur in children <4 years old.

Assessment:

- Cervical lymphadenopathy
- Exclude abdominal masses
- Fine-needle aspiration cytology (FNAC) has limited value

Lymphoma

Lymphomas are malignant neoplasms of the lymphoreticular system, most present with cervical lymphadenopathy.

Concerning features: nodes >2 cm or systemic symptoms (weight loss, fever, and organomegally).

Hodgkin's Lymphoma

Reed-Sternberg cells (large, multinucleated cells with abundant cytoplasm) are diagnostic. Can involve lower cervical, supraclavicular, and mediastinal nodes. Some subtypes are associated with Epstein-Barr virus.

Multimodal treatment preferred to single modality because there is less morbidity and mortality. Less radiotherapy required. Disease-free survival > 90% in many studies.

Non-Hodgkin's Lymphoma (NHL)

NHL accounts for 60% of pediatric lymphomas.

Found more often in males, and disease is often aggressive/disseminated. Cervical lymphadenopathy is found in 45%, and 50% are small-cell lymphomas (Burkitt and Burkitt-like).

Bone marrow involvement is common. Suspected involvement of extranodal sites is problematic.

Treatment: Multiagent chemotherapy. Consider intrathecal chemotherapy. Radiotherapy has a limited role.

Rhabdomyosarcoma

Rhabdomyosarcomas account for 60% of pediatric sarcomas, and 40% occur in the head and neck. Half occur in children <5 years old. The prognosis is extremely poor. Survival is improved with surgery (complete excision is rare) and combined multiagent chemotherapy and radiotherapy.

Histologically resembles normal fetal skeletal muscle before innervation. Two types:

- Embryonal (80%)
- Alveolar (20%); in older children, with worse prognosis

Presentation: If rhabdomyosarcoma occurs in the head and neck, it is usually orbital or in parameningeal sites (sinuses, nose, nasopharynx, middle ear). Possibly with a polypoid mass. Symptoms include pain/swelling, nasal obstruction/bloody discharge, or otalgia/bloody otorrhoea. Lymph node involvement in 3–36%. Hematogenous and lymphatic spread.

Management: Biopsy diagnosis. Full excision only if accessible polypoid lesion. Debulking rarely useful. Skull base surgery nearly always an adjunct to chemotherapy or radiotherapy.

Thyroid Cancer

- Uncommon in children. Mainly adolescents and females, higher risk if previous irradiation.
- 45% papillary carcinomas.
- 45% mixed papillary/follicular types.
- 10% follicular.
- Medullary cancer is rare. Suspect if signs of multiple endocrine neoplasia (MEN) IIa or IIb (usually found screening high-risk families). *RET* proto-oncogene on chromosome 10 or elevated calcitonin levels are indicative.
- Anaplastic and undifferentiated tumours are extremely rare.

74% have nodal involvement, 25% have distant metastases.

Thyroid function tests and calcitonin assay if medullary cancer is suspected. Ultrasound +/− FNAC if tolerated. Chest x-ray and computed tomography (CT) for regional and distal metastases.

Treatment is controversial because there is low long-term mortality but serious surgical complications. Typically slow growing with prolonged survival rates, even if extensive.

- Complete surgical excision, if possible. Some use lobectomy or subtotal lobectomy for small, isolated lesions (controversial).
- Minimum subtotal thyroidectomy if postoperative raddioiodine is required.
- Prophylactic total thyroidectomy if MEN II.

Recurrence more likely if the patient is younger or there is residual post-operative disease, typically in cervical nodes or the thyroid bed.

Neuroblastoma

Most common malignancy in children <1 year old.

From undifferentiated sympathetic nervous system precursor cells of neural crest origin. Affects adrenals, sympathetic chain, posterior mediastinum, and cervical nodes. Lymphatic spread in up to 35%. Head and neck metastases are common, primaries are not.

Presentation depends on the primary. Neck masses are associated with Horner syndrome, proptosis, periorbital ecchymosis, bilateral eye hematomas. Can involve paranasal sinuses. Urinary catecholamines (raised >90%).

Treatment is patient-dependent:

- Curative surgery for localized cervical neuroblastoma.
- Multiagent chemotherapy if incomplete resection, amplification of *MYCN* proto-oncogene, or distant metastases.
- Many tumours are radiosensitive.

Prognosis: Better if primary head and neck (compared to other sites), or present in child <1 year old. If resectable, complete excision has 90% survival rate.

Miscellaneous Tumours

Soft-tissue sarcomas are bimodal, predominantly in the head and neck in patients less than 5 years old, but in the extremities in adolescents. Treated with chemotherapy, surgery, and radiotherapy. Relatively poor prognosis.

Squamous cell carcinoma usually occurs in the nasopharynx in children and is associated with immunosuppression, irradiation, or preexisting xeroderma pigmentosum. Management is the same as for adult disease.

Malignant teratoma (germ cell tumour) is rare, and the majority are benign. Typically presents as an airway emergency at birth, but some are diagnosed in utero. Assessment: alpha-fetoprotein, beta human chorionic gonadotrophin, imaging. Airway procedure/surgical excision, may need salvage chemo/radiotherapy. Good prognosis if no metastases.

Chordoma is a rare, slow-growing, bony tumour from embryonic remnants of notochord. In head and neck, chordoma is most often found in the nasopharynx and skull base, and it is locally aggressive. Rarely is completely excisable, so post-operative radiotherapy is used, but proton-beam therapy is increasingly used.

Nonmalignant Conditions Resembling Tumours

Rosai-Dorfman disease (sinus histiocytosis): inflammatory, unknown etiology. Massive bilateral cervical lymphadenopathy, fever, malaise. Older children/adolescents. Usually benign. Spontaneous regression. Biopsy excludes lymphoma, debulk if compressive symptoms.

Langerhans cell histocytosis: lymphadenopathy, usually in a child < 5 years old. Spectrum from unifocal to multifocal multisystem disease (bone/marrow lesions, skin disease, pituitary gland lesions, chronic otitis media). Usually multifocal if cervical disease. Poor prognosis (worse in child <2 years old), aggressive treatment required.

Castleman disease: mass of enlarged nodes, histology shows B-cell lymphoproliferative disorder, possibly viral origin. Children typically have unicentric disease, while adults have multicentric disease (more aggressive). Excision. Exclude HIV.

Fibromatosis colli: sternomastoid tumour of infancy. Common, benign. Torticollis in newborns with lump in sternocleidomastoid muscle. Hip dysplasia associated. Physiotherapy to avoid disfigurement.

Cysts and Sinuses of the Head and Neck

Branchial Anomalies

Branchial anomaly presents as unilateral infected neck mass, enlarging cyst, or intermittently draining sinus. Avoid excision while it is infected.

Branchio-oto-renal syndrome: autosomal dominant, variable penetrance. Structural outer/middle/inner ear defects, branchial cleft, and renal anomalies.

First Branchial Cleft Sinuses

Are < 10% of branchial anomalies.

Superior attachment (pit) anterior to tragus, external auditory canal (EAC) floor (at osseocartilaginous junction), or, rarely, a band between meatal floor and umbo.

Cartilaginous sinus tract lined with squamous epithelium.

Present at birth, discharges sebum.
Classified by Work and Work:

- *Type I*: ectodermal origin, medial to the concha, usually superficial
- *Type II*: both ectodermal and mesodermal; opening often below angle of mandible, close to facial nerve (VII) trunk

Excision: Beware facial nerve adhesions, remove superior aspect to prevent recurrence.

Second Branchial Cleft Sinuses

Are > 90% of branchial anomalies.

Presents in young adulthood, with swelling inferior to angle of mandible, pit anterior to sternocleidomastoid muscle. Mucoid discharge (ectopic salivary tissue lines sinus). Bailey's classification:

- *Type I*: deep to platysma, anterior to sternocleidomastoid muscle
- *Type II*: abutting internal carotid artery, adherent to internal jugular vein (most common)
- *Type III*: extending between internal and external carotid arteries
- *Type IV*: abutting pharyngeal wall, to palatine tonsils, potentially extending to skull base

Treatment: excision. Consider tonsillectomy in type IV.

Third and Fourth Pharyngeal Pouch Sinuses

Are 1–2% of branchial anomalies.

Present as sinus, cyst, thyroid abscess, or fistula (pharynx to skin). Almost always treated conservatively. Airway compromise in neonates, infection in children.

Piriform sinus pit, tract passes close to/through thyroid, parathyroid, or thymus.

Third arch related to glossopharyngeal nerve, fourth to superior laryngeal nerve.

Treatment: endoscopic cautery of piriform fossa, open resection only for neonates (lower recurrence for this age).

Thyroglossal Duct Cyst

Most common congenital head and neck abnormality.

Failure of thyroglossal duct involution at 8–10 weeks' gestation; cyst may contain ectopic thyroid tissue.

Presents: Neck swelling (midline/lateral), elevates on tongue protrusion/swallowing. Infections or fistula.

Investigation: Ultrasound of neck (confirm normal thyroid gland). Treatment: excision unless very small and asymptomatic.

- Sistrunk's procedure excises duct, body of hyoid bone, mylohyoid muscle raphe, and some genioglossus muscle plus foramen cecum. Recurrence rate is 5%.
- Modified Sistrunk's procedure involves wider block dissection of infrahyoid region to isthmus.

Lingual Thyroid

Failure of thyroid descent, and 20–30% have separate thyroid tissue.

1:100,000, typically females.

Approximately one third of patients are hypothyroid.

Malignancy risk unchanged.

Typically incidental. Symptoms: dysphagia, airway obstruction, haemorrhage, or endocrine dysfunction.

Image for separate thyroid tissue (neck/ectopic). CT demonstrates lingual thyroid well, magnetic resonance imaging (MRI) reduces radiation. Technetium (^{99m}Tc) scan confirms if separate metabolically active thyroid tissue.

Treatment:

- Multidisciplinary care with lifelong thyroid monitoring.
- If small and asymptomatic, TSH suppression gives slow reduction in size.
- Excision if obstructive symptoms or hemorrhage. Transoral resection versus external approach, +/− tracheostomy.

Dermoid Cysts

Ectodermal and mesodermal origin, on lines of embryonic closure. Nasal dermoid is rare.

Presentation: nasal dorsal punctum, discharge, or hairs (pathognomonic) with cyst between columella and glabella in neonates. Occasionally tract persists. Recurrent infections can erode nasal bones.

Familial links reported.

Differential diagnosis includes glioma, encephalocele, and nasal polyposis.

Imaging: CT and MRI are used for surgical planning and to exclude intracranial extension.

Treatment: Early excision reduces bony abnormalities.

Further Reading

1. Reviewing radiological images of these conditions will further cement understanding of the condition and relevant anatomy. A useful resource can be found at https://radiologykey.com/imaging-of-the-head-and-neck-in-the-pediatric-patient/
2. The following offers a literature review of the published literature on branchial anomalies. Shenoy N, Tiwari C, Gandhi S, Dwivedi P, & Shah H. Anomalies of branchial cleft: our experience and review of literature. *Internat Surg J* 2017; 4(10): 3234–3237. http://dx.doi.org/10.18203/2349-2902.isj20174108

108. DROOLING, ASPIRATION, AND OESOPHAGEAL PROBLEMS

Drooling

Sialorrhoea (drooling) is the involuntary loss of saliva from the mouth, whilst hypersalivation is excessive production of saliva. Oral motor dyspraxia is when drooling is accompanied by dysarthria and difficulty chewing solid food.

Drooling is normal in young children <4 years old. It is due to impairment in the oral phase of swallowing, with inability to maintain lip closure, altered muscle tone, impaired oral sensation, and difficulties controlling tongue movements. General developmental and muscle control disorders are associated (e.g. cerebral palsy).

History

In a drooling child, it is key to know whether they are also aspirating. A history of coughing, choking, or frequent chest infections is important, and further assessment can be via a videofluoroscopic swallowing study (VFSS) or fibreoptic endoscopic evaluation of swallow (FEES).

If aspiration is not present, then noninvasive management strategies are used until at least 6 years of age. If aspiration is present, intervention should not be delayed, even if the child is <4 years old, to preserve long-term lung function.

Risk factors for hypersalivation include hyperkinetic oral movements, finger chewing, dental decay, reflux, medication side-effects, an open-mouth posture, and nasal obstruction.

There are numerous drooling scales, but none is commonly used. However, some clinicians find symptom questionnaires and quality of life scores useful adjuncts, because drooling has both social and physical effects.

Management

Saliva control is best managed via a multidisciplinary approach that includes paediatricians, speech and language therapists, orthodontists, and dentists (Figure 108.1).

Antimuscarinic medication is the mainstay of pharmacological management of drooling. The side-effect profile includes dry eyes, dilated pupils, constipation (with potential toxic megacolon), urinary retention, and poor seizure control. The most commonly used antimuscarinics are hyoscine hydrobromide transdermal patches, oral glycopyrronium bromide, and trihexyphenidyl hydrochloride. Hyoscine hydrobromide use can be complicated by common skin reactions to the adhesive.

Botulinum toxin injections are useful. They block release of acetylcholine from parasympathetic secretomotor nerves in the salivary glands. Onabotulinum toxin A (Botox) is the most common type used. Most clinicians inject equal amounts into the submandibular and parotid glands under ultrasound guidance. Maximal effect is at 2–6 weeks, with a median duration of response of 4 months. Transient post-injection dysphagia can occur; therefore, caution is advised for an orally fed child with a pre-existing swallowing impairment.

Children with no aspiration risk get the best long-term results with bilateral submandibular duct transfer. The ducts are re-tunneled submucosally to the inferior border of the tonsillar fossa. Risks include ranula formation and transient or persistent submandibular gland swelling. Other surgical options include four-duct ligation and submandibular gland excision. Rarely, in children with intractable aspiration, laryngotracheal separation or total laryngectomy may be considered.

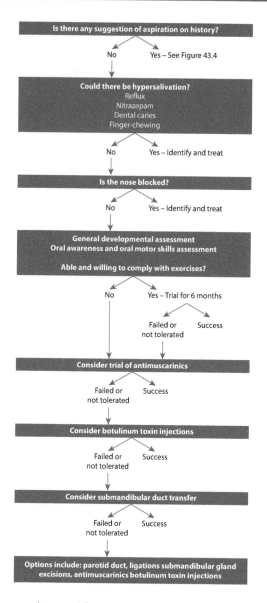

Figure 108.1 A suggested protocol for assessment and stepwise, progressive management of drooling in children.

Reflux

Gastro-oesophageal reflux (GER) occurs when stomach contents pass above the level of the lower oesophageal sphincter. The refluxate usually contains hydrochloric acid and pepsin and may include bile and pancreatic enzymes. It becomes gastro-oesophageal reflux disease (GERD) when the patient develops symptoms, signs, or histological changes. Extra-oesophageal reflux disease (EERD) is refluxate causing disease above the level of the upper oesophageal sphincter. It is important to note that patients can have EERD in the absence of GERD.

EERD is thought to be caused by the direct effect of pepsin and acid on mucosa, which is exacerbated by a low pH, causing a reduction in ciliary motility. Chemoreflexic effects may cause a vagally mediated apnoea.

BOX 108.1 POSSIBLE SYMPTOMS OF EXTRA-OESOPHAGEAL REFLUX IN CHILDREN[4]

Airway symptoms	Feeding problems	General ear, nose, and throat symptoms
Cough	Dysphagia	Nasal obstruction/congestion
Throat clearing	Odynophagia	Nasal pain
Recurrent croup	Gagging	Snoring
Wheezing	Choking	Snorting
Cyanotic spells	Globus sensation	Postnasal drip
Noisy breathing—stertor/stridor	Failure to thrive	Drooling
Hiccups		Oral sores
Recurrent pneumonia		Halitosis
Hoarseness		Taste/tongue problems
Tracheostomy problems (e.g. stomal granulations)		Otalgia
Gurgly respirations		
Apnoea		
Sleep-disordered breathing		

There are a wide range of possible symptoms associated with EER in children (Box 108.1), and therefore a thorough history is required.

In neonates, a certain degree of reflux is physiological; however, there is no threshold figure to indicate when it is pathological. Investigations include contrast swallow, pH monitoring, multichannel oesophageal intraluminal impedance testing, and gastric emptying scintigraphy. Oesophageal biopsies can help with diagnosis of eosinophilic oesophagitis, inflammatory bowel disease (IBD), coeliac disease, and Barrett's oesophagus.

Associated Conditions

Laryngomalacia is typically associated with coexisting reflux. It is unclear if it is causative, although the increased work of breathing can make it self-perpetuating. Reflux has also been linked with:

- Subglottic stenosis—gastric acid in the presence of mucosal trauma (i.e. endotracheal intubation) may lead to stenosis. This is important when considering laryngotracheal reconstruction, because reflux exposure may affect wound healing.
- Apparent life-threatening events (ALTEs).
- Recurrent croup.
- Recurrent respiratory papillomatosis (reflux is thought to affect the rate of recurrence).
- Anterior commissure web formation.

There is emerging evidence to suggest that reflux may have an impact in some cases of sinus disease, otitis media with effusion (OME), and acute otitis media (AOM). Children with GER also appear to have higher rates of post-operative complications after adenotonsillectomy.

Management

There is limited evidence for management of EER and so its management is extrapolated from the management of GERD. Management includes feeding upright, food thickeners, barrier agents, prokinetic therapy, histamine H_2 receptor antagonists, and proton pump inhibitors. If reflux is refractory to feeding changes and medical management, then surgical options, such as fundoplication, can be considered.

Eosinophilic Oesophagitis

Eosinophilic oesophagitis is an inflammatory oesophagitis related to immune-mediated eosinophilia. In children, it manifests with choking, gagging, nausea, vomiting, diarrhoea, and food refusal. Reflux may coexist. Diagnosis is confirmed on oesophageal biopsy, with more than 15 eosinophils per high-powered field seen. Eosinophilic oesophagitis is more common in men and has a strong link to atopy. The current management is swallowing of topical corticosteroids.

Congenital Abnormalities of the Oesophagus

Oesophageal Atresia

Oesophageal atresia (OA) with or without trachea-oesophageal fistula (TOF) has a prevalence between 1 in 2,000 and 1 in 5,000 live births (Figure 108.2). It is divided in to five types, with Type A accounting for 85% of cases.

Neonatal symptoms include frothing at the mouth, choking episodes, cyanosis, and respiratory distress, particularly precipitated by feeding. Diagnosis is commonly made by failure to pass an oro- or nasogastric tube, plus the presence of gas in the abdomen on x-ray. EA can be associated with other anomalies (e.g. VACTERL association). Management is surgical, with ligation of the fistula and end-to-end anastomosis of the oesophagus, through either an open extrapleural thoracotomy or a minimal access thorascopic approach. Rarely, EA and TOF can be associated with an oesophageal bronchus (i.e. bronchus that takes its origin from the oesophagus). Surgical resection is usually the treatment of choice, but angiography must be undertaken first to confirm the lung associated with the bronchus has an appropriate blood supply.

Congenital Stenosis of the Oesophagus

This is seen most commonly at the middle and distal oesophagus. In minor degrees, it can be asymptomatic, but if it is more severe, then surgical resection is required. Rarely, complete membranous oesophageal webs are described, which are indistinguishable from OA.

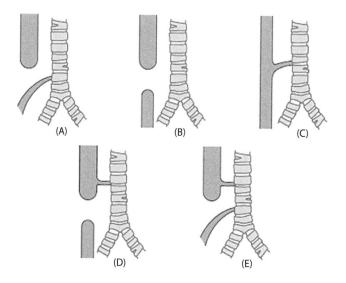

Figure 108.2 Types of oesophageal atresia (EA) with or without a tracheooesophageal fistula (TOF). Type A—OA with distal TOF, Type B—isolated OA, Type C—isolated H- or N-type TOF, Type D—OA with proximal TOF, Type E—OA with proximal and distal TOF.

Other oesophageal congenital abnormalities include oesophageal duplications which are either tubular or cystic structures. They commonly present with respiratory distress caused by cyst compression of lungs and airway. Diagnosis is usually suspected on x-ray, with follow-up computed tomography (CT) or magnetic resonance imaging (MRI). True congenital oesophageal diverticula can also occur but are rare, with false/pulsion diverticula being more common. Congenital short oesophagus is a rare anomaly in which the patient has an intrathoracic stomach and hiatal hernia. Affected babies present with failure to thrive.

Acquired Disorders of the Oesophagus

Achalasia of the cardia is a rare motility disorder that causes a functional obstruction at the level of the lower oesophageal sphincter. It is more common in teenagers, who present with vomiting, swallowing difficulties, respiratory symptoms, and occasionally chest pain. There is poor understanding of the condition and no management consensus. Options include pneumatic balloon dilatation, botulinum toxin, or surgical myotomy.

Oesophageal Injury

Most ingested foreign bodies pass through to the stomach and require no treatment (except for mini magnetic toys and button batteries, which require urgent attention). Items usually lodge at the level of the thoracic inlet, cricopharyngeus muscle, mid-oesophagus at the level of the aortic arch, and the oesophagogastric junction. More distally, the risk of perforation and mediastinitis is higher. Management is removal via rigid or flexible oesophagoscopy.

Impulsive behaviour and attention deficit hyperactivity disorder are risk factors for ingestion of caustic substances, resulting in potential airway compromise and intubation. Mucosal slough and necrosis are common; deeper injury with liquefaction of all layers of the oesophagus is also seen. Management includes hospital admission, fasting, and IV fluid administration. Neutralising fluids are not recommended because they may exacerbate the injury. Early endoscopy is indicated for assessment and nasogastric tube insertion under direct vision.

More rarely, children can be at risk of radiation-induced oesophageal injury related to radiotherapy for thoracic tumours. Mallory-Weiss tears can also occur in children, but the bleeding is usually self-limited.

Further Reading

1. Walshe M, Smith M, Pennington L. Interventions for drooling in children with cerebral palsy. *Cochrane Database Syst Rev* 2012;
2. Goyal A, Jones MO, Couriel JM, Losty PD. Oesophageal atresia and tracheo-oesophageal fistula. *Arch Dis Child Fetal Neonatal Ed* 2006; 91(5): 381–384.

109. PAEDIATRIC TRACHEOSTOMY AND PAEDIATRIC AIRWAY MANAGEMENT

Obstruction of the Upper Airway

Indications for paediatric tracheostomy are:

- To relieve upper airway obstruction (Table 109.1)
- To prevent complications of prolonged intubation
- To allow suction of tracheal secretions

Table 109.1   Examples of obstruction of the upper airway potentially requiring tracheostomy

Anatomical site	Example
Oropharynx, tongue base	Macroglossia, Treacher Collins' syndrome, Goldenhar's syndrome, cystic hygroma
Nose, nasopharynx	Choanal atresia
Supraglottis	Supraglottic cyst
Glottis	Vocal cord palsy, physical trauma
Subglottis	Subglottic stenosis, haemangioma
Trachea	Tracheomalacia, high tracheal stenosis

In practice, tracheostomies in children are nearly always performed to relieve upper airway obstruction or to allow, or to assist with, mechanical ventilation.

Perinatal Airway Obstruction (Table 109.2)

Neonates with potentially fatal airway obstruction can have good outcomes if the abnormality is recognised prenatally and the pregnancy is managed by a team with experience in interventional delivery. Prenatal and fetal imaging have improved, and airway obstruction can be identified at routine 20-week anomaly ultrasound scan. Further information may be gathered on fetal swallowing, on lung function, and for neck mass mapping via three-dimensional and four-dimensional ultrasound or magnetic resonance imaging (MRI). The fetal growth scan may also show polyhydramnios or macrosomia. A large neck lesion may compress the oesophagus and impede swallowing, leading to increased liquor volume, uterine irritability, and threatened preterm labour. Elective delivery with ex utero intrapartum treatment (EXIT) is planned if there are markers of hydrops or when the fetus is deemed mature.

Table 109.2   Causes of congenital airway obstruction

External compression	Internal blockage	Developmental
Lymphatic malformation (incidence 1 in 6,000 to 1 in 16,000)	Laryngeal web*	Laryngeal atresia*
Cervical teratoma (incidence 1 in 35,000 to 1 in 20,000)	Laryngeal stenosis*	Tracheal atresia*
Brachial cleft cyst	Laryngeal cyst*	Micrognathia (associated with Treacher Collins' syndrome, Marshall syndrome, Stickler's syndrome, 22q11 deletions, Pierre Robin syndrome)
Cervical thymic cyst	Tracheal stenosis*	
Goitre	Epignathus (oropharyngeal teratoma)	
Ectopic thyroid	Choristoma	
Sarcoma	Glioma	
Neuroblastoma	Encephalocele	
Dermoid cyst	Haemangiomata	
Granular cell tumour		
Vascular ring		

* Congenital high airway obstruction syndrome (CHAOS).

In addition to antenatal diagnosis of fetal neck anomalies, pre-operative ultrasound can be used to determine fetal position, mass location, cystic mass aspiration, and placental site prior to an EXIT procedure.

Prolonged Intubation

The long-term complications of prolonged endotracheal intubation are well recognised: ulceration at the level of the glottis and subglottis can lead to scarring and stenosis of the airway.

Long-Term and Home Ventilation

Indications for long-term ventilation include:

- Congenital central hypoventilation syndrome
- Spinal injury
- Congenital myopathy
- Airway malacia
- Chronic lung disease

Tracheal Toilet

Very few children now require tracheostomy for toilet (secretion suctioning) of the airway. Children with intractable aspiration may need regular suction, but the presence of a tracheostomy can by itself predispose to aspiration and increase the risk of respiratory tract infection.

Techniques for Surgical Tracheostomy in Children

1 The patient is positioned supine under general anaesthesia on the operating table. Neck extension is achieved with a shoulder roll.
2 A vertical skin incision is placed halfway between the cricoid ring and the sternal notch.
3 Removal of subcutaneous fat and maturation sutures (skin to tracheal incision) are used.
4 Dissection is restricted to the midline to avoid other structures. In adults and larger children, the thyroid isthmus is divided; in infants, bipolar diathermy is usually adequate to divide the isthmus of the thyroid.
5 A vertical tracheal incision is made in the midline in tracheal rings 3–4. Stay sutures are placed in the wall of the trachea on either side of the vertical tracheal incision (e.g. 4/0 Prolene), and they remain until the first tube change.
6 The tracheostomy tube is secured using the inelastic linen tapes supplied with the tube. After 7 days, the first change is undertaken, and the linen tapes may be changed. There is no standard prescribed interval at which tubes should be changed.

Suction and Humidification

Following tracheostomy, the normally warmed and humidified inspired air becomes dry, cold air, which results in an increase in airway secretions that can block the tracheostomy lumen. Humidification of inspired air and regular suctioning will reduce this tendency. The need for suctioning decreases over time. Longer-term humidification may be achieved by using a humidification moisture exchange system (HME) or a tracheostomy bib.

Indications for a cuffed tube are:

1 Significant risk of aspiration
2 A decrease in lung compliance with an intercurrent infection in a ventilated child in whom ventilation pressures need to be increased

Complications of Tracheostomy

Time after tracheostomy	Complications
General	Tube obstruction Accidental decannulation General complications of surgery and anaesthesia Death
Early	Bleeding: post-operative, wound edge Pneumothorax Subcutaneous emphysema Infection Apnoea Accidental decannulation
Late	Granulation Tube obstruction Bleeding trachea-innominate fistula Suprastomal collapse Skin complications Aphonia, speech delay Psychological disturbance Adverse effects on family Accidental decannulation Tracheocutaneous fistula (allow 6–12 months before closure)

Decision to Decannulate

Decannulation may be considered when the original condition requiring tracheostomy has improved, but the child must be able to maintain an adequate airway without the tracheostomy in place. It is essential to undertake endoscopic assessment of the airway prior to definitive decannulation. Vocal cord mobility and airway patency should be assessed at endoscopy. One should also consider comorbidity (e.g. pulmonary disease or neurological disease) and the need for further surgery. With a long-standing tracheostomy, the child may have no memory of mouth and nose breathing and the new sensation may be distressing ('decannulation panic').

Great Ormond Street Protocol for Ward Decannulation

Day	Procedure
1	Admission, downsize to 3.0 tube
2	Block for 12 hr from 8 a.m. If successful, continue overnight for a further 12 hr
3	Decannulate, occlude stoma with adhesive tape and dressing. Observe on the ward
4	Observe off the ward
5	Discharge

The U.K. National Tracheostomy Safety Project is a multidisciplinary collaboration devised to improve the management of paediatric and adult patients with tracheostomies. The recommendations of the project include:

1 An emergency minimum set of equipment (including spare tubes, suction catheters, and dressings) should accompany a tracheostomy patient at all times.
2 Bedhead documentation, including tube size and length and existing upper airway abnormalities, should be displayed at all times.
3 Emergency treatment algorithms should be provided for attending resuscitation teams.

All perinatal airway and tracheostomy cases require a multidisciplinary team, and prenatal genetic counselling is invaluable. The parents can then have an informed discussion on whether an interventional perinatal procedure is suitable for their baby in light of the probable prognosis. Congenital airway obstruction is potentially life-threatening and is associated with high mortality rates. If there is a delay in establishing an airway and ventilation in the neonate, the risks of hypoxia, acidosis, and anoxic brain injury, which are associated with neonatal morbidity and mortality, increase. In contrast, for those with effective airway access at delivery, the long-term outcome is excellent in most cases.

Interventional Delivery to Access the Fetal Airway

- Operation on placental support (OOPS).
- Performed under maternal regional anaesthesia with the fetus completely delivered through a lower-segment caesarean section. The umbilical cord is unclamped and is kept intact with the fetus. Allows 5–20 min for airway intervention.
- Ex utero intrapartum treatment (EXIT) procedure.
- The fetus is only partially delivered via a lower-segment caesarean section. This allows preservation of the uteroplacental circulation. A 50-min time frame is afforded to perform airway interventions, including establishing an airway, direct laryngoscopy and bronchoscopy, tracheostomy, surfactant administration, and resection of an obstructing mass.
- Delivery and then attempted airway intubation or tracheostomy.
- In certain circumstances, the risk of maternal haemorrhage is severe, and a rapid, safe delivery of the baby and the placenta takes precedence.

KEY POINTS

- Endotracheal intubation rather than tracheostomy is the accepted mode of management for acute obstructing airway infection in children.
- A simple vertical incision to open the trachea is associated with the lowest risk of long-term complications.
- Stay sutures in the wall of the trachea on either side of the vertical incision facilitate reintroduction of the tube in the event of accidental decannulation. Maturation sutures secure the edge of the skin incision to the tracheal wall.
- Tracheostomies in children are performed mainly to relieve upper airway obstruction or to assist with mechanical ventilation.
- Effective airway access at interventional delivery improves long-term prognosis.
- Better antenatal detection has greatly improved perinatal management of airway problems in the newborn.

Further Reading

National Tracheostomy Safety Project. Available from: http://www.tracheostomy. org.uk/Templates/Home.html

Tweedie DJ, Skilbeck CJ, Cochrane LA, et al. Choosing a paediatric tracheostomy tube: an update on current practice. *J Laryngol Otol* 2008; 122(2): 161–169.

Waddell A, Appleford R, Dunning C, et al. The Great Ormond Street protocol for ward decannulation of children with tracheostomy: increasing safety and decreasing cost. *Int J Pediatr Otorhinolaryngol* 1997; 39(2): 111–118.

110. PINNAPLASTY

Background

'Prominent ears' are a common presentation to the paediatric ENT clinic and are the most common congenital deformity of the ear, with an incidence of approximately 5–6%. They can be associated with severe psychological distress and consequently affect academic performance and social development. Therefore, it is important to address any associated psychological issues as well as manage the patient's and parent's expectations when discussing the potential outcome of surgery.

The timing of surgery remains controversial, but generally pinnaplasty is undertaken when the child is 5 years old or older.

Since Dieffenbach first performed the procedure in 1845, more than 200 different techniques of pinnaplasty have been described in the literature, indicating that no single approach is a panacea. In 1968, McDowell proposed the main objectives for a successful pinnaplasty, enabling surgeons to blend various techniques and approaches (Box 110.1).

Anatomy

The external ear develops from the first and second branchial arches during the sixth week of gestation. The six hillocks of His rotate and fuse to form the pinna (Figure 110.1).

Prominent ears are an example of first-degree dysplasia, according to the classification of auricular deformities as first described by Weerda in 1988.

BOX 110.1 OBJECTIVES FOR A SUCCESSFUL PINNAPLASTY

- Elimination of the protrusion in the upper third of the ear.
- The helical fold should be parallel to the antihelical fold but visible when viewing the patient from the front.
- The helix should have a smooth and regular contour.
- The postauricular sulcus should not be distorted.
- The auricle should be an appropriate distance away from the mastoid.
- The difference between both auricles should be within 3 mm.

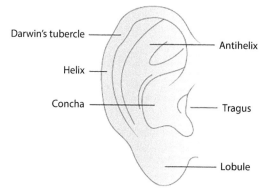

Figure 110.1   Anatomy of the pinna.

Prominent ears are commonly due to one or a combination of the following defects:

- Underdevelopment of the antihelical fold
- Hypertrophy of the conchal bowl
- Prominent lobule

The constricted ear deformity appears as a small but prominent ear due to the small circumference of the helical rim. Stahl's ear deformity consists of an additional crus that transverses the scapha.

Conservative Methods

A number of nonsurgical techniques have been developed for the treatment of protruding ears. Simple moulding or splinting devices can be considered in children up to 6 months old. The high levels of oestrogen during the neonatal period allow the cartilage to be more malleable and therefore respond to nonsurgical methods. The effectiveness of treatment is directly influenced by the age of the child; therefore, referral of neonates with external ear deformities should be encouraged. Satisfactory results can be seen in up to 90% of patients if treatment is started within the first few days of life.

Operative Techniques

Pinnaplasty can be performed under local anaesthetic or general anaesthetic as a same-day procedure, although, because most patients are children, general anaesthetic is usually the preferred option.

Before surgery takes place, it is helpful to have at least two consultations with the patient/parents to confirm the need for surgery. Photographs are essential for pre-operative planning and for medicolegal purposes.

Formation of the Underdeveloped Antihelical Fold

Two techniques define the pinnaplasty operation and can be used in isolation or in combination:

- Cartilage-sparing/suturing technique
- Cartilage-excising/scoring technique

At the start of the operation, the neo-antihelix is created by holding the helix against the mastoid. Each side of the neo-antihelix is then marked with methylene blue needle markings (Figure 110.3).

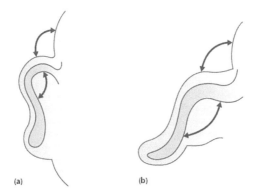

(a)   (b)

Figure 110.2   Anthropometric evaluation of a normal pinna. The aesthetically normal auricle lies with its long axis tilted posteriorly by 15°–20° (a). The top of the auricle is level with the eyebrow, and its width is approximately 60% of its height (range = 5.5–6.5 cm). A normal pinna has an auriculocephalic angle of 25°, and protruding ears have an auriculocephalic angle > 40° (b).

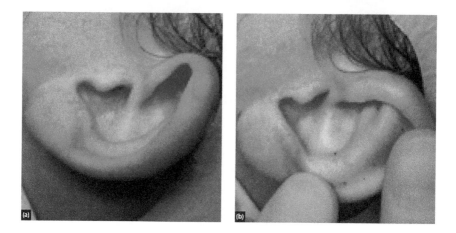

Figure 110.3 (a) A prominent ear and (b) the neo-antihelix with methylene blue markings.

An elliptical skin incision is made in the posterior sulcus, which is then excised to expose the perichondrium (Figure 110.4).

The tattoo markings are identified posteriorly (Figure 110.5) and are used as landmarks for cartilage suturing or excision.

Mustardé first described the cartilage-sparing/suturing technique in 1963.[1] Three or four non-absorbable mattress sutures are placed through the auricular cartilage and perichondrium using the methylene blue markers for precise placement (approximately 1 cm wide and 1 cm apart), thereby creating the new antihelical fold (Figure 110.6).

This technique reduces the trauma to the cartilage and, as a result, post-operative auricular irregularities rarely occur. It is widely considered to be an appropriate technique in young children with soft and malleable auricular cartilage.

It is advisable to use a non-absorbable suture to achieve a long-lasting result but with a minimum of reaction from the surrounding tissue (Figure 110.7).

Stenström described one of the initial cartilage-incising/scoring techniques.[2] The scapha cartilage is incised in a C shape and is dissected off the anterior skin and perichondrium. The cartilage is then scored by making parallel incisions caudally from the inferior crus,

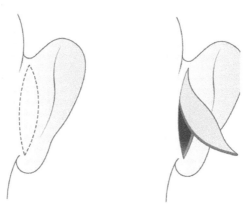

Figure 110.4 Postauricular elliptical skin excision.

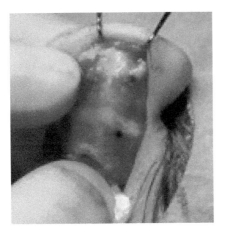

Figure 110.5   Methylene blue markings on the posterior aspect of auricular cartilage.

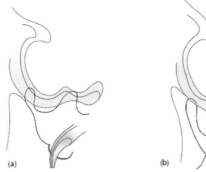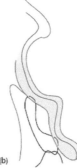

Figure 110.6   Mustardé suture.

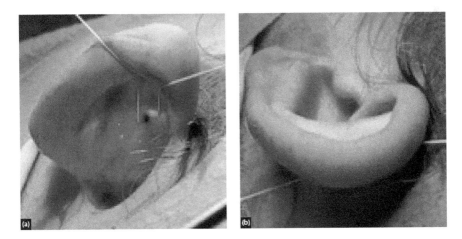

Figure 110.7   Technique of a Mustardé suture.

which allows the antihelical fold to be developed. This technique can be used even when the cartilage is thicker, as in older individuals. With this technique, there is a greater risk of haematoma formation and infection due to significant skin elevation, so intra-operative haemostasis and post-operative dressings are vital to prevent complications.

Usually, a combination of the two techniques allows for the disadvantages of the individual techniques to be minimised, thus reducing the potential for complications.

Additional techniques can be used as adjuncts to the conventional techniques. For example, a laterally based posterior auricular dermal flap or a bilateral fascioperichondrial flap can be used to prevent suture extrusion and decrease the rate of recurrence.

Without any particular gold-standard procedure, novel techniques are continuously being developed, including cartilage-sparing methods without the use of sutures and nontransfixing full-thickness incisions through the helix and antihelix that break the existing cartilaginous mould and therefore allow reshaping.

Correction of Conchal Bowl Hypertrophy

The angle between the concha and the mastoid can be reduced by a suture technique first described by Furnas in 1968 (Figure 110.8).[3] Care should be taken when placing the mastoid portion of the suture, because placing it too close to the external ear canal may narrow the meatus when the suture is tied.

If the conchal depth is more than 2.5 cm, excision of a full-thickness crescent of cartilage should be considered to correct the deformity, ideally with the excised part being taken from the region of the conchamastoid sulcus.

Reconstruction of the Lobule

A separate incision is made on the lobule to allow for a 'fishtail', 'wedge', or 'W-shaped' skin excision. The lobule can be repositioned by placing Goulian sutures (sutures that include postauricular skin, mastoid periosteum, and posterior aspect of the lobule), thereby setting the lobule back towards the mastoid.

Other Deformities

Stahl's Ear Deformity

The Kaplan and Hudson technique describes an incision being made along the helical rim and cartilage being dissected off the skin. The affected cartilage, the extra crus, is excised, and the skin is closed directly.

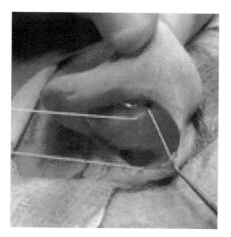

Figure 110.8   Furnas suture.

Constricted Ear Deformity
The cup-ear deformity requires elongation of the helical rim to allow the pinna to lie flat. An incision is made along the helical rim and the crus of the helix is fully mobilised and then advanced out of the concha. A standard pinnaplasty technique is then applied.

Post-Operative Care
Head bandages in the post-operative period help to keep the dressings in place and protect the ears. There is, however, no evidence to suggest that there is any clinical benefit conferred after 48 hr. Keeping the head up tends to reduce oedema.

Complications

- *Haematoma* is an early complication after pinnaplasty. It requires immediate evacuation to prevent necrosis of the cartilage. It is often signified by uncontrolled pain.
- *Infection* is a rare complication of pinnaplasty but requires early antibiotics in order to prevent chondritis and permanent deformity.
- *Keloid scarring* is a recognised complication of pinnaplasty, and patients and their families should be warned about this possibility.
- *Problems with sutures* can occur; they can extrude, and they can cause granulomas and hypertrophic scar formation.
- *Recurrence.* The rate of revision surgery is approximately 6% due to the pinna's returning to its pre-operative position.
- *Overcorrection* is the most common complication of pinnaplasty and can lead to asymmetry or further deformity.

KEY POINTS

- Prominent ears are the most common congenital deformity of the ear.
- Moulding or splinting is highly effective if commenced early and may avoid the need for surgery.
- Good quality pre-operative photography is an essential part of treatment planning.
- Timing of surgery varies, but most surgeons and parents prefer correction before the child goes to school or in the early years at school.
- Several operative techniques are available, each with benefits and drawbacks.
- Overcorrection and asymmetry may lead to poor outcomes.

Further Reading

1. Mustardé JC. The correction of prominent ears using simple mattress sutures. *Br J Plast Surg* 1963; 16: 170.
2. Stenström SJ. A 'natural' technique for correction of congenitally prominent ears. *Plast Reconstr Surg* 1963; 32: 509.
3. Furnas DW. Correction of prominent ears by conchamastoid sutures. *Plast Reconstr Surg* 1968; 42(3): 189–93.

Note: Locators in *italics* represent figures and **bold** indicate tables in the text.